Assistive Technologies for Assessment and Recovery of Neurological Impairments

Fabrizio Stasolla
University Giustino Fortunato of Benevento, Italy

IGI Global
PUBLISHER of TIMELY KNOWLEDGE

A volume in the Advances in Medical Technologies and Clinical Practice (AMTCP) Book Series

Published in the United States of America by
IGI Global
Medical Information Science Reference (an imprint of IGI Global)
701 E. Chocolate Avenue
Hershey PA, USA 17033
Tel: 717-533-8845
Fax: 717-533-8661
E-mail: cust@igi-global.com
Web site: http://www.igi-global.com

Library of Congress Cataloging-in-Publication Data

Names: Stasolla, Fabrizio, editor.
Title: Assistive technologies for assessment and recovery of neurological impairments / Fabrizio Stasolla, editor.
Description: Hershey, PA : Medical Information Science Reference, [2022] | Includes bibliographical references and index. | Summary: "This book offers research information on the use of Assistive Technology-based programs for promoting Independence and self-determination of individuals with neurological disorders"-- Provided by publisher.
Identifiers: LCCN 2021021218 (print) | LCCN 2021021219 (ebook) | ISBN 9781799874300 (hardcover) | ISBN 9781799874317 (ebook)
Subjects: MESH: Neurological Rehabilitation--methods | Autism Spectrum Disorder--rehabilitation | Nervous System Diseases--rehabilitation | Self-Help Devices
Classification: LCC RC387.5 (print) | LCC RC387.5 (ebook) | NLM WL 140 | DDC 616.8/043--dc23
LC record available at https://lccn.loc.gov/2021021218
LC ebook record available at https://lccn.loc.gov/2021021219

This book is published in the IGI Global book series Advances in Medical Technologies and Clinical Practice (AMTCP) (ISSN: 2327-9354; eISSN: 2327-9370)

British Cataloguing in Publication Data
A Cataloguing in Publication record for this book is available from the British Library.

For electronic access to this publication, please contact: eresources@igi-global.com.

Advances in Medical Technologies and Clinical Practice (AMTCP) Book Series

Srikanta Patnaik
SOA University, India
Priti Das
S.C.B. Medical College, India

ISSN:2327-9354
EISSN:2327-9370

Mission

Medical technological innovation continues to provide avenues of research for faster and safer diagnosis and treatments for patients. Practitioners must stay up to date with these latest advancements to provide the best care for nursing and clinical practices.

The **Advances in Medical Technologies and Clinical Practice (AMTCP) Book Series** brings together the most recent research on the latest technology used in areas of nursing informatics, clinical technology, biomedicine, diagnostic technologies, and more. Researchers, students, and practitioners in this field will benefit from this fundamental coverage on the use of technology in clinical practices.

Coverage

- Clinical Data Mining
- Diagnostic Technologies
- Biomechanics
- Biomedical Applications
- Nutrition
- Medical Imaging
- Patient-Centered Care
- Medical Informatics
- Telemedicine
- Nursing Informatics

IGI Global is currently accepting manuscripts for publication within this series. To submit a proposal for a volume in this series, please contact our Acquisition Editors at Acquisitions@igi-global.com or visit: http://www.igi-global.com/publish/.

The Advances in Medical Technologies and Clinical Practice (AMTCP) Book Series (ISSN 2327-9354) is published by IGI Global, 701 E. Chocolate Avenue, Hershey, PA 17033-1240, USA, www.igi-global.com. This series is composed of titles available for purchase individually; each title is edited to be contextually exclusive from any other title within the series. For pricing and ordering information please visit http://www.igi-global.com/book-series/advances-medical-technologies-clinical-practice/73682. Postmaster: Send all address changes to above address.

Titles in this Series

For a list of additional titles in this series, please visit: www.igi-global.com/book-series/advances-medical-technologies-clinical-practice/73682

Machine Learning and Data Analytics for Predicting, Managing, and Monitoring Disease
Manikant Roy (Lovely Professional University, India) and Lovi Raj Gupta (Lovely Professional University, India)
Medical Information Science Reference • © 2021 • 241pp • H/C (ISBN: 9781799871880) • US $395.00

Advancing the Investigation and Treatment of Sleep Disorders Using AI
M. Rajesh Kumar (Vellore Institute of Technology, Vellore, India) Ranjeet Kumar (Vellore Institute of Technology, Vellore, India) and D. Vaithiyanathan (National Institute of Technology, Delhi, India)
Medical Information Science Reference • © 2021 • 291pp • H/C (ISBN: 9781799880189) • US $345.00

Machine Learning in Cancer Research With Applications in Colon Cancer and Big Data Analysis
Zhongyu Lu (University of Huddersfield, UK) Qiang Xu (University of Huddersfield, UK) Murad Al-Rajab (University of Huddersfield, UK & Abu Dhabi University, UAE) and Lamogha Chiazor (University of Huddersfield, UK)
Medical Information Science Reference • © 2021 • 263pp • H/C (ISBN: 9781799873167) • US $345.00

Handbook of Research on Nano-Strategies for Combatting Antimicrobial Resistance and Cancer
Muthupandian Saravanan (Mekelle University, Ethiopia & Saveetha Dental College, Saveetha Institute of Medical and Technical Sciences (SIMATS), India) Venkatraman Gopinath (University of Malaya, Malaysia) and Karthik Deekonda (Monash University, Malaysia)
Medical Information Science Reference • © 2021 • 559pp • H/C (ISBN: 9781799850496) • US $375.00

Handbook of Research on Solving Modern Healthcare Challenges With Gamification
Ricardo Alexandre Peixoto de Queirós (uniMAD, Escola Superior de Media Artes e Design, Portugal) and António José Marques (LabRP, School of Health, Polytechnic of Porto, Portugal)
Medical Information Science Reference • © 2021 • 382pp • H/C (ISBN: 9781799874720) • US $425.00

Diagnostic Applications of Health Intelligence and Surveillance Systems
Divakar Yadav (National Institute of Technology, Hamirpur, India) Abhay Bansal (Amity University, India) Madhulika Bhatia (Amity University, India) Madhurima Hooda (Amity University, India) and Jorge Morato (Universidad Carlos III de Madrid, Spain)
Medical Information Science Reference • © 2021 • 332pp • H/C (ISBN: 9781799865278) • US $285.00

IGI Global
PUBLISHER of TIMELY KNOWLEDGE

701 East Chocolate Avenue, Hershey, PA 17033, USA
Tel: 717-533-8845 x100 • Fax: 717-533-8661
E-Mail: cust@igi-global.com • www.igi-global.com

To my Family and All the People who suffer of neurological disorders

Table of Contents

Section 4
Acquired Brain Injury and Stroke

Detailed Table of Contents

Rett syndrome is a rare genetically caused condition associated with severe disability and impaired motor functions. Local therapists typically see small numbers of affected individuals, and this limits their capacity to gain experience. Telehealth is being used increasingly to counter poor access to rehabilitation services. Moreover, there is a need to develop management plans that support individuals with Rett syndrome over their lifespan. Three projects in which telehealth support was provided by therapists experienced in Rett syndrome and supported by available local resources are presented in this chapter. The three projects responded to locally identified needs in a cost-efficient way and empowered those working with people with Rett syndrome to maintain and improve their clients' physical function and activity. This chapter will discuss the conceptual underpinnings of delivering a service using a telehealth approach and describe the results and the strategies implemented in the projects mentioned above.

Section 3
Neurodegenerative Diseases

Chapter 9
Assistive Technology for Promoting the Independence and the Quality of Life in Persons With Alzheimer's Disease: A Selective Review 173
Donatella Ciarmoli, University Giustino Fortunato of Benevento, Italy

Persons with Alzheimer's disease (AD) may present a loss of cognitive functioning, memory impairments, communication difficulties, obstacles to perform daily activities, disorientation, and challenging behaviours. Currently, there is no cure for AD. However, there are valid treatments to alleviate AD-related symptoms and to reduce the burden on carers; for example, the effectiveness of the use of assistive technology (AT) has been seen. The aim was to provide, in this chapter, an overview of the newest empirical evidences available on the use of AT-based programs to improve the independence and the quality of life of patients with Alzheimer's disease and their caregivers. A selective literature review was carried out considering Alzheimer's, assistive technologies, dementia, quality of life, and caregivers. Empirical data demonstrated the effectiveness and the suitability of the AT interventions allowing participants to improve their quality of life, as well as to mitigate the mental and physical burden of their caregivers.

Chapter 10
Assistive Technology-Based Programs and Telerehabilitation Strategies to Support Adaptive Responding of Individuals With Neurodegenerative Diseases 196
Fabrizio Stasolla, University Giustino Fortunato of Benevento, Italy
Donatella Ciarmoli, University Giustino Fortunato of Benevento, Italy

Individuals with neurodegenerative diseases (NDD) may pose serious challenges to daily life medical contexts. In fact, they commonly fail while dealing with environmental requests. To overcome this issue, one may rely on assistive technology-based programs. The COVID-19 pandemic suddenly exacerbated their clinical conditions. Telerehabilitation may be useful to profitably tackle the latter issue. A concise survey on the newest empirical contributions available was proposed. Five main categories of studies were identified. Results were satisfactory, although failures occurred. Findings were critically discussed and some useful insights for both research and practice were highlighted.

Preface

Neurological disorders broadly include any disease of the Central Nervous System. The brain, spinal cord, cranial nerves, peripherical nerves, nerve roots, autonomic nervous system, neuromuscular junctions, and muscles are usually embedded. Individuals with neurological impairments due to either a congenital or an acquired brain injury may experience different levels of intellectual disabilities, sensorial disorders, motor disorders, communication inabilities, and lack of speech. Both neurodevelopmental disorders (i.e., attention deficits hyperactivity disorders, autism spectrum disorders, cerebral palsy, rare genetic diseases), and neurodegenerative diseases (i.e., Alzheimer and Parkinson diseases, lateral amyotrophic sclerosis, and multiple sclerosis), post-coma patients either in a vegetative state, minimally conscious state or emerging from it, and patients with stroke are usually acknowledged. A common feature of the aforementioned categories of patients are their multiple disabilities which may vary between mild-moderate and severe to profound depending on their level of residual functioning. Accordingly, persons with neurological impairments forcibly rely on caregivers, families, practitioners, and professionals' daily assistance. Because they are unable to profitably cope with daily environmental requests, persons diagnosed with neurological impairments may encounter detachment, isolation, passivity, and withdrawal throughout their lifespan as a chronic clinical condition. Even if an acute clinical condition occurs, it may be deleterious for their social image and status. That is, it may seriously hamper their quality of life. In fact, their clinical conditions may have negative outcomes on caregivers, professionals, and families' burden. Recently, Covid-19 pandemic suddenly and dramatically exacerbated their precarious conditions. They were confined in their homes due to the unavailability of National Medical Services and preventive measures such as social distancing and quarantine. The vaccine's diffusion partially improved that condition worldwide. To overcome this issue, one may envisage assistive technology-based interventions (AT).

AT encompasses any piece, device, equipment or tool capable of enabling individuals affected by neurological impairments with independence and self-determination. Based on learning principles, an AT-based program provides a functional bridge between the limited human resources and high environmental requests. Consequently, an active role, positive participation, favorable occupation, and constructive engagement will be fostered. Microswitches, a basic form of AT-based interventions represent electronic sensors and tools capable of detecting small behavioral responses and provide a person affected by neurological impairments with brief periods of positive stimulation. Vocal output communication aids and/or speech generating devices may enable individuals with neurological disorders with social interactions with a caregiver. Computerized-mediated programs may ensure request and choice of desired items with leisure and occupation options. Currently, new technologies have growingly been developed. Virtual reality enables ecological validity, behavioral tracking, experimental control, and immersive environments similar to those of real life. Mobile technologies are transportable devices with internet access. Wearable technologies include basic technological solutions in the healthcare industry and have the potential to support and provide safety and assistance to both healthcare professionals and users. Serious Games promoted positive interactions and active participation. Telerehabilitation, as part of telemedicine, offers the evaluation, the recovery, and supervision of patients remotely either in a synchronous or asynchronous modality. Robots-assisted interventions may be implemented in clinical and medical settings to recovery patients with stroke. Both assessment and rehabilitative purposes may be favorably achieved.

The book is the result of two decades professional experience of the Editor in the field of multiple disabilities, cognitive-behavioral rehabilitative interventions, aided-alternative and augmentative communication strategies, and AT-based programs. It includes targeted populations such as children, adolescents, and older adults with attention deficit hyperactivity disorders, autism spectrum disorders, cerebral palsy, rare genetic syndromes, non-specified neurodevelopmental disorders, Alzheimer and Parkinson diseases, amyotrophic lateral sclerosis, multiple sclerosis, acquired brain injuries, post-coma patients, and persons with stroke. Beside empirical contributions, theoretical chapters and literature reviews were embedded. Clinicians, researchers, caregivers, professionals, teachers, users, and families may find illustrative examples of AT-based devices and programs, merged with scientific competence of the contributors who actively participated. The Volume was divided in four sections, namely (a) autism spectrum disorders, (b) special and complex needs, (c) neurodegenerative diseases, and (d) acquired brain injury and stroke. Either to evaluate the clinical severity of a diagnosis or to recovery a specific function, readers may find some useful insights for daily clinical activity, research, and practice. Cognitive and motor rehabilitation, academic and communication skills, positive participation, leisure and occupation opportunities, reduction of challenging behaviors have been empirically corroborated throughout the chapters. Narrative reviews supported clinical and practical validity of the AT-based options and/or strategies used.

Section 1 is exclusively devoted to autism spectrum disorders and includes three chapters. In Chapter 1, "Assistive Technologies for Children and Adolescents with Autism Spectrum Disorders", Leila Goosen provides readers with an overview of the latest research on assistive technologies, especially as related to children and adolescents with Autism Spectrum Disorders (ASD). While introducing and describing the general perspective of the chapter as specifically focusing on objectives in terms of children and adolescents with ASD, background that summarizes the content of this chapter as also consisting of significant results with regard to young and older adults, as well as references to other connected conditions, will be included. Issues, problems and challenges in this regard are presented, together with possible solutions and recommendations, future research directions and concluding remarks.

In Chapter 2, "Assistive Technology to Support Children With Autism Spectrum Disorder", Rishika Tiwari, Manish Shandilya, and Sonika Charak define Assistive Technology s any device or technology ranging from low to high that helps to improve functional skills of individuals with cognitive, physical or neurological disorders. These technologies are devised to improve the functional activities of persons. ATs focusing on cognitive disorders like dementia, autism spectrum disorders, etc. can be categorized as ATs for cognition (ATC) and augmentative and alternative communication (AAC). AAC interventions consist of tools that aid the challenges faced by individuals with speech impairment during communication. AAC used often are Speech Generating Devices (SGD), software programs and communication apps for efficient production of speech. ATCs include social stories and video modeling strategies. According to the authors, the use of assistive technology in Autism Spectrum Disorder (ASD) has great importance due to increased requirement for interventions in helping students. Finally, there are several lines of evidence showing the effectiveness of technology-assisted training in ASD patients.

In Chapter 3, "Assistive Technologies and Design for People With Autism Spectrum Disorders", Denise Gulino presents an overview on which assistive technology tools can be used to implement interventions for people with Autism Spectrum Disorders and what developers and designers must take into account when they want to approach to the development of these technologies. Four areas of intervention have been identified, named (a) treatment of phobias, (b) social interactions, (c) academic skills, (d) job performance. 10 contributions have been reviewed, for a total of 216 participants. Positive results and limits of various studies have been identified. In each session a specific technology was analyzed, and some general guidelines were emphasized. Some suggestions were outlined for future research.

Section 2 is devoted to children and adolescents with special and/or complex needs. Cerebral palsy, neurodevelopmental disorders, multiple disabilities, and rare genetic syndromes were featured along five chapters. In Chapter 4, "Interactive Computer Play in the Pursuit of Gait Optimization for Children With Cerebral Palsy: Home, Video Games, and Motivation", Manon Maitland Schladen, Yiannis Koumpouros, Elena America Choong, and Justine Lee Belschner describe Exercise therapy delivered through interactive computer play (ICP). The authors demonstrate its effectiveness to improve gross motor skills, and ultimately gait, in children with cerebral palsy (CP). This chapter provides an overview of CP, its impact on, gait, and the current physical therapy (PT) standard of care. The history of the home exercise program (HEP) component of standard PT care is described, along with the potential for using ICP to improve HEP. ICP systems are surveyed and their defining features discussed. The current therapeutic use of ICP is described and directions for further development to enhance therapeutic utility presented. A theoretical framework to support ICP implementation, self-determination theory (SDT) is outlined and an example of its exploration in a pilot effort provided. An example of health care system barriers to rapid uptake of ICP is presented along with alternative strategies for deployment and recommendations for further research.

In Chapter 5, "Instructional Strategies for People With Profound Intellectual and Multiple Disabilities: Overview of Approaches and Two Case Studies", Laura Roche and Jeff Sigafoos highlight an overview of three main instructional approaches that have been applied to enhance engagement and adaptive behavior functioning among people with PIMD. These approaches are: (a) Intensive Interaction, (b) Systematic Instruction, and (c) Assistive Technology. Two case studies are included to illustrate the use of assistive technology — specifically augmentative and alternative communication devices and micro-switches — with two adolescents with PIMD.

In Chapter 6, "New Technologies to Support Adaptive Responding in Children and Adolescents With Neurodevelopmental Disorders", Fabrizio Stasolla and Donatella Ciarmoli carry out an overview of the literature available on virtual reality setups, mobile devices, and wearable technologies to support adaptive skills of individuals with neurodevelopmental disorders. Some useful insights for future research and practice were highlighted. A critical comment on the empirical studies reviewed was evidenced.

In Chapter 7, "Assistive Technology to Promote Adaptive Skills in Children and Adolescents With Rett Syndrome: A Selective Review", Donatella Ciarmoli examines Rett syndrome, classified within the Rare Genetic Syndromes, characterized by intellectual delays, extensive motor impairments, lack of speech and communication difficulties, sensorial deficits and problems in adaptive responding. The use of assistive technologies, in particular microswitches, with children with RTT has been shown to effectively change the impact on their quality of life, facilitating access to recreational activities and improving their performance. A selective literature review was conducted considering Rett Syndrome, Assistive Technologies, Quality of life and Rare Genetic Syndrome. Empirical data demonstrated the effectiveness and suitability of interventions with AT, allowing participants to increase their level of independence.

In Chapter 8, "Family-Centered Telehealth Supporting Motor Skills and Activity in Individuals With Rett Syndrome", Meir Lotan, Michelle Stahlhut, Alberto Romano, Jenny Downs, and Cochavit Elefant evaluate three projects in which Telehealth support was provided by therapists experienced in Rett syndrome and supported by available local resources are presented in this chapter. The three projects responded to locally identified needs in a cost-efficient way and empowered those working with people with Rett syndrome to maintain and improve their clients' physical function and activity. The chapter argues on the conceptual underpinnings of delivering a service using a Telehealth approach and describes the results and the strategies implemented in the projects mentioned above.

Section 3 is devoted to young and older adults with neurodegenerative diseases. Alzheimer and Parkinson diseases, amyotrophic lateral sclerosis and multiple sclerosis were targeted along three chapters. In Chapter 9, "Assistive Technology for Promoting the Independence and the Quality of Life in Persons With Alzheimer's Disease: A Selective Review", Donatella Ciarmoli evidences how persons with Alzheimer Disease (AD) may present a loss of cognitive functioning, memory impairments, communication difficulties, and obstacles to perform daily activities, disorientation, and challenging behaviors. The chapter details an overview of the newest empirical evidences available on the use of AT-based programs to improve the independence, and the quality of life of patients with Alzheimer Disease and their caregivers. A selective literature review was carried out considering Alzheimer, Assistive Technologies, Dementia, Quality of life and Caregivers. Empirical data demonstrated the effectiveness and the suitability of the AT interventions allowing participants to improve their quality of life, as well as to mitigate the mental and physical burden of their caregivers.

In Chapter 10, "Assistive Technology-Based Programs and Telerehabilitation Strategies to Support Adaptive Responding of Individuals With Neurodegenerative Diseases", Fabrizio Stasolla and Donatella Ciarmoli outline microswitches, computer-mediated programs, vocal output communication aids, speech generating devices, I-PAD, I-POD, and tablets as basic tools to promote physical activities, communication skills, adaptive responding, leisure, and occupation opportunities in persons with Alzheimer and Parkinson diseases, amyotrophic lateral sclerosis, and multiple sclerosis. Telerehabilitation strategies to remotely pursue both assessment and rehabilitation purposes were additionally included.

In Chapter 11, "Using Virtual Reality for Assessment and Rehabilitation of AD and MCI Patients: A Selective Overview", Giulia Binaghi describes Alzheimer's disease (AD) as a primary cause of dementia in ageing population affecting more than 35 million people around the globe. Acquisition of information in everyday life requires memorization in complex three-dimensional environments. Emerging ICT (Information and computer technology) applications based on virtual reality (VR) environments can lead to a behavior modification as they provide a photorealistic virtual environment (VE). The chapter provides a selective overview of the empirical evidences available along last five years on the use of virtual reality (VR) to promote everyday life skills and cognitive impairment mitigation of AD patients. Virtual reality allows to identify and treat deficits memory that are relevant to everyday life yet not detectable with list learning. Articles related to virtual reality have been divided in two categories according to its use: whether for assessment and diagnostic or rehabilitative purposes. Clinical implications were critically discussed. Suggestions for future research and practice are also provided.

Section 4 includes acquired brain injuries and stroke. Four chapters describe technological-aided solutions to be used in both populations. In Chapter 12, "Cognitive Performance in Immersive Environments After Acquired Brain Injury", Ineke van der Ham evaluates the use of immersive environments such as virtual and augmented reality. For cognitive assessment and training in a neuropsychological setting, this offers a perspective for innovation and improvement of existing methods. Most of the current clinical uses of immersive environments focus on factors such as anxiety, or motor activities for physical therapy. Cognitive applications, concerning memory, attention, visuospatial processing are relatively scarce. The use of immersive environments for cognitive purposes are presented. In addition to immersion, the individual experience of immersive environments, as expressed by sense of presence will be discussed. By examining advantages and disadvantages of using immersive environments to measure and train cognitive performance, recommendations for clinical use of these methods are provided.

In Chapter 13, "The Use of Assistive Technology as a Tool for Family Support and Recovery Post Acquired Brain Injury", Khalida Akbar deals with the recovery period post Acquired Brain Injury (ABI), and emphasizes that individuals becoming vastly dependent on family support and caregivers. Theoretical data and findings suggest that there is a lack of awareness and family support structures surrounding those affected by ABI. The empirical data indicate the need for further research and development aimed at improving conditions for recovery for persons who are recovering from acquired brain injury. The chapter is aimed at creating awareness of assistive technology that can be used in conjunction with existing family support structures for people who are affected by ABI. The findings of this study have the potential to significantly contribute to practices and policies in society through research by providing a local country-contextual theoretical understanding of what needs to be done for persons with ABI and how AT can be used as a recovery tool within family support structures during the recovery process.

In Chapter 14, "Low Cost, User-Controlled Peroneal Stimulator for Foot Drop in Patients With Stroke: An Experiment in Indian Rehabilitation Set-Up", Kriti Mishra and Raji Thomas explain the foot drop as a common disabling condition following stroke, which has been conventionally managed using an ankle foot orthosis (AFO). An alternate rehabilitation option is the functional electrical stimulation (FES) systems which have undergone numerous improvisations over past few decades to make it more efficient and user friendly. This chapter aims to evaluate a prototype low-cost FES device in an Indian rehabilitation set-up to match the patients' cultural and socio-economic needs. It illustrates a pilot study designed to test the orthotic and clinical efficacy of the device in terms of dynamic ankle angle change during ambulation and comparing the walking speed and endurance with the AFO. A significant change with nearly two-third of normal ankle angle change during swing phase of the gait cycle was observed with nearly equivalent orthotic effects in terms of walking endurance and speed. In terms of receptivity, the device received a mixed response from the patients regarding its effectiveness as an orthosis.

In Chapter 15, "Motor Recovery in Stroke Rehabilitation Supported by Robot-Assisted Therapy", Alex Martino and Giovanni Morrone evidence the potential usefulness of robot-assisted therapy for motor recovery after a stroke. An overview of the available literature is performed providing up-to-date information about the use of robot-assistive technology in rehabilitation practice. Throughout the chapter the rationale for the use and the different machines in terms of basic engineering principles and the related rehabilitation possibilities were argued. Finally, clinical and rehabilitative implications of the findings are critically highlighted.

In conclusion, the book would provide the readers with practical and helpful ideas to help users and families of persons with neurological impairments in daily contexts. Assessment and Rehabilitative solutions are presented according to three basic criteria which guided all the chapters' authors, namely (a) clarity, (b) practicality, and (c) readability for daily use of technological-aided programs. To all the contributors, EAB members, and reviewers I'm extremely and sincerely grateful.

Preface

Fabrizio Stasolla
University Giustino Fortunato of Benevento, Italy

Acknowledgment

First of all, I would like to express my sincere gratitude to all the people who allow me the competition of this book. My thoughts are devoted to all the contributors, the reviewers, and the editorial advisory board members. Their encouragement, insights, and support were crucial to provide the readers with a high-quality book. I'm additionally grateful to all my colleagues who provide me with precious editorial recommendations. Last but not least, I would like to thank everyone at IGI Global who work very hard to ensure the timely production of this book. I wish to thank Ms. Jan Travers, Ms. Maria Rohde, and Mr. Eric Whalen for their continuous support throughout the editorial and production processes.

Fabrizio Stasolla
University Giustino Fortunato of Benevento, Italy

Section 1
Autism Spectrum Disorders

Chapter 1
Assistive Technologies for Children and Adolescents With Autism Spectrum Disorders

Leila Goosen
https://orcid.org/0000-0003-4948-2699
University of South Africa, South Africa

ABSTRACT

The purpose of this chapter is to provide readers with an overview of the latest research on assistive technologies, especially as related to children and adolescents with autism spectrum disorders (ASDs). While introducing and describing the general perspective of the chapter as specifically focusing on objectives in terms of children and adolescents with ASDs, background that summarizes the content of this chapter as also consisting of significant results with regard to young and older adults as well as references to other connected conditions will be included. Issues, problems, and challenges in this regard are presented, together with possible solutions and recommendations, future research directions, and concluding remarks.

INTRODUCTION

In terms of clearly stating what this chapter describes and is about, the purpose is to provide readers with an overview of the latest research on assistive technologies, especially as related to children and adolescents with Autism Spectrum Disorders (ASDs). While introducing and describing the general perspective of the chapter as specifically focusing on objectives in terms of children and adolescents with ASDs, background that summarizes the content of this chapter as also consisting of significant results with regard to young and older adults, as well as references to other connected conditions, will be included.

"Autism remains a fascinating condition, perhaps the most prolifically researched of all child psychiatric disorders" (Wolff, 2004, p. 201). The history of autism yields many lessons, but early accounts of possible cases of autism were mostly unclear, with the greatest contributions to understanding having come from the original paper by Asperger (1944) that "wished to stress that these were not just weird

DOI: 10.4018/978-1-7998-7430-0.ch001

children," who are frequently "socially isolated and relatively egocentric" (Mira, 1992, p. 14). Persons with neurological disorders, such as ASDs, may experience significant **problems**, like often being passive with few opportunities for "positive and constructive interaction with the outside world" (Stasolla, Boccasini, Perilli, Damiani, & Albano, 2015a, p. 1). They regularly need to rely on their caregivers' and families' assistance, with corresponding negative outcomes on their quality of life. As also quoted by O'Brolcháin and Gordijn (2018, p. 4), organizations like Autism Speaks Inc. (2021) are "dedicated to promoting **solutions**, across the spectrum and throughout the lifespan, for the needs of individuals with autism and their families through advocacy and support".

However, individuals with such a disability also have the potential to contribute, but since they may not be able to learn through conventional means, they are entitled to ways of overcoming these **issues** through the implementation of assistive technology-based interventions. When De Pace and Stasolla (2014, p. 285) talk about Assistive Technologies (ATs) and computer access for e.g. **motor disabilities**, they refer to all technological **solutions**, which allow people with multiple disabilities and/or severe/profound cognitive disabilities "to overcome their isolation and passivity" towards moving around the environment, by promoting environmental control, social interaction, leisure engagement and **academic performance**.

Stasolla, Boccasini and Perilli (2017) provided a literature overview on assistive technology-based programs to support the adaptive behaviors by children with autism spectrum disorders, which are broadly conceived and designed to fill the gap between human/individual capacities and/or skills and environmental **requests**. Specifically, AT builds a link to enable persons with ASDs towards independence and self-determination. By using an AT setup, people with ASDs could be capable of attaining an active role, positive participation, favorable occupation, and/or to achieve functional daily activities. Furthermore, they could be enabled towards improved social image, desirability and an enhanced status, with a reduction in families' and caregivers' burdens. Concisely, persons with ASDs would positively cope with their environment. At least two functional purposes may be pursued through an AT-based intervention, namely (a) **assessment**, and (b) recovery. In the case of autism, El Kaliouby and Robinson (2007, p. 3) indicated that assistive technologies could "be divided into two broad categories", i.e. therapeutic and prosthetic, with therapeutic technologies aimed at helping individuals to deal with impairments or particular deficiencies through teaching and intervention programs.

The **objectives** of studies, like the one by Fteiha (2017), often include investigating the effectiveness of assistive technologies in enhancing the language skills and improving the **communication skills** of children and adolescents with autism. Moreover, **physical activities** may also be fostered. A satisfactory independent role for persons with ASDs may be reached with purposeful behavior. Consequently, **challenging behaviors** may be significantly reduced. **Request and choice behaviors**, as well as opportunities for these, may be enhanced. Finally, **Virtual Reality** (VR) and/or **augmented reality** setups may be viewed as valid ecological environments, ensuring methodological control, and behavioral tracking for both **assessment** and rehabilitation purposes.

Target Audience

Similar to that of the book as a whole, scholars, researchers, families of individuals with ASDs, teachers, occupational, speech, and physiotherapists, practitioners, psychologists, educators, students, caregivers, and neurologists as interdisciplinary target audience may benefit from what is presented in this chapter.

Recommended Topics

In terms of the **recommended topics** set out for this book, this chapter will specifically focus on:

- Autism spectrum disorders,
- Academic performance,
- Alternative and augmentative communication strategies,
- Assessment,
- AT-based interventions and programs,
- Challenging behaviors,
- Communication skills,
- Intellectual, developmental and motor disabilities,
- iPad,
- iPod,
- Literacy,
- Physical activities,
- Request and choice behaviors,
- Serious games,
- Special education,
- Systematic reviews and a meta-analysis, and
- Virtual and augmented reality.

Please note that these **recommended topics** are discussed throughout the chapter, where applicable to particular sections; to highlight, these are in **bold**.

Objectives

Now that the general perspective of the chapter had been described, this section will end by specifically stating the objectives. As for the objectives of the book, those for this chapter would be to include the latest high-quality research on the use of AT-based programs for promoting the independence and self-determination of individuals with ASDs. The chapter will include theoretical and review aspects, as well as report on empirical research with evidence-based practices, including where **AT-based interventions and programs** are encouraged. VR-based setups for **assessment** and/or rehabilitation purposes in individuals with ASDs are additionally considered. The chapter is intended to provide the reader with the latest contributions available on the specific recommended topics selected from both research and practice.

Background

This section of the chapter will provide broad definitions and discussions of the topic and incorporate views of others (in the form of a *literature review*) into the discussion to support, refute, or demonstrate the author's position on the topic.

A process similar to that described by Alves, De Carvalho, Aguilar, De Brito and Bastos (2020, p. 118667) was followed: After reading through all selected references, these were tabulated and data extraction details were noted for each reference. These details included an overview of the reference, some observations with regard to "content and conclusions, as well as some basic" data, such as bibliographic particulars, publication date, summary, etc.

Autism Spectrum Disorders

In answer to the question 'What is autism?', Autism Speaks (2010) indicated that circumstances may cause a child with ASDs "to become upset and have a 'meltdown'. The child may be difficult to soothe and calm down. … Boys are more likely than" girls to be diagnosed as showing signs of ASDs (Ahmed, 2012, p. 5). With regard to a **definition** of terms, the latest "Diagnostic and Statistical Manual of Mental Disorders" (DSM-V, 2013) indicated that "several classifications of disorders exist" across the autism spectrum (Goosen, 2020, p. 85).

ASDs are related to especially children, some of whom experience atypical language development. Their emerging linguistic skills are related "to interactive competence, such as imitation. … Another behavior is joint attention" (Ahmed, 2012, p. 5). Children with ASDs typically prefer to work only with a selected group of people, who could include family members, "community members or their teachers and friends. Children with autism spectrum" disorders are also characterized by exhibiting marked difficulties in "transitioning from one activity to another", an insistence on demonstrating repetitive patterns of preservative and/or sensory behaviors, as well as possibly fixed and highly focused and/or unusual restricted sensory interests beginning early in life (Alves, et al., 2020, p. 118664; Lord, et al., 2020).

Autism spectrum disorders are considered to be common childhood, but lifelong, neurodevelopmental conditions or disabilities, affecting "how people perceive the world and interact with others" (Mansouri-Benssassi, Gomez, Boyd, Hayes, & Ye, 2018, p. 11).

In a *literature overview* on assistive technology for promoting the adaptive skills of children with autism spectrum disorders, Stasolla, et al. (2015a) indicated that many individuals with ASDs are commonly described as having a specific combination of deficits, which impact on three main areas (Fazana, et al., 2017) that may lead to significant impairments in behavioural, communicative, emotional, **intellectual** and social skills (Alzahrani, 2014).

According to Wali and Sanfilippo (2019, p. 520), autism, "also known as autism spectrum disorder" is incurable, brain-based and as a construct "refers to a wide range of complex" behaviorally **defined**, static impairments of the immature brain (Muhle, Trentacoste, & Rapin, 2004).

The disorder is of unknown aetiology, but Mold, Umar, King and Exley (2018, p. 76) suggested that it involved "both *genetic* susceptibility and environmental factors including in the latter environmental toxins." Geschwind (2009, p. 367) agreed that recent advances in terms of the genetics of autism have shown the disorder to have a strong *genetic* component: "It is not a unitary entity but a clinical syndrome, with variable deficits" with regard to social behavior and language. ASDs are "a highly heritable and heterogeneous group of neurodevelopmental *phenotypes* diagnosed in more than 1% of children. Common *genetic* variants contribute substantially to" autism spectrum disorder susceptibility (Grove, et al., 2019, p. 431), "with worldwide heritability estimates between 50% and 80%, indicating a strong *genetic* contribution to" these disorders. "There is high *phenotypic* heterogeneity, with considerable variability in the clinical presentation in terms of" symptoms (Binder, 2021, p. 11).

While a big data-based system can serve as a supportive tool in ASD analysis (Wadhera & Kakkar, 2020), leveraging 'Big data' "approaches in the form of large-scale human genomic studies have led to striking advances in" illuminating the pathobiology of autism spectrum disorder "*genetics*. Similar to many other psychiatric syndromes, advances in genotyping technology" allowed for inexpensive genome-wide assays (Quick, Wang, & State, 2021, p. 55).

"The first autism surveys were simple head counts of children already diagnosed with a severe autism *phenotype* and residing in small, circumscribed geographical areas. *Prevalence* was low, ranging from 0.4 to 2/1,000 in the 1960's and 1970's" (Fombonne, 2018, p. 717). According to Muhle, et al. (2004, p. e472), autism "is of great concern to the practicing pediatrician because of an astonishing 556% reported increase in pediatric *prevalence* between 1991 and 1997".

The rising *prevalence* of autism spectrum disorder has also "made this as one of the largest" impairment groups (Fazana, et al., 2017, p. 1). The importance of studies into the integration of assistive and wearable technologies to improve communication, social interaction and health monitoring for children with autism spectrum disorder has therefore also risen.

In a **meta-analysis** of the effectiveness of using assistive technology to enhance the social skills of students diagnosed with autism, Alzahrani (2014, p. ii) indicated that the *prevalence* of ASD was "increasing at an alarming rate and it" was therefore essential to find effective interventions for these disorders. "Numerous studies have been conducted to demonstrate that assistive technology can be useful in social skills training for individuals with" ASDs.

With regard to impairments "covered at the state and federal levels, autism and related conditions are a sharply growing *diagnostic* category among children and young adults. In education, administrators and practitioners working with affected" children are continually faced with these (Kats & Stasolla, 2021, p. xvi).

To administer the Autism *Diagnostic* Interview-Revised (ADI-R), "an experienced interviewer, following highly standardized procedures, questions a parent or caregiver. Results are scored and interpreted using a" diagnostic algorithm, a current behavior algorithm, "or both, depending on the purpose of" the **assessment** (Rutter, Le Couteur, & Lord, 2003, p. 2).

Augmentative and Alternative Communication Strategies

According to Ahmed (2012, p. 6), **Augmentative and Alternative Communication** (AAC) **strategies** "assist people with severe communication" impairments towards participating "more fully in their social roles", including care management, education, employment, and learning (Mirenda, 2001, pp. 141-151). The latter author (Mirenda, 2001) asked what was really known about autism, augmentative communication, and assistive technologies, with a focus on autism and other **developmental** impairments.

In a doctoral dissertation, McMurray (2016) provided a comparison between two types of augmentative and alternative communication systems, an **iPad** and a Picture Exchange Communication System (PECS) for children with autism spectrum disorder, in order to establish the benefits of integrating assistive technologies into the ASD classroom. According to McMurray (2016, p. ii), research has proven the benefits of integrating assistive technologies into a **special education** setting, including improving "the educational experience, as well as" optimizing "the school environment by promoting greater independence and enhancing" the "functional performance and success of" children with autism spectrum disorder.

Schlosser and Wendt (2008) provided a **systematic review** on the effects of an augmentative and alternative communication intervention on the speech production of children with autism.

MAIN FOCUS OF THE CHAPTER

Assistive Technologies

Assistive technologies are **defined** as to include any devices, equipment or pieces, which can be used to promote novel skills, improve existing behaviors, and/or reduce the negative consequences related to disabilities in patients' daily functioning (Stasolla, et al., 2015a). ATs can also provide computer-based assistance for supporting the language acquisition of an individual with ASDs. Software tracks and analyzes a student's progress, and offers help as needed, as well as suggesting and providing "logical next steps for students to take" (Ahmed, 2012, p. 6).

The *literature review* by Andersen and Jensen (2018, p. 2) was "part of a research project investigating how technologies" could be utilized to support children "with **developmental** and attention deficit" disorders "to be included in mainstream learning contexts. The review" contained "research within the field of assistive" learning technologies for learners with Attention Deficit Hyperactivity Disorder (ADHD) and ASD.

The paper by Ibrahim and Alias (2018, p. 4250) was "intended to explore published reports", journal articles, etc. "concerning the implementation of **Special Education** in Malaysia." This *literature review* targeted "the Malaysian education system, focusing on students with" Special Educational Needs (SENs), as well as on using assistive technologies to enhance social skills competence among children with autism spectrum disorders.

Recently, Alves, et al. (2020, p. 118664) provided a **systematic review** of assistive technologies, indicating Applied Behavior Analysis (ABA) as well-supported for the treatment of autism. Earlier, Nikopoulou-Smyrni, Halder, Mackeogh and Dillenburger (2012) also executed a **systematic review** of electronic assistive technologies for improving social and behavioral outcomes for individuals with autism spectrum disorders. Finally, Hong (2008) provided a *review* of high-tech assistive technologies in the language education of students with autism spectrum disorders.

The aim of the study by Pliasa and Fachantidis (2019, p. 618) was "to present some of the benefits of" mobile technologies and **serious games** for "the development of social skills in children with" autism spectrum disorders, and how these could "be enhanced when Socially Assistive Robots" (SARs) support such interventions. The use of SARs "is a promising method for improving the social skills of children with autism spectrum" disorders. "Studies conducted in this field in recent years show that the use of robots as collaborators may have positive effects on" these learners (Syriopoulou-Delli & Gkiolnta, 2020, p. 1). The latter authors provided a *review* of assistive technology in the training of children with autism spectrum disorders.

Goosen (2020) recently provided an overview of how research on technology-supported teaching and learning and Information Systems (IS) are opening new worlds for those children with autism spectrum disorders (Goosen, 2019a); (Goosen, 2019b).

Towards reducing the need for personal support among workers with autism, Gentry, Kriner, Sima, McDonough and Wehman (2015) worked on using an **iPod** touch as an assistive technology in the form of a delayed randomized control trial.

In their paper, Sula and Bushti (2014, p. 40) presented the latest research on using ATs as form of technology-based intervention to foster and promote Albanian language development in children with autism and "proposed the use of educational software 'Abetare' as a form of assistive technology aiming to assist/support children with" ASDs to learn "new language skills and improve their cognitive skills."

In another paper, Sula and Spaho (2014, p. 203) were going to propose the use of a "smart environment based on Internet of Things (IoT) and" Peer-to-Peer (P2P) technologies "as a form of assistive environment in autism care centers to support children" in the development of communication and language skills in a case study in Albania.

Assistive technologies as a predictor of general or alternate **assessment** among elementary-aged students with autism spectrum disorders were investigated by Barnard-Brak, Thompson, Wei and Richman (2014) .

The chapter by Alcantud, Alonso, Coret and Jiménez (2016, p. 895) discussed "assistive technologies applied in people with" ASDs and how these technologies promoted their adaptation. The latter authors also "analyzed different technological application areas such as detection, **assessment**, diagnosis" and intervention. Wadhera and Kakkar (2019) also offered an eye tracker as an assistive tool in the diagnosis of ASDs, while Kakkar (2019) provided diagnostic **assessment** techniques and non-invasive biomarkers for ASDs.

"The *design* and development of computer assistive technologies must be tied to the needs and goals of end users and must take into account their capabilities and preferences. In" their paper, Hervás, Francisco, Méndez and Bautista (2019, p. 85) presented MeDeC@, a user-centered "Methodology for the Development of" Computer-based assistive technologies for individuals with autism.

The conference paper by Sampath, Agarwal and Indurkhya (2013, p. 325) described and discussed their experiences of developing assistive technologies for children with autism and lessons for interaction *design*, as well as "AutVisComm, an assistive communication system developed on ubiquitous tablets, and Autinect, a set of activities to teach social skills" as "two applications designed for children with autism to aid them in communication and learning social skills" (Sampath, et al., 2013, p. 332).

The journal article by O'Brolchain and Gordijn (2020, p. 607) aimed to explore the role that assistive technologies "might play in helping people with autism spectrum disorder … and a concomitant responsibility deficit become more morally responsible. Toward this goal, the" latter authors discussed the philosophical concepts of responsibility-enhancing assistive technologies for people with autism.

According to Conn, Liu, Sarkar, Stone and Warren (2008b, p. 365), investigations "into technology-assisted intervention for children with autism spectrum" disorders had gained momentum. "Therapists involved in interventions must overcome the communication impairments generally exhibited by children with" ASDs towards affect-sensitive assistive intervention technologies for children with autism.

The study by Ahmed (2012, p. 5) could help to "effectively educate children with autism spectrum" disorders. It provided "information about the effects of" assistive technologies versus manual communication aids on the vocabulary development of children with autism and pointed out that there are advantages and disadvantages to both methods.

In a case study of pupils with autism, Almami, Patel, Koay, Juric and Everiss (2012) worked towards identifying teaching practices using assistive technologies through ontological reasoning.

In their paper, Ringland, Wolf, Boyd, Baldwin and Hayes (2016, p. 39) explained that those with impairments "have long adopted, adapted, and appropriated collaborative systems to serve as assistive devices." Minecraft was "imbued with and built on the values of enabling customization through building and creating." Against this background, Ringland, et al. (2016, p. 33) presented "the results of a digital ethnography in a Minecraft **virtual** world for children with autism, specifically examining how this community" appropriated Minecraft as an assistive technology for youth with autism. In moving from virtuality to **reality**, Moore, Cheng, McGrath and Powell (2005) considered avatars, autism, and assistive technologies.

Ensino em Realidade Aumentada (E.R.A.) "**Augmented Reality** Teaching is a developed product that assists autistic children to learn how to read and write through" **augmented reality** technology. "E.R.A. is capable of overcoming the digital and physical apart-feeling", which could be found in such a relationship (Cirino, Fernandes, e Silva, & Serra, 2020, p. 405).

Most individual students with autism spectrum disorder need help in terms of supporting their writing skills through assistive technologies. Coffin, Myles, Rogers and Szakacs (2016, p. 59) pointed out that the "elements of written expression require a set of complicated skills that go beyond the act of holding a pencil and putting words on paper and encompass … complex interaction among physical, cognitive, and sensory systems."

"Adults with Autism Spectrum Conditions" (ASCs) experience marked difficulties in recognizing "the emotions of others and responding appropriately. The clinical characteristics of" ASCs mean that face-to-face "or group interventions may not be appropriate" (Cassidy, et al., 2016, p. 193). The latter authors therefore looked at expressive *visual* text-to-speech as an assistive technology for individuals with autism spectrum conditions. In terms of a classroom-based assistive technology, Cramer, Hirano, Tentori, Yeganyan and Hayes (2011) investigated the collective use of interactive *visual* schedules by students with autism.

According to Mitchell, Engleman and Linden (2012, p. 2), it "is known that young children with autism" spectrum disorders "require specialized support in order to make educational progress. It has been reported that children with autism are also *visual* learners and that their interactions with technology are sometimes more motivating than" other interactions. The latter authors investigated the effectiveness of assistive technologies (TAP-it® and VizZle®) for enhancing the progress of such children.

The chapter by Lang, et al. (2014, p. 157) reviewed "research involving the use of assistive technology in the education and treatment of people with" ASDs. Their chapter was organized into "three sections corresponding to the most common uses of" assistive technologies for this population.

The goal of the study by Fan (2012, p. 5) was "to understand the effective learning of the **iPad** and the use of the system to assist elementary-age students with learning. The research literature" promoted different types of assistive technologies used for learning and suggested a few applications towards enhancing learning with the use of assistive technology for children on the autism spectrum.

As most people with ASDs "have some degree of a learning disability", students with ASDs "cannot learn in the same way as typically developing children do and they need special treatment to learn a concept. The purpose of" the paper by Radwan and Cataltepe (2016, p. 112) was to investigate using assistive technology to enhance teaching for students with autism spectrum disorders. In their paper, Radwan and Cataltepe (2016, p. 120) also presented "an analysis and visualization of the data collected using a web application during" learning sessions.

Kenney (2013, p. xiii) used a "single subject study with multiple baselines across participants … to explore the effect of" providing young students, with moderate forms of "autism, and documented difficulties with written language" with "access to picture-to-text software for writing". The impact of using assistive technology on the writing productivity of young writers with autism was thus established.

The importance of assistive technologies in the classroom for males and females with autism spectrum disorders lies in maximizing "the school environment by enhancing the functional performance of" such students (McMurray & Pierson, 2016, p. 59). "Advancements in technology has supported males and females with" autism spectrum disorders to make "academic and social gains in the school setting."

The research methods used in the study by Fteiha (2017, p. 36) entailed twelve children with autism, with a mean age of eight years being "randomly assigned to either experimental groups or a control group", while Schafer, et al. (2016) presented assistive technology evaluations of a remote-microphone technology for children with autism spectrum disorders.

While Chandler (2014) presented a course on 'Assistive Technology and Communication for Students with Autism Spectrum Disorders (ASD)', other references on the use of assistive technologies in the education of children with autism spectrum disorders include Cuhadar (2008) and Koch (2012). Kulkarni (2017) not only considered assistive technologies for autism, but also for cerebral palsy, multiple disabilities, and **intellectual** disabilities.

The study by Stasolla, et al. (2015b, p. 69) proposed the use of assistive technology "to promote communication and leisure opportunities" for three children with Traumatic Brain Injury "(TBI). Furthermore, it assessed the effects of such" technologies on indices of positive participation.

Issues, Problems, Challenges

This subsection of the chapter will present the author's perspective on issues, gaps, problems, challenges, risks, difficulties, limitations, etc., as these relate to the theme and arguments supporting the author's position. It will further compare and contrast with what has been, or is currently being, done as it relates to the specific topic of the chapter and the main theme of the book.

"It is important to explore" key factors, because these could help researchers and technology developers to address "issues and gaps in a meaningful way when developing specific products or services for Chinese" individuals with autism spectrum disorders in the future (Deng & Rattadilok, 2020, p. 3).

Hashim and Yussof (2017, p. 374) pointed out that humanoids "as a form of assistive technologies have been shown to have positive effects on the social-cognitive behavior of brain-impaired children, particularly those with" ASDs. However, a gap was identified in that more evidence was needed "on the socio-economic benefits of assistive technologies for social-skill training on brain-impaired children with autism as preparation for adulthood.

Another gap is indicated by the fact that although much "of autism research has focused on the social, communication and cognitive difficulties associated with the condition", autism remains "a complex neurodevelopmental condition, and little is known about its neurobiology" (Robertson & Baron-Cohen, 2017, p. 671). "The reasons autism occurs are not understood, and researchers are looking for answers, as well as ways to prevent" these disorders. (Autism Speaks, 2010).

As camouflaging "of autistic characteristics in social situations is" hypothesized "as a common social coping strategy for adults with" autism spectrum conditions (Hull, et al., 2017, p. 2519), such camouflaging "may impact diagnosis, quality of life, and long-term outcomes, but little is known about" this.

The updated edition of a book by Frith (2003) on explaining the enigma of autism provided "a psychological account of what happens in the mind of a person with" ASDs. The book proposed that key problems included "an inability to recognize and think about thoughts (theory of mind) and an inability to integrate pieces of information".

According to Mansouri-Benssassi, et al. (2018, p. 11), wearable assistive technologies for autism present both opportunities and challenges. "Challenges with typical social engagement, common in the autism experience, can have a significant negative impact on the quality of life of individuals". "Assistive technologies for social skills learning in general and" Wearable Assistive Technologies (WATs) in particular have therefore become "a popular research topic in recent years" (Mansouri-Benssassi, et al., 2018, p. 19).

The chapter by Christopher (2018) focused on addressing how ATs "can be used by teachers to foster inclusion and participation" for students with high functioning autism spectrum disorder. "Core deficits of" autism spectrum disorder challenges were also briefly outlined.

"Many children with autism have language delays and language and communication impairments. To overcome these challenges, a series of interventions is needed", "and the use of assistive technologies is often one of" these (Sula & Bushti, 2014, p. 33).

ASDs have "a significant impact on the social development and educational achievement of affected students. In the Kingdom of Saudi Arabia (KSA), students with ASD still face a number of challenges, including *stigmatization*" (Jamal, 2020, p. 1). In such a context of **special education** and *rehabilitation*, the study by the latter author looked at developing the language ability of children with autism spectrum disorder using assistive technology and a picture exchange communication system by adapting elements of "success attributed to the Australian educational environment on inclusive public schools in the" KSA (Jamal, 2020, pp. 31-32).

The short paper by O'Brolcháin and Gordijn (2017, p. 265) presented "a philosophical analysis of the ways in which assistive technologies" can result in the *stigmatization* of users with ASDs. It framed their "discussion in the context of the medical and social models of" impairment and outlined the risks of *stigmatization* resulting from assistive technologies for people with autism spectrum disorder.

Assistive technologies are "being developed for cohorts of vulnerable people, including persons with autism spectrum" disorders. The paper by O'Brolcháin and Gordijn (2018, p. 1) focused on and discussed the risks, which "the development of ATs for persons with ASD might lead to", increasing risks of *stigmatization*.

The agreement of autistic and non-autistic adults with scientific knowledge about ASDs, "how they define autism, and their endorsement of *stigmatizing* conceptions of autism" had not previously been examined. Gillespie-Lynch, Kapp, Brooks, Pickens and Schwartzman (2017, p. 1) used an online survey to assess evidence of autistic adults as critical autism experts on autism knowledge.

In their book on educating children with autism, the National Research Council (2001) indicated that autism is a word most are familiar with. But is there really an understanding of "what it means? Children with autism are challenged by the most essential human behaviors. They have difficulty interacting with other people-often failing to see people as people rather than simply objects".

According to Stanger, Mims, Wood and Ahlgrim-Delzell (2016, p. 51), education "professionals are challenged with re-evaluating the learning capacity of students with **developmental**" impairments, such as **intellectual** disabilities and autism. Assistive technologies provide both the means for the "delivery of instruction and the measure of outcomes". The latter authors incorporated such assistive technologies for supporting the **literacy** achievement of students with **intellectual** disabilities and autism through curricular programs.

In terms of background, persistent disparities exist in the early identification of autism spectrum disorder "among children from low-income families who are racial and/or ethnic minorities and where English is not the primary language. Parental **literacy**" in the context of validation of the **developmental** check-in tool for low-**literacy** autism screening were considered (Harris, Janvier, Mandell, & Cidav, 2021).

The risk of Substance Use Disorder (SUD) in patients with autism spectrum disorder remains unclear. The objective of Huang et al. (2021) was to "investigate the risk of SUD in patients with ASD and its associations with comorbidities," Psychotropic Agents (PAs), and mortality.

In terms of importance, there is still "limited evidence supporting an association of" ASDs "with suicidality and the risk factors for suicide attempt and suicide among people with" ASDs. Existing research highlighted "the need for national cohort studies." Amongst the objectives of Kõlves, Fitzgerald, Nordentoft, Wood and Erlangsen (2021, p. 1) was such an assessment of suicidal behaviors among individuals with autism spectrum disorder in Denmark.

The promise and limitations of using innovative assistive technologies to benefit children on the autism spectrum was looked at by Andersen, Levenson and Blumberg (2014).

Baron-Cohen (2009, p. 68) suggested the Empathizing-Systemizing (ES) theory, as the "mind-blindness theory of autism spectrum conditions has been successful in explaining the social and communication difficulties that characterize these conditions but cannot explain the" non-social "features (the narrow interests, need for sameness, and attention to detail)."

As mental "health difficulties are highly prevalent in individuals on the autism spectrum", the study by Cage, Di Monaco and Newell (2018, p. 473) "examined how experiences and perceptions of autism acceptance could impact on the mental health of ... 111 adults on the autism spectrum", who completed an online survey.

"A large number of people in China have been affected by" autism spectrum disorders. "However, different factors associated with" the need for and "barriers to accessing external support" and using assistive technologies among individuals with ASDs "in China have been identified" (Deng & Rattadilok, 2020, p. 1).

In terms of techniques to include users with autism in the *design* of assistive technologies, "tools are often paper-based and can be bulky", while there was "an increasing number of possible technology platforms, such as personal digital assistants and mobile phones, and a wide variety of techniques available to the designer to involve the user in the design" (Francis, 2004, p. i).

The conference paper by Francis, Firth and Mellor (2005, p. 1104) reported on an investigation, which "found that conventional techniques for including users in technology *design* are likely to fail if the user has autism. The heterogeneity of autistic symptomatology across cognitive, social", behavioral and communication domains need to be considered towards reducing the risk of abandonment of assistive technologies for people with autism.

The paper by Moktar, et al. (2014, p. 172) depicted the prominence of culture in the adoption of assistive technologies, "in terms of *design*, which are particularly anticipated for autism" treatments. The latter researchers believed that cultural aspects "should be considered in designing assistive" technologies and therefore extended a cultural model of assistive technology design for autism treatment.

While Khan (2021) looked at balancing non-discrimination and **risk** management in mental health legislation for autism, de Villiers (2021) and Courtenay (2021) respectively presented the case against and for removing **intellectual** disability and autism from the Mental Health Act.

Deleterious Copy Number Variants "(CNVs) are identified in up to 20% of individuals with autism. However, levels of autism risk conferred by most rare CNVs remain unknown." Douard, et al. (2021, p. 78) "recently developed statistical models to estimate the effect" sizes of deletions and duplications on autism risk across the genome.

According to Manoli and State (2021, p. 30), recent "progress in the identification of genes and genomic regions contributing to autism spectrum disorder ... has had a broad impact on" understanding "the nature of genetic risk for a range of psychiatric disorders," as well as understanding ASD biology.

SOLUTIONS AND RECOMMENDATIONS

This section of the chapter will discuss solutions and recommendations in dealing with the issues, problems, etc. presented in the preceding section.

Solutions

It "is important to note that ASD is very heterogeneous, so the difficulties encountered when working with this impairment can be very different depending on the specific users. Different **solutions** have been tried to overcome" limitations in this regard (Hervás, et al., 2019, p. 4).

The first of two groups into which "most common existing assistive technologies for people with" ASDs in the workplace can be divided includes Personal Digital Assistants (PDAs), which are "mostly used for the purpose of reducing the need" for personal support "and being able to manage different tasks independently" (Wali & Sanfilippo, 2019, p. 10). "PDAs are pocket-size, easily accessible and economical when compared to other solutions."

Francis, Mellor and Firth (2009, p. 67) "investigated issues surrounding the direct involvement of people with autism in the *design* of digital assistive" technologies and found that in terms of solutions, "there was no clear 'winner' among the techniques examined, as all would need some modification and management." Earlier, Francis (2004, p. 54) had indicated that a "good way to identify problems and suggest solutions" is to compile "a list of the key issues in" information systems management.

A participatory "approach to software *design* actively involves the end users of the software product in the design process to better understand their needs and requirements and is considered the de-facto standard for developing solutions for users with special needs" (Sampath, et al., 2013, p. 326).

Assistive technologies offer a range of solutions for "people who cannot speak or hear speech" (Fan, 2012, p. 18).

Experts "on software development and programming with ten years of industrial experience" developed solutions in terms of, for example, "Linux technologies, and mobile and web applications" (Alves, et al., 2020, p. 118672).

According to Mansouri-Benssassi, et al. (2018, p. 12), recent work had "leveraged technological advances to create wearable solutions for real-world social interactions with the support of real-time sensing, inference, and delivery of *in situ* social cues via multimodal feedback."

An overview of state-of-the-art assistive technology "solutions for assisting people with autism spectrum" disorders in their day-to-day work and in everyday life "by considering different sensor channels" was presented by Wali and Sanfilippo (2019, p. 10).

"Observing and working to understand what" Do-It-Yourself (DIY) practices children were already implementing "to address their own needs, administrators can then open up yet more possibilities for creation and modification", "as well as developing similar solutions to those offered by" children to the wider community (Ringland, et al., 2016, p. 39).

With regard to repetitive DNA and next-generation sequencing, Treangen and Salzberg (2012) investigated computational challenges and solutions.

Recommendations

An increasing number "of technology platforms offer opportunities to develop new visual assistive aids for people with autism. However, their involvement in the *design* of such aids is critical to" short-term uptake and longer-term "use. Using a three-round Delphi study", Francis, et al. (2009, p. 57) explored techniques and recommendations for the inclusion of users with autism in the design of assistive technologies. The Delphi study used by Francis, et al. (2005) also ran for three rounds and with the involvement of seven panelists that was consistent with recommendations.

The Telematics Applications Supporting Cognition (TASC) project was cited by Francis (2004, p. 11) as having made "recommendations for the design of interview questions and the use of visual communication tools for less-verbal users in designer-user interviews", which emphasized "the importance of careful sequencing and delivery of simple sentence structures that avoid the use of abstract concepts."

Two of the healthcare practitioners interviewed by Deng and Rattadilok (2020, p. 7) "suggested that the development of assistive technologies can focus on the provision of the most current and advanced therapeutic recommendations to parents of ASD individuals based on their symptoms so that parents can obtain professional advice and treatment recommendations at home."

In a special supplement, Parens and Asch (1999) provided a disability rights critique of reflections and recommendations, while in terms of diagnosis, Quick, et al. (2021, p. 64) pointed out that the "specific workup for an individual is influenced both by presentation and discipline-specific recommendations".

FUTURE RESEARCH DIRECTIONS

This section of the chapter will discuss future and emerging trends and provide insight about the future of the theme of the book from the perspective of the chapter focus. The viability of a paradigm, model, implementation issues of proposed programs, etc., may also be included in this section. It will further suggest future research opportunities within the domain of the topic.

Emerging trends in assistive technologies implementation for individuals with ASDs show that the "majority of technologies supporting students with ASD capitalize on their visual strengths" (Spence-Cochran & Pearl, 2012, p. 295).

The chapter by Beals (2017, p. 160) surveyed and critiqued existing and emerging trends with regard to "remediation technologies and assistive technologies targeted at verbal communication deficits in individuals with autism spectrum disorders. Focusing on deficits in grammar/syntax and pragmatics (language use)" served towards supporting the education of children with autism.

Mansouri-Benssassi, et al. (2018) discussed numerous future research directions with regard to wearable assistive technologies for autism, while Alves, et al. (2020, p. 118670) mentioned several references, the research in which "may be considered *technological* and may be replicable" in future. The research by Francis, et al. (2009) also suggested a number of avenues in terms of future research directions.

In the near future, Hervás, et al. (2019, p. 20) planned for their work "to evolve in two different" research directions.

The paper by Conn, Liu, Sarkar, Stone and Warren (2008a, p. 442) presented an overview of their "work on the investigation of an affect-sensitive system to be applied in future autism" interventions. "A physiology-based affect-inference and adaptation framework was proposed, which" should allow for an individual-specific approach towards affect-sensitive assistive intervention technologies for children with autism.

Information and Communication Technologies (ICTs) "offer new opportunities to people with" impairments to develop "autonomy and independence in their daily life activities. However, more research should be done in order to comprehend how" mobile devices as assistive technologies for ASD affects experiences in the classroom (Roldán-Álvarez, Gomez, Márquez-Fernández, Martín, & Montoro, 2016, p. 187).

Assistive technologies "aimed at improving the life quality of persons with Autism Spectrum Disorder and/or **Intellectual** Disability (ASD/ID) is an important research area. Few have examined how this population use and experience AT or their vision for future uses of" these (O'Neill, Smyth, Smeaton, & O'Connor, 2020, p. 251). The latter authors therefore worked on developing an understanding of the needs and experiences of such individuals in Ireland and the United Kingdom.

CONCLUSION

This final section will provide a discussion of the overall coverage of the chapter and concluding remarks.

The purpose of this chapter was to introduce an overview and summary of the latest research on assistive technologies for especially children and adolescents with autism spectrum disorders. Similar to that of Jamal (2020), the subsequent sections of this chapter provided background by reviewing relevant scholarly literature, explained the methodologies, which had been adopted by applicable studies, and outlined and discussed these studies' results.

While Francis, et al. (2005, p. 1107) concluded that it was "possible to include users with autism" or Asperger's Syndrome (AS) "directly in the *design* process," the latter authors warned that care "must be taken to conduct a thorough **assessment** of the user and their abilities, motivators and" behaviors "prior to commencement of the design process, no matter which technique" was adopted. Including such users directly was also dependent on three conclusions regarding "thorough **assessment** and planning by a designer experienced with the target group and with the user" (Francis, 2004, p. 43). "Taking into account the conclusions obtained in the *design* phase, a completely functional instance of the plug-in was implemented" (Hervás, et al., 2019, p. 16).

According to Deng and Rattadilok (2020, p. 10), it was evident that individuals with ASDs "have special needs and barriers when considering using assistive technologies in their daily" lives, while as a conclusion, Hashim and Yussof (2017, p. 377) pointed out that "the socio-economic benefits gained by having assistive technologies", such as humanoid robots "to assist special needs children in preparation for adulthood" were significant.

Fan (2012, p. 31) discussed solutions to improve on the academic, language and social skills, as well as executive functioning, of children with autism and made "appropriate recommendations for the improvement of the current situation",

In terms of future research directions and conclusions, Conn, et al. (2008b, p. 384) indicated that there was "increasing consensus in the autism community that development of assistive tools that exploit advanced" technologies will likely make the application of intensive interventions for children with ASDs more readily accessible, while in their paper, Sula and Spaho (2014, p. 211) "proposed the use of the smart environment based on P2P technology and IoT in the Regional Center for Autism in Tirana",

Albania "as a form of assistive technology aiming to assist/support children with" ASDs to improve their communication and language skills.

"In conclusion, new interactive technologies" will continue to rapidly advance and are therefore promising intervention tools for improving the emotional processing and attention skills of adults with ASCs (Cassidy, et al., 2016, p. 199).

REFERENCES

Ahmed, R. (2012). *The Effects of Assistive Technology Versus Manual Communication Aids on the Vocabulary Development of Children With Autism* (Doctoral dissertation). San Marcos, CA: California State University.

Alcantud, F., Alonso, Y., Coret, J., & Jiménez, E. (2016). Assistive Technologies and Autism Spectrum Disorders. In Human-Computer Interaction: Concepts, Methodologies, Tools, and Applications (pp. 895-924). IGI Global. doi:10.4018/978-1-4666-8789-9.ch041

Almami, E., Patel, F., Koay, N., Juric, R., & Everiss, C. (2012, June). Towards identifying teaching practices using assistive technologies through ontological reasoning: A Case Study of Pupils with Autism. In *Proceedings of the 17th International Conference on Society for Design and Process Science (SDPS)*, (pp. 10-14). Academic Press.

Alves, F. J., De Carvalho, E. A., Aguilar, J., De Brito, L. L., & Bastos, G. S. (2020). Applied behavior analysis for the treatment of autism: A systematic review of assistive technologies. *IEEE Access: Practical Innovations, Open Solutions*, *8*, 118664–118672. doi:10.1109/ACCESS.2020.3005296

Alzahrani, N. S. (2014). *Meta analysis of the effectiveness of using assistive technology to enhance social skills with students diganosed with autism (Master of Special Education Diagnostician Program).* Lamar University.

Andersen, H. V., & Jensen, R. H. (2018). Assistive Learning Technologies for Learners with ADHD and ASD: A Review 2006-2016. *Læring og Medier*, *11*(19). Advance online publication. doi:10.7146/lom.v11i19.109755

Andersen, K., Levenson, L., & Blumberg, F. C. (2014). The Promise and Limitations of Assistive Technology Use among Children with Autism. In N. R. Silton (Ed.), *Innovative Technologies to Benefit Children on the Autism Spectrum* (pp. 1–19). IGI Global. doi:10.4018/978-1-4666-5792-2.ch001

Asperger, H. (1944). Die 'Autistischen Psychopathen' im Kindesalter [Autistic Psychopathy of Childhood] [Archives of Psychiatry and Clinical Neuroscience]. *Archiv für Psychiatrie und Nervenkrankheiten*, *117*(1), 76–136. doi:10.1007/BF01837709

Autism Speaks. (2010, April). *What is autism?* Retrieved November 17, 2011, from https://www.educateiowa.gov/sites/files/ed/documents/Parent-Factsheets_April2010_Autism.pdf

Autism Speaks Inc. (2021). Retrieved October 13, 2016, from https://www.autismspeaks.org/about-us

Barnard-Brak, L., Thompson, S., Wei, T., & Richman, D. (2014). Assistive technology as a predictor of general or alternate assessment among elementary-aged students with autism spectrum disorders. *Assistive Technology*, *26*(2), 81–87. doi:10.1080/10400435.2013.833557 PMID:25112052

Baron-Cohen, S. (2009). Autism: The Empathizing-Systemizing (ES) Theory. *Annals of the New York Academy of Sciences*, *1156*(1), 68–80. doi:10.1111/j.1749-6632.2009.04467.x PMID:19338503

Beals, K. (2017). Remediation and Assistive Technologies for Communication Deficits in Autism Spectrum Disorders. In *Supporting the Education of Children with Autism Spectrum Disorders* (pp. 160–183). IGI Global. doi:10.4018/978-1-5225-0816-8.ch009

Binder, E. B. (2021). Genotype-Phenotype Predictions in Autism: Are We There Yet? *The American Journal of Psychiatry*, *11-12*(1), 11–12. Advance online publication. doi:10.1176/appi.ajp.2020.20111589 PMID:33384006

Cage, E., Di Monaco, J., & Newell, V. (2018). Experiences of autism acceptance and mental health in autistic adults. *Journal of Autism and Developmental Disorders*, *48*(2), 473–484. doi:10.100710803-017-3342-7 PMID:29071566

Cassidy, S. A., Stenger, B., Van Dongen, L., Yanagisawa, K., Anderson, R., Wan, V., Baron-Cohen, S., & Cipolla, R. (2016). Expressive visual text-to-speech as an assistive technology for individuals with autism spectrum conditions. *Computer Vision and Image Understanding*, *148*, 193–200. doi:10.1016/j.cviu.2015.08.011 PMID:27375348

Chandler, W. G. (2014, June). *Assistive Technology and Communication for Students with Autism Spectrum Disorders (ASD).* Retrieved from https://www.wku.edu/cebs/peu/documents/course-syllabi/sped/sped-619.pdf

Christopher, D. (2018). Assistive Technologies, Inclusion, and Participation for Students with High Functioning ASD. In *Technology and the Curriculum.* Retrieved from https://techandcurriculum.pressbooks.com/chapter/assistive-tech-and-asd/

Cirino, C. B., Fernandes, A. C., Silva, J. D., & Serra, H. P. (2020, July). ERA-Augmented Reality Teaching-Assistive Technology Developed for the Literacy Process of Children with ASD. In *International Conference on Human-Computer Interaction* (pp. 405-414). Cham: Springer.

Coffin, A. B., Myles, B. S., Rogers, J., & Szakacs, W. (2016). Supporting the writing skills of individuals with autism spectrum disorder through assistive technologies. In *Technology and the treatment of children with autism spectrum disorder* (pp. 59–73). Springer. doi:10.1007/978-3-319-20872-5_6

Conn, K., Liu, C., Sarkar, N., Stone, W., & Warren, Z. (2008a). Affect-sensitive assistive intervention technologies for children with autism: An individual-specific approach. In *RO-MAN 2008-The 17th IEEE International Symposium on Robot and Human Interactive Communication* (pp. 442-447). Munich: IEEE.

Conn, K., Liu, C., Sarkar, N., Stone, W., & Warren, Z. (2008b). Towards affect-sensitive assistive intervention technologies for children with autism. In *Affective computing: Focus on emotion expression, synthesis and recognition* (pp. 365–390). IntechOpen. doi:10.5772/6171

Courtenay, K. (2021). The case for removing intellectual disability and autism from the Mental Health Act. *The British Journal of Psychiatry*, *218*(1), 64–65. doi:10.1192/bjp.2020.183 PMID:33541473

Cramer, M., Hirano, S. H., Tentori, M., Yeganyan, M. T., & Hayes, G. R. (2011). Classroom-based assistive technology: collective use of interactive visual schedules by students with autism. In *Proceedings of the SIGCHI Conference on Human Factors in Computing Systems* (pp. 1-10). Vancouver: Association for Computing Machinery (ACM). 10.1145/1978942.1978944

Cuhadar, S. (2008). Use of assistive technologies in the education of the children with autism. *The 8th International Educational Technology Conference.* Retrieved from http://ietc2008.home.anadolu.edu.tr/ietc2008/187.doc

De Pace, C., & Stasolla, F. (2014). Promoting environmental control, social interaction, and leisure/academy engagement among people with severe/profound multiple disabilities through assistive technology. In *Assistive technologies and computer access for motor disabilities* (pp. 285–319). IGI Global. doi:10.4018/978-1-4666-4438-0.ch010

de Villiers, J. (2021). The case against removing intellectual disability and autism from the Mental Health Act. *The British Journal of Psychiatry*, *218*(1), 63. doi:10.1192/bjp.2020.181 PMID:33541476

Deng, L., & Rattadilok, P. (2020). The need for and barriers to using assistive technologies among individuals with Autism Spectrum Disorders in China. *Assistive Technology*, 1–12. doi:10.1080/10400435.2020.1757787 PMID:32310026

Diagnostic and Statistical Manual of Mental Disorders (DSM-V) (5th ed.). (2013). American Psychiatric Association (APA).

Douard, E., Zeribi, A., Schramm, C., Tamer, P., Loum, M. A., Nowak, S., ... Moreau, C. (2021). Effect sizes of deletions and duplications on autism risk across the genome. *The American Journal of Psychiatry*, *178*(1), 87–98. doi:10.1176/appi.ajp.2020.19080834 PMID:32911998

el Kaliouby, R., & Robinson, P. (2007). *Therapeutic versus prosthetic assistive technologies: The case of autism.* Retrieved from Computer Laboratory, University of Cambridge: https://www.cl.cam.ac.uk/~pr10/publications/at07.pdf

Fan, T. (2012, May). *Enhancing Learning with the Use of Assistive Technology for Children on the Autism Spectrum* (Master of Science in Education). San Rafael, CA: Dominican University of California.

Fazana, F., Alsadoon, A., Prasad, P. W., Costadopoulos, N., Elchouemi, A., & Sreedharan, S. (2017, July). Integration of assistive and wearable technology to improve communication, social interaction and health monitoring for children with autism spectrum disorder (ASD). In *Region 10 Symposium (TENSYMP)* (pp. 1-5). Cochin: IEEE. 10.1109/TENCONSpring.2017.8070018

Fombonne, E. (2018). The rising prevalence of autism. *Journal of Child Psychology and Psychiatry, and Allied Disciplines*, *59*(7), 717–720. doi:10.1111/jcpp.12941 PMID:29924395

Francis, P. (2004, October). *Techniques to include users with autism in the design of assistive technologies* (Honor's thesis). University of Melbourne.

Francis, P., Firth, L., & Mellor, D. (2005, September). Reducing the risk of abandonment of assistive technologies for people with autism. In *International Federation for Information Processing (IFIP) Conference on Human-Computer Interaction* (pp. 1104-1107). Berlin: Springer.

Francis, P., Mellor, D., & Firth, L. (2009). Techniques and recommendations for the inclusion of users with autism in the design of assistive technologies. *Assistive Technology, 21*(2), 57–68. doi:10.1080/10400430902945561 PMID:19715250

Frith, U. (2003). *Autism: Explaining the enigma* (2nd ed.). Blackwell Publishing. Retrieved from https://psycnet.apa.org/record/2003-00578-000

Fteiha, M. A. (2017). Effectiveness of assistive technology in enhancing language skills for children with autism. *International Journal of Developmental Disabilities, 63*(1), 36–44. doi:10.1080/20473869.2015.1136129

Gentry, T., Kriner, R., Sima, A., McDonough, J., & Wehman, P. (2015, March 1). Reducing the need for personal supports among workers with autism using an iPod touch as an assistive technology: Delayed randomized control trial. *Journal of Autism and Developmental Disorders, 45*(3), 669–684. doi:10.100710803-014-2221-8 PMID:25212414

Geschwind, D. H. (2009). Advances in autism. *Annual Review of Medicine, 60*(1), 367–380. doi:10.1146/annurev.med.60.053107.121225 PMID:19630577

Gillespie-Lynch, K., Kapp, S. K., Brooks, P. J., Pickens, J., & Schwartzman, B. (2017, March 28). Whose expertise is it? Evidence for autistic adults as critical autism experts. *Frontiers in Psychology, 8*. Advance online publication. doi:10.3389/fpsyg.2017.00438 PMID:28400742

Goosen, L. (2019a). Research on Technology-Supported Teaching and Learning for Autism. In L. Makewa, B. Ngussa, & J. Kuboja (Eds.), *Technology-Supported Teaching and Research Methods for Educators* (pp. 88–110). IGI Global. doi:10.4018/978-1-5225-5915-3.ch005

Goosen, L. (2019b). Information Systems and Technologies Opening New Worlds for Learning to Children with Autism Spectrum Disorders. Smart Innovation, Systems and Technologies, 111, 134-143. doi:10.1007/978-3-030-03577-8_16

Goosen, L. (2020). Technology Opening New Worlds for Those with Autism – an Overview. In M. Clasquin-Johnson, D. Mahlo, & M. Clasquin-Johnson (Eds.), *Autism: Perspectives from Africa* (Vol. 1, pp. 135–168). UNISA Press.

Grove, J., Ripke, S., Als, T. D., Mattheisen, M., Walters, R. K., Won, H., ... Awashti, S. (2019). Identification of common genetic risk variants for autism spectrum disorder. *Nature Genetics, 51*(3), 431–444. doi:10.103841588-019-0344-8 PMID:30804558

Harris, J. F., Janvier, Y. M., Mandell, D., & Cidav, Z. (2021, January). Validation of the developmental check-in tool for low-literacy autism screening. *Pediatrics, 147*(1), e20193659. Advance online publication. doi:10.1542/peds.2019-3659 PMID:33303635

Hashim, R., & Yussof, H. (2017, October). Preparation for adulthood: Benefits of assistive technologies in social skills training of children with autism. In *International Symposium on Robotics and Intelligent Sensors (IRIS)* (pp. 374-378). Ottawa: IEEE. 10.1109/IRIS.2017.8250151

Hervás, R., Francisco, V., Méndez, G., & Bautista, S. (2019, September). A User-Centred Methodology for the Development of Computer-Based Assistive Technologies for Individuals with Autism. In *IFIP Conference on Human-Computer Interaction* (pp. 85-106). Cham: Springer. 10.1007/978-3-030-29381-9_6

Hong, J. A. (2008). A review on high-tech assistive technologies in language education for the students with autism spectrum disorders. *Special Education Research, 7*(1).

Huang, J. S., Yang, F. C., Chien, W. C., Yeh, T. C., Chung, C. H., Tsai, C. K., Tsai, S.-J., Yang, S.-S., Tzeng, N.-S., Chen, M.-H., & Liang, C. S. (2021, January 4). Risk of Substance Use Disorder and Its Associations with Comorbidities and Psychotropic Agents in Patients with Autism. *JAMA Pediatrics, 175*(2), e205371. Advance online publication. doi:10.1001/jamapediatrics.2020.5371 PMID:33394019

Hull, L., Petrides, K. V., Allison, C., Smith, P., Baron-Cohen, S., Lai, M. C., & Mandy, W. (2017). "Putting on my best normal": Social camouflaging in adults with autism spectrum conditions. *Journal of Autism and Developmental Disorders, 47*(8), 2519–2534. doi:10.100710803-017-3166-5 PMID:28527095

Ibrahim, Z., & Alias, M. (2018). A review on using assistive technology to enhance social skills competence among children with autism spectrum disorder (ASD). *Advanced Science Letters, 24*(6), 4250–4254. doi:10.1166/asl.2018.11582

Jamal, H. A. (2020, May). Developing the Language Ability of Children with Autism Spectrum Disorder (ASD) Using Assistive Technology and a Picture Exchange Communication System (PECS) through Adapting Elements of the Australian Educational Environment on Inclusive Public Schools. *Journal of Special Education and Rehabilitation, 10*(36), 1–47. doi:10.12816/0055786

Kakkar, D. (2019). Diagnostic assessment techniques and non-invasive biomarkers for Autism Spectrum Disorder. *International Journal of E-Health and Medical Communications, 10*(3), 79–95. doi:10.4018/IJEHMC.2019070105

Kats, Y., & Stasolla, F. (Eds.). (2021). *Education and Technology Support for Children and Young Adults With ASD and Learning Disabilities*. IGI Global. doi:10.4018/978-1-7998-7053-1

Kenney, S. (2013). *The Impact of Using Assistive Technology on Writing Productivity of Young Writers with Autism* (Ph.D. thesis). Fairfax, VA: George Mason University. Retrieved January 22, 2021, from https://www.learntechlib.org/p/119919/

Khan, M. (2021). Balancing non-discrimination and risk management in mental health legislation for autism. *The British Journal of Psychiatry, 218*(1), 63–64. doi:10.1192/bjp.2020.182 PMID:33541470

Koch, A. (2012). *Assistive technologies for children with autism spectrum disorders*. Division of Science and Mathematics, University of Minnesota.

Kõlves, K., Fitzgerald, C., Nordentoft, M., Wood, S. J., & Erlangsen, A. (2021, January 12). Assessment of Suicidal Behaviors Among Individuals With Autism Spectrum Disorder in Denmark. *JAMA Network Open*, *4*(1), e2033565. Advance online publication. doi:10.1001/jamanetworkopen.2020.33565 PMID:33433599

Kulkarni, M. (2017, January 15). *Assistive technologies for autism, cerebral palsy, multiple disabilities, and intellectual disabilities.* An invited report submitted to The National Trust, Ministry of Social Justice and Empowerment, Government of India. Retrieved from https://repository.iimb.ac.in/handle/2074/13855

Lang, R., Ramdoss, S., Raulston, T., Carnet, A., Sigafoos, J., Didden, R., & O'Reilly, M. F. (2014). Assistive technology for people with autism spectrum disorders. In *Assistive Technologies for People with Diverse Abilities* (pp. 157–190). Springer. doi:10.1007/978-1-4899-8029-8_6

Lord, C., Brugha, T. S., Charman, T., Cusack, J., Dumas, G., Frazier, T., ... Taylor, J. L. (2020, January 16). Autism spectrum disorder. *Nature Reviews. Disease Primers*, *6*(5), 1–23. doi:10.103841572-019-0138-4 PMID:31949163

Manoli, D. S., & State, M. W. (2021). Autism Spectrum Disorder Genetics and the Search for Pathological Mechanisms. *The American Journal of Psychiatry*, *178*(1), 30–38. doi:10.1176/appi.ajp.2020.20111608 PMID:33384012

Mansouri-Benssassi, E., Gomez, J. C., Boyd, L. E., Hayes, G. R., & Ye, J. (2018). Wearable assistive technologies for autism: Opportunities and challenges. *IEEE Pervasive Computing*, *17*(2), 11–21. doi:10.1109/MPRV.2018.022511239

McMurray, K., & Pierson, M. R. (2016). The importance of assistive technology in the classroom for males and females with autism spectrum disorder. *Journal of Gender and Power*, *5*(1), 59–78.

McMurray, K. R. (2016). *A comparison of two types of augmentative and alternative communication systems (iPad and PECS) for children with autism spectrum disorder: The benefits of integrating assistive technology into the ASD classroom* (Doctoral dissertation). Fullerton, CA: California State University.

Mira, M. (1992). Book Review: Autism and Asperger syndrome. *Focus on Autistic Behavior*, *7*(3), 13–15. doi:10.1177/108835769200700302

Mirenda, P. (2001). Autism, augmentative communication, and assistive technology what do we really know? *Focus on Autism and Other Developmental Disabilities*, *16*(3), 141–151. http://foa.sagepub.com/content/16/3/141.short. doi:10.1177/108835760101600302

Mitchell, L. C., Engleman, M., & Linden, M. T. (2012). *The effectiveness of assistive technology (TAP-it® and VizZle®) to enhance progress of young children with autism spectrum disorders.* Retrieved from https://www.teachsmart.org/pdf/the-effectiveness-of-assistive-technology-to-enhance-progress-of-young-children-with-autism-spectrum-disorders.pdf

Moktar, M. N., Fikry, A., Musa, R., Hassan, H., Ahmad, S. S., Ismail, Z., ... Hashim, R. (2014, December). Extending cultural model of assistive technology design for autism treatment. In *International Symposium on Robotics and Manufacturing Automation (ROMA)* (pp. 172-175). Kuala Lumpur: IEEE. 10.1109/ROMA.2014.7295882

Mold, M., Umar, D., King, A., & Exley, C. (2018). Aluminium in brain tissue in autism. *Journal of Trace Elements in Medicine and Biology*, *46*, 76–82. doi:10.1016/j.jtemb.2017.11.012 PMID:29413113

Moore, D., Cheng, Y., McGrath, P., & Powell, N. (2005). Avatars and Autism, Assistive Technologies. In A. Pruski & H. Knops (Eds.), *Virtuality to Reality* (pp. 442–448). IOS Press.

Muhle, R., Trentacoste, S. V., & Rapin, I. (2004). The genetics of autism. *Pediatrics*, *113*(5), e472–e486. doi:10.1542/peds.113.5.e472 PMID:15121991

National Research Council. (2001). *Educating children with autism*. National Academies Press.

Nikopoulou-Smyrni, P., Halder, S., Mackeogh, T., & Dillenburger, K. (2012). *Registration for a Systematic Review: Electronic Assistive Technology for Improving Social and Behavioral Outcomes for Individuals with Autism Spectrum Disorder (ASD)*. Retrieved from Campbell Systematic Reviews: https://www.campbellcollaboration.org/lib/project/248/

O'Brolcháin, F., & Gordijn, B. (2017, January). Risks of Stigmatisation Resulting from Assistive Technologies for People with Autism Spectrum Disorder. *Studies in Health Technology and Informatics*, *242*, 265–268. PMID:28873808

O'Brolcháin, F., & Gordijn, B. (2018). Risks of stigmatisation resulting from assistive technologies for persons with autism spectrum disorder. *Technologies*, *6*(1), 27. Advance online publication. doi:10.3390/technologies6010027

O'Brolcháin, F., & Gordijn, B. (2020). Responsibility-enhancing assistive technologies and people with autism. *Cambridge Quarterly of Healthcare Ethics*, *29*(4), 607–616. doi:10.1017/S0963180120000353 PMID:32892779

O'Neill, S. J., Smyth, S., Smeaton, A., & O'Connor, N. E. (2020). Assistive technology: Understanding the needs and experiences of individuals with autism spectrum disorder and/or intellectual disability in Ireland and the UK. *Assistive Technology*, *32*(5), 251–259. doi:10.1080/10400435.2018.1535526 PMID:30668926

Parens, E., & Asch, A. (1999). Special Supplement: The Disability Rights Critique of Prenatal Genetic Testing Reflections and Recommendations. *The Hastings Center Report*, *29*(5), S1–S2. doi:10.2307/3527746 PMID:10587809

Pliasa, S., & Fachantidis, N. (2019, October). Mobile Technologies Serious Games for the Development of Social Skills in Children with Autism Spectrum Disorders. In *Interactive Mobile Communication, Technologies and Learning* (pp. 618–628). Springer.

Quick, V. B., Wang, B., & State, M. W. (2021). Leveraging large genomic datasets to illuminate the pathobiology of autism spectrum disorders. *Neuropsychopharmacology*, *46*(1), 55–69. doi:10.103841386-020-0768-y PMID:32668441

Radwan, A., & Cataltepe, Z. (2016). Using assistive technology to enhance teaching for students with autism spectrum disorders. *International E-Journal of Advances in Education*, *2*(4), 112–121. doi:10.18768/ijaedu.15760

Ringland, K. E., Wolf, C. T., Boyd, L. E., Baldwin, M. S., & Hayes, G. R. (2016, October). Would you be mine: Appropriating minecraft as an assistive technology for youth with autism. In *Proceedings of the 18th International ACM SIGACCESS Conference on Computers and Accessibility* (pp. 33-41). Reno: ACM. 10.1145/2982142.2982172

Robertson, C. E., & Baron-Cohen, S. (2017, September 29). Sensory perception in autism. *Nature Reviews. Neuroscience*, *18*(11), 671–684. doi:10.1038/nrn.2017.112 PMID:28951611

Roldán-Álvarez, D., Gomez, J., Márquez-Fernández, A., Martín, E., & Montoro, G. (2016, July). Mobile devices as assistive technologies for ASD: Experiences in the classroom. In *International Conference of Design, User Experience, and Usability* (pp. 187-197). Cham: Springer.

Rutter, M., Le Couteur, A., & Lord, C. (2003). *Autism diagnostic interview-revised.* Western Psychological Services. Retrieved from https://www.academia.edu/download/2163587/8j7zpy2k00w44i8.pdf

Sampath, H., Agarwal, R., & Indurkhya, B. (2013, September). Assistive technology for children with autism-lessons for interaction design. In *Proceedings of the 11th Asia Pacific Conference on Computer Human Interaction* (pp. 325-333). Bangalore: ACM. 10.1145/2525194.2525300

Schafer, E. C., Wright, S., Anderson, C., Jones, J., Pitts, K., Bryant, D., Watson, M., Box, J., Neve, M., Mathews, L., & Reed, M. P. (2016). Assistive technology evaluations: Remote-microphone technology for children with Autism Spectrum Disorder. *Journal of Communication Disorders*, *64*, 1–17. doi:10.1016/j.jcomdis.2016.08.003 PMID:27592101

Schlosser, R. W., & Wendt, O. (2008, August). Effects of augmentative and alternative communication intervention on speech production in children with autism: A systematic review. *American Journal of Speech-Language Pathology*, *17*(3), 212–230. doi:10.1044/1058-0360(2008/021) PMID:18663107

Spence-Cochran, K., & Pearl, C. (2012). Assistive technology to support people with autism spectrum disorders. In *Educating students with autism spectrum disorders: Research-based principles and practices* (pp. 295–311). Routledge.

Stanger, C., Mims, P., Wood, L., & Ahlgrim-Delzell, L. (2016). Supporting Literacy Achievement for Students with Intellectual Disability and Autism through Curricular Programs that Incorporate Assistive Technology. *Assistive Technology Outcomes & Benefits*, *10*(1), 51–73.

Stasolla, F., Boccasini, A., & Perilli, V. (2017). Assistive Technology-Based Programs to Support Adaptive Behaviors by Children with Autism Spectrum Disorders: A Literature Overview. In Y. Kats (Ed.), *Supporting the Education of Children with Autism Spectrum Disorders* (pp. 140–159). IGI Global. doi:10.4018/978-1-5225-0816-8.ch008

Stasolla, F., Boccasini, A., Perilli, V., Damiani, R., & Albano, V. (2015a). Assistive technology for promoting adaptive skills of children with autism spectrum disorders: A literature overview. *International Journal of Psychology and Psychoanalysis*, *1*(2). Advance online publication. doi:10.23937/2572-4037.1510008

Stasolla, F., Caffò, A. O., Damiani, R., Perilli, V., Di Leone, A., & Albano, V. (2015b). Assistive technology-based programs to promote communication and leisure activities by three children emerged from a minimal conscious state. *Cognitive Processing*, *16*(1), 69–78. doi:10.100710339-014-0625-1 PMID:25077461

Sula, A., & Bushti, J. (2014, February). Using Assistive Technologies (AT) as form of technology based intervention to foster and promote Albanian language development in children with autism. *International Journal of Science, Innovation & New Technology*, *1*(9), 33–41.

Sula, A., & Spaho, E. (2014). Using assistive technologies in autism care centers to support children develop communication and language skills. A case study: Albania. *Academic Journal of Interdisciplinary Studies*, *3*(1), 203–212. doi:10.5901/ajis.2014.v3n1p203

Syriopoulou-Delli, C. K., & Gkiolnta, E. (2020). Review of assistive technology in the training of children with autism spectrum disorders. *International Journal of Developmental Disabilities*, 1–13. doi: 10.1080/20473869.2019.1706333

Treangen, T. J., & Salzberg, S. L. (2012). Repetitive DNA and next-generation sequencing: Computational challenges and solutions. *Nature Reviews. Genetics*, *13*(1), 36–46. doi:10.1038/nrg3117 PMID:22124482

Wadhera, T., & Kakkar, D. (2019). Eye Tracker: An Assistive Tool in Diagnosis of Autism Spectrum Disorder. In Emerging Trends in the Diagnosis and Intervention of Neurodevelopmental Disorders (pp. 125-152). IGI Global.

Wadhera, T., & Kakkar, D. (2020). Big Data-Based System: A Supportive Tool in Autism Spectrum Disorder Analysis. In Interdisciplinary Approaches to Altering Neurodevelopmental Disorders (pp. 303-319). IGI Global. doi:10.4018/978-1-7998-3069-6.ch017

Wali, L. J., & Sanfilippo, F. (2019, September). A Review of the State-of-the-Art of Assistive Technology for People with ASD in the Workplace and in Everyday Life. In *Conference on e-Business, e-Services and e-Society* (pp. 520-532). Cham: Springer. 10.1007/978-3-030-29374-1_42

Wolff, S. (2004). The history of autism. *European Child & Adolescent Psychiatry*, *13*(4), 201–208. doi:10.100700787-004-0363-5 PMID:15365889

KEY TERMS AND DEFINITIONS

Assistive Technologies (ATs): Are defined as to include any devices, equipment, or pieces, which can be used to promote novel skills, improve existing behaviors, and/or reduce the negative consequences related to disabilities in patients' daily functioning.

Augmentative and Alternative Communication (AAC) Strategies: Are meant for assisting persons with severe communication disabilities towards participating more fully in particular social roles, including care management, education, employment, and learning.

Autism Spectrum Disorders (ASDs): Autism spectrum disorders are related to especially children, some of whom experience atypical language development. Children with ASDs typically prefer to work only with a selected group of people, who could include family members. Autism spectrum disorders are considered to be common childhood, but lifelong, neurodevelopmental conditions or disabilities. These disorders are also characterized by exhibiting marked difficulties, including an insistence on demonstrating repetitive patterns of preservative and/or sensory behaviors, as well as possibly fixed and highly focused and/or unusual restricted sensory interests beginning early in life. Many individuals with ASDs are commonly described as having a specific combination of deficits, which impact on three main areas that may lead to significant impairments in behavioral, communicative, emotional, intellectual, and social skills. As a construct, ADSs are incurable, brain-based, and behaviorally defined static impairments of the immature brain.

Chapter 2
Assistive Technology to Support Children With Autism Spectrum Disorder

Rishika Tiwari
National Brain Research Centre, India

Manish Shandilya
Amity University, Haryana, India

Sonika Charak
National Brain Research Centre, India

ABSTRACT

Assistive technology (AT) is defined as any device or technology ranging from low to high that helps to improve functional skills of individuals with cognitive, physical, or neurological disorders. These technologies are devised to improve the functional activities of persons. ATs focussing on cognitive disorders like dementia, autism spectrum disorders, etc. can be categorized as ATs for cognition (ATC) and augmentative and alternative communication (AAC). AAC interventions consist of tools that aid the challenges faced by individuals with speech impairment during communication. AACs used often are speech-generating devices (SGD), software programs, and communication apps for efficient production of speech. ATCs include social stories and video modeling strategies. The use of assistive technology in autism spectrum disorder (ASD) has great importance due to increased requirement for interventions in helping students. There are several lines of evidence showing the effectiveness of technology-assisted training in ASD patients.

1. AUTISM SPECTRUM DISORDER

The WHO defines Autism spectrum disorder (ASD) as a range of conditions characterized by some degree of impaired social behavior, communication and language, and a narrow range of interests and

DOI: 10.4018/978-1-7998-7430-0.ch002

activities that are both unique to the individual and carried out repetitively. ASD symptoms also include impairment in motor skills. The characteristics of the Autism Spectrum Disorders patients can be divided into three categories:

- Social skills and behavioral impairments: Individuals with ASD face difficulties in making friends, interacting with people, maintaining eye contact, and reading body gestures and facial expressions. Instead of interacting with human beings, ASD patients prefer interacting with the surrounding objects.
- Communication impairments: The ASD patients also face problems in speech production and comprehension. They are also known to repeat a word or a phrase in a conversation. Some patients cannot produce speech at all or have limited speech.
- Repetitive movements and behaviors: The individuals, mostly children with ASD show inappropriate behaviors such as hand flapping, screaming, falling on the ground, and repeating sounds and phrases.

These characteristics are known as the 'Triad of impairments' together. The available epidemiological data suggests that approximately 1 in 54 children in the United States are diagnosed with an autism spectrum disorder (ASD), and ASD affects all racial, ethnic, and socioeconomic groups (Centres for Disease Control and Prevention [CDC], 2020). Furthermore, the prevalence of this spectrum of disorders has been increasing globally in the past 50 years; this may also be a result of increasing awareness among common citizens, improved diagnostic tools and a better understanding of the disorders with time. Although autism can occur in people with a high IQ, more than half the individuals with autism suffer from intellectual disability (defined as an IQ below 70) (Investigators, 2012).

Screening of autism spectrum disorders is a challenge because most of the diagnostic tools involve the detection of behavioral symptoms which include social interaction, aggression, attention deficits, gait patterns, and sensory processing, and the developmental traits of the subject which have to be carefully observed by an expert to reach at the conclusion (Wadhera et al., 2019). One major drawback of these diagnosis techniques is that they are not useful for early diagnosis. Another drawback is that the questionnaires are designed by the experts and the response of the children needs to be recorded and analyzed by the experts; this makes the process tedious and time-consuming (Wadhera & Kakkar, 2019). Some recent advancements in the diagnostic tools include:

Eye Tracker system: This system detects the gaze patterns and cognitive abilities of individuals and assists the analysis of eye movements using a deep learning system, which makes this process objective instead of subjective such as during the manual interpretation (Wadhera & Kakkar, 2019).

Multiple biometrics identification system: Biometrics is a pattern recognition system that distinguishes between individuals based on unique characteristics like fingerprints, gait, facial pattern, and iris pattern. Wadhera et al. had described that a combination of a biometrics system is useful in the early diagnosis of ASD by analyzing the morphology of the face and fingers (Wadhera et al., 2019).

Big-data-based system: Big Data is recently gaining more attention for the detection and treatment of ASD. It is an information hub with a large number of data points from different individuals suffering from ASD. These data points may consist of structured or unstructured data; structured data includes phenotypes, International Codes for Diseases (ICD) codes, etc. and unstructured data includes information about the environmental factors, clinical prescriptions, etc. The data is so huge that even the variations due to minute factors can be tracked (Wadhera & Kakkar, 2020).

2. AT FOCUSSING ON DIFFERENT DEVELOPMENTS IN CHILDREN WITH ASD

The technologies play a vital role in learning for the students suffering from impairments. Assistive technology (AT) is defined as any device that assists people in certain tasks and helps to improve the functional skills of individuals with cognitive, physical or neurological disorders. AT also promotes some objectives of inclusive education such as a sense of being similar to the peers and balanced education. These can also be categorized as low, mid, and high technologies (Bouck, 2010). Low AT refers to the technology that uses simple tools or techniques operated without using batteries or electricity and does not require any training, mid AT tools can be battery operated and require little training, and high AT are highly specialized and complex tools requiring extensive training for their usage. These tools are usually powered by electricity and have more features that mean consultation and training are a must while using these high-tech tools.

These technologies are devised to improve the functional activities of persons. ATs focussing on neurological disorders like dementia, autism spectrum disorders, etc. can be categorized as ATs for cognition (ATC) and augmentative and alternative communication (AAC) (Gupta et al., 2018). ATCs include social stories and video modeling strategies whereas the AAC interventions consist of tools

Table 1. AT Interventions for social skills

Type of intervention	Name of intervention	Examples and links
Low-tech	Social stories	https://carolgraysocialstories.com/social-stories/ https://www.autismparentingmagazine.com/social-stories-for-autistic-children/
	Power cards	https://www.amazon.com/Power-Cards-Interests-Motivate-Children/dp/1931282013 https://www.erinoakkids.ca/ErinoakKids/media/EOK_Documents/Autism_Resources/Power-Cards.pdf https://www.ocali.org/project/resource_gallery_of_interventions/page/power_cards
	Comic strips	https://erinoakkids.ca/ErinoakKids/media/EOK_Documents/Autism_Resources/Comic-Strip-Conversations.pdf https://sparkingspeech.com/2020/06/27/understanding-the-unwritten-rules-comic-strip-conversations/ http://www.smcacademy.co.uk/wp-content/uploads/2018/09/comicstrip-conversations-booklet.pdf
	Social scripts	https://www.andnextcomesl.com/p/social-scripts.html https://starautismsupport.com/simple-social-scripts-work https://www.teacherspayteachers.com/Browse/Search:social%20scripts%20autism
Mid tech	Video modeling	https://www.youtube.com/watch?v=QuukBPccAeE https://www.youtube.com/channel/UCrsqgUJmRCGQZyK698hETIA http://www.watchmelearn.com/
High tech	Multi touch table top games	https://www.rug.nl/staff/f.cnossen/2009_vanveen_devries_cnossen.pdf https://www.cnet.com/news/infinity-game-table-hands-on-touch-screen-table-gives-classic-board-games-new-spin/ http://www.sciencedirect.com/science/article/pii/S1877050912007855/pdf?md5=accc2b164126da64cd7373dd1033e0b1&pid=1-s2.0-S1877050912007855-main.pdf
	Computer/ Mobile-phone based interventions	http://www.facesay.com/ https://reu.uncc.edu/sites/reu.uncc.edu/files/media/cMotion_2008.pdf https://web.uvic.ca/~carte/facemaze.html https://www.revelian.com/employer/product/emotify/
	Social robots	Keepon: https://beatbots.net/keepon-pro Kaspar: https://www.herts.ac.uk/kaspar/meet-kaspar NAO: https://www.robotlab.com/store/nao-power-v6-standard-edition KIBO: https://kinderlabrobotics.com/at-home/

that aid the challenges faced by individuals with speech impairment during communication. AAC used often are Speech Generating Devices (SGD), software programs and communication apps for efficient production of speech. The use of assistive technology in Autism Spectrum Disorder (ASD) has great importance due to the increased requirements for interventions in helping students. There are several lines of evidence showing the effectiveness of technology-assisted training in ASD patients.

2.1 Social Skills and Behavior Development

Skills that are used while interacting with each other are known as social skills. Interaction can be verbal or nonverbal via different facial expressions, body language and personal appearances. The use of the same AT to all ASD-affected children is challenging and is not a prudent idea as each ASD-affected individual has a different type of impairment as discussed earlier. Appropriate AT interventions needs modifications or alterations depending upon the situation of the ASD affected person characteristics. It is well known that different social situations have different unwritten guidelines.

Assistive technology-based interventions along a continuum from low- to high-technology are used for developing social skills is represented in figure 1.

Figure 1.

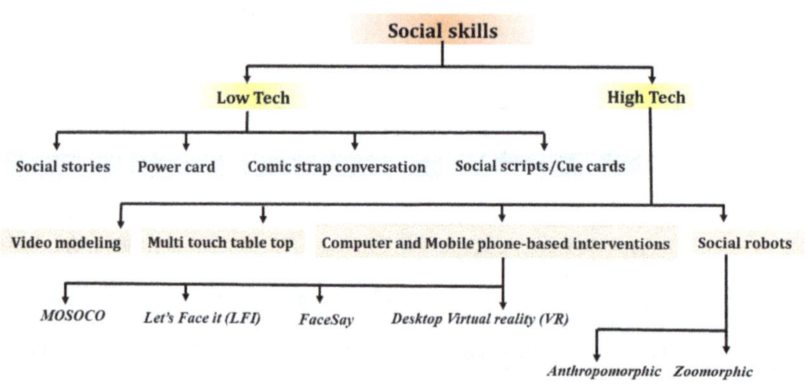

Low AT techniques like telling social stories, social scripts, playing turn-taking cards with different icons, pictures and symbols. Mid AT tools like video modeling have a positive impact on ASD children in developing social skills. **High AT** tools involve the usage of different computer software, apps for developing social skills as discussed in the upcoming sections (Table 1).

2.1a Low-Tech AT for Social Skill Development

1. Social Stories

These are short descriptions of a particular situation, event, or activity, and define appropriate responses. Components of the social story make them appropriate for ASD intervention. Social stories consist of three types of sentences, descriptive, directive, and perspective. Descriptive sentences provide information about the social situation and how people are dealing with the situation in the stories. These assist children in focusing on relevant cues. Directive statements are a list of expected responses in a target situation. Perspective sentences describe the reaction of other people involved in the situation to the expected response of the child. **Generic social stories** outline the situations that are common to almost all autistic children and consist of mostly descriptive sentences. For example, going to a restaurant and ordering food is a common situation. Not only did the children learn general social skills like greeting teachers and parents, sharing toys, and turn-taking, the social stories are also successfully used to decrease inappropriate behaviors such as hand flapping, falling on the floor, talking/humming to self, aggression (Adams et al., 2004; Khantreejitranon, 2018).

2. Power Card Strategy

It is a visual aid developed by trainers and parents to assist individuals with autism in understanding social situations, routines, and non-verbal language. It is a small version of social stories in which the trainer determines the favorite character of the child from any movie, comic, game. The trainer then explains a particular social situation to the child and asks them to imagine how their favorite character will react to that situation. Based on the behavior assessment, the trainer instructs the child how to react in those situations and thus helps in improving social skills deficits. However, the drawback of this power card strategy is it cannot be implemented to those children who cannot read. The power card strategy has been useful to decrease challenging behaviors like whining, screaming and running away while being talked with (Spencer et al., 2008).

3. Comic Strip Conversation

It is a variation of a social story and it is suitable for children with limited communication skills, especially for younger children, as they mostly rely on visual cues. Simple figures and symbols in a comic strip format are incorporated in a socially relevant story. This type of conversation helps autistic children to improve interpersonal relationships and thereby decreasing the feeling of loneliness and social dissatisfaction (Glaesar et al., 2003) .

4. Social Scripts/Cue Cards

These are used to facilitate communication by introducing a prepared list including initiating phrases, comments on a particular topic, and phrases to end the interaction. Each script can be written according to the needs of the student and social situation. It improves the conversational skills of autistic children and enhances social interaction and generalizes to other social situations as well (Benson, 2020).

2.1b Mid Tech Interventions for Social Skill Development

Video modeling is a type of video-based intervention that integrates the principles of modeling and visual learning. Video displaying an adult or peers engaging in the particular activity is shown to the child before performing the target skill. The participant is then provided with opportunities to perform the skills displayed in the video and ask them to imitate the behavior of the model. It is an evidence-based practice for improving social communication skills in children with ASD (Qi et al., 2017). This intervention allows to focus on target skills and eliminates the irrelevant cues, minimizes adult supervision, and encourages independence. Social skills such as social initiation, i.e. any initiating any social activity, reciprocal play, purchasing skills, questioning, perspective taking, i.e. the ability to determine the mental state of other people and predict their behavior, maintaining eye contact and smiling (Nikopoulos & Keenan, 2004), complex sequences of social behavior involving social initiation, reciprocal play, object engagement, and imitative response (Nikopoulos & Keenan, 2007), sequences of scripted verbalizations and play actions (Macdonald et al., 2005), greeting peers (Alhuzimi, 2020), can be successfully learned by using video modeling strategies.

2.1c High Tech Interventions for Social Skill Development

Research shows that children with ASD tend to enjoy and benefit significantly from computerized interventions such as cartoons, video modeling, computer-assisted instruction, computer games, and virtual worlds (Grynszpan et al., 2014).

1. Multi-Touch Table-Top

It is a kind of technology that can be programmed to enhance social interaction, the use of vocabulary, and the communication abilities of children and adults with ASD. These devices allow simultaneous interaction by multiple users on the same large screen-like surface. People with ASD vary in sensory tolerance and motor ability levels. For those who have difficulties in motor coordination, the direct touch input of tabletop technology has advantages because it allows individualized and unmediated control over the interface.

Different multiuser table-top games are known to enhance social skills like negotiation, turn taking, active listening, perspective-taking by using a game called SIDES, social interaction in both low-functioning and high-functioning ASD children by the Collaborative puzzle game, problem-solving and collaboration in children with PDD-NOS (Pervasive Developmental Disorder- Not Otherwise Specified), or atypical autism in particular by Raketeer game, mutual planning, display of sharing skills by using Join-in Suite interface (Chen, 2012), reduction of stereotyped ASD-associated behaviors by employing StoryTable game (Gal et al., 2016).

2. Computer and Mobile Phone-Based Interventions

MOSOCO is an android-based application that motivates autistic children to sustain suitable spatial boundaries while taking a turn, share their interests with the partner, disperse appropriately after the interaction, identify potential communication partners, and eye-gaze directing (Escobedo et al., 2012).

Let's Face it (LFI) is a computer-based intervention that curriculum designed to train children with ASD in basic face processing skills. LFI targets skills involved in the identification, interpretation of facial expressions and attention to eye gaze through a set of diagnostic assessments as well as a set of training exercises. The study demonstrated significant improvements in their analytic recognition of mouth features and holistic recognition of a face based on its eyes features (Tanaka et al., 2010).

Face Say is a computer-based assistive software that teaches recognition and social skills such as face processing to children with ASD. Studies suggest that children show improved capabilities, especially face processing, after being trained with the intervention (Rice et al., 2015).

Desktop Virtual reality (VR) is a computer-generated three-dimensional simulation of real-life environments that are explored and interacted with by real-time users. A **virtual reality (VR)** based learning environment allows participants to practice social skills in a safe, realistic, controllable, and diversifiable

Figure 2.

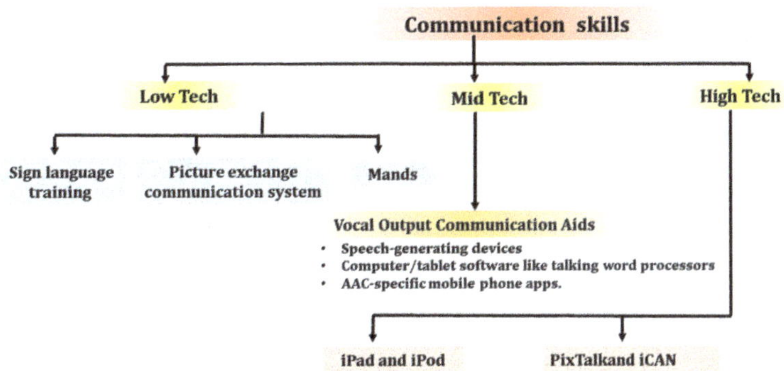

environment. Using VR tools, serious games are designed which support training on many different skills and they favor interactions in diverse contexts and situations, some of which may resemble real-life. Collaborative virtual environments (CVE) allow multiple users in remote locations to interact within a shared virtual setting using a computer network. They can navigate and control the shared virtual world as well as communicate (verbally or nonverbally) to share information, which enhances social interaction. Children with ASD show improved performance of eye contact, listening to others, and social empathy during both verbal and nonverbal communication with the three-dimensional virtual characters (Cheng et al., 2010). The children also show improved social skills such as turn-taking, appreciation expression, social initiation, greeting, ending a conversation, and observational learning (Ke et al., 2020). An intelligent agent was designed by Zhang et al, 2020 to play collaborative puzzle games with children with ASD and measure cooperation and verbal communication skills (Zhang et al., 2020). ECHOES (Smith & Bernardini, 2014), hand-in-hand is a communication enhancement collaborative virtual reality system (Zhao et al., 2018), and CoMove (Zhang et al., 2018) are some virtual reality systems that are effective interventions for the enhancement of social skills in children with ASD.

3. Social Robots

These are known to encourage more engagement and motivation to perform better because of their physical presence, more than a virtual agent or a video model (Leyzberg et al., 2012). It is hypothesized that interacting with robots is easier for children with ASD than with humans because robots are highly predictable, and simpler (David et al., 2019). Two categories of social robots are used in ASD intervention: **anthropomorphic and zoomorphic**. Zoomorphic robots are animal-like robots used for analyzing the behavior of an ASD child. Example: "Keepon" robot (Kozima et al., 2007) is known for its simple and friendly appearance which aids positive social interaction with ASD children. Human-like robots are called anthropomorphic robots. Examples are "KASPAR" and NAO.

Anthropomorphic robots can play a vital role in significantly improving the child's behavior due to their matching appearance with humans. The distinguishing characteristics of the robots are their high repeatability and willingness to interact without any complaints and fatigue. Some studies suggest that the use of robot-assisted intervention is more effective than a human therapist (Vanderborght et al., 2012) and computer-display strategies (Pop et al., 2013). A study that compared the robot-enhanced therapy and standard human therapy suggest that both therapies have an equivalent effect in teaching the turn-taking skills to children with ASD, however, RET was more suitable for behavioral activation

Table 2. AT Interventions for communication skills

Type of intervention	Name of intervention	Examples and links
Low-tech	Sign language	American sign language for the deaf: https://www.nad.org/resources/american-sign-language/learning-american-sign-language/ Comprehensive signed dictionary: http://gupress.gallaudet.edu/3051.html
	PECS	https://pecsusa.com/pecs/ https://nationalautismresources.com/the-picture-exchange-communication-system-pecs/
	FCT (Functional communication training)	https://raisingchildren.net.au/autism/therapies-guide/fct https://www.appliedbehavioranalysisedu.org/how-is-functional-communication-training-used-in-applied-behavior-analysis/
	SL (Statistical learning)	https://doi.org/10.3389/fpsyg.2016.01245 https://doi.org/10.1007/s10803-018-3625-7
Mid tech	Dedicated SGDs	BIGmack: https://www.ablenetinc.com/bigmack MessageMates: http://www.aactechconnect.com/images/products/pdf/3.pdf Cheap Talk: https://enablingdevices.com/product/cheap-talk-4-in-line-direct/ BIG step-by-step communicator: https://www.ablenetinc.com/big-step-by-step-with-levels
High tech	Computer and Mobile-phone based inerventions	www.Proloquo2Go.com https://apps.apple.com/us/app/sono-flex/id463697022 https://www.ablenetinc.com/soundingboard/ https://apps.apple.com/us/app/gotalk-now/id454176457 https://apps.apple.com/us/app/speak-for-yourself/id482508198

(David et al., 2019). Upon interaction with a robot, Eye-gaze, joint attention, and imitation skills improve (Scassellati et al., 2018), along with verbal communication and physical contact (Valadão et al., 2016) and the ability to interact with multiple people at a time (Ali et al., 2019).

2.2 Communication

The problem in communicating is a common feature observed in all autistic people. Communication consists of two parts receptive and expressive. Receptive language means a person understands based on listening whereas expressive language is the ability of the person to speak to others. Persons with ASD disease might have a problem in the receptive part or the expressive part or both communication areas. Proper analysis of the person is done to understand the area in which the problem is there.

Low AT to high AT tools are used in creating communication skills are displayed in the figure 2.

Low AT devices are without voice output and can be further characterized into unaided and aided communications methods. Unaided communications methods involve gestures, signs/symbols or body language used to improve communications skills in autistic people. Aided communication methods involve a device or object other than the operator's body. Examples of aided communications are paper cards, symbols on a particular topic, different pictures demonstrating a specific topic. **Mid AT** tools are with voice output and include digitized speech, static display, text, and speech devices. **High AT** devices contains recorded computerized speech, dynamic display where the user has options to change the display (Table 2). Three technologies can produce speech outputs: dedicated Speech generating devices, computer/tablet software like talking word processors, and AAC-specific mobile phone apps. Speech Generating Devices (SGDs) or Vocal Output Communication Aids (VOCA) are portable electronic devices that produce digitized or synthetic output. The SGDs are classified as dedicated and non-dedicated speech-generating devices. Dedicated SGDs are exclusively designed and used for the assistance in speech generation and are a type of mid AT, whereas non-dedicated devices include a computer, iPad, tablet, android, etc. and these devices can be utilized to perform like dedicated devices by installing the communication features like speech generation in these devices. These are a part of high AT.

2.2a Low-Tech Assistive Technology for Communication

1. *Sign Language Training*

It had been helpful for non-verbal autistic children until the recent developments of high-tech interventions. Some studies suggest that similar neuroanatomical areas and high-level neural integration systems are involved in processing both signs and speech (Willems et al., 2007). Therefore, sign language training has greater chances of enhancing speech production. The basic task in this type of training is to teach the child to make a specific sign on the sight of a specific object, i.e. labeling. This can be done by using any available sign language dictionaries; the most frequently used one is the American Sign Language for the deaf (https://www.nad.org/resources/american-sign-language/learning-american-sign-language/) and the comprehensive signed English dictionary. The child should be presented simultaneously with visual and auditory stimuli. Example: When a therapist picks up an apple in his hand, he says "apple". The therapist should now employ prompting, that is, hold the hand of the child and mold it to the sign meaning apple, and say the word "apple". Next, the child learns to produce the signs without prompts; he will be able to produce the hand sign when the therapist just picks up the apple and says "apple". This behavior is reinforced by a social reward such as appreciation, but not physical rewards like food or toy. The sign is considered as properly learned when the child could produce it perfectly for 10 successive trials. These above steps can be exploited to teach new signs to the child, to discriminate between the signs of several objects.

2. *Picture Exchange Communication System (PECS)*

It is a communication training system developed within the Delaware Autistic Program (DAP) (Winterling, 2013). The trainer and the communication board are nearer to the child and then gradually distance away so that the child learns to pick up the picture and approach the trainer with time. After further training, non-preferred pictures can also be added to the communication board to enhance discriminability. If the child handover these new pictures to the trainer, he/she gestures them towards the preferred pictures. Next, pictures of different categories can be color-coded and placed on the board. By placing a card saying phrases like "I want" or "I see" on the top left corner of the board, a sentence strip is formed. The child has to put the picture in front of that card, completing the sentence. Now he can request the object to the trainer using a sentence strip. The trainer can prompt the behavior. The child can similarly learn to label. Recent work elaborates the usefulness of PECS in improving speech utterance (Jusoh & Majid, 2017), social communication such as initiating mands and responding to peer mands (Doherty et al., 2018), personal health care such as tooth-brushing (Al-Batayneh et al., 2020), and also led to a reduction in problematic behavior (Charlop-Christy et al., 2002).

3. *Functional Communication Training (FCT)*

Mands (a verbal form of demands and requests) are necessary for the child to convey its needs. Many children with ASD often show problem behavior like screaming or hitting to get their needs fulfilled. Functional communication training (FCT) is a procedure often used in the treatment of severe problem behavior that involves teaching appropriate mands to replace inappropriate behaviors that served the same function (Durand, 1999). The inappropriate behavior should not be reinforced by the provision of the needs of the children so that they should learn to produce proper mands (Tiger et al., 2008).

4. *Statistical Learning (SL)*

This is a type of implicit learning during which the experience is gained by observing repetitive patterns through different sensory modalities such as touch, hearing, visualizing or a combination of all. This type of learning is necessary for the development of prediction ability, social skills, and cognitive skills. A recent study had suggested that not only is the statistical learning ability intact in the children with ASD, it also leads to stable learning which is retained even after removal of training (Kakkar & Tanu, 2018). The SL was reported to be beneficial for artificial grammar learning and speech learning for children with ASD (Obeid et al., 2016).

2.2b Mid Tech Assistive Technology Intervention for Communication

Dedicated SGDs are the electronic devices that are committed to assisting the user in expressing themselves through a speech by producing the digitized or synthetic output. There are two varieties of speech output: digitized speech and synthesized speech.

Digitized speech is produced by recording a human voice, followed by its conversion into digits by sampling the speech waveform at equal intervals (analog to digital conversion) and storing it in the form of a series of numbers, converting them back to speech output when instructed (digital to analog conversion). The intelligibility of digitized speech produced at a higher sampling rate is similar to that of natural speech but its major drawback is that communication output is limited to a set of pre-stored messages. Synthesized speech refers to text-to-speech conversion that involves the production of unlimited spontaneous speech by converting alphabets, digits, words, and sentences into speech output using a set of algorithmic rules. However, the synthesized speech is less intelligible than natural speech.

Some popular and user-friendly dedicated VOCAs include BIG mack, BIG step-by-step communicator, Tech/Talk, Cheap Talk, Speak Easy, Black hawk, Easy Talk, Alpha Talker, Vanguard, Delta talker, Pathfinder, Dynavox, Parakeet 15 by Zygo industries.

Studies suggest that the utility of VOCAs increases by the participants with time and the choice of VOCA varies with the participants, some might prefer one type of VOCA and others might prefer another; however, it was found that VOCAs were preferred over communication boards (Sigafoos et al., 2005). Additionally, children who use VOCA are capable of learning more complex communicative repertoires (Shillingsburg et al., 2019). VOCAs are used by the trainers to teach mands for requesting as well as information, such as "what", "where", "when" and "how" (Shillingsburg et al., 2019).

Table 3. AT Interventions for cognitive skills

Type of intervention	Name of intervention	Examples and links
Low-tech	Social stories	https://carolgraysocialstories.com/social-stories/ https://www.autismparentingmagazine.com/social-stories-for-autistic-children/
	Photographic activity schedule	https://www.yourtherapysource.com/blog1/2016/11/02/evidence-based-practice-visual-activity-schedules/ https://asatonline.org/for-parents/learn-more-about-specific-treatments/activity-schedules/ https://www.appliedbehavioranalysisprograms.com/faq/what-is-visual-scheduling/
	Statistical learning	https://link.springer.com/article/10.1007/s10803-018-3625-7 https://www.emerald.com/insight/content/doi/10.1108/AIA-06-2018-0022/full/html
Mid tech	Video modeling	http://www.watchmelearn.com/ https://www.youtube.com/watch?v=JpxGV11wRSY https://www.speechandlanguagekids.com/using-video-modeling-with-autistic-and-low-functioning-kids/
High tech	Augmented reality	https://www.atandme.com/?p=976 https://technologyforlearners.com/augmented-reality-in-the-classroom/ https://www.aiga.org/aiga-design-futures/bridging-digital-and-physical-experiences/
	Computer/Mobile-phone based interventions	https://www.educationalappstore.com/app/iprompts-pro https://apps.apple.com/us/app/upad-for-icloud/id401643317 https://apps.apple.com/us/app/ireward/id324643198 https://apps.apple.com/in/app/iconnect-by-timex-2/id1475728681

2.2c High Tech AT Interventions for Communication

iPad and iPod- With the release of the Apple iPad1 in April 2010, thousands of applications have been developed to use with this technology (www.apple.com/iPad). One application that was developed to assist those with difficulty speaking is the Proloquo2GoTM application for the Apple iPhone1, iTouch1, and iPad1 (www.Proloquo2Go.com). Using a device such as an iPad™ as an SGD may be less stigmatizing for a person with a disability than other interventions as it is a common consumer product (Lorah et al., 2013). Because iPads® function through applications, there is versatility and an endless possibility of options for integrating iPads® in work with children.

The non-dedicated SGDs include applications on iPads and iPod touch. Research reveals that across 17 studies, 93% of individuals improved their ability to communicate by using an iPad or iPod as a multi-functional speech-generating device (SGD) (Lorah et al., 2013) . Children with ASD can successfully learn how to initiate requests, respond to questions, and made more frequent social comments after a few weeks' training on an SGD iPad app, SonoFlex, Proloque2Go software, Sounding Board, Speak For Yourself and GoTalkNow. Besides assisting speech production, the Proloque2Go application aids in teaching Picture and word matching tasks, which is important from an academic point of view (van der Meer et al., 2014) and reducing echolalia speech utterances (Alrusayni, 2017).

PixTalk communication system and **iCAN** has been demonstrated as an important teaching tool and is also said to have a positive effect on the children's behavior such as motivation, stability, and cognitive growth (Chien et al., 2015; De Leo et al., 2011). **Talking Hands** is an innovative, user-friendly, wearable device that can partially translate sign language (SL) to voice. Simultaneous speech and sign production facilitate speech utterance in children with limited speech. Therefore, it is possible to attain speech utterance without constant attention from a trainer while using talking hands (Pezzuoli et al.,

2020). Since talking hands is a more recent advancement, it is not evidence-based and more research is required to observe its advantages and drawbacks among the target users.

2.3 Cognitive Development

Cognition refers to the mental action of the person involved in attaining knowledge through understandings from past experiences. Cognition encompasses various aspects like thinking, intellectual ability, the formation of memory, remembering past, judgment and evaluation, problem-solving, etc. AT interventions for children with ASD target to improve complex attention, emotional recognition and its self-regulation, executive-functions skills like planning of a goal-driven behavior and cognitive flexibility (Margari et al., 2016). These AT assist children in the planning and execution by guiding daily routines (Desideri et al., 2020). Low technology includes all non-digital artifacts that may help thinking and to remember (e.g., written notes); mid technology encompasses devices that have electronic components but are not computerized (e.g., calculators), while high technology includes computerized devices such as personal computers, smartphones or smartwatches, tablets, and robots [Table 3 and Figure 3].

Figure 3.

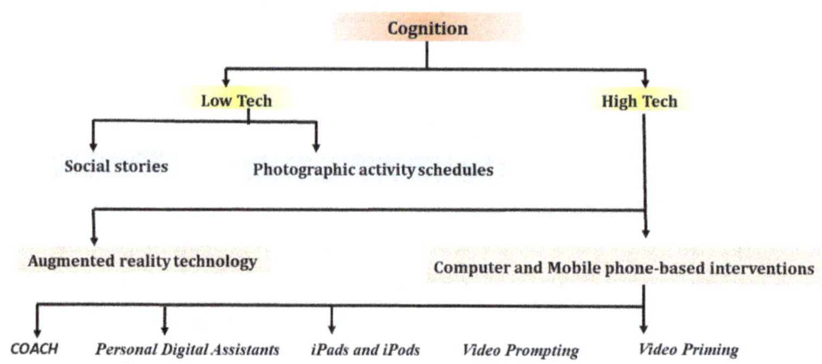

2.3a Low Technology Interventions for Cognition

a. **Social stories:** Variants of social stories such as curriculum stories and checklist stories are useful low-tech interventions. Curriculum stories are the type of social stories in which a part of the academic curriculum, for example, writing or maths, such as counting the number of children in a picture, may be introduced. Checklist stories teach the children to follow a routine. Each page in the story describes a step of the routine. On the last page, there is a checklist of all the steps in the routine, the child has to check the step as it is completed in the story. If one page is removed, a step is missing and the child is encouraged to recall that step. After some experience, the child can be given the task to arrange the step according to the routine.

b. **Photographic activity schedules:** These are similar to the cue cards used for teaching social skills. People with autism have difficulty acquiring lengthy response chains, for example, an autistic child may have learned to brush his teeth, get dressed, and go to breakfast, but he may not complete this sequence without prompts for the initiation of each activity. An activity schedule is a visual support system that combines photographs, images, or line drawings in a sequential format to represent a targeted sequence of activities in the child's schedule. The acquisition of schedule-following skills using photographic cues enables these children to display lengthy response chains (MacDuff et al., 1993), improved play behaviors (Morrison et al., 2002) and decreased transition time between two tasks (Dooley et al., 2001).

c. **Statistical Learning:** Risk-prediction ability in children with ASD is impaired due to an impaired action prediction. It was suggested by research that SL allows these children to learn to discriminate the risk and this knowledge is retained by the children after the removal of training and exposure to the risk (Kakkar & Tanu, 2018).

2.3b Mid Technology Interventions for Cognition

1. **Video modeling** is an intervention that can be used via computers and mobile technology. VM was successfully used to teach several different types of behaviors including eye contact, a library task, furniture assembly, making copies, sending fax, making coffee, grocery shopping, toileting, hand washing, and toy clean-up. A meta-analysis on video modeling use for individuals with ASD classified it as highly effective for individuals with ASD (Mason et al., 2012).
2. **Video self-modeling** was found to be effective for the improvement of various target behaviors of the participants with ASD including social initiations, responding to questions, making copies, sending fax, packaging first aid kits, greeting peers, and spontaneous requests (Buggey & Ogle, 2012), and vocational task achievement (Cullen et al., 2017).
3. **Video Prompting (VP)** is a simplified form of video modeling that breaks down a task into smaller component steps. VP is useful when the targeted skill involves many sub-steps. VP has been used to teach learners with ASD self-help skills (Norman et al., 2001). VP provides instructions for various daily activities such as table setting, ATM money withdrawal, laundry washing, emergency exiting skills, cleaning, mopping, and dishwashing (Banda et al., 2011).
4. **Video Priming** introduces an individual with ASD to an event or situation, creates familiarization and predictability, and effectively increases comfort with the specific activity before the real-life experience (Koegel et al., 2003). Ma, 2009 identified video priming to be a highly effective intervention for individuals with ASD (Ma, 2009).

2.3c High Technology Interventions for Cognition

a. Augmented Reality (AR) Technology

AR is defined as a real-time view of the actual environment with some additional virtual information. Augmented reality superimposes virtual objects on real objects. AR applications can stimulate problem-solving skills for cognitive empowerment in typically or atypically developing children, as well as promoting inclusion and social integration as would be desirable in educational and group rehabilitation settings (Lorusso et al., 2018). AR rehabilitation approaches have been growing in recent years promoting the increase in selective and sustained attention (Escobedo et al., 2014), reading (Howorth et al., 2019), and improvements in performance and reaction time skills (Anta˜o et al., 2020). Some mobile-phone-based AR systems like Aura come with modules that assist children with ASD to recognize some basic shapes, learn to draw, write, and also learn empathy towards people (Lumbreras et al., 2018), whereas others like Mobis (Mobile Object Identification System) increase the attention and focus of the child and elicit positive emotions (Escobedo et al., 2014). Several AR-based tools have also proven to be useful for improvements in the body postures and balance (Tentori et al., 2015). Moreover, the researchers plan to design a smart environment by using AR and computer-based technologies for the individuals with autism. Such an environment can promote independence in these individuals and lead to increased positive behavior, and better attention span (Tentori et al., 2015). This has led to research interests in a range of everyday adaptive living situations, including living tasks, such as brushing their teeth independently, pretend play, enhance social communication, and promotion of greeting skills (Lee et al., 2018).

b. Computer and Mobile-Based Interventions

These interventions are mostly used for assessing the self-monitoring attention-related behaviors by the students (Desideri et al., 2020). GPS is most commonly used for navigation by the general public and it is also useful for the children with ASD.

COACH (Cognitive Orthosis for Assisting aCtivities in the Home) is a computer-based multifunctional system to support time management (i.e., task initiation), insight (i.e., self-monitoring of activities), and organization and planning (i.e., providing step-by-step instructions to complete the task) (Bimbrahw et al., 2012).

Personal Digital Assistants (PDA) are used for task management (Gentry et al., 2010), independent task completion (Mechling et al., 2010), time management by setting reminders and digital calendars, cognitive flexibility (Palmen et al., 2012), and vocational support to improve work performance (Gentry et al., 2015).

iPads and iPods also provide several applications to increase task independence using Upad lite app, support activity planning and execution, remediation of social cognitive skills (Fage et al., 2018), providing training for transitioning from one task to other using iPrompts app (Ben-Avie et al., 2014), self-management of homework skills using wunderlist and iRewards apps (Hampshire & Allred, 2018), improve the on-task behaviors by Iconnect app (Huffman et al., 2019), classroom engagement by the Iconnect app and decrease in stereotypic behaviour (Rosenbloom et al., 2016), and organization and planning (Gentry et al., 2015).

3. BARRIERS OF THE AT USE FOR THE SUPPORT OF CHILDREN WITH ASD

Despite having innumerable AT tools for supporting ASD patients, these techniques remain unimplemented. Lack of resources and time for training is the most common barrier against the practice of AT interventions for children with autism in the school and personal settings (Barry et al., 2020). Inconsistency in the usage of the tools is also a problem faced during the training. This lead to a lack of generalization of the AT use. Lack of professional trainers who could teach autistic children about the use of AT is also a roadblock. A systematic review by Moorcroft et al., (2018) provides insights on how personal and environmental factors both can act as barriers and facilitators for the implementation of AAC interventions. Personal factors include the cultural and socioeconomic status of the sufferer. Environmental factors include the personal caretakers, relatives, teachers, and education and health organizations. As reported by Barry et al., (2020), the lack of awareness of the immediate acquaintances of the ASD patients about the disorder as well as the AT tools were found to be a major hurdle in applying AT interventions (Moorcroft et al., 2018).

4. CONCLUSION

ASD is a neurological developmental disorder characterized by impairments in social, communication, emotional, challenging behavior. Several AT devices are created focusing on specific impaired skills like social, communication and cognitive behavior in autistic children. The development of these devices has enhanced the quality of life of the users by correcting the impaired behaviors making them self-reliant in taking all small or big decisions. Studies suggest that technology-based interventions have a significantly positive effect on the target outcomes in the children with ASD. The interventions that are highlighted in this chapter are not only applicable for the ASD-suffering children, but these are also applicable for the children suffering from other learning disabilities like ADHD (Attention Deficit Hyperactivity Disorder) because some symptoms like poor organizational skills, social skills deficits, problems in reading and writing etc. are common.

The goal of categorization of AT tools into low, mid, and high tech tools in each section was to accentuate the availability of these tools to all the people. For example, the low-tech interventions mentioned in all the categories are inexpensive and easily applicable without professional support also, therefore these can be handy for most people regardless of their economic status. Similarly, nowadays the mid-tech video modeling strategies can be executed with the help of smartphone, tablets, and computer, which are commonly used tools. The price to accomplish video modeling is lesser as compared to the application of high-tech interventions. The high tech interventions involve buying some ‘apps’ and tools like iPad and iPods, which are user-friendly, but might be expensive for some users. For example, an app called *Proloque2Go* is one of the most common apps among users with ASD and costs 249.99 US dollars on the apple store. Nevertheless, it is also true that nowadays having a smartphone is common and affordable to most customers. Therefore, the AT tools should be easy to be brought into practice.

However, there are many obstacles in the implementation of the AT tools. Sometimes, the support personnel are unaware and untrained for the execution of a certain AT tool and sometimes they don’t prefer using an appropriate tool due to the lack of knowledge about the research behind it. Thus, the healthcare professionals and supporters should be aware and updated about the constant rigorous research going on to provide support to the children with ASD. One major hindrance that is observed is the lack of awareness of the disorder itself. In most of the developing countries, people barely know about neurological disorders, let alone the technology to treat or support the patients. It is the responsibility of the aware people to enhance the awareness of others.

In terms of research, only Naturalistic Developmental Behavioral Intervention (NDBI) has enough quality evidence to be considered promising for supporting children with ASD to achieve a range of developmental outcomes. Thus, assistive technology is an emerging intervention in the case of autism spectrum disorders. More research is required to confirm the effectiveness of these interventions for children with autism spectrum disorders. More research in this field needs to be accompanied by an increase in the production and supply of the AT tools, along with the constant advertisement of the availability of these tools to increase awareness about it.

REFERENCES

Adams, L., Gouvousis, A., Vanlue, M., & Waldron, C. (2004). Social Story Intervention: Improving Communication Skills in a Child With an Autism Spectrum Disorder. *Focus on Autism and Other Developmental Disabilities*, *19*(2), 87–94. doi:10.1177/10883576040190020301

Al-Batayneh, O. B., Nazer, T. S., Khader, Y. S., & Owais, A. I. (2020). Effectiveness of a tooth-brushing programme using the picture exchange communication system (PECS) on gingival health of children with autism spectrum disorders. *European Archives of Paediatric Dentistry; Official Journal of the European Academy of Paediatric Dentistry*, *21*(2), 277–283. doi:10.100740368-019-00485-x PMID:31628661

Alhuzimi, T. (2020). Efficacy of Video Modelling (VM) in Developing Social Skills in Children with Autism Spectrum Disorder (ASD) at School in Saudi Arabia. *International Journal of Disability Development and Education*, 1–15. doi:10.1080/1034912X.2020.1716962

Ali, S., Mehmood, F., Dancey, D., Ayaz, Y., Khan, M. J., Naseer, N., Amadeu, R. D. E. C., Sadia, H., & Nawaz, R. (2019). An Adaptive Multi-Robot Therapy for Improving Joint Attention and Imitation of ASD Children. *IEEE Access: Practical Innovations, Open Solutions*, *7*, 7. doi:10.1109/ACCESS.2019.2923678

Alrusayni, N. (2017). *The Effectiveness of the High-Tech Speech-Generating Device with Proloquo2Go App in Reducing Echolalia Utterances in a Student with Autism*. Academic Press.

Anta˜o, J. Y. F. de L., Abreu, L. C., de, Barbosa, R. T. de A., & Crocetta, T. (2020). Use of Augmented Reality with a Motion-Controlled Game Utilizing Alphabet Letters and Numbers to Improve Performance and Reaction Time Skills for People with Autism Spectrum Disorder. *Cyberpsychology, Behavior, and Social Networking*, *23*(1), 16–22. doi:10.1089/cyber.2019.0103 PMID:31976770

Banda, D. R., Dogoe, M. S., & Matuszny, R. M. (2011). Review of Video Prompting Studies with Persons with Developmental Disabilities. *Education and Training in Autism and Developmental Disabilities*, *46*(4), 514–527. http://www.jstor.org/stable/24232363

Barry, L., Holloway, J., & Mcmahon, J. (2020). A scoping review of the barriers and facilitators to the implementation of interventions in autism education. *Research in Autism Spectrum Disorders*, *78*, 101617. Advance online publication. doi:10.1016/j.rasd.2020.101617

Ben-Avie, M., Newton, D., & Reichow, B. (2014). Using Handheld Applications to Improve the Transitions of Students with Autism Spectrum Disorders. In N. R. Silton (Ed.), *Innovative Technologies to Benefit Children on the Autism Spectrum* (pp. 105–124). IGI Global. doi:10.4018/978-1-4666-5792-2.ch007

Benson, A. (2020). *Math Problem Solving Discussions : Increasing Communication for Students with Autism*. Academic Press.

Bimbrahw, J., Boger, J., & Mihailidis, A. (2012). Investigating the Efficacy of a Computerized Prompting Device to Assist Children with Autism Spectrum Disorder with Activities of Daily Living. *Assistive Technology*, *24*(4), 286–298. doi:10.1080/10400435.2012.680661

Bouck, E. C. (2010). Chapter 6 Technology and students with disabilities: Does it solve all the problems. In F. E. Obiakor, J. P. Bakken, & nthony F. Rotatori (Eds.), Current Issues and Trends in Special Education: Research, Technology, and Teacher Preparation (Vol. 20, pp. 91–104). Emerald Group Publishing Limited. doi:10.1108/S0270-4013(2010)0000020009

Buggey, T., & Ogle, L. (2012). Video self-modeling. *Psychology in the Schools*, *49*(1), 52–70. doi:10.1002/pits.20618

Charlop-Christy, M. H., Carpenter, M., Le, L., LeBlanc, L. A., & Kellet, K. (2002). Using the Picture Exchange Communication System (Pecs) With Children With Autism: Assessment of Pecs Acquisition, Speech, Social-Communicative Behavior, and Problem Behavior. *Journal of Applied Behavior Analysis*, *35*(3), 213–231. doi:10.1901/jaba.2002.35-213 PMID:12365736

Chen, W. (2012). Multitouch Tabletop Technology for People with Autism Spectrum Disorder : A review of the Literature. *Proceedings of the 4th International Conference on Software Development for Enhancing Accessibility and Fighting Info-Exclusion*, *14*(1877), 198–207. 10.1016/j.procs.2012.10.023

Cheng, Y., Chiang, H., Ye, J., & Cheng, L. (2010). Enhancing empathy instruction using a collaborative virtual learning environment for children with autistic spectrum conditions. *Computers & Education*, *55*(4), 1449–1458. doi:10.1016/j.compedu.2010.06.008

Chien, M. E., Jheng, C. M., Lin, N. M., Tang, H. H., Taele, P., Tseng, W. S., & Chen, M. Y. (2015). iCAN: A tablet-based pedagogical system for improving communication skills of children with autism. *International Journal of Human-Computer Studies*, *73*, 79–90. doi:10.1016/j.ijhcs.2014.06.001

Cullen, J. M., Alber-Morgan, S. R., Simmons-Reed, E. A., & Izzo, M. V. (2017). Effects of self-directed video prompting using iPads on the vocational task completion of young adults with intellectual and developmental disabilities. *Journal of Vocational Rehabilitation*, *46*(3), 361–375. doi:10.3233/JVR-170873

David, D. O., Costescu, C. A., Matu, S., Szentagotai, A., & Dobrean, A. (2019). Effects of a Robot-Enhanced Intervention for Children With ASD on Teaching Turn-Taking Skills. *Journal of Educational Computing Research*, *58*(1), 29–62. doi:10.1177/0735633119830344

De Leo, G., Gonzales, C. H., Battagiri, P., & Leroy, G. (2011). A smart-phone application and a companion website for the improvement of the communication skills of children with autism: Clinical rationale, technical development and preliminary results. *Journal of Medical Systems*, *35*(4), 703–711. doi:10.100710916-009-9407-1 PMID:20703781

Desideri, L., Di Santantonio, A., Varrucciu, N., Bonsi, I., & Di Sarro, R. (2020). Assistive Technology for Cognition to Support Executive Functions in Autism: A Scoping Review. *Advances in Neurodevelopmental Disorders*, *4*(4), 330–343. doi:10.100741252-020-00163-w

Doherty, A., Bracken, M., & Gormley, L. (2018). Teaching Children with Autism to Initiate and Respond to Peer Mands Using Picture Exchange Communication System (PECS). *Behavior Analysis in Practice*, *11*(4), 279–288. doi:10.100740617-018-00311-8 PMID:30538902

Dooley, P., Wilczenski, F. L., & Torem, C. (2001). Using an activity schedule to smooth school transitions. *Journal of Positive Behavior Interventions*, *3*(1), 57–61. doi:10.1177/109830070100300108

Durand, V. M. (1999). Functional Communication Training Using Assistive Devices: Recruiting Natural Communities of Reinforcement. *Journal of Applied Behavior Analysis, 32*(3), 247–267. doi:10.1901/jaba.1999.32-247 PMID:10513023

Escobedo, L., Nguyen, D. H., Boyd, L., Hirano, S., Rangel, A., Garcia-Rosas, D., Tentori, M., & Hayes, G. (2012). MOSOCO: A Mobile Assistive Tool to Support Children with Autism Practicing Social Skills in Real-Life Situations. *Proceedings of the SIGCHI Conference on Human Factors in Computing Systems*, 2589–2598. 10.1145/2207676.2208649

Escobedo, L., Tentori, M., Quintana, E., Favela, J., & Garcia-Rosas, D. (2014). Using Augmented Reality to Help Children with Autism Stay Focused. *IEEE CS*, 38–46.

Fage, C., Consel, C. Y., Balland, E., Etchegoyhen, K., Amestoy, A., Bouvard, M., & Sauzéon, H. (2018). Tablet apps to support first school inclusion of children with autism spectrum disorders (ASD) in mainstream classrooms: A pilot study. *Frontiers in Psychology, 9*, 2020. doi:10.3389/fpsyg.2018.02020 PMID:30405498

Gal, E., Lamash, L., Bauminger-Zviely, N., Zancanaro, M., & Weiss, P. L. (2016). Using Multitouch Collaboration Technology to Enhance Social Interaction of Children with High-Functioning Autism. *Physical & Occupational Therapy in Pediatrics, 36*(1), 46–58. doi:10.3109/01942638.2015.1040572 PMID:26422262

Gentry, T., Kriner, R., Sima, A., McDonough, J., & Wehman, P. (2015). Reducing the Need for Personal Supports Among Workers with Autism Using an iPod Touch as an Assistive Technology: Delayed Randomized Control Trial. *Journal of Autism and Developmental Disorders, 45*(3), 669–684. doi:10.100710803-014-2221-8 PMID:25212414

Gentry, T., Wallace, J., Kvarfordt, C., & Lynch, K. B. (2010). Personal digital assistants as cognitive aids for high school students with autism: Results of a community-based trial. *Journal of Vocational Rehabilitation, 32*(2), 101–107. doi:10.3233/JVR-2010-0499

Glaesar, B. C., Pierson, M. R., & Fritschmann, N. (2003). Comic Strip Conversations: A positive behavioral support strategy. *Teaching Exceptional Children, 36*(2), 14–19. doi:10.1177/004005990303600202

Grynszpan, O., Weiss, P. L. T., Perez, F., & Gal, E. (2014). Innovative technology-based interventions for autism spectrum disorders : A meta-analysis. *Autism, 18*(4), 346–361. doi:10.1177/1362361313476767 PMID:24092843

Gupta, S., Mishra, C., Katyayan, P., & Joshi, N. (2018). Assistive Technology for Neurological Disorders. SSRN *Electronic Journal, January*. doi:10.2139/ssrn.3166499

Hampshire, P. K., & Allred, K. W. (2018). A Parent-Implemented, Technology-Mediated Approach to Increasing Self-Management Homework Skills in Middle School Students with Autism. *Exceptionality, 26*(2), 119–136. doi:10.1080/09362835.2016.1216848

Howorth, S. K., Rooks-ellis, D., Flanagan, S., & Ok, M. W. (2019). Augmented Reality Supporting Reading Skills of Students with Autism Spectrum Disorder. *Intervention in School and Clinic, 55*(2), 71–77. doi:10.1177/1053451219837635

Huffman, J. M., Bross, L. A., Watson, E. K., Wills, H. P., & Mason, R. A. (2019). Preliminary Investigation of a Self-monitoring Application for a Postsecondary Student with Autism. *Advances in Neurodevelopmental Disorders, 3*(4), 423–433. doi:10.100741252-019-00124-y

Investigators, A. and D. D. M. N. S. Y. 2008 P. (2012). Prevalence of Autism Spectrum Disorders — Autism and Developmental Disabilities Monitoring Network, 14 Sites, United States, 2008. *Morbidity and Mortality Weekly Report: Surveillance Summaries, 61*(3), 1–19. http://www.jstor.org/stable/24806043

Jusoh, W., & Majid, R. A. (2017). Using Picture Exchange Communication System To Improve Speech Utterance Among Children With Autism. *Journal of ICSAR, 1*(1), 46–49. doi:10.17977/um005v1i12017p046

Kakkar, D., & Tanu, T. (2018). Strengthening risk prediction using statistical learning in children with autism spectrum disorder. *Advances in Autism, 4*(3), 141–152. doi:10.1108/AIA-06-2018-0022

Ke, F., Moon, J., & Sokolikj, Z. (2020). Virtual Reality–Based Social Skills Training for Children With Autism Spectrum Disorder. *Journal of Special Education Technology*, 1–14. doi:10.1177/0162643420945603

Khantreejitranon, A. (2018). Using a social story intervention to decrease inappropriate behavior of preschool children with autism. *Kasetsart Journal of Social Sciences, 39*(1), 90–97. doi:10.1016/j.kjss.2017.12.019

Koegel, L. K., Koegel, R. L., Frea, W., & Green-Hopkins, I. (2003). Priming as a method of coordinating educational services for students with autism. *Language, Speech, and Hearing Services in Schools, 34*(3), 228–235. doi:10.1044/0161-1461(2003/019) PMID:27764324

Kozima, H., Nakagawa, C., & Yasuda, Y. (2007). Children–robot interaction: a pilot study in autism therapy. In C. von Hofsten & K. B. T.-P. In B. R. Rosander (Ed.), *From Action to Cognition* (Vol. 164, pp. 385–400). Elsevier. doi:10.1016/S0079-6123(07)64021-7

Lee, I.-J., Chen, C.-H., Wang, C.-P., & Chung, C.-H. (2018). Augmented Reality Plus Concept Map Technique to Teach Children with ASD to Use Social Cues When Meeting and Greeting. *The Asia-Pacific Education Researcher, 27*(3), 227–243. doi:10.100740299-018-0382-5

Leyzberg, D., Spaulding, S., Toneva, M., & Scassellati, B. (2012). The Physical Presence of a Robot Tutor Increases Cognitive Learning Gains. *Proceedings of the Annual Meeting of the Cognitive Science Society, 34*(34).

Lorah, E. R., Tincani, M., Dodge, J., Gilroy, S., Hickey, A., & Hantula, D. (2013). *Evaluating Picture Exchange and the iPad ™ as a Speech Generating Device to Teach Communication to Young Children with Autism.* doi:10.1007/s10882-013-9337-1

Lorusso, M. L., Giorgetti, M., Travellini, S., Greci, L., Zangiacomi, A., Mondellini, M., Sacco, M., & Reni, G. (2018). Giok the Alien: An AR-Based Integrated System for the Empowerment of Problem-Solving, Pragmatic, and Social Skills in Pre-School Children. In Sensors (Vol. 18, Issue 7). doi:10.339018072368

Lumbreras, M. A. M., de Lourdes, M.-T. M., & Ariel, S.-R. (2018). Aura: Augmented Reality in Mobile Devices for the Learning of Children With ASD – Augmented Reality in the Learning of Children With Autism. In G. R. Ruiz & M. H. Hernández (Eds.), *Augmented Reality for Enhanced Learning Environments* (pp. 142–169). IGI Global. doi:10.4018/978-1-5225-5243-7.ch006

Ma, H.-H. (2009). The effectiveness of intervention on the behavior of individuals with autism: A meta-analysis using percentage of data points exceeding the median of baseline phase (PEM). *Behavior Modification, 33*(3), 339–359. doi:10.1177/0145445509333173 PMID:19282505

Macdonald, R., Clark, M., Garrigan, E., & Vangala, M. (2005). Using video modeling to teach pretend play to children with autism. *Behavioral Interventions, 20*(4), 225–238. doi:10.1002/bin.197

MacDuff, G. S., Krantz, P. J., & McClannahan, L. E. (1993). Teaching Children With Autism To Use Photographic Activity Schedules: Maintenance and Generalization of Complex Response Chains. *Journal of Applied Behavior Analysis, 26*(1), 89–97. doi:10.1901/jaba.1993.26-89 PMID:8473261

Margari, L., Craig, F., Margari, F., Legrottaglie, A., Palumbi, R., & De Giambattista, C. (2016). A review of executive function deficits in autism spectrum disorder and attention-deficit/hyperactivity disorder. *Neuropsychiatric Disease and Treatment, 12*, 1191. doi:10.2147/NDT.S104620 PMID:27274255

Mason, R. A., Ganz, J. B., Parker, R. I., Burke, M. D., & Camargo, S. P. (2012). Moderating factors of video-modeling with other as model: A meta-analysis of single-case studies. *Research in Developmental Disabilities, 33*(4), 1076–1086. doi:10.1016/j.ridd.2012.01.016 PMID:22502832

Mechling, L. C., Gast, D. L., & Seid, N. H. (2010). Evaluation of a personal digital assistant as a self-prompting device for increasing multi-step task completion by students with moderate intellectual disabilities. *Education and Training in Autism and Developmental Disabilities*, 422–439.

Moorcroft, A., Scarinci, N., & Meyer, C. (2018). A systematic review of the barriers and facilitators to the provision and use of low-tech and unaided AAC systems for people with complex communication needs and their families. *Disability and Rehabilitation. Assistive Technology, 0*(0), 1–22. doi:10.1080/17483107.2018.1499135 PMID:30070927

Morrison, R. S., Sainato, D. M., Benchaaban, D., & Endo, S. (2002). Increasing play skills of children with autism using activity schedules and correspondence training. *Journal of Early Intervention, 25*(1), 58–72. doi:10.1177/105381510202500106

Nikopoulos, C. K., & Keenan, M. (2004). Effects of Video Modelling on Training and Generalisation of Social Initiation and Reciprocal Play by Children With Autism. *European Journal of Behavior Analysis, 5*(1), 1–13. doi:10.1080/15021149.2004.11434227

Nikopoulos, C. K., & Keenan, M. (2007). Using Video Modeling to Teach Complex Social Sequences to Children with Autism. *Journal of Autism and Developmental Disorders, 37*(4), 678–693. doi:10.100710803-006-0195-x PMID:16897375

Norman, J. M., Collins, B. C., & Schuster, J. W. (2001). Using an instructional package including video technology to teach self-help skills to elementary students with mental disabilities. *Journal of Special Education Technology, 16*(3), 5–18. doi:10.1177/016264340101600301

Obeid, R., Brooks, P. J., Powers, K. L., Gillespie-lynch, K., & Lum, J. A. G. (2016). Statistical Learning in Specific Language Impairment and Autism Spectrum Disorder : A Meta-Analysis. *Frontiers in Psychology, 7*, 1–18. doi:10.3389/fpsyg.2016.01245 PMID:27602006

Palmen, A., Didden, R., & Verhoeven, L. (2012). A personal digital assistant for improving independent transitioning in adolescents with high-functioning autism spectrum disorder. *Developmental Neurorehabilitation, 15*(6), 401–413. doi:10.3109/17518423.2012.701240 PMID:23030628

Pezzuoli, F., Tafaro, D., Pane, M., Corona, D., & Corradini, M. L. (2020). Development of a New Sign Language Translation System for People with Autism Spectrum Disorder. *Advances in Neurodevelopmental Disorders, 4*(4), 439–446. doi:10.100741252-020-00175-6

Pop, C. A., Simut, R. E., Pintea, S., Saldien, J., Rusu, A. S., Vanderfaeillie, J., David, D. O., Lefeber, D., & Vanderborght, B. (2013). Social robots vs. computer display: Does the way social stories are delivered make a difference for their effectiveness on ASD children. *Journal of Educational Computing Research, 49*(3), 381–401. doi:10.2190/EC.49.3.f

Qi, C. H., Barton, E. E., Collier, M., & Lin, Y. (2017). A Systematic Review of Single-Case Research Studies on Using Video Modeling Interventions to Improve Social Communication Skills for Individuals With Autism Spectrum Disorder. *Focus on Autism and Other Developmental Disabilities*, ●●●, 1–9. doi:10.1177/1088357617741282

Rice, L. M., Wall, C. A., Fogel, A., & Shic, F. (2015). Computer-Assisted Face Processing Instruction Improves Emotion Recognition, Mentalizing, and Social Skills in Students with ASD. *Journal of Autism and Developmental Disorders, 45*(7), 2176–2186. Advance online publication. doi:10.100710803-015-2380-2 PMID:25694364

Rosenbloom, R., Mason, R. A., Wills, H. P., & Mason, B. A. (2016). Technology delivered self-monitoring application to promote successful inclusion of an elementary student with autism. *Assistive Technology, 28*(1), 9–16. doi:10.1080/10400435.2015.1059384 PMID:26151808

Scassellati, B., Boccanfuso, L., Huang, C. M., Mademtzi, M., Qin, M., Salomons, N., Ventola, P., & Shic, F. (2018). Improving social skills in children with ASD using a long-term, in-home social robot. *Science Robotics, 3*(21), eaat7544. Advance online publication. doi:10.1126cirobotics.aat7544 PMID:33141724

Shillingsburg, M. A., Marya, V., Bartlett, B. L., & Thompson, T. M. (2019). Teaching mands for information using speech generating devices: A replication and extension. *Journal of Applied Behavior Analysis, 52*(3), 756–771. doi:10.1002/jaba.579 PMID:31157409

Sigafoos, J., Reilly, M. O., Ganz, J. B., Lancioni, G. E., & Schlosser, R. W. (2005). Supporting self-determination in AAC interventions by assessing preference for communication devices. *Technology and Disability, 17*(3), 143–153. doi:10.3233/TAD-2005-17302

Smith, T. J., & Bernardini, S. (2014). ECHOES : An intelligent serious game for fostering social communication in children with autism. *Information Sciences, 264*, 41–60. doi:10.1016/j.ins.2013.10.027

Spencer, V., Simpson, C. G., Day, M., Buster, E., Spencer, V. G., & Simpson, C. G. (2008). Using the Power Card Strategy to Teach Social Skills to a Child with Autism. *TEACHING Exceptional Children Plus, 5*(1), 1–10.

Tanaka, J. W., Wolf, J. M., Klaiman, C., Koenig, K., Cockburn, J., Herlihy, L., Brown, C., Stahl, S., Kaiser, M. D., & Schultz, R. T. (2010). Using computerized games to teach face recognition skills to children with autism spectrum disorder: The Let's Face It! program. *Journal of Child Psychology and Psychiatry, and Allied Disciplines*, *51*(8), 944–952. doi:10.1111/j.1469-7610.2010.02258.x PMID:20646129

Tentori, M., Escobedo, L., & Balderas, G. (2015). A Smart Environment for Children with Autism. *IEEE Pervasive Computing*, *14*(2), 42–50. doi:10.1109/MPRV.2015.22

Tiger, J. H., Hanley, G. P., & Bruzek, J. (2008). Functional communication training: A review and practical guide. *Behavior Analysis in Practice*, *1*(1), 16–23. doi:10.1007/BF03391716 PMID:22477675

Valadão, C. T., Goulart, C., Rivera, H., Caldeira, E., Bastos Filho, T. F., Frizera-Neto, A., & Carelli, R. (2016). Analysis of the use of a robot to improve social skills in children with autism spectrum disorder. *Revista Brasileira de Engenharia Biomédica*, *32*(2), 161–175. doi:10.1590/2446-4740.01316

van der Meer, L., Achmadi, D., Cooijmans, M., Didden, R., Lancioni, G. E., O'Reilly, M. F., Roche, L., Stevens, M., Carnett, A., Hodis, F., Green, V. A., Sutherland, D., Lang, R., Rispoli, M., Marschik, P. B., & Sigafoos, J. (2014). An iPad-Based Intervention for Teaching Picture and Word Matching to a Student with ASD and Severe Communication Impairment. *Journal of Developmental and Physical Disabilities*, *27*(1), 67–78. doi:10.100710882-014-9401-5

Vanderborght, B., Simut, R., Saldien, J., A. Pop, C., Rusu, A. S., Pintea, S., Lefeber, D., & David, D. O. (2012). Using the social robot probo as a social story telling agent for children with ASD. *Interaction Studies. Social Behaviour and Communication in Biological and Artificial SystemsInteraction Studies / Social Behaviour and Communication in Biological and Artificial SystemsInteraction Studies*, *13*(3), 348–372. doi:10.1075/is.13.3.02van

Wadhera, T., & Kakkar, D. (2019). Eye Tracker: An Assistive Tool in Diagnosis of Autism Spectrum Disorder. In S. K. Gupta, S. Venkatesan, S. P. Goswami, & R. Kumar (Eds.), *Emerging Trends in the Diagnosis and Intervention of Neurodevelopmental Disorders* (pp. 125–152). IGI Global. doi:10.4018/978-1-5225-7004-2.ch007

Wadhera, T., & Kakkar, D. (2020). Big Data-Based System: A Supportive Tool in Autism Spectrum Disorder Analysis. In T. Wadhera & D. Kakkar (Eds.), *Interdisciplinary Approaches to Altering Neurodevelopmental Disorders* (pp. 303–319). IGI Global. doi:10.4018/978-1-7998-3069-6.ch017

Wadhera, T., Kakkar, D., Kaur, G., & Menia, V. (2019). Pre-Clinical ASD Screening Using Multi-Biometrics-Based Systems. In D. R. Kisku, P. Gupta, & J. K. Sing (Eds.), *Design and Implementation of Healthcare Biometric Systems* (pp. 185–211). IGI Global. doi:10.4018/978-1-5225-7525-2.ch008

Willems, R. M., Özyürek, A., & Hagoort, P. (2007). When language meets action: The neural integration of gesture and speech. *Cerebral Cortex*, *17*(10), 2322–2333. doi:10.1093/cercor/bhl141 PMID:17159232

Winterling, V. (2013). *Delaware Autism Program BT.* In F. R. Volkmar (Ed.), *Encyclopedia of Autism Spectrum Disorders* (pp. 854–856). Springer New York. doi:10.1007/978-1-4419-1698-3_381

Zhang, L., Amat, A. Z., Zhao, H., Swanson, A., Weitlauf, A., Warren, Z., & Sarkar, N. (2020). Design of an Intelligent Agent to Measure Collaboration and Verbal-Communication Skills of Children with Autism Spectrum Disorder in Collaborative Puzzle Games. *IEEE Transactions on Learning Technologies*, 1–15. doi:10.1109/TLT.2020.3029223

Zhang, L., Fu, Q., Swanson, A. M. Y., Weitlauf, A. M. Y., Warren, Z., & Sarkar, N. (2018). Design and Evaluation of a Collaborative Virtual Environment (CoMove) for Autism Spectrum. *ACM Transactions on Accessible Computing*, *11*(2), 1–22. doi:10.1145/3209687

Zhao, H., Swanson, A. R., Weitlauf, A. S., Warren, Z. E., Sarkar, N., & Member, S. (2018). Hand-in-Hand: A Communication-Enhancement Collaborative Virtual Reality System for Promoting Social Interaction in Children With Autism Spectrum Disorders. *IEEE Transactions on Human-Machine Systems*, *48*(2), 1–13. doi:10.1109/THMS.2018.2791562

Chapter 3
Assistive Technologies and Design for People With Autism Spectrum Disorders:
A Selective Overview

Denise Gulino
University Giustino Fortunato of Benevento, Italy

ABSTRACT

This chapter has the aim to provide a concise overview of which assistive technology tools can be used to implement interventions for people with autism spectrum disorders and what developers and designers must take into account when they want to approach to the development of these technologies. Four areas of intervention have been identified: (1) treatment of phobias, (2) social interactions, (3) academic skills, (4) job performance. Ten contributions have been reviewed for a total of 216 participants. Positive results and limits of various studies have been identified. In each session a specific technology will be analyzed, and some general guidelines will be provided. Some suggestions will be emphasized for future research.

INTRODUCTION

Autism is a disorder characterized by behavioral and physical symptoms. There is not a unanimous consensus concerning the etiopathogenesis currently unknown. Autism onset in the developmental age, during the first three years of life (ICD-10). Autism is described as an atypical condition of neurological development, depending on genetic predisposition and environmental factors. There are multiple dimensions of autism and the characteristics of the various individuals are clinically heterogenous, so the disorder is considered within a 'spectrum'. But generally speaking, the Autism Spectrum Disorders (ASD) concern a severe and generalized impairment of two macro areas of development: one related to communication skills and social interactions and the other related to the sphere of interests and activities. The various symptoms of the ASD are grouped in these two domains both in the fifth edition of the *American Psychiatric Association's Diagnostic and Statistical Manual of Mental Disorders* (DSM-5)

DOI: 10.4018/978-1-7998-7430-0.ch003

and in the *International Classification of Disorders-10* (ICD-10). The seriousness of the deficits must be such as to compromise various important areas of a person's life (family, education, school/work, social sphere). The difficulties are pervasive and are observable in all the contexts. Therefore, knowing the different areas affected by autism, it is possible understand in which fields to intervene and which the most appropriate tools are to guarantee to the person and his family the achievement of goals to improve their lives.

According to the Centers for Disease Control and Prevention (CDC), a constant tendency toward the increase of cases of autism of around 10% is evident: in the U.S.A., the prevalence increases from a child every 59 in 2014 to a child every 54 in 2016 (Maenner, Yeargin-Allsopp, Van Naarden Braun, Christensen & Schieve, 2016); furthermore the disorder is three times more common in males than females (Loomes, Hull & Mandy, 2017).

The aim of the chapter is to examine the use of some Assistive Technologies (ATs). In particular applications, Virtual Reality (VR), Augmented Reality (AR), and robots, were listed to provide a selective overview on the empirical evidences available between 2014 to 2020, selected in the electronic databases such as PubMed, Scopus, ResearchGate. The evaluated studies allow to understand how these technologies can be used in rehabilitative interventions for autism in the following areas: (a) treatment of phobias, (b) improvement of social interactions, (c) strengthening of academic skills, (d) job performance. The studies concern AT-based programmes for people with autism, in particular children and young adults.

Another goal is to provide some suggestions to whom intended to approach the development of 'autism-friendly' technologies. The technology that aims at the social inclusion of people with ASD should be thought so as to simulate everyday situations that represent a challenge for those who are involved. In the planning of interfaces and scenarios of VR, the designers should take into account, for instance, the hypersensitivity of children with ASD to tactile, verbal and visual stimuli (Takahashi et al., 2014). Additionally the use of a methodology considering clear utterances, insertion of descriptive button, use of a simple layout in the interactive interfaces process it should be acknowledged. To exhaustively tackle features and needs of children with ASD specifics guidelines for each technology-aided setup or device are mandatory and highly recommended. Towards a desirable increase of life quality and expectancy, AT could be the new starting point for implementation of treatments aimed at guaranteeing the autonomy to the autistic individual and at improving the various cognitive domains in which they are impaired.

So the chapter is aimed at caregivers, professional (such as doctors, therapists, psychomotor therapists, educators, teachers) and the entire social network inside the community. However, a valid contribution to the implementation of the interventions for people with autism using various technologies can be given by developers and designers.

1. BACKGROUND

The term AT 'means any item, piece of equipment, or product system, whether acquired commercially off the shelf, modified, or customized, that is used to increase, maintain, or improve functional capabilities of a child with a disability' (Acts, 1998). The goal of the ATs is to provide to people with development delays tools to increase independence and self-determination. The intervention with ATs for people with ASD considers the use of strategies that allow the self-management of environmental events (Stasolla & Passaro, 2020). Also considering the literature, the treatment with the employment of a computer exceeds in terms of effectiveness, attention and motivation a merely behavioral programme (Di Pietro, Kelemen, Liang & Sik-Lanyi, 2019).

This research tried to provide professionals working with autistic people an overview clarifying the ATs indicated for the major areas affected by ASD. Interventions that based their programs on AT were evaluated. The categorization of the areas, and consequently of the ATs identified in the various studies, has allowed to clarify the possibilities of intervention in particular at the disposal of children and young adults with ASD. Additionally, guidelines for developers and designers approaching the development of 'autism-friendly' technologies have been identified.

In the following section, the criteria used to pursue the research have been indicated.

2. METHOD

The chapter is based on a computer research of journal articles, conference documents within database such as PubMed, Scopus, ResearchGate published between 2014 and 2020. The keywords used for the research were: ASD, AT, treatments, VR, AR, robot, children, adolescents, anxiety disorder, social interactions, academic performance, job performance, User Experience (UX) design, universal design, guidelines. A manual search of article in UX specialized website was also made. The examined research concerns only some of the areas of functioning for which the intervention for autism are implemented. The inclusion of the other areas would have determined an excess compared to the declared aims.

To identify studies in support of the discussion, the included criteria were: (a) studies with children and young adults with ASD as participants, (b) presence of at least one rehabilitation programme based on AT, (c) studies concerning the considered functioning areas, (d) studies starting from 2014 (supporting literature excluded). The exclusion criteria were: (a) studies with adult participants only (considering adults people who are over 30 years), (b) absence of a rehabilitation programme, (c) participants with exclusively development disability different than ASD, (d) studies concerning impaired areas not included in the overview. 10 studies were analyzed, for a total of 216 interested participants, children and young adults. The studies were gathered based on practical matters considering some of the functioning areas impaired in the ASD. In particular: (a) treatment of phobias, (b) social interactions, (c) academic skills, (d) job performance. Within each section, illustrative studies have been delineated. For each it was indicated: participants' number, age and characteristics, rehabilitation goals, used procedures, obtained results and observed limits. For each section, from time to time, indications will be provided for the development and design of the ATs used in the indicated studies. For this topic, the following research criteria were included: (a) specific guidelines for ASD, (b) ATs development and design, (c) specific indications for the technologies contained in the above-mentioned studies. Instead, the exclusion criteria were: (a) specific guidelines exclusively for disorders different than ASD, (b) non-AT, (c) indications for ATs not presented in the indicated studies.

3. LITERATURE OVERVIEW

A teamwork capable of taking into account all the aspects related to the intervention with an autistic person is essential. It should be considered the support given to the person with autism by caregivers, professionals (such as doctors, therapists, psychomotor therapists, educators, teachers) and by the entire social network inside the community. Further, adequate tools to carry on care, assistance, education, autonomy task for autistic people are fundamental. To be effective and valid ATs need to be customized: every disorder has its peculiarities and necessities. For this reason, firstly general indication for technology development and then the studies (listed in Table 1) were provided. These studies allow to understand how specific technologies can be used for the treatment of different functioning areas.

Before approaching the design for autism, designers and developers should deepen their knowledge about ASD. Understood autism spectrum, designers and developers can address their actions keeping in mind characteristics and preferences. Since no suitable designs are available for all the user groups (Darejeh & Singh, 2013), clear ideas about who will use the technology are essential. Following, some general indications to be applied in the various types of technologies to make them 'autism-friendly' were provided .

1. **Atypical sensorial symptoms**: atypical sensorial symptoms in ASD, in particular hyperreactivity and hyporeactivity to sensorial symptoms (DSM-5), are common. Already Frith (1989), with the weak central coherence theory (WCC), suggested that the individuals with ASD have a better perception of details. This leads them to pay minor attention to global information and, thus, to difficulties in the elaboration of the information of the context.
    a. **Colours**: children with ASD are visual thinkers (Frauenberger, Good, Alcorn, & Pain, 2012). So, it does not matter the type of technology to develop, chromatic preference of people with ASD should be taken into account. The perceptual categorization of colours is regulated by the same mechanism in people with ASD and without ASD, but hypersensitivity to colour seems to influence colour perception. This would lead to an aversion by people with ASD to some colours. In one study conducted on 29 children with ASD and 28 typical children, aged between 4 and 17, the following was noticed: in the typical children the preferred colours were (in order) red, blue and yellow; the children with ASD preferred green and brown and they tended to avoid yellow, hardly tolerable for children with ASD (Grandgeorge & Masataka, 2016). The obsession for green colour by children with ASD, compared to the classic primary colours preferred by typical children, is documented in other studies (Higashida, 2013; Silberman, 2015).
    b. **Sounds**: in people with ASD, the most evident anomalies at the auditive level concern the greater elaboration of tone and the greater sensitivity to volume. Further another anomaly is the reduced attention to more complex auditive stimulus. For more information please take a look to O'Connor (O'Connor, 2012). In general, in the development of ATs for people with autism, it would be preferable avoiding too strong and sudden sounds, giving more time between an instruction and another to avoid auditive excess loads, reducing auditory distraction.
2. **Predictable interactions and control**: keeping in mind children with ASD find it difficult to deal with unpredictability of others' behavior, the predictability is attractive for them (Alcorn et al., 2019). Furthermore, repeatability allows them to master a skill and to provide control of the learning rate (Carlier, Van der Paelt, Ongenae, De Backere, De Turck, 2020).
3. **Uniqueness**: each person is unique, any kind of support should be thought taking into account the person, the family and the context, the strengths and weaknesses.

In the following session different areas of intervention were identified, and specific indications concerning ATs used for each of the areas were provided.

3.1 Academic Performance

Rosello, Berenguer, Baixauli, Colomer & Miranda (2018) explored the literature concerning learning behaviors. The authors highlighting how, in children with ASD, different deficits are present related to the comprehension of linguistic expressions (such as metaphors, figures of speech), problem solving, conceptual learning and abstract learning (typical of mathematics), reading, and text comprehension. The improvement of learning and of academic performance is one of the most relevant challenges for the intervention in the autistic population. Providing learning opportunities to all students is essential to guarantee the accessibility already during the design phase. Cerga-Pashoja, Gaete, Shishkova & Jordanova (2019) investigated the use of AT for the comprehension of written documents. According to the authors, people with ASD experience several language deficits, including comprehension of speech and writing and complex instructions. Since the small number of trials based on a experimental design or including a large sample involving non-child participants, the authors focused on adolescents and adults. Their study considers a technology, called Open Book, capable of converting written texts into more simple forms: using this technology, texts are more comprehensive for people with ASD because the software reduces the sentences, it substitutes and solves metaphors and figures of speech, it replaces particularly difficult words with images, it uses functions such as the 'magnify', that highlights phrases to facilitate attention and support; moreover, the software provides the possibility to gather and save documents using folders and labels.

The participants (divided in groups of English, Spanish and Bulgarian adults and adolescents) were 243, of which 90 adolescents between 12 and 17 years with diagnosis of ASD and score ≥70 in a measure in an intelligence test. To read a text for 10 minutes and answer to some multiple choice questions was asked to the adolescents. Then, using a Likert scale from 1 (very easy) to 5 (very difficult), a self-report on the complexity of the text was proposed. According to the results, the responses of participants in the simplified texts compared to the original ones were more accurate. More specifically, the responses of adolescents to the questions about the simplified contents compared to the questions about the original texts were more exact. Furthermore, in the self-reports the simplified texts were evaluated easier than the original texts from all participants. In spite of the encouraging results, it is necessary to consider some limitations of the study: the long-term effects on the reading skills and in the functioning of the participants were not possible to determine; and the generalization of the data to other people with ASD was not possible to verify.

Another tool analyzed for the support to academic performance is the touch-screen, in particular the hardware tablet. These tools can support skills such as touch, gesture, pointing (Flewitt, Kucirkova & Messer, 2014). Also the possibility to customize provided by these tools should be considered relevant. For instance, the apps based on the PECS (Picture Exchange Communication System) may allow the instant creation of catalogue of photographic images of real objects, whenever the tablet is equipped of incorporated camera (Allen, Hartley & Cain, 2016). Moreover, considering the technical specifications (including the possibility to connect to the internet, storage capacity, dimension of the device, accessibility), tablet can be considered as a proper tool for teaching in class and an adequate device for innovative educational intervention using apps. The literature on the effectiveness of employment of the iPad in this field is various and in some cases discordant. Lorah, Parnell, Schaefer Whitby & Hantula (2015) took into account 17 studies for a total of 57 participants. 53 of them were able to acquire the ability to communicate in the educational context using iPod and iPad such as SGD (Speech Generating Device).

However, other studies were not able to demonstrate, in terms of effectiveness, the supremacy of these tolls compared to the more traditional ones or to alternative interventions.

Little research has explored the ability of people with ASD and severe language impairments to understand and learn from symbolic information via tablets. In addition, there is a lack of guidance as to how to maximize the functionality of electronic apps to facilitate learning in people with ASD (Allen et al., 2016). However, ascertaining the level of understanding the symbolic role of pictures, and how people with ASD might learn from them is important. With their study, Allen et al. (2016) tried to understand whether the use of an iPad can influence the extension of words learned via pictures to real objects in children with ASD and severe language impairments. For this reason, they carried out a study on 16 minimally-verbal children with ASD between 3 and 9 years. They were already exposed to interventions based on images and to iPad in educational context. The researchers tried to understand if symbolic learning changes whether the images are presented on an iPad or on another traditional tool, such as an illustrated book. According to the results, there was not a substantial difference between the two tools in terms of learning.

O'Malley, Lewis, Donehower & Stone (2014) wondered whether technological devices can improve academic skills and at the same time the independence of students with ASD and moderate to severe developmental disabilities. They conducted a study evaluating the difference between traditional teaching and use of the iPad, focusing on: (a) improvement of basic mathematics skills, (b) reduction of non-complaint behaviors, (c) completion of independent activities, (d) advantage from the use of technology. Seven students, aged between 10 and 13, with ASD and developmental delays from moderate to severe in different areas (communication, socialization and behavior) took part to the study. The single subject research methodology and the ABAB design were used. To evaluate the development of basic mathematics skills, items of Cognitive Domain subtest of the Learning and Achievement Profile-3 (LAP-3) were selected. The results are extremely conflicting. In the specific, it was not registered an increase of the number of completed mathematics tasks between baseline and intervention phase; however, the rough scores of five children on the LAP-3 showed an improvement. The mixed results were highlighted in the intervention for the reduction of non-compliant behaviors. The results related to the completion of independent activities proved moderate effects, while the test of the single students showed, for some of them, the non-effectiveness of intervention in this field. Concerning the advantages, it appears that: (a) the necessity of support and the solicitation on the part of the teachers has decreased, (b) it was possible an educational differentiation for each students, (c) the overall non-compliant behaviors have decreased, (d) teachers evaluated acceptable and effective the tool for teaching in class, (e) there were clear progresses towards goals of learning and that were not reached yet, (f) an improvement of the teaching skills and of the students' interest for the contents was perceived. Thus, despite of the teachers' positive perception in the use of the iPad, it required a high ratio between stuff and students and an elevated technological support; furthermore, the necessity to provide an higher level training to improve teachers' competences in the use of technology is highlighted from the study.

3.1.1 Applications

The first thing to be considered is the User Interface (UI). Because the UI defines the experience of the user, the UI design is predictive of the success of the developed software or application (Pavlov, 2014). But an engaging design, with easy interaction and simple system that make possible a greater productivity and user satisfaction, are not enough for the technologies thought for ASD. Pavlov (2014) has provided different indications on how building an UI for people with ASD. As the symptoms and their seriousness in people with ASD vary, the software should be customized. In general, to be disposable for people with ASD, UI should aim at: (a) simplicity, (b) possibility of customization, (c) ease of reading, (d) assistance, (e) possibility to save document for subsequent access, (f) use of intermediaries and assistants.

Language interaction and visual experience prove to be fundamental: images (drawings, pictures or other images) should be clear, easy to understand and located on the left side. Beside the image, on the right side, words should be inserted, also easy to understand (possibly written in Arial, dimension 14) and related to the image. The sentences should be short (max 15 words), the documents less than 20 pages. More and specific indications are reported in 'Make it Simple: European Guidelines for the Production of Easy- to-Read Information for People with Learning Disability for authors, editors, information providers, translators and other interested persons' report (Freyhoff et al., 1998). To these indications, it is possible to add some principles:

1. **Clearness, coherence, simplicity**: the design should be clear, coherent and simple. The content should be appropriate, well labeled, grouped according to the topics. The text field should be separated from the content, images as text background should be avoid and clear calls to action should to used. Web surfing, ideal if it follows the clustering principle, is helped by an architecture and a hierarchy.
2. **Avoiding ambiguity**: It is necessary to use a literal and simple language without the metaphors, proverbs or expressions.
3. **Colours**: keeping in mind colour, avoiding strong contrasts, reducing brightness and luminance of colours, using natural and soft colours.
4. **Avoiding sudden interactions**: such as pop-up.
5. **Control**: Allowing a greater control on execution time, on the interaction with the contents, using customization (e.g. font size, contrast)
6. **Flow**: designing pages according to a flow idea, considering the accessibility not of single page, but of the entire digital path; simplifying the flows and password management; adding feedback and reinforcement (Rusakova, 2021).

3.2 Treatment of Phobias

ASD is characterized by the presence of anxiety and common phobias. In a meta-analysis on anxiety disorders in children and young adults with ASD under 18 years, 39,6% of them presents a comorbidity with anxiety disorder, in particular specific phobia (29,8%), obsessive-compulsive disorder (17,4%) and social anxiety disorder (16,6%) (van Stenseel, Zegers, & Bögels, 2016). In children with autism 92 different fears were observed, including the most common, such as fear of animals or of the darkness, and other less common, such as fear of mechanical objects (Mayes et al., 2013). Anxiety can be managed learning some strategies of coping that enable to obtain some improvement concerning scholastic attendance and performance, social participation and preparation for a future employment (Drahota, Wood, Sze & Van Dike, 2011). The best intervention for the treatment of specific fears and phobias is the exposure (Craske, Treanor, Conway, Zbozinek & Vervliet, 2014). However, the production and control of imaginary scenes, necessary also for imaginative desensitization, results difficult for people with ASD. Furthermore, to understand which thoughts are stimulated by the exposure or to evaluate the intensity of the reaction to the phobic stimulus for the therapists is impossible (Maskey, Lowry, Rodgers, McConachie & Parr, 2014).

Maskey et al. (2014) tried to investigate how to adapt traditional approaches to treating specific phobias/fears through the use of Virtual Reality Environment (VRE) to increase accessibility for people In their study, 9 verbally fluent children, between 7 and 13 years, have been subjected to a treatment with VR. Each of the children had a phobia and each of them was subjected to a personalized treatment, using the exposure therapy technic. For the treatment, the 'Blue Room' immersive technic was used, an immersive VRE inside which the participants could move in the room and see the scenarios with a 360° vision. Conducted by a cognitive-behavioral psychologist, the study consisted of 4 sessions of 20-30 minutes that exposed the child to a phobic stimulus in this immersive VRE. 8 children out of 9 were able to face the phobic stimulus, 4 of them overcame the phobia. The results have been maintained for 12-16 months after the treatment. Moreover, the involved families had the possibility to learn coaching technic used in real-life situations (e.g. shopping or taking the bus). This contributed to the generalization of the ability to manage the child anxiety, thereby improving in other daily situations.

Another study (Maskey et al., 2019) confirmed the results obtained by Maskey et al. (2014). Based on the assumption of the efficacy of Cognitive-Behavioral Treatment (CBT) and VR in facilitating exposure to the phobic stimulus, the authors argued the importance of evaluating the combination of a VRE environment with CBT provided by the therapist to reduce anxiety. The study involved a sample of 32 verbally fluent young people (8-14 years) with ASD and with a specific phobia. Four treatment sessions were made. Each of the sessions consisted in two intervention of 20 minutes conducted by an expert in ASD and/or CBT. Comparing to the children of the control group, an improvement of phobia management and in daily activities in a third of the people undergoing the CBT with the support of the 'Blue Room' VRE has shown. The group control received the treatment later obtaining similar results to the children of the immediate treatment group (Maskey et al., 2019).

Thanks to the employment of VR is possible to recreate environments provoking anxiety in the participants but with several advantages. For example, the therapist working with the autistic child manage the interaction while the child is quiet and attentive. This allows the maintenance of low level of anxiety. The child can use visual stairs to convey their inner state, reducing language to a minimum, and exposing himself to the anxiety-inducing agent according to his pace. The scene can be repeated once or more times and consistently, giving to the child the sensation of control because there will be nothing unexpected. Furthermore, this does not need a verbal exchange, unpleasant for the child. The therapist shares the same scenario, and he can address the participant towards learning strategies of positive coping. Finally, another advantage is provided by the intrinsic characteristics of the tools used: the ATs motivate the child more, are adequate for the reinforcement of learning, can be developed by adapting them to people's needs (e.g. management of auditive and visual stimulus). The size of the sample, the potential placebo effect of the self-assessment, the potential impartiality of the parents reporting the updates on participants' functioning are the limits of this study. Moreover, anxiety levels should be considered as they may affect treatment. Finally, a research able to study the impact of this treatment on the various anxiety disorder subtypes is desirable (Maskey et al., 2014).

3.2.1 Virtual Reality

The VR is a tool that recreate a scenario providing a sensorial input and interacting with the user. It can be used through system that project the scenarios in a room, as in Maskey's study, in which the 'Blue

Room' is used; or through wearable devices, for example, the Head Mounted Displays (HMDs) or an enable tracking display (Cheng, Huang & Yang, 2015).

Although conducted on a restricted sample of children with ASD, a study carried out by Halabi et al. (2017) allows to deduce different useful indications to understand which tools should be developed and used to support VR. In particular, using adequate the user can interact in a virtual environment through a guiding display based on what the user sees.

Effective in the field of intervention with VR are the speech recognition applications. Involving the use of a wearable microphone, the answers given by user to the virtual characters of the virtual scenario are recognized; gesture recognition applications can also facilitate the identification of non-verbal communicative answers. The use of customized avatars is extremely useful because each of them contributes to the scenario. In the Halabi's study (2017), a VR scenario recreates a classroom environment and greeting activity. The teacher-avatar is similar in the appearance to a scholastic role model of the student with autism and it undertakes actions similar to those of the reality. So the replicability of the real conversational skills in daily life has allowed. The scenarios should be recreated in specific and customized environment, allowing to the student to browse in the virtual environment (Halabi et al., 2017).

3.3 Social Interactions

ATs have also been developed to overcomes social limitations of people with ASD. Indeed, people with autism score lower than people without ASD in autonomous assessments involving subdomains that typically refer to social cognition: social perception, emotion recognition, and theory of mind (Morrison et al., 2019).

Cheng et al. (2015) evaluated the impact of using immersive equipment in learning skills related to non-verbal communication and social cognition in subjects with ASD. Using HMDs within VRE, a 3D social comprehension system (3D-SU) was developed. The system interacted with HMD technology to promote the social comprehension in 3 young people aged between 10 and 13 with ASD. While browsing in the VRE, the users could isolate themselves or interact with other virtual objects and humans. The selected scenarios were those often observed by the participants, in particular the classroom and the bus stop. The system read some questions and brought back some auditive and visual reinforcement, adopting useful approaches to develop behaviors and maintain them over time, such as modelling, promotion, reinforcement and guide. The scenes seen by the participants were projected on a big scream. In this way, teachers and researchers could know what the participants were watching. This study showed how the comprehension and social skills can be improved if virtual situations with realism features are used. The virtual environment, in fact, gives the possibility to explore and involve with social events. The 3D animations and scenarios have motived the learning of target behaviors, they have helped the participants to perform behaviors appropriate to the real life context, using competences learned during the intervention. In addition, the study confirmed the results already obtained by Cheng, Chiang, Ye & Cheng (2010). According Cheng et al. (2010), the immersive VRE enables people with difficulties to improve their learning skills of social abilities, also thanks to the visual assistance of mutual interaction and repeated practice. However, some limitations should be emphasized. In particular, the restricted number of participants, their high functioning and the absence of evaluation of the general use of the learnt behaviors, necessitating the collection of new evidence (Cheng et al., 2015).

Another extremely useful AT is the Augmented Reality (AR). Considering the necessity of a research based on more rigorous methodologies and a more representative sample, Berenguer, Baixauli, Gomez,

Andrés & De Stasio (2020) presented a review on the use of AR technology. The review showed how several abilities, including social interaction, verbal and non-verbal social communication, facial expression recognition, improve thanks to AR. The cognitive-behavioral intervention for children and teenagers with ASD can benefit from the support of this technology.

Whereas the fictional game is the basis of development of different skills, Bai, Blackwell & Coulouris (2015) examined the use of AR in gaming. The starting point was to understand if children with ASD simply imitate the modeled behaviors or if they form original play intentions. The study was a single-subject design with multiple probes. It was conducted on 12 participants with ASD between 4 and 7 years. The researchers claimed that the AR may be considered as a support to mental representation because the combination of reality and virtual contents allows a better understanding of the surrounding environment. Aided by visual representation, children can manipulate imaginary scenarios and undertake actions in non-real situations. In particular, all children easily adapted themselves to the AR mirrored display, except a child with selective mutism that took more time. Two children were not able to perform episodes game theme-based on the AR system due to severe language and attention impairment. For this reason they were excluded from the main results. The AR proved to be useful to increase the regularity and duration of pretend play (although the percentage of time in constructive games was higher in the non-AR condition). The participants broadened their interests and showed more consistent ideas of game. Moreover, the parents, in the majority of cases, rated their children as improving in the AR condition. However, this study does not test the potential effect of generalization; in addiction, the researchers examined the AR only for solitary pretend play, while it may be useful to investigate the development of pretend play within a social context. Finally, it must be reported that the majority of the participants were male, resulting in a gender prejudice (Bai et al., 2015).

Di Nuovo, Conti, Trubia, Buono & Di Nuovo (2018) promoted a study that investigates how to improve RMI (Robot-Mediated Intervention) via an automatic personalization of the robot behavior. The study integrates the use of robot and the TEACCH approach (Treatment and Education of Autism and related Communication Handicapped Children) in a standard treatment, focusing the attention on the use of eye contact as a method to understand the attention at the interaction level. The involved participants were 6 children with ASD and ID (Intellectual Disability). The ability of the child to direct his gaze to the robots, seen as interaction partner, was considered a method to evaluate the involvement level in the therapy. First, a human therapist carried out a baseline study to preliminary evaluate the ability of the child to perform some imitation tasks. Then, 3 tasks that the children were not able to do were proposed, for a total of 3 sessions each of 6-8 minutes (each session for a task) during every meeting, for a total of 14 meetings in a month. Thanks to the extraction of frames from the videos recorded during the sessions of therapy, the moments of ‘attention’ and of ‘distraction’ were labeled. In the study, several approaches were used including the VJ (The Viola-Jones Framework for Face Detection), the T-CNN (Faster Convolution Neural Networks with Region Proposal) and the MTCNN (Multitask Cascated Convolution Networks for Face Detention and Landmark Estimation) (Di Nuovo et al., 2018). The children reacted differently to the various approaches. The highest precision was reached through the MTCNN approach, although there is the necessity to examine in depth the results due to the poor performance of some children (Di Nuovo et al., 2018). The results showed that even today the study on robotic interventions is severely limited by the equipment, by the low resolution, by the need to improve the algorithms and to support them with adequate hardware.

Before 2010, the majority of the studies in this field examined the interest and the sympathy that the individuals with ASD may feel towards a robot or its features. Instead, after 2010 the studies have focused more on the efficiency of the intervention with robots for people with ASD. According to these studies, the RMI does not seem to be capable to teach and modify behaviors, even though it is able to modify the participants' target behaviors during or after the RMI. Few experimental studies based on robot-mediated intervention satisfy clinical standard (Begum, Serna & Yanco, 2016). Thus, it is not possible to provide a totally positive opinion on the efficiency of the intervention that involves the use of robots for teaching new abilities or for removing maladaptive behaviors.

3.3.1 Augmented Reality

Besides the VR, also the study with AR has given encouraging results providing non-traditional learning environment (Cunha, Brandão, Vasconcelos, Soares & Carvalho, 2016; Lumbreras, Méndez-Trejo, & Sanluis-Ramírez, 2018). In the AR technology, virtual and real elements are merged, creating an interactive environment. Computer-generated artificial information overlaps with the reality (Craig, 2013).

Promising results have been obtained: (a) using children favorite characters and (b) combining various multimedia contents, especially video and audio. Indeed, starting from the studies of Rosset et al. (2008) and Mokashi, Yarosh & Abowd (2013), Abou El-Seoud, Halabi & Geroimenko (2019) showed the usefulness of the employment of virtual assistants. They should have the feature of a character choose by child (possibly alone) among his favorite cartoons, comics or computer games. In their research, the authors used a marker employing a camera and a visual marker capable of generating multimedia contents, with the possibility to use singularly or to combine 3D animation, audio, images and video. In particular, the merging of the video in the real world and the employment of sound-only files attached to markers implicating the increase of the audio of objects and of real world environment showed to be effective.

3.4 Job Performance and Self-Efficacy

The AT can be used in a perspective of inclusion in the labor market, taking into account that less than 1 out of 5 people with disability works receiving, in the 70% of cases, a minimum salary or no compensation. The rate of employment decreases to 10% for people with ASD under 20 years. Therefore disability causes impoverishment and marginality. Moreover, it has an impact on exclusion from the labor market, self-fulfillment and loss of earnings (Waisman-Nitzan, Schreuer, Gal, 2020).

The VR may enable to compensate some of the major limitations encountered by a person with ASD and, in general, with disability. To overcome the job interview is the first limitations for the person with ASD. Especially in this field, the lack of social introduction abilities penalize autistic people (Strickland, Coles & Southern, 2013). In part the limitation is due to the poor support of services in obtaining a job (Gerhardt & Lainer, 2011). Furthermore, the training takes place on-the-job, and the number of hours used is unfavourable for the employers both in terms of direct (expenditure for the training) and indirect costs (loss of productivity) (Lattimore, Parsons & Reid, 2008). With VR, high-functioning young people can learn skills related to job interviews, such as verbal and non-verbal skills required for the interaction (eye contact, proper language) and social skills. Using VR and undergoing a training, autistic people can learn or improve those abilities useful for potential hiring. For example, high-functioning people with ASD can receive explicit instructions to recognize his own and others' state of mind, to be directed to repeat situations that presume several social skills, to learn how to behave inside artificial universe (Venturoli, 2016).

Smith et al. (2015) intend to find a method to overcome the job interview for high-functioning adolescents and adults with ASD. They published a report highlighting the results obtained through the implementation of various interventions with regards to the employment of people with disorders. The programme simulated job interviews and it was based on repetition and hierarchic learning. The use of this programme, called Virtual Reality Job Interview Training (VR-JIT), was initially tested by the designers on adults with psychiatric disability and young adults with ASD. The study highlighted a clear improvement of the interview skills (Smith et al., 2014). So the researchers implemented another intervention direct to high-functioning young adults with ASD. The participants were 26 people with autism, between 18 and 31 years, actively seeking employment. Thanks to the VR-JIT application, the interns interacted with a virtual representative simulating an interview for the hiring in a department store. Using algorithms based on customized features and taking into account answers given by the intern, the human resources virtual representative created answers that simulated a job interview. After six months, the VR-JIT interns have been invited to participate to a follow-up investigation. It was completed by 23 of them. Participants' self-esteem and the previous rate of paid employment increased. Also, the probability to accept a job offer for a competitive position increased by 7,82%. This results were confirmed by Smith et al. (2017) through a study conducted on 79 individuals including people with ASD. After identifying the relevant contents for a successful job interview and highlighting goals for the performance of an interview, the virtual representative proposed various virtual interview with different level of difficulties. The post-test performances were evaluated after an interview with two professional actors. The results showed a correlation between repeated virtual interview and obtained job offers. In particular, to obtain a clear improvement is enough to complete a number of sessions from 3 to 5 in order. The limits of this study, recognized by the researchers themselves, are the conduction in a lab environment (therefore it would be necessary to evaluate the generalization of the competences), the restricted number of participants and the necessity that they needed a sixth grade reading level to use the VR-JIT (Smith et al., 2017).

The improvement of the competences acquired by people with disability in view of a real world interaction is potentially made possible by the implementation of interventions seeing the person and the robot interacting inside a virtual environment stimulating the learning (Warren et al., 2015). In this regard, Kumazaki et al. (2017) employed an android robot with human features and movements in order to allow a 3D learning experience. The authors also evaluated the effectiveness of the use of an android robot for the presentation to a job interview in the perspective of reinforcing self-esteem and reducing the levels of stress related to the need to interact with a human during the job interview. The participants were 15 young adults with ASD, between 18 and 25 years, actively seeking employment. The method to evaluate the stress, considered effective and not invasive, was the control of the level of the salivary cortisol compared to the control condition. The participants were randomly divided in two groups, the android robot-mediated group and the independent study group. On the first and fifth day, both for the baseline study and the post-test, a human confederate interview were proposed to both of the groups. During the three central days of the intervention, only the participants of the android robot-mediated group faced a fake job interview conducted by the android robot. Exposure to android robot-mediated interview procedures contributed to an improvement in self-esteem levels and confidence (although it did not reach the statistical minimum threshold) and a reduction in stress / anxiety indicators in young adults. These trends were assessed using a self-reporting questionnaire for self-esteem and tests on the salivary cortisol. However, the study has several limitations, including the small number of participants, low levels of symptoms of anxiety and medium cognitive skills in participants, a very short period of time.

3.4.1 Robot

Regarding the employment of robot for the RMI, the researchers consider the following indications fundamental:

1. **Humanoid form**: robots interacting with people with ASD should have a humanoid form, but they should be less detailed and complex than humans (Robins, Dautenhahn & Dubowski, 2006). This indication has been confirmed by Kumazaki et al. (2019). A study to evaluate interview training for people with autism involved 33 people with ASD (age, 17-35 years). According to the authors, greater is the feeling of humanity given by the robot lower is the motivation for interview training for people with ASD.
2. **Colours**: as already mentioned, the proper use of colours is fundamental: bright lights and contrasting colours may distract the child and undermine the robot effectiveness.
3. **Facial expressions**: robot facial expressions should be simple and not too realistic. Otherwise there is the risk to obtain a disturbing 'uncanny effect', according to which going beyond a certain threshold of anthropomorphism corresponds a curve of negative reactions (Reuten, van Dam & Naber, 2018).
4. **Dimension**: the dimension gives the possibility to the robot to have an involving and not threatening appearance. The size of a child for a robot is the most recommended. Indeed, besides facilitating skills, such as imitation, shared attention and role-playing game, this size could facilitate the generalization (Giullian et al, 2010).
5. **Movements**: according to Kumazaki et al. (2019), the motivation of the individuals with ASD may depend on the regulation of the degree of implementation and extension of autonomous action. As indicated by Scassellati et al. (2012), the levels of biological movement are extremely important: a robot with higher degrees of freedom of movement may show a range of different expressions, move the arm in manner more similar to a human, so reaching various goals of interaction.

4. DISCUSSION

This selective review has tried to outline an overview on the range of ATs that can be used in the intervention with people with ASD in order to improve different aspects of the life of these people and of their families. Indeed, an AT-based intervention take into account the needs of the people and of their families and of the professionals that work to improve the quality of their life. Furthermore, professionals can to act in a targeted and customized manner. The devices available to reach goals, also considering the accessibility, the cost, the timing, the individual characteristics are the best choice. The analyzed studies are broadly encouraging in claiming the validity of many tools. However, in some cases, some failures were reported and there were some intrinsic limitations to the studies themselves. For this reasons, the results can be extended to the whole autistic population. Concerning the use of the tablet, the examined studies did not lead to the conclusion that a very common equipment, such as an iPad, and for which hundreds of apps exist (also considering the prerequisites of the children, of the set objectives and cost), increases promptly the learning and the communication compared to other tools (also not technologic). However, it is not detrimental for the learning. In the light of this, Allen et al. (2016) focus their atten-

Table 1. Reviewed studies grouped according to the intervention area

Authors	Participants	Age	Intervention Area	AT	Results
O'Malley et al. (2014)	7	10 - 13	Academic Performance	App	Improvement of math skill: mixed results between baseline and intervention phases; moderated effects on independent activities.
Allen et al. (2016)	16	3 - 9	Academic Performance	App	No differences between iPad and illustrated book.
Cerga-Pashoja et al. (2019)	90	12 - 17	Academic Performance	App	More accurate answers in simplified texts compared to the original ones using AT.
Maskey et al. (2014)	9	7 – 13	Anxiety Disorder	VR	8/9 participants faced the phobic stimulus; 4 participants overcome the phobia.
Maskey et al. (2019)	32	8 – 14	Anxiety Disorder	VR	Statistically significant greater improvement on Target Behaviour ratings.
Bai et al. (2015)	12	4 – 7	Social Interaction	AR	Significantly higher frequency and duration of pretend play in AR condition; more constructive play in the non-AR condition.
Cheng et al. (2015)	3	10 – 13	Social Interaction	VR	Effective intervention system in improving the target behaviors.
Di Nuovo et al. (2018)	6	Non-specified	Social Interaction	Robot	Best result achieved with MTCNN approach (highest accuracy on the test set, 88,2%).
Smith et al. (2015)	26	18 - 31	Job Performance	VR	Increase in self-esteem and in the previous rate of paid employment.
Kumazaki et al. (2017)	15	18 - 25	Job Performance	Robot	Self-reported increases in confidence; reductions in biological indicators of stress/anxiety.

tion on the possibilities of the iPads to reduce the environmental stress related to social interactions. The saved cognitive resources could be allocate to learning by children with ASD.

The impact on academic skills should be examined, but also on the levels of involvement and the positive effects that these have on learning following the use of the iPad, including greater commitment, time dedicated to activity, reduction of behaviors of challenge. The selection of the tool should mainly be evaluated based on the person necessity and availability. There are also some interventions that are already more valid than others. The professionals should have the knowledge and experience in using the various tools to make the intervention effective. Considering the treatment of anxiety disorder through VR, it is crucial to be able to identify, as an example, the scenarios useful for the treatment of specific phobias using environments that replicate as much as possible the reality. Also, the person with ASD should have the possibility to face real-life situations and to train in a safe, protect and controlled environment (Maskey et al., 2014).The VR exposure has already many advantages at the level of time, cost, safety, need of less organization.

In addition, a better acceptance of the treatment by the person should be kept in mind, reducing the risk of drop-out (Wechsler, Kümpers & Mühlberger, 2019). Finally, it is necessary to consider that the VR gives the possibility of a control and flexibility that go beyond reality, also in terms of appropriate adaptations to the therapeutic considerations (Botella, Fernández-Álvarez, Guillén, García-Palacios & Baños, 2017). Also, the AR proved itself to be a very promising technology in the involvement of the participants and in the stimulation of specific cognitive activities as in the pretend play (Bai, Blackwell

& Coulouris, 2015). However, there is the risk to overcrowd the play areas with AR and non-AR objects and this leads to problems of usability. Also, the motivational merits of the innovations introduced by the AR technology could disappear with the time, thus, the intervention with the AR technology should remove the specific deficit from a mechanism level (Bai et al., 2015). The other technology frontier with a considerable potential to analyse in-depth is the RMI. The use of robot for assistive interventions is a widespread topic in literature, but the high cost, the not advanced equipment, the use of algorithms not yet improved and not supported by hardware makes this field to be implemented and improved (Di Nuovo et al., 2018). In this chapter, the use of robot for the improvement of the social interactions of the children with ASD was probed. In the clinical context of ASD, the robot may support and assist the therapist reducing the workload, for instance monitoring and registering the activities of the child. Probing the contribution provided by robots in supporting people with ASD in environment different from those merely educative or related to the period of development could be extremely profitable. The constant increase of the cases of ASD must necessarily be translated in an increase of the population with ASD growing into adulthood. According to Shattuck et al. (2012), the ID has an economic impact on families both at a direct level (e.g. treatment cost) and indirect (e.g. impossibility for the caregiver to go to work). Moreover, the ID is related to a risk of unemployment and poverty. Preventive intervention on teenagers and young adults, could prepare them to a potential entry to the labor market. Indeed, the use of robots has proved that it is possible to intervene to increase self-esteem and feeling of self-efficacy, as well as to reduce the anxiety related to the job interview (Kumazaki et al., 2017). Despite of the potentialities, there is still a long way to go. Today, few experimental studies based on the RMI satisfy the clinical standard. Thus, it is not possible to give fully positive opinion on the effectiveness of the interventions involving the use of robots for the teaching of new skills or the removal of maladaptive behaviors (Begum et al., 2016).

5. CONCLUSION

People with ASD can use a variety of AT that support them in varies areas of their life (Boucenna et al. 2014). The studies taken into account have examined the different types of technologies and environments that can be extensively used as part of the interventions aimed at people with ASD. The results of the studies were positive in the majority of cases. However, caution in their evaluation is fundamental. Indeed, the studies considered are characterized by limits concerning the choice of the sample, or the technology employed. In the first case: (a) most of the inquiries are carried out on high-functioning people with ASD, (b) in most of the studies the sample were small in size, indeed only one study involved a sample of more than 50 people, (c) due to the small size cannot be excluded the influence of variety of individual abilities and limits making the autistic population not very heterogeneous, (d) the analysed studies focused on how and if the individuals have generalized the results. In the second case, it is important to consider that the technologies available today for the therapeutic intervention are various (Chia, Anderson, McLean, 2018) . So, it is mandatory to know the disorder and the main treatment that can be implemented. But also, it is necessary to have an overview of the technologies, of how they can be used, and which are those that best fit the individual to undergo the treatment. Given the limitations, and the caution in interpreting the results derived from the available literature, first of all, it is fundamental to extend the activity of research. Later, evaluating which technologies is more adequate to reach the objectives set by the therapist with a view to the peculiarities of the individual is mandatory

(Zervogianni et al., 2020). Finally, the literature review brought out four types of ATs used for people with ASD that are needed to reach several rehabilitative goals to promote the skills and competences deficient in people with ASD. But the use of the various ATs by the professionals imposed a previous competence that makes valid the tools themselves (Groba et al., 2021). Indeed, those that work on the development and design of the ATs for the people with ASD cannot disregard the knowledge of the disorder: only looking at the specific needs of the individual and of the therapist it is possible to design and implement valid and effective tools.

6. FUTURE RESEARCH

In the lights of what mentioned above, it is good to look to the future and to the prospects provided by the tech world to the therapeutic intervention and, in this case, to the intervention with people with ASD. A first effort of research may be made to extend the ATs to a broader sample of population. It is necessary to consider the heterogeneity of the disorder, the comorbidities possibly present, the socio-educational context in which the interventions are distributed. Professional working for people with ASD should outline their availability in terms of (a) access and use of the equipment, (b) customization possibility, (c) involvement at various levels of the whole team and of the caregivers. Furthermore, the contribution of those who implement and support the technology by making it 'autism-friendly' and, above all, customizable should be taken into account. 'Autism-friendly' technology means a more accessible and usable technology for people with ASD in line with the principles of the Universal Design and of the User Experience Design. For instance, the implementation of a robotic device gives the possibility to involve the child in a proactive way. Also, it could adapt the levels of intervention individually based on the child (Esteban, 2017). It would be possible to use technologies of computational intelligence to favor adaptability and flexibility in view of the integration of robots of various therapeutical and rehabilitative context (Di Nuovo et al., 2018). A further consideration with a view to a future research is the one related to the side effects of the virtual technologies, e.g. the VR sickness. This problem is more relevant than ever. The research concerning it should be implemented, especially considering a population such as the autistic one, that strongly favors the technologies. The comprehension of the side effects could be useful to improve the technology and the experience of the users and to establish safety protocols (Szpak, Michalski, Saredakis, Chen & Loetscher, 2019).

REFERENCES

Alcorn, A. M., Ainger, E., Charisi, V., Mantinioti, S., Petrović, S., Schadenberg, B. R., Tavassoli, T., & Pellicano, E. (2019). Educators' Views on Using Humanoid Robots With Autistic Learners in Special Education Settings in England. *Frontiers in Robotics and AI*, *6*, 107. doi:10.3389/frobt.2019.00107 PMID:33501122

Allen, M. L., Hartley, C., & Cain, K. (2016). IPads and the Use of 'Apps' by Children with Autism Spectrum Disorder: Do They Promote Learning? *Frontiers in Phycology*, *7*, 1305. doi:10.3389/fpsyg.2016.01305 PMID:27625621

Bai, Z., Blackwell, A. F., & Coulouris, G. (2015). Using Augmented Reality to Elicit Pretend Play for Children with Autism. *IEEE Transactions on Visualization and Computer Graphics*, *21*(5), 598–610. doi:https://doi.org/10.1109/TVCG.2014.2385092

Begum, M., Serna, R. W., & Yanco, H. A. (2016). Are Robots Ready to Deliver Autism Interventions? *International Journal of Social Robotics*, *8*, 157–181.doi:https://doi.org/10.1007/s12369-016-0346-y

Berenguer, C., Baixauli, I., Gomez, S., Andrés, M. d., & De Stasio, S. (2020). Exploring the Impact of Augmented Reality in Children and Adolescents with Autism Spectrum Disorder: A Systematic Review. *International Journal of Environmental Research and Public Health*, *17*(17), 6143.doi: https://doi.org/10.3390/ijerph17176143

Botella, C., Fernández-Álvarez, J., Guillén, V., García-Palacios, A., & Baños, R. (2017). Recent Progress in Virtual Reality Exposure Therapy for Phobias: A Systematic Review. *Current Psychiatry Reports*, *19*, 42.doi:https://doi.org/10.1007/s11920-017-0788-4

Boucenna, S., Narzisi, A., Tilmont, E., Muratori, F., Pioggia, G., Cohen, D., & Chetouani, M. (2014). Interactive technologies for autistic children: A review. *Cognitive Computation*, *6*(4), 722–740. doi:10.100712559-014-9276-x

Carlier, S., Van der Paelt, S., Ongenae, F., De Backere, F., & De Turck, F. (2020). Empowering Children with ASD and Their Parents: Design of a Serious Game for Anxiety and Stress Reduction. *Sensors (Basel)*, *20*(4), 966. https://doi.org/10.3390/s20040966

Cerga-Pashoja, A., Gaete, J., Shishkova, A., & Jordanova, V. (2019). Improving Reading in Adolescents and Adults With High-Functioning Autism Through an Assistive Technology Tool: A Cross-Over Multinational Study. *Frontiers in Phychiatry, 10*, 546. doi:10.3389/fpsyt.2019.00546

Cheng, Y., Chiang, H.-C., Ye, J., & Cheng, L.-h. (2010). Enhancing empathy instruction using a collaborative virtual learning environment for children with autistic spectrum conditions. *Computer Education*, *55*(4), 1449–1458.doi:https://doi.org/10.1016/j.compedu.2010.06.008

Cheng, Y., Huang, C.-L., & Yang, C.-S. (2015). Using a 3D immersive virtual environment system to enhance social understanding and social skills for children with autism spectrum disorders. *Focus on Autism and Other Development Disabilities, 30*, 4. doi:10.1177/1088357615583473

Chia, G. L. C., Anderson, A., & McLean, L. A. (2018). Use of Technology to Support Self-Management in Individuals with Autism: Systematic Review. *Review Journal of Autism and Developmental Disorders*, *5*(2), 142–155.https://doi.org/10.1007/s40489-018-0129-5

Craig, A. B. (2013). *Understanding Augmented Reality: Concepts and Applications*. Morgan Kaufmann Publishers.

Craske, M. G., Treanor, M., Conway, C. C., Zbozinek, T., & Vervliet, B. (2014). Maximizing exposure therapy: An inhibitory learning approach. *Behaviour Research and Therapy*, *58*, 10–23. https://doi.org/10.1016/j.brat.2014.04.006

Cunha, P., Brandão, J., Vasconcelos, J., Soares, F., & Carvalho, V. (2016). Augmented reality for cognitive and social skills improvement in children with ASD. In 13th International Con- ference on Remote Engineering and Virtual Instrumentation (REV). IEEE. https://doi.org/10.1109/REV.2016.7444495.

Darejeh, A., & Singh, D. (2013). A review on user interface design principles to increase software usability for users with less computer literacy. *Journal of Computational Science*, *9*(11), 1443–1450. doi:https://doi.org/10.3844/jcssp.2013.1443.1450

Di Nuovo, A., Conti, D., Trubia, G., Buono, S., & Di Nuovo, S. (2018). Deep Learning Systems for Estimating Visual Attention in Robot-Assisted Therapy of Children with Autism and Intellectual Disability. *Robotics*, *7*(2), 25.doi:https://doi.org/10.3390/robotics7020025

Di Pietro, J., Kelemen, A., Liang, Y., & Sik-Lanyi, C. (2019). Computer- and Robot-Assisted Therapies to Aid Social and Intellectual Functioning of Children with Autism Spectrum Disorder. *Medicina (Kaunas, Lithuania)*, *55*(8), 440. https://doi.org/10.3390/medicina55080440

Drahota, A., Wood, J. J., Sze, K. M., & Van Dyke, M. (2011). Effects of cognitive behavioral therapy on daily living skills in children with high-functioning autism and concurrent anxiety disorders. *Journal of Autism and Developmental Disorders*, *41*(3), 257–265.doi:https://doi.org/10.1007/s10803-010-1037-4

El-Seoud, S. A., Halabi, O., & Geroimenko, V. (2019). Assisting Individuals with Autism and Cognitive Disorders: An Augmented Reality-Based Framework. *International Journal of Online Biomedical Engineering*, *15*(04), 28.doi:http://dx.doi.org/10.3991/ijoe.v15i04.9835

Esteban, P. B. (2017). How to Build a Supervised Autonomous System for Robot-Enhanced Therapy for Children with Autism Spectrum Disorder. *Paladyn: Journal of Behavioral Robotics*, *8*(1), 18–38. doi:https://doi.org/10.1515/pjbr-2017-0002

Flewitt, R., Kucirkova, N., & Messer, D. (2014). Touching the virtual, touching the real: iPads and enabling literacy for students experiencing disability. *Australian Journal of Language and Literacy*, *37*(2), 107–116.

Frauenberger, C., Good, J., Alcorn, A., & Pain, H. (2012). Supporting the design contributions of children with autism spectrum conditions. In IIDC '12: Proceedings of the 11th International Conference on Interaction Design and Children. Association for Computing Machinery. https://doi.org/10.1145/2307096.2307112.

Freyhoff, G., Hess, G., Kerr, L., Menzel, E., Tronbacke, B., & Van Der Veken, K. (1998). *Make it Simple - European Guidelines for the Production of Easy-to-Read Informationfor People with Learning Disability for authors, editors, information providers,translators and other interested persons.* Brussels: ILSMH European Association. Retrieved from https://moodle2.units.it/pluginfile.php/303860/mod_resource/content/1/ILSMH%201998%20or%20Freyhoff%20Make%20it%20simple.pdf

Frith, U. (1989). *Autism: Explaining the Enigma*. Blackwell Publishing.

Gerhardt, P. F., & Lainer, I. (2011). Addressing the Needs of Adolescents and Adults with Autism: A Crisis on the Horizon. *Journal of Contemporary Psychotherapy*, *41*, 37–45. doi:10.100710879-010-9160-2

Giullian, N., Ricks, D., Atherton, A., Colton, M., Goodrich, M., & Brinton, B. (2010). Detailed Requirements for Robots in Autism Therapy. In *International Conference on Systems, Man and Cybernetics* (pp. 2595-2602). Istanbul: IEEE. doi:10.1109/ICSMC.2010.5641908

Grandgeorge, M., & Masataka, N. (2016). Atypical Color Preference in Children with Autism Spectrum Disorder. *Frontiers in Psychology, 7*. doi:10.3389/fpsyg.2016.01976

Groba, B., Nieto-Riveiro, L., Canosa, N., Concheiro-Moscoso, P., Miranda-Duro, M., & Pereira, J. (2021). Stakeholder Perspectives to Support Graphical User Interface Design for Children with Autism Spectrum Disorder: A Qualitative Study. *International Journal of Environmental Research and Public Health, 18*(9), 4631. https://doi.org/10.3390/ijerph18094631

Halabi, O., El-Seoud, S. A., Alja'am, J. M., Alpona, H., Al-Hemadi, M., & Al-Hassan, D. (2017). Design of Immersive Virtual Reality System to Improve Communication Skills in Individuals with Autism. *International Jouranl of Emerging Technologies in Learning, 12*(5), 50. doi:10.3991/ijet.v12i05.6766

Higashida, N. (2013). *Jump: The Inner Voice of a Theirteen-Year-Old Boy with Autism.* New York: Penguin Random House.

IDEA. (n.d.). https://sites.ed.gov/idea/statute-chapter-33/subchapter-i/1401

Kumazaki, H., Muramatsu, T., Yoshikawa, Y., Matsumoto, Y., Miyao, M., Ishiguro, H., ... Kikuchi, M. (2019). How the Realism of Robot Is Needed for Individuals With Autism Spectrum Disorders in an Interview Setting. *Frontiers in Psychiatry, 10*, 486.doi:https://doi.org/10.3389/fpsyt.2019.00486

Kumazaki, H., Warren, Z., Corbett, B. A., Yoshikawa, Y., Matsumoto, Y., Higashida, H., ... Kikuchi, M. (2017). Android Robot-Mediated Mock Job Interview Sessions for Young Adults with Autism Spectrum Disorder: A Pilot Study. *Frontiers in Psychiatry, 8*, 169.doi:https://doi.org/10.3389/fpsyt.2017.00169

Lattimore, L. P., Parsons, M. B., & Reid, D. H. (2008). Simulation Training of Community Job Skills for Adults with Autism: A Further Analysis. *Behavior Analysis in Practice, 1*, 24–29.doi:https://doi.org/10.1007/BF03391717

Loomes, R., Hull, L., & Mandy, W. (2017). What Is the Male-to-Female Ratio in Autism Spectrum Disorder? A Systematic Review and Meta-Analysis. *Journal of the American Academy of Child and Adolescent Psychiatry, 56*(6), 466–474. https://doi.org/10.1016/j.jaac.2017.03.013

Lorah, E. R., Parnell, A., Schaefer Whitby, P., & Hantula, D. (2015). A systematic review of tablet computers and portable media players as speech generating devices for individuals with autism spectrum disorder. *Journal of Autism and Developmental Disorders, 45*(12), 3792–3804. doi:10.100710803-014-2314-4

Lumbreras, M. A., Méndez-Trejo, M. d., & Sanluis-Ramírez, A. (2018). Aura: Augmented Reality in Mobile Devices for the Learning of Children With ASD – Augmented Reality in the Learning of Children With Autism. In *Augmented Reality for Enhanced Learning Environments* (pp. 142–169). IGI Global. doi:10.4018/978-1-5225-5243-7.ch006

LuxAI. (n.d.). https://luxai.com/blog/robot-for-autism-hardware-design/

Maenner, M. J., Yeargin-Allsopp, M., Van Naarden Braun, K., Christensen, D. L., & Schieve, L. A. (2016). Development of a Machine Learning Algorithm for the Surveillance of Autism Spectrum Disorder. *PLoS One*, *11*(12), e0168224. doi:10.1371/journal.pone.0168224

Maskey, M., Lowry, J., Rodgers, J., McConachie, H., & Parr, J. R. (2014). Reducing specific phobia/fear in young people with autism spectrum disorders (ASDs) through a virtual reality environment intervention. *PLoS One*, *9*(7).https://doi.org/10.1371/journal.pone.0100374

Maskey, M., Rodgers, J., Grahame, V., Glod, M., Honey, E., Kinnear, J., ... Parr, J. R. (2019). A Randomised Controlled Feasibility Trial of Immersive Virtual Reality Treatment with Cognitive Behaviour Therapy for Specific Phobias in Young People with Autism Spectrum Disorder. *Journal of Autism and Developmental Disorders*, *49*(5), 1912–1927.doi:https://doi.org/10.1007/s10803-018-3861-x

Mayes, S. D., Calhoun, S. L., Aggarwal, R., Baker, C., Mathapati, S., Molitoris, S., & Mayes, R. D. (2013). Unusual fears in children with autism. *Research in Autism Spectrum Disorders*, *7*, 151–158. doi:https://doi.org/10.1016/j.rasd.2012.08.002

Mokashi, S., Yarosh, S., & Abowd, G. D. (2013). Exploration of videochat for children with autism. In IIDC '13: Proceedings of the 12th International Conference on Interaction Design and Children. Association for Computing Machinery. https://doi.org/10.1145/2485760.2485839.

Morrison, K. E., Pinkham, A. E., Kelsven, S., Ludwig, K., Penn, D. L., & Sasson, N. J. (2019). Psychometric Evaluation of Social Cognitive Measures for Adults with Autism. *Autism Research: Official Journal of the International Society for Autism Research, 12*(5), 766–778. doi:10.1002/aur.2084

O'Connor, K. (2012). Auditory processing in autism spectrum disorder: a review. *Elsevier, 36*, 836-854. doi:10.1016/j.neubiorev.2011.11.008

O'Malley, P., Lewis, M. E., Donehower, C., & Stone, D. (2014). Effectiveness of Using iPads to Increase Academic Task Completion by Students with Autism. *Universal Journal of Educational Research*, *2*(1), 90–97. doi:10.13189/ujer.2014.020111

Pavlov, N. (2014). User interface for people with autism spectrum disorders. *Journal of Software Engineering and Applications*, *7*(2), 7. doi:10.4236/jsea.2014.72014

Reuten, A., van Dam, M., & Naber, M. (2018). Pupillary Responses to Robotic and Human Emotions: The Uncanny Valley and Media Equation Confirmed. *Frontiers in Psychology*, *9*, 774. https://doi.org/10.3389/fpsyg.2018.00774

Robins, B., Dautenhahn, K., & Dubowski, J. (2006). Does appearance matter in the interaction of children with autism with a humanoid robot? *Interaction Studies: Social Behaviour and Communication in Biological and Artificial Systems*, *7*(3), 479–512.doi:https://doi.org/10.1075/is.7.3.16rob

Rosello, B., Berenguer, C., Baixauli, I., Colomer, C., & Miranda, A. (2018). ADHD symptoms and learning behaviors in children with ASD without intellectual disability. A mediation analysis of executive functions. *PLoS One*, *13*(11).doi: https://doi.org/10.1371/journal.pone.0207286

Rosset, D. B., Rondan, C., Da Fonseca, D., Santos, A., Assouline, B., & Christine, D. (2008). Typical emotion processing for cartoon but not for real faces in children with autistic spectrum disorders. *Journal of Autism and Developmental Disorders*, *38*(5), 919–925.doi:https://doi.org/10.1007/s10803-007-0465-2

Rusakova, I. (2021). *Designing for the autistic community*. Retrieved from UX Collective: https://ux-design.cc/inclusive-design-guide-7-principles-of-designing-for-the-autistic-community-1e6dcd4bae85

Scassellati, B., Admoni, H., & Matarić, M. (2012). Robots for Use in Autism Research. *Annual Review of Biomedical Engineering*, *14*, 275–294. https://www.annualreviews.org/doi/abs/10.1146/annurev-bioeng-071811-150036

Shattuck, P. T., Roux, A. M., Hudson, L. E., Lounds Taylor, J., Maenner, M. J., & Trani, J.-F. (2012). Services for adults with an autism spectrum disorder. *Canadian Journal of Psychiatry*, *57*(5), 284–291. doi:10.1177/070674371205700503

Silberman, S. (2015). *NeuroTribes: The Legacy of Autism and the Future of Neurodiversity*. Avery Pub Group.

Smith, M. J., Fleming, M. F., Wright, M. A., Losh, M., Boteler Humm, L., Olsen, D., & Bell, M. D. (2015). Brief report: Vocational outcomes for young adults with autism spectrum disorders at six months after virtual reality job interview training. *Journal of Autism and Developmental Disorders*, *45*(10), 3364–3369.doi:https://doi.org/10.1007/s10803-015-2470-1

Smith, M. J., Ginger, E. J., Wright, K., Wright, M. A., Lounds Taylor, J., Boteler Humm, L., ... Fleming, M. F. (2014). Virtual reality job interview training in adults with autism spectrum disorder. *Journal of Autism and Developmental Disorders*, *44*, 2450–2463.doi:https://doi.org/10.1007/s10803-014-2113-y

Smith, M. J., Smith, J. D., Fleming, M. F., Jordan, N., Brown, H. C., Humm, L., ... Bell, M. D. (2017). Mechanism of Action for Obtaining Job Offers With Virtual Reality Job Interview Training. *Psychiatric Services (Washington, D.C.)*, *68*(7), 747–750.doi:https://doi.org/10.1176/appi.ps.201600217

Stasolla, F., & Passaro, A. (2020). Enhancing Life Skills of Chidren and Adolescents with Autism Spectrum Disorders and Intellectual Disabilities through Technological Supports: A selective overview. In T. Wadhera & D. Kakkar (Eds.), *Interdisciplinary Approaches to Altering Neurodevelopmental Disorders* (pp. 41–62). IGI Global. doi:10.4018/978-1-7998-3069-6.ch004

Strickland, D. C., Coles, C. D., & Southern, L. B. (2013). JobTIPS: A transition to employment program for individuals with autism spectrum disorders. *Journal of Autism and Developmental Disorders*, *43*(10), 2472–2483.doi:https://doi.org/10.1007/s10803-013-1800-4

Szpak, A., Michalski, S. C., Saredakis, D., Chen, C. S., & Loetscher, T. (2019). Beyond Feeling Sick: The Visual and Cognitive Aftereffects of Virtual Reality. *IEEE Access: Practical Innovations, Open Solutions*, *7*, 130883–130892. doi:10.1109/ACCESS.2019.2940073

Takahashi, H., Nakahachi, T., Komatsu, S., Ogino, K., Iida, Y., & Kamio, Y. (2014). Hyperreactivity to weak acoustic stimuli and prolonged acoustic startle latency in children with autism spectrum disorders. *Molecular Autism*, *5*, 23.doi:https://doi.org/10.1186/2040-2392-5-23

UX Collective. (n.d.). https://uxdesign.cc/inclusive-design-guide-7-principles-of-designing-for-the-autistic-community-1e6dcd4bae85

van Stenseel, F. J., Zegers, V., & Bögels, S. M. (2016). Predictors of Treatment Effectiveness for Youth with ASD and Comorbid Anxiety Disorders: It all Depends on the Family? *Journal of Autism and Developmental Disorders*, *47*, 636–645. doi:10.100710803-016-2956-5

Venturoli, A. (2016). *Autismo e lavoro. Una breve rassegna bibliografica internazionale.* Rome: ISFOL. Retrieved from https://isfoloa.isfol.it/xmlui/handle/123456789/1268

Waisman-Nitzan, M., Schreuer, N., & Gal, E. (2020). Person, environment, and occupation characteristics: What predicts work performance of employees with autism? *Research in Autism Spectrum Disorders*, *78*, 101643. https://doi.org/10.1016/j.rasd.2020.101643

Warren, Z., Zheng, Z., Das, S., Young, E. M., Swanson, A., Weitlauf, A., & Sarkar, N. (2015). Brief Report: Development of a Robotic Intervention Platform for Young Children with ASD. *Journal of Autism and Developmental Disorders*, *45*, 3870–3876.doi:https://doi.org/10.1007/s10803-014-2334-0

Wechsler, T. F., Kümpers, F., & Mühlberger, A. (2019). Inferiority or Even Superiority of Virtual Reality Exposure Therapy in Phobias?—A Systematic Review and Quantitative Meta-Analysis on Randomized Controlled Trials Specifically Comparing the Efficacy of Virtual Reality Exposure to Gold Standard in vivo Exp. *Frontiers in Psychology*, *10*, 1758. doi:10.3389/fpsyg.2019.01758

Zervogianni, V., Fletcher-Watson, S., Herrera, G., Goodwin, M., Pérez-Fuster, P., Brosnan, M., & Grynszpan, O. (2020). A framework of evidence-based practice for digital support, co-developed with and for the autism community. *Autism*, *24*(6), 1411–1422. https://doi.org/10.1177/1362361319898331

ADDITIONAL READING

Bradley, R., & Newbutt, N. (2018). Autism and virtual reality head-mounted displays: A state of the art systematic review. *Journal of Enabling Technologies*, *12*(2), 101–113. Advance online publication. doi:10.1108/JET-01-2018-0004

Conti, D., Di Nuovo, S., Buono, S., Trubia, G., & Di Nuovo, A. (2015). Use of robotics to stimulate imitation in children with Autism Spectrum Disorder: A pilot study in a clinical setting. *Proceedings of the 24th IEEE International Symposium on Robot and Human Interactive Communication*, Kobe, Japan. 10.1109/ROMAN.2015.7333589

Kamaruzaman, M. F., Rani, N. M., Nor, H. M., & Azahari, M. H. H. (2016). Developing user interface design application for children with autism. *Procedia: Social and Behavioral Sciences*, *217*, 887–894. doi:10.1016/j.sbspro.2016.02.022

Kumazaki, H., Warren, Z., Muramatsu, T., Yoshikawa, Y., Matsumoto, Y., Miyao, M., Nakano, M., Mizushima, S., Wakita, Y., Ishiguro, H., Mimura, M., Minabe, Y., & Kikuchi, M. (2017). A pilot study for robot appearance preferences among high-functioning individuals with autism spectrum disorder: Implications for therapeutic use. *PLoS One*, *12*(10), e0186581. doi:10.1371/journal.pone.0186581 PMID:29028837

Park, M. J., Kim, D. J., Lee, U., Na, E. J., & Jeon, H. J. (2019). A Literature Overview of Virtual Reality (VR) in Treatment of Psychiatric Disorders: Recent Advances and Limitations. *Frontiers in Psychiatry*, *10*, 505. doi:10.3389/fpsyt.2019.00505 PMID:31379623

Riva G. (2020). Virtual Reality in Clinical Psychology. Reference Module in Neuroscience and Biobehavioral Psychology, B978-0-12-818697-8.00006-6. https://doi.org/ doi:10.1016/B978-0-12-818697-8.00006-6

Stasolla, F., Damiani, R., & Caffò, A. O. (2014). Promoting constructive engagement by two boys with autism spectrum disorders and high functioning through behavioral interventions. *Research in Autism Spectrum Disorders*, *8*(4), 376–380. doi:10.1016/j.rasd.2013.12.020

KEY TERMS AND DEFINITIONS

Academic Performance: Intellectual ability and skills of students reached in the academic context.

Assistive Technology: Any item, piece, equipment, or device used to increase, maintain, or improve functional capacities of persons with disabilities.

Autism Spectrum Disorder: Developmental disorder characterized by repetitive and characteristic pattern of behaviour and by persistent challenges with social communication and social interaction.

Job Performance: Sum total of a worker's execution of assigned tasks.

Phobia: Anxiety disorder characterized by abnormal and irrational fear of situations, activities, animal, people, or objects.

Social Interaction: Process of reciprocal stimulation or response between two or more people.

Social Skills: Any competence facilitating communication and interaction with others where social rules and relations are created, communicated, and managed in verbal and nonverbal ways.

User Experience Design: Process aiming at increasing the satisfaction and loyalty of the user improving the usability, ease of use and the interaction pleasure with the product.

Section 2
Special and Complex Needs

Chapter 4
Interactive Computer Play in the Pursuit of Gait Optimization for Children With Cerebral Palsy:
Home, Video Games, and Motivation

Manon Maitland Schladen
https://orcid.org/0000-0001-8783-6721
The Catholic University of America, USA

Yiannis Koumpouros
https://orcid.org/0000-0001-6912-5475
University of West Attica, Greece

Elena America Choong
U.S. Food and Drug Administration, USA

Justine Lee Belschner
Children's National Hospital, USA

ABSTRACT

Exercise therapy delivered through interactive computer play (ICP) has been shown to be effective for improving gross motor skills, and ultimately gait, in children with cerebral palsy (CP). This chapter provides an overview of CP, its impact on, gait and the current physical therapy (PT) standard of care. The history of the home exercise program (HEP) component of standard PT care is described, along with the potential for using ICP to improve HEP. ICP systems are surveyed, and their defining features discussed. The current therapeutic use of ICP is described and directions for further development to enhance therapeutic utility presented. A theoretical framework to support ICP implementation, self-determination theory (SDT), is outlined, and an example of its exploration in a pilot effort is provided. An example of healthcare system barriers to rapid uptake of ICP is presented along with alternative strategies for deployment and recommendations for further research.

DOI: 10.4018/978-1-7998-7430-0.ch004

INTRODUCTION

Physical (physio-) therapy (PT) improves gait in children with cerebral palsy (CP) as they mature (Franki et al., 2012). However, deciding which PT intervention will provide the greatest benefit to any individual child, at a given developmental stage, and in what dosage (frequency and intensity) is a multifactorial process and currently as much art as science. A limited ability to measure intervention inputs against outcomes, both immediate and longitudinal, figures prominently among the barriers to precision therapy.

Measurement implies instrumentation which, in PT, ranges from standardized and normed tests, for example, the Gross Motor Function Measure (GMFM, Alotaibi, Long, Kennedy, & Bavishi, 2014) Timed Up and Go (TUG, Carey, Martin, Combs-Miller, & Heathcock, 2016), and Six Minute Walk Test (6 MWT, Maher, Williams, & Olds, 2008) to electro-mechanical devices (for example, goniometers and hand-held dynamometers) to survey tools (for example, clinical questionnaires). Under the current standard system of care, measurement tools largely reside with the therapist in the clinic. The child with CP goes to the clinic to receive therapy, details of interventions are recorded, and progress over time is measured. The difficulties inherent in coordination of family and clinical schedules, and the inevitable vagaries of daily life result in unintended gaps in a child's therapy record and increase uncertainty of measurement. Home exercise programs (HEP) are a commonly prescribed adjunct to in-clinic therapy to enhance a child's progress toward therapy goals. However, families' reports of adherence are unverifiable, so the informative potential of HEP is not currently available to add power to intervention measurement and evaluation.

The research on HEP described in this chapter provides a window into the interpersonal dynamics and vulnerabilities experienced in families of children with CP. The home environment may have greater potential than the clinic to provide flexible blocks of time for a child to practice therapeutic exercise. In actual experience however, uncertainty about how exercises should be done, conflicting motivations among family members, and other factors have diffused the promise of HEP. Exercises performed during interactive computer play (ICP), using general market technologies such as the Nintendo Wii as well as custom-engineered systems, has been shown to be effective for improving gross motor outcomes. There is also preliminary evidence that use of ICP in HEP reduces parental apprehension and thus may increase the attractiveness of HEP and hence the feasibility of effectively extending therapy into the home. Use of computer technologies in HEP also provides the potential to leverage the information captured by these devices to more precisely measure therapy and use those measurements to improve therapeutic planning and outcomes.

Chapter Organization

The sections that follow provide background on CP and the current standard of care for gross motor therapy to improve gait. Research on the factors involved in generic HEP adherence are reviewed and a theoretical framework widely endorsed for understanding these factors, self-determination theory (SDT), is summarized. Subsequently, the application of ICP in HEP for children with CP is explored. ICP and conceptually-related systems are surveyed and their use in therapy for children with CP described. A section on measurement comes next. The state of knowledge relative to the effectiveness of ICP (with a strong focus on virtual reality (VR) systems) for improving physiological measures supportive of gait is presented. A discussion of dosage effect for therapy delivered via ICP follows. The potential for real-time monitoring of ICP-mediated exercise is explored and examples from research in progress presented.

A tentative adaptation of SDT to the evaluation of HEP/ICP is also explored. The chapter concludes with a survey of barriers to deployment of ICP in HEP as experienced in the health care system in the United States.

Recommendations for facilitation of HEP deployment and suggestions for further research follow. Authors bring perspectives from technology development and assessment, human factors research, patient/consumer-centered design, clinical service delivery and program implementation to the chapter.

BACKGROUND

Cerebral Palsy

Cerebral palsy (CP) is the clinical description of a constellation of developmental disorders that arise secondary to a perinatal, non-progressive neurologic injury (Novak et al., 2017). Such injuries align to a variety of diagnoses, for example, periventricular leukomalacia, peri/intraventricular hemorrhage, perinatal stroke, and migration abnormalities (Hadders-Algra, Boxum, Hielkema, & Hamer, 2017). While the neurologic injury itself is non-progressive, the musculoskeletal and neuromuscular impairments that result from it can progress and fluctuate throughout the lifespan. Occurring in an estimated 11 out of 1,000 births, (Oskoui, Coutinho, Dykeman, Jetté, & Pringsheim, 2013), CP is the most commonly identified neuromotor disorder affecting children worldwide.

Deficits in postural control and purposeful movement are common in the developing child with CP. Secondary to impairments in muscle tone and force production, altered mechanics in both the swing and stance phases of gait are also common and provide a key area of focus for physical therapy, PT (Wright & Palisano, 2017). The cascade of problems flowing from impaired gait place improvement and/or maintenance of lower extremity function high among the priorities for supporting a person with CP's wellbeing. Explained using the framework provided by the International Classification of Functioning, Disability and Health (ICF, World Health Organization, 2021), gait therapy is a priority in treating children with CP because difficulty in walking negatively impacts their activities and participation, engagement with peers, physical and emotional safety (Hutton, Colver, & Mackie, 2000), and hence, overall quality of life. Gait impairments, along with other neurological problems associated with CP, negatively impact social integration during childhood and on into the adult years (Williams, 2008).

Standard of Care for Gait Therapy in CP

Standard lower extremity PT care for children with CP typically focuses on exercise designed to promote strength and balance, and may also include serial casting to increase range of motion, as well as the use of orthotic devices to increase lower limb stability and function during walking and other mobility tasks (Moreau et al., 2016). Although there are no *definitive* guidelines for decision making around the optimal frequency, intensity, and duration of services (Bailes, Reder, & Burch, 2009), PT sessions at an outpatient clinic are a common addition to the routines of families of children with CP and visits frequently continue after the child with CP becomes an adult (O'Neil et al., 2006).

Episodic Care

PT service delivery is typically *episodic*, with episode length varying according to the needs of the individual child and the nature of the therapy of being delivered. Strengthening programs for children with CP, for example, have been found to range from five to 40 weeks; functional training, from six to eight weeks; treadmill training, from two to 12 weeks, and neurodevelopmental treatment, from six to 16 weeks (Dodd, Taylor, & Damiano, 2002).

Frequency and Intensity of PT Intervention

Like the length of an episode of care, the frequency with which PT services are delivered within a defined episode also varies. Children with CP have been reported to receive PT as often as four to five times per week, as well as in ranges varying from bi-weekly to every six months (Benedetto, Bailes, Pandya, Edwards, & Booker-Feister, 2017; Christiansen & Lange, 2008; Ustad, Sorsdahl, & Ljunggren, 2009). There is no widely accepted evidence for determining the length (maximum or minimum) of individual PT sessions (Benedetto et al., 2017). Decision making at the PT visit level is based on the therapist's experience, practice setting, and reimbursement constraints (Ulrich, Lloyd, Tiernan, Looper, & Angulo-Barroso, 2008). The American Physical Therapy Association (APTA) recommends that therapists consider the feasibility of intensity of services, types of outcome measures, and the inclusion of longitudinal follow up in structuring service delivery (Benedetto et al., 2017).

Skill Practice Outside of the Clinic

Part of standard PT care includes the practice of skills at home: a home exercise program (HEP). PT is usually implemented in an outpatient setting with additional practice prescribed for the child and family at least one hour per week at home (Novak, 2014; O'Neil et al., 2006). Because timing of therapy is critical to positive outcomes (Gannotti, 2017), and the logistics of clinic access and scheduling can be challenging, practicing prescribed exercises at home between PT visits provides an important failsafe for meeting therapy objectives.

The goal of a HEP is to assure (or increase) a child's *dosage* of individually tailored exercise therapy. Home practice also provides opportunities to train skills in their natural environment to promote task carryover to real-life situations and skill generalization (Steenbergen, van der Kamp, Verneau, Jongbloed-Pereboom, & Masters, 2010). The ability to successfully extend practice beyond clinic sessions opens options for titrating exercise frequency, duration, and intensity in a way not feasible in the usual clinic environment. Yet, adherence, doing one's exercises at home as often and in the form prescribed, has been a major barrier to successful HEP implementation (Lillo-Navarro et al., 2015; Lord, Rapley, Marcroft, Pearse, & Basu, 2018; Taylor, Dodd, McBurney, & Graham, 2004). Lack of confidence in how and to what degree a child adheres to his/her exercise regimen at home adds uncertainty to measurement of therapeutic effect and makes it difficult for the therapist to 1) interpret how well the prescribed exercise program is working for the child with CP and 2) interject appropriate course corrections if needed.

The Home Exercise Program (HEP)

Traditional, Technology-Naïve Model

The traditional, technology-naïve, model of HEP has involved a therapist prescribing exercises to target specific physical limitations which contribute to the functional limitations experienced by the child with CP (Lillo-Navarro et al., 2015; Lord et al., 2018; Medina-Mirapeix et al., 2017; Taylor et al., 2004). These exercises are typically hands-on, requiring the parent to manually stretch and manipulate the child's body according to the exercise protocol. Effective execution of an exercise depends on the therapist's skill in teaching and the reciprocal ability of the parent to learn how to perform the exercise correctly. Communication, support, and teaching style on the part of the therapist and the agility of the parent in coping with the challenge of serving as the therapist's proxy in the home, emerged as key themes in the traditional model. Further, managing a HEP competes with other life demands in the family of a child with CP. How and whether a HEP gets carried out is a function of the value the child with CP, his/her parents, and other family stakeholders place on it (Wigfield & Eccles, 2000). This valuation calculus, based on personal and situational factors continually in flux, is non-deliberate and subject to change over time.

A synthesis of the literature from January 1989 to May 2017 reporting on 17 parent-delivered therapy interventions (i.e., HEP) for children with CP identified three themes supporting HEP adherence: building trusting relationships, enabling parents to cope, and seeing the intervention as a priority (Lord et al., 2018). Lord and colleagues' further analysis yielded a model of three interrelated concepts: empowerment, motivation, and trust. This model describes a relational triad composed of therapist, parent, and child. Each person in the triad acts, at the core, in accordance with his/her internal motivation. Coping strategies also form part of the parent's internal schema. Each person influences the motivation of every other person in the triad. The therapist, uniquely, empowers the parent.

Consonant with Lord et al.'s model, physical activity (PA, of which home exercise is a type) researchers have also observed that a parent's personal feelings about PA influence his/her support of the PA of their child with motor delay (Columna, Prieto, Elias-Revolledo, & Haegele, 2020). Columna and colleagues also found the reciprocal, however: that children's motivation with respect to PA also influenced their parents' decision to support or not support activities. The importance of the therapist's contribution to parental empowerment and coping strength is echoed in other research identifying five effective coaching practices used by therapists to support parental HEP adherence: joint planning, observation, practice, reflection, and feedback (Gmmash, Effgen, Skubik-Peplaski, & Lane, 2021). In addition to these specific practices, Gmmash and colleagues also observed that the fit of therapeutic activities to the home environment, the degree to which the child found the activity enjoyable, and the parent's overall self-efficacy also promoted adherence.

Introduction of Computing Technology Into HEP

At least three of the 17 studies in Lord et al.'s 2018 synthesis involved use of interactive computer play (ICP) technology in carrying out the parent-controlled home therapy program. However, Lord et al. did not. and colleagues did not report any differences in experience across the parent-child-therapist triad based on the technology factor. A later study compared two models of CP HEP that did not involve computer-augmented interventions (Lillo-Navarro et al., 2015; Taylor et al., 2004) to the experience of a computerized, robotic and game-based home exercise platform for ankle therapy (Schladen et al.,

2020). The most pronounced difference in technology-mediated therapy versus therapy delivered hands-on by the parent, was the parent's high degree of confidence that the therapeutic maneuvers were being executed correctly. Schladen and colleagues observed that families had little concern about competent execution of exercise tasks when the system program ran the HEP routine and the system robot guided the child's alignment during exercise When interviewed, parents denied they felt any need to check in with the supervising therapist to monitor how the intervention was going.

The interaction among the motivations of parent and child modeled by Lord et al. (2018) was also observed in a comparison of the robotic ankle therapy HEP experience previously described with a parallel robotic home therapy targeting hand function in adults after stroke (Schladen, Koumpouros, & Lum, 2021). In both applications, technology removed most of the uncertainty surrounding how to carry out the exercise program. In both cases as well, decisional dyads were formed: parent-child and spouse-stroke survivor. Investigators observed that the positive intentions to adhere to therapy by one member of the dyad were frequently canceled by the negative intentions of the other and vice versa forming a pattern reminiscent of the reciprocating motivation described by Columna et al. (2020).

A Theoretical Framework for Adherence in HEP

Though Lord et al. do not explicitly cite their 2018 model in the context of Self-Determination Theory (SDT, Ryan & Deci, 2000), the focus on relations, motivation, and empowerment fit SDT well. Several other studies have used SDT as a framework for understanding what motivates adherence to therapeutic activity, both broadly conceived and in the specific contexts of CP and computer-interactive HEP (Biddiss, Chan-Viquez, Cheung, & King, 2021; D'Arrigo, Ziviani, Poulsen, Copley, & King, 2017; Sandlund, Dock, Häger, & Waterworth, 2012; Schladen, Koumpouros, et al., 2021; Tatla et al., 2013). Through a sub-theory of *organismic integration*, SDT identifies three intrinsic human needs that motivate all choices made: relatedness, autonomy, and competence. Motivation (always understood against the backdrop of the three intrinsic needs) comes in two basic flavors: intrinsic, where a pursuit is valued in and of itself; and extrinsic, where a pursuit is undertaken for some other cause. Autonomy, in the sense it is employed in SDT, refers to voluntariness, not independence. Voluntariness measures the degree one's actions are "self-determined," and self-determination maps to a motivational continuum from amotivation at one pole, through varying degrees of extrinsic motivation, to intrinsic motivation at the opposite pole.

As SDT has developed over time, four, increasingly more self-determined categories of extrinsic motivation have been defined: external regulation, introjected regulation, and integrated regulation. As individuals mature, they internalize social norms and increasingly adopt behaviors that they "want to do" versus "have to do." The various motivation constructs, or levels of self-determination, correspond to qualitatively different forms of behavioral regulation. Amotivation is the state in which the individual has yet to engage with a target activity such as performing therapeutic exercise at home. Metaphorically, the individual has not yet begun climbing the motivation *ladder*. See Figure 1. External regulation corresponds to the level where motivation is exclusively external and regulated by compliance, external rewards, and punishments. The next level is introjected regulation, where motivation is driven by self-control, efforts to protect one's ego, and internal rewards. Identified regulation comes next. It is the level where motivation is based on conscious values that are important to the individual. The final and highest level of extrinsic motivation is integrated regulation, where the desire to be self-aware guides an individual's behavior. Intrinsic motivation, where the activity is desired for its innately satisfying properties alone, lies at the summit of the extrinsic motivation hierarchy.

Figure 1. Self-Determination Theory motivation hierarchy

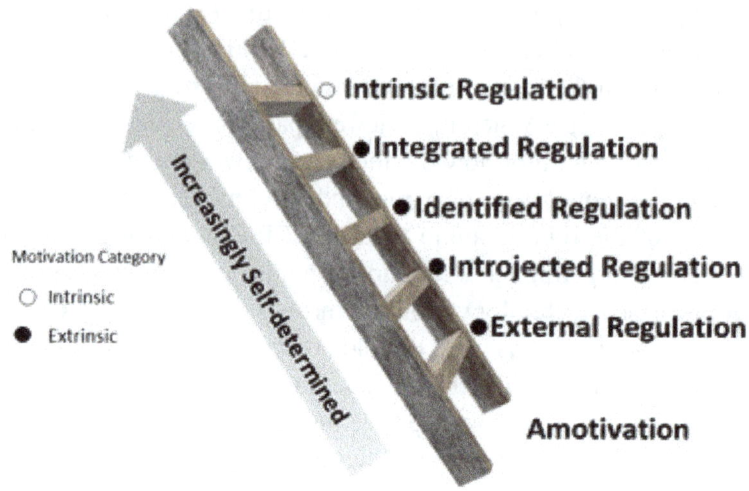

This developmental framework and the instruments created to measure where individuals fall along the motivational continuum for any given focus, may be useful for understanding the dynamics in the homes of children with CP in the context of effective HEP prescription, particularly in determining which children and families are likely to benefit from which technologies. SDT aligns with Gibson's original idea that technology *affordance* lies not so much in the technology as it does in the match between technology and user (Greeno, 1994).

INTERACTIVE, COMPUTER-BASED HEP FOR CHILDREN WITH CP

Challenges

As set forth in the Background section, three broad challenges lie on the path to helping children with CP maximize their gait potential as they grown. First, there is the logistical challenge of reliably connecting children with the therapy they need in a timely fashion. Second, and relatedly, is the uncertainty surrounding not only the match of intervention/exercise to child, but how often and with what intensity the child should perform the prescribed exercise. Computing technology, deployed in the home, provides a promising tactic for tackling both these challenges.

The third challenge arises from the HEP model itself, and is inherent in the model's defining strategy of increasing a child's therapeutic interactions by extending them beyond the clinic into the child's home. The personal and environmental dynamics of the home, outside of the clinical environment where the therapist has significant and immediate control, brings a host of new variables to bear on the objective of providing a child with CP the optimal therapeutic support. Computer-mediated home therapy systems inherit that challenge from the overarching model of HEP. A match between child and therapeutic technology does not guarantee a match between the technology and the home environment in all its complexity. This section first provides a descriptive overview and general taxonomy of interactive computing technology systems as they have been leveraged in exercise programs for children with

CP. Subsequently the subject of measurement is explored: 1) in the context of reported gross motor outcomes following interactive computer-based therapy, 2) in the nascent potential for process monitoring and course correction inherent in the technology, and 3) in the context of user-technology engagement.

Systems Overview and Taxonomy

At the highest level of abstraction, in a HEP that incorporates interactive computing technology, the child with CP interacts with a computer to practice maneuvers (exercises) that support improvement or maintenance of gait. *Interaction* is the key concept. Different researchers have parsed the computers-in-therapy landscape somewhat differently. The term *interactive computer play,* (ICP), appears to have been coined in a systematic review of the literature (January, 1995 to May, 2008) investigating the effects of interactive, computer-mediated therapy on children with sensorimotor impairments (Sandlund, McDonough, & Häger-Ross, 2009). Other researchers have carried the ICP construct forward (Biddiss et al., 2021; Fehlings, Switzer, Findlay, & Knights, 2013; Levac, Rivard, & Missiuna, 2012). Other terms to describe the technology have been *motion interactive* (Sandlund, Waterworth, & Hager, 2011) and *active video games* (AVG, Fehlings et al., 2013). *Video* and *game* are particularly important constructs in computer-based therapy.

The choice of the term AVG to describe computer-based therapy systems makes it clear that video is a defining characteristic of the genre. However, the criteria for *how* video is best used in therapy are not clear. Most noticeably, the terms, *video games* (VG) and *virtual reality* (VR) are not well differentiated in studies (Fehlings et al., 2013) and no standard definition is in broad use for describing therapeutic interventions. This blurring of the differences may be problematic if the active ingredients (see, Levac et al., 2012) of the two forms are not the same and result in different therapeutic outcomes.

The principal differentiator along the VR spectrum is the degree of immersion a system produces (Fehlings et al., 2013). At one end of the spectrum, VR takes the form of "an immersive and interactive three-dimensional (3D) computer experience occurring in real time" (Pimentel & Teixeira, 1995, as cited by Reid, 2002). Among the characteristics of this concept of VR is the use of cameras to capture and respond to the user's movements, providing a realistic sense of being inside the virtual environment (Reid, 2002). A more liberal description admitting more subjectivity, states that VR "typically refers to the use of interactive simulations created with computer hardware and software to present users with opportunities to engage in environments that appear to be and feel similar to real world objects and events." (Weiss, Rand, Katz, & Kizony, 2004, p. 1).

At the other end of the spectrum, a less exacting definition of VR plays down the importance of immersion and describes VR as "an interactive computer-based environmental system that presents artificially generated sensory information" (Laufer & Weiss, 2011). VR always falls under the ICP umbrella, the original definition of which was "any kind of computer game or virtual reality (VR) technology where the individual can interact and play with virtual objects in a computer-generated environment" (Sandlund et al., 2009, p. 173). An ICP system, however, does not always meet the criteria of strictly construed VR.

It has been hypothesized that the older the child with CP, the less interest he or she has in conventional therapy (Chiu, Ada, & Lee, 2018) whereas a survey of the activities of adolescents with CP revealed video gaming as their number one preference for recreation (Shikako-Thomas et al., 2015). Putting these two ideas together, one might conclude that therapy using AVG (inclusive of VR) might be a productive approach for engaging teens with CP with therapy. There is some evidence however that older children (adolescents in particular) have finely tuned expectations for the AVG they choose to play. Adolescents piloting a game-based, robotic ankle therapy system in their homes reported that the games younger children in the study received with enthusiasm did not engage them at all and one 13-year-old participant explicitly asked for immersive VR to bring the intervention game to a level she might find interesting (Schladen et al., 2020). Aligning with these qualitative findings, a meta-analysis of the effects of VR (without reference to its quality) on ambulation reported a significant negative linear relationship between the age of the child with CP and effect size: the younger the child, the greater the effect (Y. Chen, Fanchiang, & Howard, 2018).

Adolescent dissent aside, interactive computer-based systems have also been labeled *motivational interventions* (Tatla, Sauve, Jarus, Virji-Babul, & Holsti, 2014; Tatla et al., 2013) placing the focus on the potential they may have to motivate children and their families to engage in therapeutic activities. Engagement refers to both the state of being engaged and the process of becoming engaged, the latter of which may be facilitated though the SDT (Ryan & Deci, 2000) framework (D'Arrigo et al., 2017). Hypothetically, computer-interactive systems create an experience that is intrinsically motivating (fun) such that children will want to engage in the activities they provide (implicitly, the AVG) and therapy gets done as a by-product. The construct of game is as omnipresent as that of video in computer-based therapy systems targeting children with CP. Game play is closely associated with engagement (Deutsch & Westcott McCoy, 2017). Framing exercise in a (serious) game format may increase motivation (Lopes et al., 2018), promote adherence to therapy, and facilitate positive outcomes.

A potential difficulty of this approach is that it separates the game (intrinsically motivating, engaged for its own sake) from its purpose, therapy (extrinsically motivating, engaged as a means to maintaining or improving function) and introduces tension between the two. Children with CP playing games on a system designed to provide ankle therapy expressed frustration when the system "made them miss," by increasing resistance as part of prescribed strength training (Schladen et al., 2020). Considerable skill (and/or computing power) is needed to design a system that continually matches a child's abilities with the right amount of challenge to maintain a sense of *flow* (Csikszentmihalyi, 1990) in the activity, a criterion that is believed to be important to sustaining engagement (Boyle, Connolly, Hainey, & Boyle, 2012).

Commercial Off-the-Shelf Versus Engineered Systems

A core group of commercial off-the-shelf (COTS) AVG home systems have been used to provide gait therapy to children with CP. Three recent SR/meta-analyses (Y. Chen et al., 2018; Lopes et al., 2018; Ren & Wu, 2019) suggest that the Nintendo Wii platform, including the Wii Fit and Balance Board, is the most frequently used system. The now deprecated Microsoft Xbox Kinect and the Sony Playstation EyeToy (in various releases over time) follow in frequency of use. Computer-interactive virtual cycling systems, such as the ElotonSimCycle, also have a history of use in lower extremity home therapy for children with CP (C. L. Chen et al., 2013). More costly, custom-engineered systems have appeared in the literature less frequently, though a meta-analysis of 19 randomized controlled trials determined that custom-built systems had a stronger effect overall on therapy outcomes than did COTS systems (Y. Chen et al., 2018).

COTS AVG employed for gait therapy work by creating a scenario that induces the child to execute therapeutic maneuvers. In the most typical applications, there is no control on a child's movement beyond his or her own proprioceptive reactions. The home balance and mobility training described by Chiu et al. (2018) leveraging the Wii Fit balance board provides a good illustration. Children drove their onscreen avatar by shifting their weight on the balance board which detected their action and moved the character accordingly. In other games (Balance Bubble, Table Tilt, Perfect 10, and Super Hula Hoop) children, again, shifted their weight forward, backward, or sideways, to play the game. Children played a final set of games (Obstacle Course, Ultimate Obstacle Course, Ski Jump, and Basic) by marching in place, squatting, extending their legs, or stepping up and down, forward and backward, off the balance board. This type of exercise allows for measurement of therapeutic outcomes such as strength, balance, and walking speed, but not changes over the course of therapeutic game play that might provide just-in-time adjustment to optimize outcomes.

Custom-engineered systems, on the other hand, have greater facility to incorporate ancillary devices, such as robots, to guide practice of specific exercise maneuvers, for example, ankle dorsiflexion. The robot interacts directly with the child, reacting to how he or she is performing in the game and providing assistance if needed or resistance to increase challenge and the quality of exercise (Monfaredi et al., 2018). Such systems are currently being piloted in the homes of children with CP (Cleary et al., 2019) and are positioned to take advantage of innovations in ankle therapy robotics developed in non-gaming and adult-focused therapeutic contexts (for example, stroke. See Dong et al., 2021)

Measurement

Three main areas are of central interest in the measurement of computer-based HEP: 1) therapeutic outcomes, 2) the real-time therapeutic process, and 3) process engagement. Therapeutic outcomes (1) relate to the goals underlying the HEP prescribed for the child with CP. They track changes in gait parameters as measured by standard clinical instruments and are sampled at pre-determined intervals, for example, pre- and post-episode of engagement with a new HEP program. Measurement of the therapeutic process as it unfolds in real-time (2) is uniquely enabled through computer-based therapy. It can provide information, for example, on the child's level of effort during or across sessions. Measuring the child's engagement with the HEP (3) can be direct, through inquiry or survey, or indirect, inferred from real-time performance data.

Lower Extremity Outcomes of ICP/VR Therapy in Children with CP

For all the reviews and meta-analyses described in this section, research focuses on the computer-based intervention itself, neglecting, for the moment, whether there is an effect of being deployed in the home versus the clinic or lab. Several studies directly address changes in gross motor function as quantified using the Gross Motor Function Measure (GMFM), a standard clinical tool to evaluate change in specific aspects of lower extremity function over time or with intervention. Major constructs in the GMFM, such as activity and participation, have their basis in the ICF (Park, 2016). This linkage supports the importance of working to increase gross motor function in children with CP.

Evidence of positive outcomes for lower extremity, gross motor control or function, in children with CP following use of ICP in therapy was beginning to emerge as early as 2012 (Fehlings et al., 2013).. Based on analysis of 9 studies (114 children with CP) published in English prior to December, 2012, Fehlings and colleagues reported that there was American Academy of Neurology (Gronseth et al., 2017) level B (probable) evidence for ICP interventions to improve gross motor outcomes.

Five years later, a systematic review of randomized controlled trials (RCTs), published in English or Chinese between 2002 and 2016, retrieved 19 studies involving a total of 504 children with CP who participated in VR game-based therapy (Y. Chen et al., 2018). These studies, as a whole, scored in the fair to good range on the 11-point Physiotherapy Evidence Database (PEDro, Macedo et al., 2010) quality scale that rates methodological criteria such as random allocation, concealment of allocation, baseline equivalence, blinding procedure, intention to treat analysis, adequacy of follow-up, between-group analysis, and consideration of data variability (Y. Chen et al., 2018, p.4) . Eight studies addressed ambulation outcomes. Meta-analysis initially found a medium-to-large effect size (see Cohen, 1988) for VR, 0.755 [95% CI = 0.348–1.161]. However, a medium level of heterogeneity was also detected in the studies, along with publication bias. Heterogeneity, for example, differing technologies implemented in different ways, decreases confidence that study outcomes can be meaningfully compared. Publication bias further complicates finding the true effect size of an intervention since positive and negative outcomes may not be equally reported. In this particular meta-analysis, these defects caused Chen and colleagues to shift the effect down to 0.378, denoting a small to medium effect. A further 10 studies addressed the outcome of postural control for which a large effect size, 1.003 [95% CI = 0.503–1.502], was calculated. Authors detected large heterogeneity among this set of studies, though no publication bias. A revision to the initial large effect size for VR relative to postural control was not reported.

A further systematic review and meta-analysis was published the next year focused on VR and its impact on multiple factors involved in supporting gait in children with CP (Ghai & Ghai, 2019). This study retrieved 16 studies, RCTs or controlled clinical trials, published before July 2018 in English, German, Hindi, Punjabi, or Sanskrit. The average PEDro scale (Macedo et al., 2010) rating of these 16 studies was good. There were 274 children with CP involved across the 16 studies, which authors grouped according to outcomes reported for the specific gait parameters of velocity (12), stride length (5), cadence (3), stride width (4), and gross motor function (6).

VR showed a large effect, 0.76 [95% CI = 0.44-1.07] on increasing gait velocity, with negligible heterogeneity among studies. It demonstrated a medium effect in extending stride length, 0.20 [95% CI = 0.40-1.01], with no heterogeneity. There was a medium effect of VR on cadence, 0.66 [95% CI = -0.52-1.84] with negligible heterogeneity between the studies. VR had a small effect on reducing stride width, -0.07 [95% CI = -0.57-0.43]. Finally, a medium effect on increasing children's gross motor function, 0.44 [95% CI = 0.06-0.83] was detected.

Later in 2019, a further meta-analysis, restricted to RCTs with a focus on the effect of VR games on gross motor skills in children with CP, was conducted (Ren & Wu, 2019). Nine RCT reports, published between 2014 and 2019, in English or Chinese, including data from 234 children with CP, were included in the meta-analysis. All studies were evaluated as good according to the PEDro scale (Macedo et al., 2010).A small effect, 0.23 [95% CI = 0.04, 0.41, p = 0.02], for VR game-based versus traditional therapy was detected. Authors concluded that VR game interventions could be effective for improving gross motor skills in children with CP (Ren & Wu, 2019).

That the effect sizes calculated by Ren and Wu (2019) differ from those reported by Ghai and Ghai (2019) would not be unexpected considering that the analyses were performed on different studies with very little overlap. Taken together, the two meta-analyses cast a very wide net, embracing the Western literature as well as the Indian and Chinese. The direction of the effect (positive) is consistent between the meta-analyses, and the overall methodological quality of their constituent studies was good. These results support the effectiveness of ICP/VR-mediated therapy for achieving improved gross motor outcomes.

Moderating Effects

The meta-analyses of Ghai and Ghai (2019) and Ren and Wu (2019) both investigated the effect of VR game dosage on therapy outcomes. Moderators of effect include such variables as the time a child spends in a single VR game session, how often (times per week) s/he plays the therapy game, how long the episodes of therapy using a given program last, and the total time the child has accumulated in training overall.

Ren and Wu reported that there was no significant effect associated with any *single* dosage parameter. However, when the child spent 17-40 minutes in each VR session, engaged with VR therapy more than five times per week over a period longer than 12 weeks and, additionally, logged more than 1,000 minutes in VR therapy time, the effect of the VR intervention on gross motor skills was increased (Ren & Wu, 2019).

Ghai and Ghai (2019) reported the effect of VR game session length on gross motor function and suggested that the hypothesis that more training is better for motor gain may not be the case. They found that sessions lasting 20-30 minutes were associated with a medium effect size, 0.56 (95% CI = 0.05-1.07) whereas longer sessions lasting from 40-45 minutes produced only a small effect size, 0.14 [CI = -0.50-0.78]. They noted similar findings with respect to the impact of number of sessions per week on gait velocity where the most gain was seen when sessions were limited to four or fewer. Conversely, training outcomes overall saw greater effects when continued for at least eight weeks (0.83) versus stopped sooner (0.65).

It is perhaps notable that the upper bound of session length for positive effect on gross motor function reported by Ren and Wu (2019), 40 minutes, corresponds to the threshold reported by Ghai and Ghai (2019) for effect drop off. As dosage-effect relationship data continues to emerge from ICP/VR therapies, children with CP stand to benefit from therapists' increased ability to individualize and optimize their care plans.

Process Monitoring Potential

Knowledge about the dosage and timing effects of computer-based therapy at the group level can provide guidance for tailoring the HEP programs of individual children with CP. A research question that arises from findings across groups is whether the computing power of a child's therapy system, sampling the child's performance in real-time, might not be useful for providing personalized HEP prescriptions to optimize training balance for maximal therapeutic effect. Personalized HEP aligns conceptually with personalized medicine, where a patient's own data, increasingly aggregated via wearables, is used to understand him/her at an increasing level of detail and use that understanding to more precisely target interventions (Ho et al., 2020).

Wearable, COTS activity monitors have been used by children with CP to provide feedback about their activity level during prescribed post-operative therapeutic exercise (Sharan, Rajkumar, & Balakrishnan, 2016). A child with CP who engages with a computer-based HEP does not "wear" the therapy system per se. However, referring back to the centrality of the concept of action in ICP/AVG/VRG system descriptions, it is clear that the record of the child's interaction is *imprinted* on the computer-based therapy system during each session and has the potential to be captured and used in therapeutic decision making, asynchronously, and ultimately synchronously (i.e., in real-time) as well.

Figure 2. In-home setup of PedBotHome

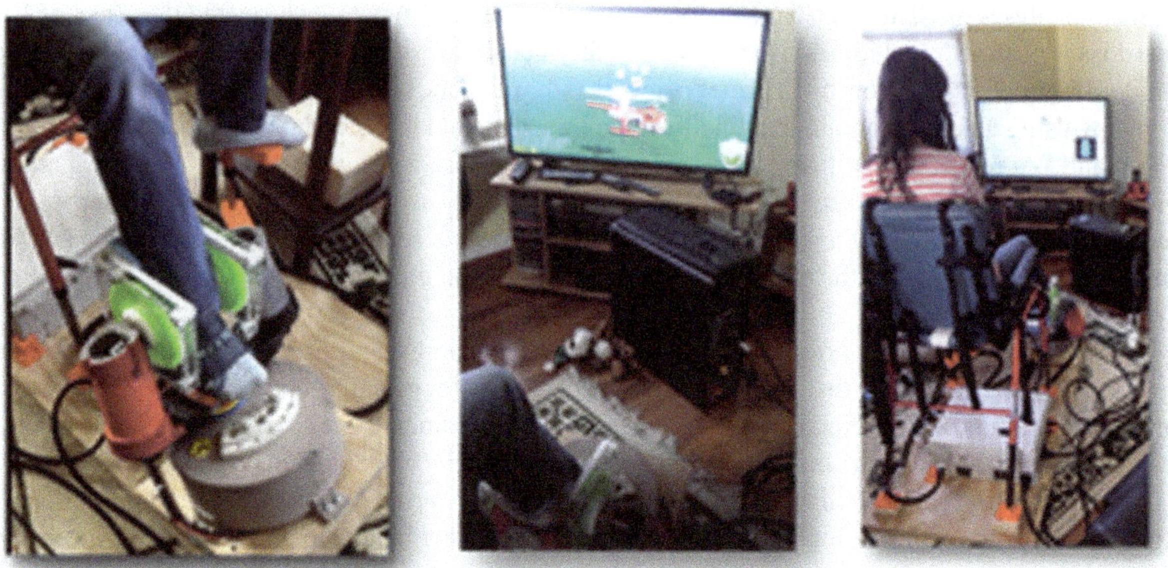

A B C

Note.
Image A: The child's ankle movements drive avatar actions in-game through a robotic controller. Image B: An exemplar game, airplane acrobatics. Image C: Typical in-home system setup. A portable therapy chair is used to help align the child's body and lower extremity for proper execution of therapeutic maneuvers.

PedBotHome2 (PBH2) is the second build of the game-based, robotic, ankle therapy system referenced earlier in this chapter (See Figure 2. For a technical description of PedBotHome, see Cleary et al., 2019). PBH2 tracked the movements of adolescents with CP over 90 days as they pilot-tested the system in a therapist-prescribed and remotely monitored HEP aimed at increasing ankle strength and flexibility to improve gait (Schladen & Choong, 2021). Ankle range-of-motion (ROM) was calculated at the beginning and end of each PBH2 therapy session for the three degrees of ankle rotation freedom. During each PBH2 therapy session, the participating teen with CP played non-immersive AVG using a set of therapist-designed ankle maneuvers, to control the system using a robot-interfaced footplate. Therapeutic maneuvers were mapped to the maneuvers required to drive avatars and objects in the game: dorsiflexion-plantarflexion controlled avatar/object pitch; inversion-eversion effected rolling motions; and abduction-adduction of the forefoot produced yaw. See Figure 2 for an illustration of in-home, system setup. In additional to pre-/post-session ROM, PBH2 also captured time in game, time in each of the three maneuvers (pitch, roll, yaw), and game score.

Initial exploration of the data suggested that the trace of pre- and post-session ROM could be used to provide the player with CP meaningful feedback on performance over longer periods of time, for example, weeks or months. Longitudinally, upward, downward or plateauing trends could be visualized with relative ease. See Figure 3. Day-to-day feedback, however, proved "noisy" and not useful for monitoring short-term progress, or gaining useful insight into such factors as fatigue and readiness to do ankle training. The interpretation of increase or decrease in ROM from the beginning to the end of a single session is ambiguous.

Figure 3. Ankle abduction-adduction range of motion after and before PedBotHome exercise sessions

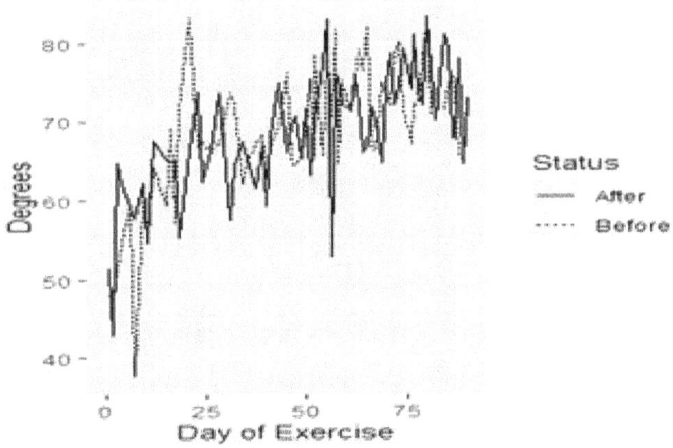

Over the course of a PBH2 session, the teen with CP played multiple prescribed games requiring the execution of pitch, yaw, or roll maneuvers. The system captured the cumulative time the teen had spent practicing each maneuver (angle) and plotted each successive time increment against the teen's score in the game currently in play. Figure 4 shows the game scores (y axis) in two levels of the Spaceship Game that the teen earned over the course of a dozen session of play. The x axis shows how much time (in seconds) the teen had been playing when she earned that score. When asked what the data suggested to her, the teen with CP interpreted the trace as warm up, peak performance, fall back, and finally, fatigue (Schladen & Choong, 2021). This very early exploration suggests that a custom-engineered system has the capacity to provide multiple data points describing a child with CP's trajectory of play, and that this data holds promise for incorporating greater precision into therapy prescriptions.

Engagement

As described earlier, computer-interactive therapy systems have been framed as motivational rehabilitation interventions with a corresponding need for robust measures of motivation to guide their use with children with CP (D'Arrigo et al., 2017; Tatla et al., 2013). Engagement is not a foreign concept in technology acceptance research, with Gibson's foundational work (Greeno, 1994), also previously noted, grounded in the idea that the characteristics of a technology itself are only half of the uptake equa-

Figure 4. Game score vs. time practicing ankle abduction-adduction to maneuver an avatar in two levels of a Spaceship Game

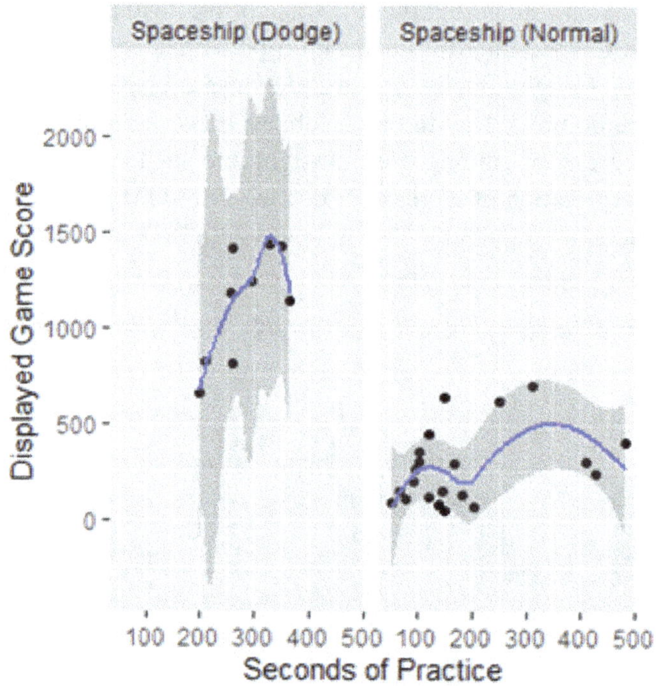

tion; the characteristics of the technology user form the other half. Conceptual frameworks supporting engagement through the development of instruments focused on the user's subjective assessment of a technology may be improved by casting an eye back on the user him-/herself. SDT (Self-determination Theory, Ryan & Deci, 2000) has been recommended for this purpose by many of the researchers whose work has been described in this chapter (Biddiss et al., 2021; D'Arrigo et al., 2017; Sandlund et al., 2012; Schladen, Koumpouros, et al., 2021; Tatla et al., 2013).

SDT is a long-standing framework with an active community of adherents working to refine and extend it (CSDT: Center for Self-Determination Theory, 2021). Further, it has been applied in numerous domains that might be informative for developing measures of motivation in computer-mediated HEP, for example, healthcare, technology, parenting and exercise. In the latter instance, a family of Behavioral Regulation in Exercise Questionnaires (BREQ) has evolved grounded in the continuum concept of extrinsic and intrinsic motivation described within the organismic integration theory that identifies the three basic human needs for relatedness, competence, and autonomy (Deci & Ryan, 1985; Ryan & Deci, 2000).

The BREQ-3, latest in the series, was targeted to the specific application of understanding the motivation of families who agreed to participate in a 90-day HEP mediated by the PBH2 gamified, robotic ankle therapy system (Schladen & Choong, 2021). As an initial exploration of how SDT might be incorporated in understanding HEP engagement and family adherence, two different, 24-item questionnaires were adapted from the single BREQ-3 instrument, one for the adolescents with CP participating in home therapy and another for the parents who facilitated the engagement. Since the BREQ-3 has published reliability and validity data, strong efforts were made to make as few changes to item text as possible. The questions on the adolescent questionnaire were focused to capture the child's motivation surrounding doing ankle therapy generally, irrespective of the ICP intervention. The questions on the parents' questionnaire were focused to capture their motivation to support their child's ankle therapy, again, irrespective of the use of PBH2. Like the original BREQ-3, the questionnaire presented four items measuring each of six gradations of motivation along the continuum from amotivation through the four stages of extrinsic motivation, to the final construct of intrinsic motivation. The questionnaire was administered privately by mobile phone to individuals in two families: 1) a father-son dyad; and 2) a mother-daughter dyad. Figures 4 and 5 shows the results.

Figure 5. Two adolescents' motivation to do ankle exercise as measured by a questionnaire adapted from the BREQ-3

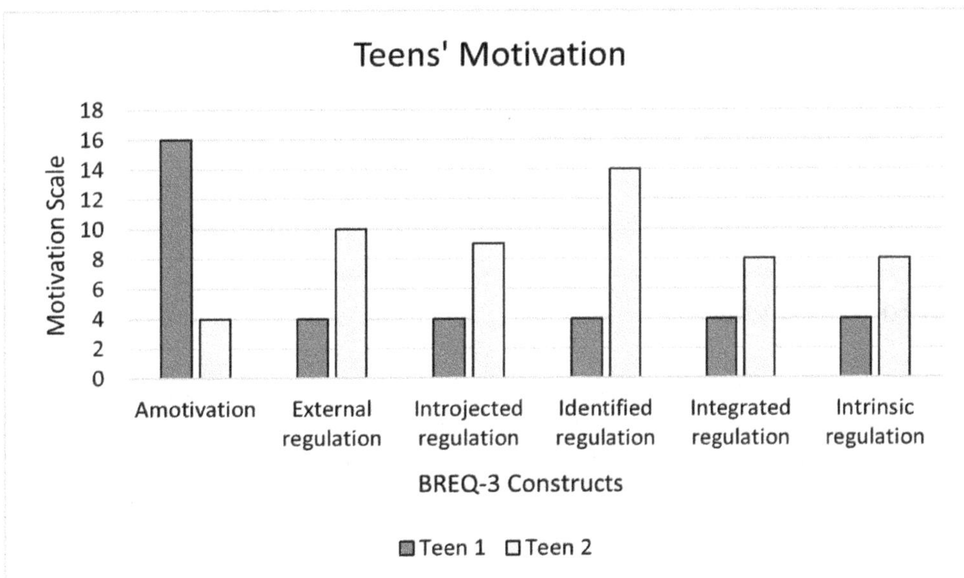

The item clusters are ordered from least to most self-determined. (See also Figure 1, which depicts the Motivation Hierarchy.) The more self-determined one's motivation, the more likely one is to persist. Teen 1 appears largely unmotivated to do ankle exercise. Teen 2 scores high in identified regulation, signifying that she does her ankle exercise because she identifies with that behavior, not because she finds it pleasurable. Both parents found supporting their children's ankle therapy intrinsically rewarding, it contained an element of fun for them, slightly more so for parent 1 than for parent 2. See Figure 6. Readers are left to draw their own conclusions as to which teen engaged more frequently with PBH2 during the 90-day home trial. The ability to measure a CP family's motivational temperature at HEP initiation may help therapists create a better fit between family, therapy, and mediating technology. Adapting valid instruments such as the BREQ-3 from one-off domains such as general population exercise may be an efficient means to achieving that end.

Figure 6. Parents' motivation to support their teens' ankle exercise as measured by a questionnaire adapted from the BREQ-3

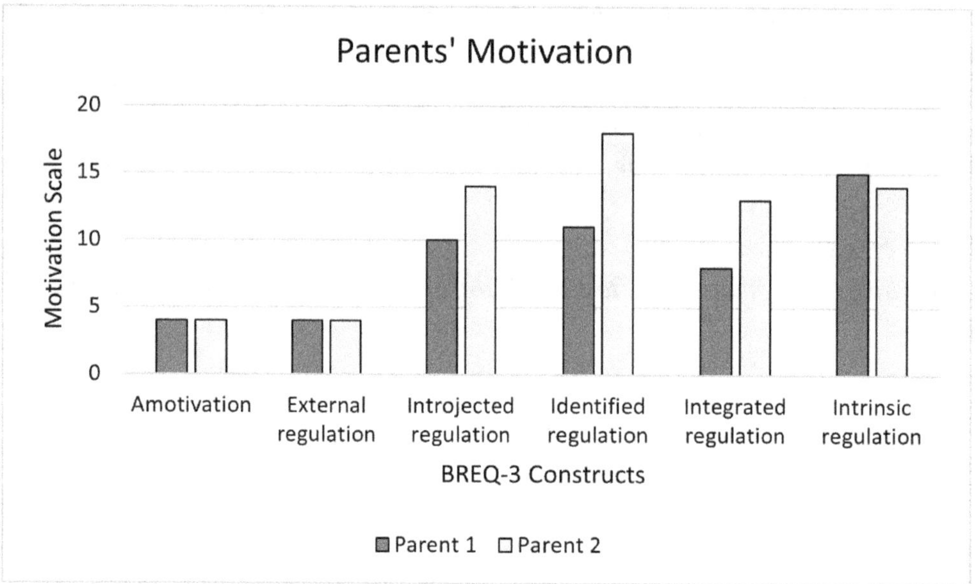

Pragmatics for Deployment

The "hard" challenge of determining which exercises in which formats work best to support gait in any given child and the "soft" challenge of understanding the personal and familial dynamics that facilitate or impede engagement are met with a third, external challenge rooted in the regulatory and reimbursement system in which PT is delivered. Globally, the priorities individual jurisdictions place on providing health and disability support to their citizens differ and result in widely varying policies. Within the legal framework of the European Union, for example, health care policy and organization remain among the exclusive competences of each Member State, and European countries differ in the models they use for healthcare and social services (STOA, Scientific Foresight Unit, 2018), The current (2021) situation in the United States where private, state, and federal agencies all potentially play a role in the care a child with CP ultimately receives, provides one case study of the types of challenges that may be encountered when clinicians seek to leverage technology in CP gait therapy.

In the United States, before health care technologies (devices) can be put in use (brought to market), they pass through a multi-stage vetting process managed by the U.S. Food and Drug Administration (FDA, Fau, 2020). If the device being evaluated is not *substantially equivalent* to a device already approved (known as a "predicate" device), the developer must demonstrate its safety and efficacy. Substantial equivalence means that the new device is as safe and effective as the predicate device. In comparison to the predicate device, a new device is considered substantially equivalent if the device has the same intended use and the same technological characteristics as the predicate or has the same intended use as the predicate and has different technological characteristics that do not raise different questions of safety and effectiveness (U.S. Food & Drug Administration, 2017, 2020). Such demonstrations may involve clinical trials which are very costly to carry out. Notably, devices targeting children face a higher level of scrutiny prior to approval due to the innate vulnerability of that population. The device submission should incorporate the proposed indications for use of the device for the diseases or conditions that the device is intended to treat, diagnose, or cure, as well as an estimated number of affected pediatric patients in the U.S. who suffer from the disease or conditions that the proposed device is intended to treat, diagnose, or cure (Center for Devices and Radiologial Health, 2014).

Once the FDA approves a device, private health insurers in the U.S. will, at their discretion and subject to their internal rules, reimburse its cost. In practice, however, private insurers typically follow the lead of the U.S. national insurer, Medicare, whose mission focus is on adults (specifically, adults over 65) and their health care needs. The Centers for Medicare and Medicaid Services (CMS) set rules with fee schedules governing which types of devices the programs will reimburse. The second program referenced in the CMS acronym, Medicaid, is administered individually by the various states in the U.S. and, like private insurers, might optionally reimburse a device to support therapy in a child with CP (For a case study of the U.S. device reimbursement network, see Schladen, Rounds, et al., 2021.) The interpretive and discretionary nature of reimbursement in the U.S. makes it difficult to shop for an insurance provider based on coverage of therapy devices since the standard procedure is to purchase a health plan, submit a claim, and then discover whether the insurer will agree to reimburse the chosen device.

A unique barrier pediatric devices face is that CMS will not include them in their coding system unless the device has a demonstrated *adult* application (Peiris, 2020). As previously described, there is some evidence that computer interactive therapy that suits younger children with CP is not developmentally appropriate for engaging older children/adolescents. Designing an intervention that provides effective gait training to both young children and older adults can be seen as a high hurdle for developers and serves to suppress the flow of technologies to a market where there is perhaps need but no clear channel for payment.

Various strategies have been proposed to address the external challenge of market viability for promising therapeutic devices. The National Institute on Disability, Independent Living, and Rehabilitation Research (NIDILRR), through its sponsorship of the IMPACT Center at the University of Pittsburgh ("IMPACT: Training Featuring Real Case Studies," 2021), programmatically supports the process of positioning rehabilitation technologies to facilitate their market uptake and availability to individuals with disabilities. The repurpose of low-cost, COTS systems previously described is one strategy to make home gait therapy systems financially viable. Since therapy systems using COTS may be less effective than engineered systems (Y. Chen et al., 2018), a business-to-business (B2B) strategy where developers target systems to clinics and clinics, in turn, lease them to families (business-to-business-to-consumer, B2B2C) for therapy (For an illustration, see Children's National, 2020). The episodic nature of therapy and evidence that there is an optimal periodicity to engagement, may recommend the B2B2C approach. It minimizes a family's initial investment in technology and creates a further economy by allowing serial replacement of a system that may have been appropriate for a child with CP at an earlier stage of development with one that fits his/her current developmental level.

SOLUTIONS AND RECOMMENDATIONS

That ICP is not currently reimbursable for families with children with CP in therapy is a barrier to uptake in the United States. Limited utilization is itself a further barrier to expanded discovery and development of what has emerged from research as a promising approach to improving gross motor outcomes. U.S. PT clinics can moderate this problem by purposively incorporating ICP into the clinical program and further, by implementing a leasing program such as was described in the previous section, *Pragmatics for Deployment*.

Given the suggestion that COTS systems produce inferior outcomes compared to engineered systems, more support for the development of custom-engineered ICP should be included in the funding priorities of federal and private sponsors with an interest in improving therapies for children with CP.

As the ambiguity over degree of immersion in any given AVG/VRG demonstrated, comparing the active ingredients of any two interactive play therapy interventions often contained an inescapable element of uncertainty. The situation could be improved through the development checklists and scales to provide a more granular understanding of the effects of system characteristics.

FUTURE RESEARCH DIRECTIONS

Future research directions mentioned in the chapter are listed below.

- Explore the translation of instruments developed in the exercise domain (specifically, the SDT-grounded Behavioral Regulation of Exercise Questionnaire series) for use in gaging the motivation of families prescribed ICP HEP for carrying out the program.
- Explore the characteristics of the interaction trajectories of children with CP using ICP. Possible applications include visual feedback to the child to help him/her gage progress, information to the system to moderate system program in response to the child's changing status.
- Better define the active ingredients in ICP, both in terms of motivation and in terms of neurologic changes that might be associated with ICP interaction.
- Differentiate the needs and preferences for ICP of younger children and adolescents.

CONCLUSION

There is evidence that therapies delivered in the course of interactive computer play, ICP/VR, are effective for improving gross motor outcomes for children with CP. Multi-national systematic reviews and meta-analyses suggest that the effects of the ICP/VR approach transcend national boundaries and culture and may provide better outcomes for some children than the standard approach to care. The active ingredients in ICP/VR interventions that drive outcomes, as well as those that promote training persistence (adherence) are not well-understood. Further, the specific effects of ICP/VR deployment as HEP in families with children with CP is relatively unexplored. Theoretical frameworks, such as SDT (Self-determination theory) may be useful in promoting continuity of therapy through better understanding, and measurement, of factors underlying child and family motivation and engagement.

Information on therapeutic dosage is beginning to emerge and it does not appear to be linear: more is not always better. Leverage of the child's own training data captured during an ICP/VR therapy session is just beginning to be mined for its potential to more precisely inform exercise prescription and, potentially, course corrections delivered via a computer-based therapy platform in real-time. The potential of ICP/VR therapy is limited by the need to conform gross motor therapies to the formats that work using relatively low-cost, general population, COTS systems for lack of a mechanism for funding (specifically in the U.S.) through established health care reimbursement channels.

DISCLAIMER

The views expressed in this chapter are solely those of the authors and not of any federal government agency.

ACKNOWLEDGMENT

This work was supported, in part, by the Rehabilitation Engineering Research Center on Patient-centered, Home-based Technologies to Assess and Treat Motor Impairment in Individuals with Neurologic Injury (RERC-DC), Grant #90REGE0004 from the National Institute on Disability, Independent Living, and Rehabilitation Research.

REFERENCES

Alotaibi, M., Long, T., Kennedy, E., & Bavishi, S. (2014). The efficacy of GMFM-88 and GMFM-66 to detect changes in gross motor function in children with cerebral palsy (CP): A literature review. *Disability and Rehabilitation*, *36*(8), 617–627. doi:10.3109/09638288.2013.805820 PMID:23802141

Bailes, A., Reder, R., & Burch, C. (2009). Development of guidelines for determining frequency of therapy services in a pediatric medical setting. *Pediatric Physical Therapy*, *20*(2), 194–198. doi:10.1097/PEP.0b013e3181728a7b PMID:18480720

Benedetto, M., Bailes, A., Pandya, S., Edwards, P., & Booker-Feister, C. (2017). *Section on Pediatrics Fact Sheet: Intensity of Service in an Outpatient Setting for Children with Chronic Conditions*. American Physical Therapy Association.

Biddiss, E., Chan-Viquez, D., Cheung, S. T., & King, G. (2021). Engaging children with cerebral palsy in interactive computer play-based motor therapies: Theoretical perspectives. *Disability and Rehabilitation*, *43*(1), 133–147. doi:10.1080/09638288.2019.1613681 PMID:31104517

Boyle, E. A., Connolly, T. M., Hainey, T., & Boyle, J. M. (2012). Engagement in digital entertainment games: A systematic review. *Computers in Human Behavior*, *28*(3), 771–780. doi:10.1016/j.chb.2011.11.020

Carey, H., Martin, K., Combs-Miller, S., & Heathcock, J. C. (2016). Reliability and Responsiveness of the Timed Up and Go Test in Children With Cerebral Palsy. *Pediatric Physical Therapy*, *28*(4), 401–408. doi:10.1097/PEP.0000000000000301 PMID:27661230

Center for Devices and Radiologial Health. (2014). *Providing Information about pediatric Uses of Medical Devices: Guidance for Industry and Food and Drug Administration Staff.* Washington, DC: U.S. Department of Health and Human Services Retrieved from https://www.fda.gov/regulatory-information/search-fda-guidance-documents/providing-information-about-pediatric-uses-medical-devices

Chen, C. L., Chen, C. Y., Liaw, M. Y., Chung, C. Y., Wang, C. J., & Hong, W. H. (2013). Efficacy of home-based virtual cycling training on bone mineral density in ambulatory children with cerebral palsy. *Osteoporosis International*, *24*(4), 1399–1406. doi:10.100700198-012-2137-0 PMID:23052930

Chen, Y., Fanchiang, H. D., & Howard, A. (2018). Effectiveness of Virtual Reality in Children With Cerebral Palsy: A Systematic Review and Meta-Analysis of Randomized Controlled Trials. *Physical Therapy*, *98*(1), 63–77. doi:10.1093/ptj/pzx107 PMID:29088476

Children's National (Producer). (2020). *PedBot & PedBotHome*. Retrieved from https://drive.google.com/file/d/1sB3t1FuFO6-UFSjs453ST2Kdsn9XZQ5m/view?usp=sharing

Chiu, H. C., Ada, L., & Lee, S. D. (2018). Balance and mobility training at home using Wii Fit in children with cerebral palsy: A feasibility study. *BMJ Open*, *8*(5), e019624. doi:10.1136/bmjopen-2017-019624 PMID:29764871

Christiansen, A. S., & Lange, C. (2008). Intermittent versus continuous physiotherapy in children with cerebral palsy. *Developmental Medicine and Child Neurology*, *50*(4), 290–293. doi:10.1111/j.1469-8749.2008.02036.x PMID:18279411

Cleary, K., Monfaredi, R., Salvador, T., Talari, H. F., Coley, C., Kovelman, S., . . . Evans, S. H. (2019). *Pedbothome: Robotically-Assisted Ankle Rehabilitation System For Children With Cerebral Palsy*. Paper presented at the 2019 IEEE 16th International Conference on Rehabilitation Robotics (ICORR). 10.1109/ICORR.2019.8779468

Cohen, J. (1988). *Statistical Power Analysis for the Behavioral Sciences*. Erlbaum.

Columna, L., Prieto, L., Elias-Revolledo, G., & Haegele, J. A. (2020). The perspectives of parents of youth with disabilities toward physical activity: A systematic review. *Disability and Health Journal*, *13*(2), 100851. doi:10.1016/j.dhjo.2019.100851 PMID:31679949

CSDT. (2021). *Center for Self-Determination Theory*. Self-Determination Theory.

Csikszentmihalyi, M. (1990). *Flow: The Psychology of Optimal Experience*. Harper & Row.

D'Arrigo, R., Ziviani, J., Poulsen, A. A., Copley, J., & King, G. (2017). Child and parent engagement in therapy: What is the key? *Australian Occupational Therapy Journal*, *64*(4), 340–343. doi:10.1111/1440-1630.12279 PMID:26831473

Deci, E. L., & Ryan, R. M. (1985). *Intrinsic motivation and self-determination in human behavior*. Plenum Press. doi:10.1007/978-1-4899-2271-7

Deutsch, J. E., & Westcott McCoy, S. (2017). Virtual Reality and Serious Games in Neurorehabilitation of Children and Adults: Prevention, Plasticity, and Participation. *Pediatr Phys Ther*, *29*(S3), S23-S36. doi:10.1097/PEP.0000000000000387

Dodd, K. J., Taylor, N. F., & Damiano, D. L. (2002). A systematic review of the effectiveness of strength-training programs for people with cerebral palsy. *Archives of Physical Medicine and Rehabilitation*, *83*(8), 1157–1164. doi:10.1053/apmr.2002.34286 PMID:12161840

Dong, M., Zhou, Y., Li, J., Rong, X., Fan, W., Zhou, X., & Kong, Y. (2021). State of the art in parallel ankle rehabilitation robot: A systematic review. *Journal of Neuroengineering and Rehabilitation*, *18*(1), 52. doi:10.118612984-021-00845-z PMID:33743757

Fau, D. (2020). *FDA U.S. Food & Drug & Devices Administration*. Retrieved from https://wku.edu/research/documents/covid-19_nih_an_fda_afternoon_webinar.pdf

Fehlings, D., Switzer, L., Findlay, B., & Knights, S. (2013). Interactive computer play as "motor therapy" for individuals with cerebral palsy. *Seminars in Pediatric Neurology*, *20*(2), 127–138. doi:10.1016/j.spen.2013.06.003 PMID:23948687

Franki, I., Desloovere, K., De Cat, J., Feys, H., Molenaers, G., Calders, P., ... Van Broeck, C. (2012). The evidence-base for conceptual approaches and additional therapies targeting lower limb function in children with cerebral palsy: A systematic review using the ICF as a framework. *Journal of Rehabilitation Medicine*, *44*(5), 396–405. doi:10.2340/16501977-0984 PMID:22549647

Gannotti, M. E. (2017). Coupling Timing of Interventions With Dose to Optimize Plasticity and Participation in Pediatric Neurologic Populations. *Pediatr Phys Ther, 29* (S3), S37-S47. doi:10.1097/PEP.0000000000000383

Ghai, S., & Ghai, I. (2019). Virtual Reality Enhances Gait in Cerebral Palsy: A Training Dose-Response Meta-Analysis. *Frontiers in Neurology*, *10*, 236. doi:10.3389/fneur.2019.00236 PMID:30984095

Gmmash, A. S., Effgen, S. K., Skubik-Peplaski, C., & Lane, J. D. (2021). Parental Adherence to Home Activities in Early Intervention for Young Children With Delayed Motor Development. *Physical Therapy*, *101*(4), pzab023. Advance online publication. doi:10.1093/ptj/pzab023 PMID:33481991

Greeno, J. G. (1994). Gibson's affordances. *Psychological Review*, *101*(2), 336–342. doi:10.1037/0033-295X.101.2.336 PMID:8022965

Gronseth, G. S., Cox, J., Gloss, D., Merillat, S., Dittman, J., Armstrong, M. J., & Getchius, T. S. D. (2017). *Clinical Practice Guideline Process Manual*. American Academy of Neurology.

Hadders-Algra, M., Boxum, A. G., Hielkema, T., & Hamer, E. G. (2017). Effect of early intervention in infants at very high risk of cerebral palsy: A systematic review. *Developmental Medicine and Child Neurology*, *59*(3), 246–258. doi:10.1111/dmcn.13331 PMID:27925172

Ho, D., Quake, S. R., McCabe, E. R. B., Chng, W. J., Chow, E. K., Ding, X., Gelb, B. D., Ginsburg, G. S., Hassenstab, J., Ho, C.-M., Mobley, W. C., Nolan, G. P., Rosen, S. T., Tan, P., Yen, Y., & Zarrinpar, A. (2020). Enabling Technologies for Personalized and Precision Medicine. *Trends in Biotechnology*, *38*(5), 497–518. doi:10.1016/j.tibtech.2019.12.021 PMID:31980301

Hutton, J. L., Colver, A. F., & Mackie, P. C. (2000). Effect of severity of disability on survival in north east England cerebral palsy cohort. *Archives of Disease in Childhood*, *83*(6), 468–474. doi:10.1136/adc.83.6.468 PMID:11087278

IMPACT. (2021). *Training Featuring Real Case Studies*. Retrieved from https://idea2impact.org/

Laufer, Y., & Weiss, P. L. (2011). Virtual reality in assessment and treatment of children with motor impairments: A systematic review. *Journal, Physical Therapy Education*, *25*(1), 59–71. doi:10.1097/00001416-201110000-00011

Levac, D., Rivard, L., & Missiuna, C. (2012). Defining the active ingredients of interactive computer play interventions for children with neuromotor impairments: A scoping review. *Research in Developmental Disabilities*, *33*(1), 214–223. doi:10.1016/j.ridd.2011.09.007 PMID:22093667

Lillo-Navarro, C., Medina-Mirapeix, F., Escolar-Reina, P., Montilla-Herrador, J., Gomez-Arnaldos, F., & Olivera-Sousa, S. L. (2015). Parents of children with physical disabilities perceive that characteristics of home exercise programs and physiotherapists' teaching styles influence adherence: A qualitative study. *Journal of Physiotherapy*, *61*(2), 81–86. doi:10.1016/j.jphys.2015.02.014 PMID:25804826

Lopes, S., Magalhães, P., Pereira, A., Martins, J., Magalhães, C., Chaleta, E., & Rosário, P. (2018). Games Used With Serious Purposes: A Systematic Review of Interventions in Patients With Cerebral Palsy. *Frontiers in Psychology*, *9*, 1712. doi:10.3389/fpsyg.2018.01712 PMID:30283377

Lord, C., Rapley, T., Marcroft, C., Pearse, J., & Basu, A. (2018). Determinants of parent-delivered therapy interventions in children with cerebral palsy: A qualitative synthesis and checklist. *Child: Care, Health and Development*, *44*(5), 659–669. doi:10.1111/cch.12592 PMID:30033521

Macedo, L. G., Elkins, M. R., Maher, C. G., Moseley, A. M., Herbert, R. D., & Sherrington, C. (2010). There was evidence of convergent and construct validity of Physiotherapy Evidence Database quality scale for physiotherapy trials. *Journal of Clinical Epidemiology*, *63*(8), 920–925. doi:10.1016/j.jclinepi.2009.10.005 PMID:20171839

Maher, C. A., Williams, M. T., & Olds, T. S. (2008). The six-minute walk test for children with cerebral palsy. *International Journal of Rehabilitation Research. Internationale Zeitschrift fur Rehabilitationsforschung. Revue Internationale de Recherches de Readaptation*, *31*(2), 185–188. doi:10.1097/MRR.0b013e32830150f9 PMID:18467936

Medina-Mirapeix, F., Lillo-Navarro, C., Montilla-Herrador, J., Gacto-Sánchez, M., Franco-Sierra, M., & Escolar-Reina, P. (2017). Predictors of parents' adherence to home exercise programs for children with developmental disabilities, regarding both exercise frequency and duration: A survey design. *European Journal of Physical and Rehabilitation Medicine*, *53*(4), 545–555. doi:10.23736/S1973-9087.17.04464-1 PMID:28466627

Monfaredi, R., Fooladi, H., Tabrizi, P. R., Kovelman, S., Salvador, T., Coley, C., . . . Evans, S. (2018). *PedBot: Robotically assisted ankle robot and video game for children with neuromuscular disorders*. Paper presented at the SPIE Medical Imaging Conference. 10.1117/12.2295031

Moreau, N. G., Bodkin, A. W., Bjornson, K., Hobbs, A., Soileau, M., & Lahasky, K. (2016). Effectiveness of rehabilitation interventions to improve gait speed in children with cerebral palsy: Systematic review and meta-analysis. *Physical Therapy*, *96*(12), 1938–1954. doi:10.2522/ptj.20150401 PMID:27313240

Novak, I. (2014). Evidence-based diagnosis, health care, and rehabilitation for children with cerebral palsy. Journal of child neurology. *Journal of Child Neurology*, *29*(8), 1141–1156. doi:10.1177/0883073814535503 PMID:24958005

Novak, I., Morgan, C., Adde, L., Brunstrom-Hernandez, J., Blackman, J., Boyd, R. N., & Badawi, N. (2017). *Early Detection and Diagnosis of Cerebral Palsy and "High-Risk of Cerebral Palsy" International Clinical Practice Guideline*. Academic Press.

O'Neil, M. E., Fragala-Pinkham, M. A., Westcott, S. L., Martin, K., Chiarello, L. A., Valvano, J., & Rose, R. U. (2006). Physical therapy clinical management recommendations for children with cerebral palsy - spastic diplegia: Achieving functional mobility outcomes. *Pediatric Physical Therapy*, *18*(1), 49–72. doi:10.1097/01.pep.0000202099.01653.a9

Oskoui, M., Coutinho, F., Dykeman, J., Jetté, N., & Pringsheim, T. (2013). An update on the prevalence of cerebral palsy: A systematic review and meta-analysis. *Developmental Medicine and Child Neurology, 55*(6), 509–519. doi:10.1111/dmcn.12080 PMID:23346889

Park, E.-Y. (2016). Effect of physical therapy frequency on gross motor function in children with cerebral palsy. *Journal of Physical Therapy Science, 28*(6), 1888–1891. doi:10.1589/jpts.28.1888 PMID:27390440

Pimentel, L., & Teixeira, K. (1995). *Virtual reality: Through the new looking glass*. McGraw Hill.

Reid, D. T. (2002). Benefits of a virtual play rehabilitation environment for children with cerebral palsy on perceptions of self-efficacy: A pilot study. *Pediatric Rehabilitation, 5*(3), 141–148. doi:10.1080/1363849021000039344 PMID:12581476

Ren, Z., & Wu, J. (2019). The Effect of Virtual Reality Games on the Gross Motor Skills of Children with Cerebral Palsy: A Meta-Analysis of Randomized Controlled Trials. *International Journal of Environmental Research and Public Health, 16*(20), 3885. Advance online publication. doi:10.3390/ijerph16203885 PMID:31614990

Ryan, R. M., & Deci, E. L. (2000). Self-determination theory and the facilitation of intrinsic motivation, social development, and well-being. *The American Psychologist, 55*(1), 68–78. doi:10.1037/0003-066X.55.1.68 PMID:11392867

Sandlund, M., Dock, K., Häger, C. K., & Waterworth, E. L. (2012). Motion interactive video games in home training for children with cerebral palsy: Parents' perceptions. *Disability and Rehabilitation, 34*(11), 925–933. doi:10.3109/09638288.2011.626489 PMID:22066685

Sandlund, M., McDonough, S., & Häger-Ross, C. (2009). Interactive computer play in rehabilitation of children with sensorimotor disorders: A systematic review. *Developmental Medicine and Child Neurology, 51*(3), 173–179. doi:10.1111/j.1469-8749.2008.03184.x PMID:19191834

Sandlund, M., Waterworth, E. L., & Hager, C. K. (2011). Using motion interactive games to promote physical activity and enhance motor performance in chldren with cerebral palsy. *Developmental Neurorehabilitation, 14*(1), 15–21. doi:10.3109/17518423.2010.533329 PMID:21241174

Schladen, M. M., & Choong, E. A. (2021). Preferences of adolescents with CP for design of performance feed from a gamified, robotic home ankle therapy system. Manuscript in Process. Department of Biomedical Engineering. The Catholic University of America.

Schladen, M. M., Cleary, K., Koumpouros, Y., Monfaredi, R., Salvador, T., Talari, H. F., Slagle, J., Coley, C., Kovelman, S., Belschner, J., & Evans, S. H. (2020). Toward Evaluation of the Subjective Experience of a General Class of User-Controlled, Robot-Mediated Rehabilitation Technologies for Children with Neuromotor Disability. *Informatics (MDPI), 7*(4), 45. Advance online publication. doi:10.3390/informatics7040045

Schladen, M. M., Koumpouros, Y., & Lum, P. (2021). *Factors Mediating Use of Advanced Rehabilitation Technologies in the Home.* Paper presented at the Advances in Human Factors and Ergonomics in Healthcare and Medical Devices, Cham.

Schladen, M. M., Rounds, A. K., McManus, T., Bennewith, A., Claypool, H., & Groah, S. L. (2021). Intermittent Catheter Reimbursement in the United States: The Experience of Nine Stakeholders Through the Lens of Actor-Network Theory. *Qualitative Report, 26*(2), 443–464. doi:10.46743/2160-3715/2021.4660

Scientific Foresight Unit. (2018). *Part IV: Legal and socio-ethical perspectives*. Retrieved from https://www.europarl.europa.eu/RegData/etudes/IDAN/2018/603218/EPRS_IDA(2018)603218(ANN4)_EN.pdf

Sharan, D., Rajkumar, J. S., & Balakrishnan, R. (2016). Efficacy of an activity monitor as a biofeedback device in cerebral palsy. *Journal of Rehabilitation and Assistive Technologies Engineering, 3*. doi:10.1177/2055668316676032 PMID:31186915

Shikako-Thomas, K., Shevell, M., Lach, L., Law, M., Schmitz, N., Poulin, C., & Majnemer, A. (2015). Are you doing what you want to do? Leisure preferences of adolescents with cerebral palsy. *Developmental Neurorehabilitation*, *18*(4), 234–240. doi:10.3109/17518423.2013.794166 PMID:23869565

Steenbergen, B., van der Kamp, J., Verneau, M., Jongbloed-Pereboom, M., & Masters, R. S. (2010). Implicit and explicit learning: Applications from basic research to sports for individuals with impaired movement dynamics. *Disability and Rehabilitation*, *32*(18), 1509–1516. doi:10.3109/09638288.2010.497035 PMID:20575752

Tatla, S. K., Sauve, K., Jarus, T., Virji-Babul, N., & Holsti, L. (2014). The effects of motivating interventions on rehabilitation outcomes in children and youth with acquired brain injuries: A systematic review. *Brain Injury: [BI]*, *28*(8), 1022–1035. doi:10.3109/02699052.2014.890747 PMID:24661000

Tatla, S. K., Sauve, K., Virji-Babul, N., Holsti, L., Butler, C., & Van Der Loos, H. F. (2013). Evidence for outcomes of motivational rehabilitation interventions for children and adolescents with cerebral palsy: An American Academy for Cerebral Palsy and Developmental Medicine systematic review. *Developmental Medicine and Child Neurology*, *55*(7), 593–601. doi:10.1111/dmcn.12147 PMID:23550896

Taylor, N. F., Dodd, K. J., McBurney, H., & Graham, H. K. (2004). Factors influencing adherence to a home-based strength-training programme for young people with cerebral palsy. *Physiotherapy*, *90*(2), 57–53. doi:10.1016/j.physio.2003.09.001

Ulrich, D. A., Lloyd, M. C., Tiernan, C. W., Looper, J. E., & Angulo-Barroso, R. M. (2008). Effects of intensity of treadmill training on developmental outcomes and stepping in infants with Down syndrome: A randomized trial. *Physical Therapy*, *88*(1), 114–122. doi:10.2522/ptj.20070139 PMID:17940103

U.S. Food & Drug Administration. (2017). *Deciding When to Submit a 510(k) for a Change to an Existing Device: Guidance for Industry and Food and Drug Administration Staff*. Washington, DC: Center for Devices and Radiological Health, Center for Biologics Evaluation and Research Retrieved from https://www.fda.gov/media/99812/download

U.S. Food & Drug Administration. (2020). *Premarket Notification 510(k)*. Retrieved from https://www.fda.gov/medical-devices/premarket-submissions/premarket-notification-510k#s

Ustad, T., Sorsdahl, A. B., & Ljunggren, A. E. (2009). Effects of intensive physiotherapy in infants newly diagnosed with cerebral palsy. *Pediatric Physical Therapy*, *21*(2), 140–148. doi:10.1097/PEP.0b013e3181a3429e PMID:19440122

Weiss, P. L., Rand, D., Katz, N., & Kizony, R. (2004). Video capture virtual reality as a flexible and effective rehabilitation tool. *Journal of Neuroengineering and Rehabilitation*, *1*(1), 12. doi:10.1186/1743-0003-1-12 PMID:15679949

Wigfield, A., & Eccles, J. S. (2000). Expectancy-Value Theory of Achievement Motivation. *Contemporary Educational Psychology*, *25*(1), 68–81. doi:10.1006/ceps.1999.1015 PMID:10620382

Williams, J. (2008). Children with disability grow into adults with a disability. *Developmental Medicine and Child Neurology*, *50*(3), 163. doi:10.1111/j.1469-8749.2008.00163.x PMID:18302633

World Health Organization. (2021). *International classification of functioning, disability, and health (ICF)*. Retrieved from https://www.who.int/classifications/international-classification-of-functioning-disability-and-health

Wright, M., & Palisano, R. J. (2017). Cerebral Palsy. In R. J. Palisano, M. N. Orlin, & J. Schreiber (Eds.), *Campbell's Physical Therapy for Children* (pp. 447-487). St. Louis, MO: Elsevier.

ADDITIONAL READING

Lord, C., Rapley, T., Marcroft, C., Pearse, J., & Basu, A. (2018). Determinants of parent-delivered therapy interventions in children with cerebral palsy: A qualitative synthesis and checklist. *Child: Care, Health and Development*, *44*(5), 659–669. doi:10.1111/cch.12592 PMID:30033521

Schladen, M. M., Cleary, K., Koumpouros, Y., Monfaredi, R., Salvador, T., Talari, H. F., Slagle, J., Coley, C., Kovelman, S., Belschner, J., & Evans, S. H. (2020). Toward Evaluation of the Subjective Experience of a General Class of User-Controlled, Robot-Mediated Rehabilitation Technologies for Children with Neuromotor Disability. *Informatics (MDPI)*, *7*(4), 45. Advance online publication. doi:10.3390/informatics7040045

KEY TERMS AND DEFINITIONS

Affordance: The alignment between the features and functionalities of a technology and the needs and characteristics of a user and that work together to enable and sustain a satisfactory use experience.

Cerebral Palsy: A non-progressive, neuromotor disorder secondary to a perinatal brain injury associated with a heterogeneous group of diagnoses.

Commercial-off-the-Shelf (COTS): General market technologies repurposed for therapeutic purposes.

Engagement: The quality and strength of a user's entrainment with a technology during interaction.

Gross Motor Function: The aggregate of complementary physiological measures of lower extremity capacity that impact activity, participation, and quality of life.

Home Exercise Program (HEP): Therapeutic exercise carried out in the home and under the control of the individual or family.

Interactive Computer Play (ICP): Therapeutic exercise carried out in the course of a play (game) activity mediated by computing technology.

Motivation: The impetus of an individual to engage in an activity.

Self-Determination Theory (SDT): A framework for understanding human motivation.

Virtual Reality (VR): A computer simulation of scenarios that look and feel real and create an experience providing some degree of immersion.

Chapter 5
Instructional Strategies for People With Profound Intellectual and Multiple Disabilities:
Overview of Approaches and Two Case Studies

Laura Roche
The University of Newcastle, Australia

Jeff Sigafoos
Victoria University of Wellington, New Zealand

ABSTRACT

Educating people with profound intellectual and multiple disabilities (PIMD)creates a number of challenges. One general challenge relates to identifying and successfully implementing instructional programs for developing and enhancing the person's adaptive behavior, such as teaching communication and social skills and increasing their overall level of engagement. The purpose of this chapter is to provide an overview of three main instructional approaches that have been applied to enhance engagement and adaptive behavior functioning among people with PIMD. These approaches are (1) intensive interaction, (2) systematic instruction, and (3) assistive technology. Two case studies are included to illustrate the use of assistive technology—specifically augmentative and alternative communication devices and micro-switches—with two adolescents with PIMD. This overview and the case studies suggest that the use of systematic instructional tactics to establish functional use of assistive technology can be an effective instructional approach for people with PIMD.

DOI: 10.4018/978-1-7998-7430-0.ch005

INTRODUCTION

The general perspective of this chapter is that people with profound intellectual and multiple disabilities (PIMD) can benefit from educational and habilitation efforts. While providing an effective instruction to such individuals can be challenging due to the significant nature of their intellectual and physical impairments, there is some evidence to support the use of a number of different instructional approaches. For people with PIMD, it is generally the case that explicit, deliberate, and often intensive instruction is required to develop and enhance their communication and social skills, levels of engagement, and more generally improve their overall level of adaptive behavior functioning. This chapter provides background on the characteristics associated with PIMD and the challenges that arise in providing effective instruction to people with PIMD. Following this background section is an overview of three instructional approaches that have been applied for the purposes of supporting the engagement and adaptive behavior functioning of individuals with PIMD. These instructional approaches are (a) Intensive Interaction, (b) Systematic Instruction, and (c) Assistive Technology. The consideration of assistive technology interventions focuses on the use of augmentative and alternative communication (AAC) devices, specifically speech-generating devices (SGDs) and related microswitch technology. The use of such technology is illustrated by presenting two case studies in which two adolescents with PIMD were supported through the application of systematic instruction and assistive (AAC/SGD) technology. This overview and the illustrative case studies suggest that the use of systematic instructional tactics to establish functional use of assistive technology appears to be a promising approach for enabling people with PIMD to develop effective communication and social skills and increase their engagement in a range of functional activities.

BACKGROUND

The term PIMD describes a population that presents with severe to profound intellectual disability and significant physical impairment (Bellamy, Croot, Bush, Berry, & Smith, 2010; Maes, Lambrechts, Hostyn, & Petry, 2007). Such individuals also often have additional sensory impairments, such as limited sight and impaired hearing. They may also have serious health problems, such as having seizures and requiring tube feeding or ventilation.

The combination of intellectual and physical impairments can severely restrict the person's learning and the acquisition and performance of communication, self-care, daily living, academic, social, and recreation/leisure skills. The presence of additional sensory and/or medical problems can further complicate instructional efforts and, in turn, their overall level of functioning and quality of life (Gulati & Sondhi, 2018). An additional factor complicating educational efforts is the observation that many such individuals often appear to be passive and seemingly under-responsive to learning opportunities and environmental stimulation (Arthur, 2003; Arthur-Kelly, Foreman, Maes, Colyvas, & Lyons, 2018). Furthermore, persons with PIMD present with very little or no speech and language development. The lack of responsivity and limited speech and language are likely to severely limit their ability to interact with others and their engagement in meaningful social activity (Atkin & Lorch, 2014; Belva, Matson, Sipes, & Bamburg, 2012; Greathead et al., 2016; Lancioni et al., 2019; Schweigert, 2012).

Teaching people with PIMD can also often be further complicated because of problems involving a seeming lack of motivation and a general level of under-responsiveness (Sigafoos, Roche, & Tait, 2021). Thus, a major issue for educators relates to effectively engaging students with PIMD and creating effective opportunities for engagement and the learning of new adaptive skills. Furthermore, once students are engaged and responsive to learning opportunities, it remains difficult to identify the best way to provide effective instruction to enhance the adaptive abilities of adolescents with PIMD (Lancioni et al., 2019). One approach that might help to improve engagement and increase levels of alertness for individuals with PIMD is to support these people to acquire skills that will enable them to more actively participate within their current environment (Arthur-Kelly et al., 2018; Lancioni et al., 2019; Roche et al., 2015). For example, identifying preferences and teaching students to request access to their preferred stimuli could be suggested as an initial step in helping to motivate people with PIMD to participate and benefit from learning opportunities aimed at enhancing their adaptive behavior (Lancioni et al., 2019; Roche et al., 2015).

The next section of this chapter provides an overview of three instructional approaches that have been implemented in efforts to teach people with PIMD, and to illustrate this approach through two case studies.

OVERVIEW OF INSTRUCTIONAL APPROACHES

A number of instructional approaches for enhancing adaptive skills and engagement of persons with PIMD have been developed and evaluated. Three such approaches will be reviewed in greater detail next with the aim of highlighting the strengths and limitations of each approach. These three approaches are (a) Intensive Interaction, (b) Systematic Instruction, and (c) Assistive Technology.

Intensive Interaction

Intensive interaction (II: Nind & Hewett, 1988) is promoted as a style of interaction that is intended to evoke and enhance the communication and social skills of individuals with PIMD. This approach aims to engage individuals in a one-on-one interaction that focuses on increasing the person's levels of alertness and providing sensory and social stimulation. II is is typically implemented in the context of what are hoped to be preferred and engaging activities, such as during play routines. The central component to this approach is the notion that any communicative behavior exhibited by the individual should be interpreted (or over-interpreted) as conveying a meaningful message for that individual (Nakken, & Vlaskamp, 2009; Nind, & Hewett, 2005, 2012). Trainers and participants engage in a positive and sensitive manner during an intensive interaction that aims to (a) increase attention span and concentration; (b) enhance the participants ability to learn and follow sequences of activities; (c) increase opportunities for turn taking and exchanges of behavior and vocalizations; (d) increase the use of appropriate eye gaze, facial expression, physical contact; (e) increase the trainers understanding of the participants non-verbal communication including idiosyncratic behaviors; and (f) to maintain and regulate arousal levels (Nind & Hewett, 2005, 2012).

Although studies adopting II have shown increases in engagement for persons with PIMD and this appears to be a low-resource option for many educators, the lack of methodological rigor and minimal direct adaptive behavior gains seen from this approach would seem to suggest that II is somewhat limited in terms of its supporting evidence. Its potential to improve engagement and skill acquisition is somewhat unclear (see a recent systematic review of II efficacy: Hutchinson & Bodicoat, 2015). However, instructional approaches that incorporate a range of methods, including elements of II, might be used in an effective way to enhance the skills of persons with PIMD. Specifically, increasing carer responsiveness to persons with PIMD during communication attempts would seem to be of potential value of enhancing social communicative interactions, strengthening communication responses, and reducing the social isolation for these individuals. Further, the establishment of a more sensitive care role could be seen as one way to provide a more intensive and responsive environment for the individual. They may thus experience greater instances of constructive interaction and achieve higher engagement levels (Arthur-Kelly et al., 2018). At the present time additional research that addresses the methodological limitations is necessary to establish the efficacy of II.

Systematic Instruction

Systematic instruction (SI) is a method of teaching involving identifying specific responses or skills to teach, creating opportunities to evoke the skill, using response prompts to ensure the responses occur at the right time, fading out prompts over time, and providing reinforcing consequences and corrective feedback for responses (Snell, 1987). SI involves the use of a number of well-established instructional procedures, including modeling, prompting, and reinforcement. Modeling is often required for those with PIMD where a new more complex skill is taught and requires the trainer to visually and/or physically demonstrate the desired response. Prompting and fading involves the use of verbal cues, gestural cues, graduated guidance, hand-over-hand instruction, and time delay procedures to ensure responses occur and can then be reinforced. A further critical component in SI is the use of response contingent reinforcement to strengthen responses. SI results in the opportunity for quantifiable performance- based data collection and precise and reliable data analysis. It can also allow for opportunities to program for generalization and maintenance (Drasgow, Wolery, Chezan, Halle & Hajiaghamohseni, 2017). Additionally, procedures implemented repetitively and continuously over a certain timeframe can lead to faster skill acquisition, especially for those with PIMD and developmental disabilities who may benefit from repeated learning opportunites (Drasgow et al., 2017; Kennedy, 2005; Snell, 1987). In a recent randomized study, Brock, Barczak and Dueker (2020) taught 17 paraprofessionals (15 females) to use SI to enhance the skills of individuals with severe disabilities. Participants were randomly assigned to a either a control group, which received written training materials, or an experimental group, involving group training across four 1-hour sessions (i.e., 4 hours in total). SI for the control group in this study involved a checklist for developing effective use of response prompting methods. The experimental group received training in these same prompting methods in addition to using didactic instruction, modeling and performance feedback. The results showed that the quality of implementation and fidelity of implementation was higher for the experimental group. Furthermore, students receiving SI from the paraprofessionals who received the group training made more progress in comparison to students taught by those from the control group. These results provide additional support for the use of SI for students with severe and complex disabilities and indicate that group training can be effective. Overall, SI has consistently proven to be effective in enhancing the adaptive skills of persons with PIMD (Brock et al., 2020; Canella-Malone & Schaefer, 2017; Spooner et al., 2019). Recently, researchers have been interested in combining SI with assistive technology in order to enable persons with PIMD to accomplish a range adaptive functions, including communicative functions.

Assistive Technology

It has been said that for "…people without disabilities technology makes things easier, but for people with disabilities technology makes things possible" (Bryant et al., 2010, p 203). Various types of assistive technology, such as speech-generating devices (SGDs), have been used to enhance the communication skills of persons with PIMD (Lancioni et al., 2013; Stasolla, Perilli & Boccasini, 2019). For those with PIMD, the use of assistive technology can offer an opportunity to become an active participant within their environment through the use of behavioral responses or natural gestures, that already exist within their motor repertoire (Calculator, 1988; Lancioni et al., 2013; Lancioni et al., 2019; Schweigert & Rowland, 1992).

A microswitch is a type of assistive technology that is designed to enable individuals with minimal motor skills to produce functional responses that are feasible within their existing motor repertoire. Responses of this type might enable them to have a positive impact on their immediate environment through active participation, the control of specific stimulation, and constructive engagement within their immediate context (Lancioni et al., 2013; Stasolla et al., 2019). Microswitches can be effective tools in translating motor behavior into functional active responses when motor skills already present within the user's repertoire are targeted for intervention, as opposed to attempting to teach a new motor behavior in order to activate the microswitch (Lancioni et al., 2019; Stasolla, Perilli & Boccasini, 2019). By capturing a feasible motor movement already possessed by the learner, microswitches might be a more appropriate option for those with limited physical skills as opposed to other AAC options that are often implemented to enhance communication skills. Examples of microswitches include a pressure switch/button that when pressed or activated produces a pre-recorded voice message, for example requesting access to an item, or producing a social greeting. Other microswitches involve motion detection via position and optic microswitches (Lancioni et al., 2006; Lancioni et al., 2007), where a specific movement breaks a sensor and activates a pre-programmed message or sensory stimulation.

As summarized by Lancioni et al. (2013), four common empirically validated components of SI are often incorporated into instructional strategies when teaching individuals with PIMD to use assistive technology including: (a) the creation of structured opportunities for the execution of a target response, (b) specific response prompting strategies, such as graduated physical guidance, (c) the systematic fading of the response prompting strategies, and (d) providing reinforcement contingent upon a target response (Lancioni et al., 2013).

Microswitch technology taught using SI has documented efficacy in increasing functional skills and creating opportunities to increase self-determination and promote adaptive behavior in individuals with PIMD (Lancioni et al., 2019). For example, a recent study aimed to enhance the locomotion skills of six girls (aged from 13 to 17 years of age) with Rett Syndrome and PIMD (Stasolla, Caffo & Perilli, 2018). A microswitch device, comprised of one round photocell and one rectangular reflector panel both attached to the girls' walkers and linked to a control unit, was set-up to provide positive reinforcement (in the form of music, lights and vibrations) to the girls upon performing the target response, gait fluency (defined as 4 steps forward within a 3-s time-period). The study followed an ABABCBC single case experimental design where A represented baseline (no teaching phase), B represented the contingent reinforcement phase (where 3-s of positive reinforcement was provided contingent upon correct gait performance), and C represented a non-contingent control phase (where positive reinforcement was provided for the full 5-min session regardless of gait performance). Results reported improved gait performance during the B phase for all six girls, with all girls demonstrating an awareness for the contingent vs non-contingent phases. Results from several reviews of the use of microswitch interventions to enhance adaptive behavior (Lancioni., 2019; Roche et al., 2015; Stasolla et al., 2015) noted the critical importance of appropriately matching a microswitch to a learner's existing motor skill level and motivational state when designing and implementing microswitch-based interventions. Furthermore, what is unique about these behavioral interventions is the ability to translate minimal motor movements into functional acts.

AAC, SGDs, and Microswitches

The coupling of microswitch technology with AAC modes, such as a speech-generating device (SGD), has opened the door for more elaborate and possibly more effective communicative messaging by those with PIMD. By linking a microswitch (via a Bluetooth or wireless connection), a minimal motor response of hitting a switch, can now be transformed into synthesized speech producing a range of messages programmed onto a user's SGD.

Lancioni et al. (2008a, 2008b), for example, taught two participants in the first study, and three participants in the second, to activate microswitches and SGDs to access desired environmental stimuli and request social interaction from carers. Both studies adopted modified multiple-probe experimental designs where the microswitches were taught for the purpose of controlling desired environmental stimuli, followed by the introduction of the SGD to request social interaction. Following this, both the microswitch and the microswitch-activated SGDs were available for use, allowing the participants to choose between the stimuli or social interaction. By the end of intervention, all participants from both studies had gained proficiency in operating the microswitches and the SGDs to request and obtain sensory stimuli and social contact (Lancioni et al., 2008b; 2008c).

In a recent review, Simacek et al. (2018) summarized 25 studies into the provision of AAC and other additional assistive technology for persons with PIMD. Variables of interest in this study included (a) participant demographics and diagnoses; (b) type of device used; (c) communicative function targeted; (d) study design and reports of reliability and treatment fidelity; and (e) dosage parameters. Overall, across a total of 59 participants, 30 participants received training in using a microswitch to communicate. Largely, studies targeted communicative functions such as requesting for tangibles and social attention with few studies targeting commenting or rejecting non-preferred stimuli. The authors concluded that the provision of AAC is feasible and useful for those with PIMD, however, studies lacked adequate reporting of dosage parameters, generalization, maintenance, and the discrimination of communicative skills (Simacek et al., 2018).

Ovverall it could be seen that there is promising evidence that documents the successful outcomes of assistive technology, including microswitch-activated SGDs for improving communication and other adaptive behaviors of persons with PIMD (Lancioni et al., 2019; Lancioni et al., 2013; Simacek et al., 2018; Stasolla, Perilli & Boccasini, 2019). Empirical research in this literature provides instructional procedures, such as SI, which demonstrate successful outcomes in enhancing adaptive behaviors for persons with PIMD. However, due to the heterogeneity that exists within this population of learners, individualization regarding the design of such teaching programs is warranted. Furthermore, effective communication interventions not only require the learner to acquire new skills, but that the environment is equipped to encourage and enhance communication opportunity, and that communication partners are more able to consistently respond in an appropriate way, which may indicate the value of incorporating elements of II into SI and assistive technology-based interventions.

The following two case studies are intended to illustrate methods to first identify potential communicative acts and consistent natural gestures in two adolescents with PIMD, and then evaluate the outcomes of implementing a beginning microswitch-activated SGD intervention to enhance their natural use of gestures to request further access to preferred stimuli.

CASE STUDIES

The two case studies describe evaluation methods to assess the overall level of functioning and communicative abilities of two male adolescents with PIMD and identify instructional procedures that might enhance their communication skills. Specifically, the participants' communication skills and adaptive behaviors were first assessed using the *Vineland Adaptive Behavior Scales* (VABS: Sparrow, Balla & Cicchetti, 2005) and the *Inventory of Potential Communicative Acts* (IPCA: Sigafoos et al., 2000). An additional assessment was undertaken as well to validate the IPCA assessment findings. Intervention for these two adolescents involved assigning appropriate assistive technology connected to a SGD, loaded with speech generating software. The aim of this technology set-up was to transform the participants prelinguistic behaviors into more effective forms of communicative requests.

Case Study 1: Thomas

Thomas was an 18-year-old male with a diagnosis of profound intellectual disability and severe physical disability (quadriplegia). Thomas also experienced severe visual impairment due to a detached retina with limited vision in his left eye and extreme short sightedness in his right eye. Thomas was described as being tactile resistant with possible craniofacial syndrome. To communicate his basic wants and needs, Thomas would typically produce loud stereotypical vocalizations and would repeat the word 'Hi' when people would approach him or during a social interaction. Thomas did not have functional use of his legs or hands but would 'hook' desired items within his reach using his wrist and/or elbow to bring them closer to him. Often Thomas would become upset and scream loudly. Staff were often not aware of the specific triggers for these outbursts. Typically, Thomas would spend the majority of his day within his wheelchair, except for specific periods of his day where he was placed on the floor to move around. He appeared to enjoy these sessions. Thomas had difficulty swallowing and was fed through a tube, he also required full support with all of his daily cares including toileting.

Assessment data were collected, using the Vineland Adaptive Behavior Scales (VABS: Sparrow, Balla & Cicchetti, 2005), the Inventory of Potential Communicative Acts (IPCA: Sigafoos et al., 2000), and a variation of the IPCA, known as the Behavior Indication Assessment Scale (BIAS: Sigafoos et al., 2006) to identify Thomas' level of adaptive behavior functioning and his communicative inventory. The Communication domain standard score from the Vineland for Thomas was 34, indicating a low adaptive level. In the receptive sub-domain, Thomas had a raw score of 13, which corresponded to a low adaptive level and an age equivalency of 1:2 (years: months) and in the expressive sub-domain, Thomas's raw score was 14 indicating his adaptive level was low, and his age equivalency was 0:9. In the Daily living skills domain standard score, Thomas scored 25, indicating his adaptive level was low. In the Socialization domain standard score, Thomas scored 42 indicating his adaptive level was low. Similarity, Thomas' score in the Motor skills domain was 34, corresponding to a low adaptive level.

Thomas' results from the IPCA indicated that he reportedly used a total of 33 different behaviors for a range of functions. Specifically, to request access to objects Thomas would move in his wheelchair, make noises and vocalize. To request more of something, he would vocalize and make noises, and to access toys he wanted when he was out of his wheelchair, Thomas would bum shuffle towards the item. The BIAS is an assessment tool that is intended to provide supplementary information to support assessment information gathered using the IPCA and more specifically highlights isolated manding (i.e., requesting and/or rejecting) behaviors relating to positive and negative reinforcement in similarly non-verbal persons (Sigafoos et al., 2006). Results from the BIAS are presented in Table 1.

To verify the results of the BIAS assessment and identify a consistent requesting behavior from Thomas, discrete trials adopting the following procedures were implemented: (a) the trainer provided social interaction; (b) the trainer paused the social interaction and said 'Let me know if you want more'; (c) the trainer waited for a response for 15 seconds and; (d) the trainer re-engaged in social interaction after the response delay. Thomas demonstrated reaching behaviors during 80% of these interruptions and this appeared to indicate that he wanted to re-engage with the communication partner and/or that he wanted the interrupted social interaction and sensory stimulation activity to be continued. These results suggest that the social interaction and sensory stimulation activity was a motivating activity for Thomas, and that he had the capacity to produce consistent prelinguistic behaviors (PLBs) to request the reinstatement of preferred activities when those activities were interrupted.

Thomas' PLB of reaching for preferred items was identified as a consistent response, therefore Thomas was taught to 'request social interaction' via hitting a switch located within reach. When he hit the switch, this activated a synthesized speech-output request of 'please play with me'. A pressure sensor microswitch, was used for Thomas. The switch was a highly sensitive round red colored microswitch called an iPad wireless switch #1164 from the Enabling Devices Company (www.enablingdevices.com). Activations of the switch would produce voice output from the iPad loaded with the GoTalk app via a wireless Bluetooth connection. An iPad-mini® loaded with iOS7 capability was used to video record all sessions. For Thomas, a handheld vibrating massager was used as the preferred type of sensory stimulation in addition to social interaction with the interaction partner (first author). The study was conducted according to three phases each involving multiple sessions, with sessions lasting 10-minute in duration. In the first phase (teaching) most-to-least prompting was implemented to instruct Thomas on how to activate the microswitch to request access to social interaction. During this phase, the trainer provided four interaction interruptions and produced the verbal prompt '*Let me know what you want*' followed by a 15-second response delay. Activation of the switch during this phase resulted in the synthesized SGD output '*please play with me*'. In the next phase, the microswitch was placed within reach, but no synthesized SGD message was produced during an activation. During this phase, the trainer provided no interruptions to the play for the whole 10-minute session. The aim of this phase was to determine if the output and resulting reinforcement was in fact maintaining responding. In the final phase, procedures were identical to the first teaching phase where interaction was interrupted and Thomas was prompted to request continuation of the interaction. Treatment integrity and inter-observer agreement data were collected for 30% of sessions across all three phases of this study and were reported at above 80%.

The results of the evaluation approach implemented to enhance Thomas's communication skills are presented in Figure 1 as the percentage of independent microswitch activations per interruption during each session, and the frequency of additional activations per session, across the three phases. As shown in Figure 1, during the first interruption phase, Thomas showed an increasing percentage of correct responses over sessions. He reached the 75% correct level during the fourth session and maintained this high level over the final three sessions of this phase. However, there were an average of 15.7 additional activations per session in this phase. This finding prompted a move to a second (no interruption) phase. During his first session of the no interruption phase, Thomas produced four additional switch activations and during the next two sessions he produced zero and six additional switch activations. This decrease in additional switch activations is in contrast to the previous phase and as these frequencies were lower than 10 additional activations, a decision was made to return to the use of the interruption procedure in a final phase. During this final phase, Thomas was consistently at or above 75% for percent of correct, responses (except during the second session). During this final phase he averaged 6.4 additional activations per session.

Table 1. BIAS results for Thomas

	Communicative Functions		
Behaviours	**Attention**	**Request**	**Reject**
Problem behaviours	×	×	×
Intentional eye gaze	×	×	□
Vocalising	×	×	×
Reach, touch, grab	×	×	×
Move body	×	×	×
Guide another's' hand	×	×	×
Point with finger	×	×	□
Use electronic device	×	×	□

×= present; □ = absent

Figure 1. The percentage of microswitch activations (MSA) and additional activations (AA) produced by Thomas during the intervention (Int) and no intervention (no Int) phases

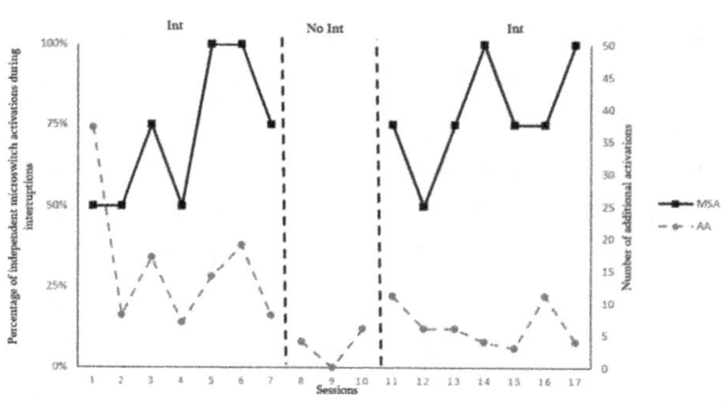

Case Study 2: Blake

Blake was a 17-year-old male with a diagnosis of profound intellectual disability and epilepsy. To communicate basic wants and needs, Blake would typically produce loud stereotypical noises and reach for items that were close by. Blake could walk around his classroom unaided and would occasionally go outside to the playground during break times at his school. Mostly Blake spent his day at school sitting in his chair, chewing on his t-shirt, and vocalizing loudly. Additionally, he sometimes engaged in maladaptive behaviors such as putting his hands down his trousers and hitting his head or his legs with his open hand or closed fist. Blake often seemed largely unresponsive to staff interactions and would fall in and out of a state of sleep regularly during the day. Blake was fed orally by staff and relied on staff for support with all of his daily cares including toileting.

Consistent with Thomas, the VABS (Sparrow, Balla & Cicchetti, 2005) and IPCA (Sigafoos et al., 2000) were administered to identify Blakes' level of adaptive behavior functioning and his repertoire of prelinguistic communication responses. In the Communication domain standard score, Blake scored 28. Blake had a raw score of 12 in the receptive sub-domain, which corresponded to a low adaptive level and an age equivalency of 1:1 (years: months) as shown in table 1.1. In the expressive sub-domain, Blake's raw score was 15, his adaptive level was low, and his age equivalency was 0:9. In the Daily living skills domain standard score, Blake scored 25. In the Socialization domain standard score, Blake scored 23. In the Motor skills domain, Blake's domain standard score was 54.

Blakes' results from the IPCA indicated that he used a total of 26 different behaviors for a range of communicative functions. Specifically, to request access to objects Blake would bang his hands on the table, vocalize, and make noises. He would bang his hands on the table make noises and take an item of food that he wanted and would make noises and take an item that he wanted more of. Similarly to Thomas, the BIAS was used to supplement specific information from the IPCA and results are presented in Table 2.

To verify the results of the BIAS, and to identify a consistent requesting behavior from Blake, discrete trials adopting the following procedures were implemented: (a) the trainer provided access to the preferred edible (bowl of potato chips); (b) the trainer removed access to the edible and prompted 'Let me know if you want more'; (c) the trainer waited for a response for 15 seconds and; (d) reinstated access to the edible after the response delay. During these trials, Blake demonstrated reaching behaviors during 100% of these interruptions that appeared to indicate that he wanted further access to the potato chips. These results suggest that access to the potato chips was a highly motivating snack for Blake, and that he had the capacity to produce a consistent prelinguistic behavior (PLB) to request further access to this snack item.

Blake's PLB of reaching for his preferred snack item was considered a consistent motor response, therefore Blake was taught to 'request further access to preferred snack item' via hitting a switch located within reach, which activated a synthesized speech-output request of 'More please'. A pressure sensor microswitch, was used for Blake (the same switch as used with Thomas). Activations of the switch would produce voice output from the iPad loaded with the GoTalk app via a wireless Bluetooth connection. An iPad-mini® loaded with iOS7 capability was used to video record all sessions. During Blake's sessions, a small bowl filled with preferred snacks (potato chips) were used as the preferred type of sensory stimulation. The study was conducted according to three phases each involving sessions of 5-min duration. In the first phase, the microswitch was placed within reach, but no prompting was provided by the trainer. In the second phase (teaching) most-to-least prompting was implemented to instruct Blake on how to activate the microswitch to request access to his preferred snack item. During this phase, the trainer provided an initial verbal prompt '*Let me know if you want more*'. During this phase, if Blake reached for the bowl of chips, the trainer would direct his hand to the switch and physically support him to activate the switch. This physical prompt was systematically faded over time. Activation of the switch during this phase resulted in the synthesized SGD output '*more please*'. In the final phase, procedures were identical to the first phase where no prompting was provided. Treatment integrity and inter-observer agreement data were collected for 30% of sessions across all three phases of this study and were above 80%.

The results of the intervention implemented to enhance Blake's communication skills are presented in Figure 2. Figure 2 displays the frequency of reaching and microswitch activations across sessions during each phase of the intervention. During the first three sessions of the first phase, Blake reached for the preferred item once during each of the sessions, and independently hit the microswitch a maximum of two times per session. During the 10 sessions when microswitch use was prompted, Blake's frequency of reaching decreased as the number of independent microswitch activations increased from one during the first session, to three in the fifth session. Over the remaining five sessions, Blake pushed the microswitch an average of 4.6 times per 5-min session. During the last no-prompt phase, Blake maintained a high frequency of microswitch activations across the three sessions resulting in nine switch activations during the first two sessions, and 12 switch activations during the final session. The frequency of Blake's reaching averaged two reaches per each 5-min session during this final phase.

Table 2. BIAS results for Blake

	Communicative Functions		
Behaviours	**Attention**	**Request**	**Reject**
Problem behaviours	□	□	×
Intentional eye gaze	×	×	□
Vocalising	×	×	×
Reach, touch, grab	×	×	×
Move body	×	×	×

×= present; □ = absent

Figure 2. The frequency of microswitch activities (MSA) and reaching responses by Blake during the no prompting and prompting phases

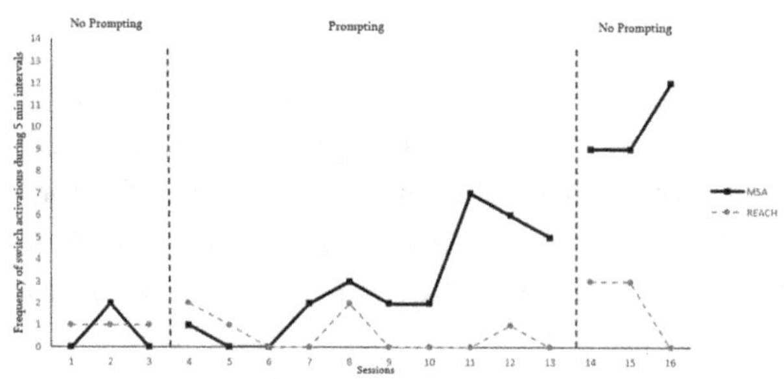

CONCLUSION

These case studies illustrate an initial intervention approach that could be useful for some people with PIMD. The approach might be indicated when the individual presents with low levels of alertness and a lack of clear functional responses prove challenging for educators to devise and plan for effective learning opportunities. The general approach adopted with Thomas and Blake involved using systematic instructional tactics to establish their functional use of appropriately configured assistive technology.

The positive results from these case studies should be considered in light of the following limitations. Firstly the designs of these case studies lack experimental rigor in that no follow-up phases were conducted, nor were complete reversal experimental designs implemented. Secondly, these case studies involved only two male adolescents who were taught one communicative function of requesting. These limitations are, however, not unique to this field whereby recent reviews have identified that studies often only target simple communicative functions involving small sample sizes of learners with PIMD (Lancioni et al., 2019; Simacek et al., 2018).

There are several evidenced based instructional approaches that are effective in enhancing the adaptive behavior functioning of individuals with PIMD. In order to effectively enhance specific functional skills, such as effective communication skills to increase engagement levels for individuals with PIMD, the use of systematic instruction combined with microswitch technology appears to be favorable for a wide population of those with PIMD and has been utilized successfully to teach a wide variety of skills (Lancioni et al., 2019; Simacek et al., 2018).

An initial starting point for implementing microswitch-based communication interventions, using an SGD to produce a synthesized speech message, is illustrated in two case examples. Here, basic requesting skills were taught to two male adolescents with PIMD and varying degrees of alertness/engagement. The two adolescents presented in the case studies illustrate the complexities involved in beginning a communication intervention for persons with PIMD. Thomas and Blake had varying degrees of alertness/responsivity and physical ambulatory skills yet shared some common characteristics. Both engaged in some problematic behaviors (Blake would chew on his T-shirt and often rip his diapers from his pants, Thomas would often become upset and scream during class time), and both lacked an effective method by which they could express clear communicative functions. Moreover, neither of the two boys had any prior experience in using assistive technology to produce functional communicative requests.

The combination of the microswitch and the SGD provided a feasible communication option that adopted a consistent PLB that was within each participant's motor repertoire, ensuring that a new motor response was not needed. The synthesized speech message was clear and effective and the act of pressing the microswitch to activate the speech out-put appeared to be pleasing to both participants. The level of direct engagement with the trainer increased over the duration of the sessions for both participants, which was especially significant for Blake as during a typical school day, he tended to fluctuate between levels of low and high alertness. By providing multiple sessions per day for Blake whereby he was able to independently access his preferred snack and engage with the trainer, time periods where Blake was in a state of high arousal or high alertness was enhanced, increasing the time Blake spent in a state of arousal that was optimal for learning (Arthur-Kelly et al., 2018; Johnson, Rahn, & Bricker, 2015). This may have had positive flow-on effects for the rest of Blake's time spent in his classroom.

The positive results from these case studies must be considered with caution however due to methodological limitations and a lack of follow-up data. To extend these results for these participants for example, teaching rejection of non-preferred stimuli or activities would be a logical next step to enhance Blake and Thomas' functional communication repertoire. However, in light of these limitations these case studies do illustrate a starting point for those working with adolescents with PIMD to begin an intervention within a classroom to enhance existing PLBs using AAC.

REFERENCES

Arthur, M. (2003). Socio-communicative variables and behavior states in students with profound and multiple disabilities: Descriptive data from school settings. *Education and Training in Developmental Disabilities, 38*, 200–219.

Arthur-Kelly, M., Foreman, P., Maes, B., Colyvas, K., & Lyons, G. (2018). Observational data on socio-communicative phenomena in classrooms supporting students with profound intellectual and multiple disability (PIMD): Advancing theory development on learning and engagement through data analysis. *Advances in Neurodevelopmental Disorders, 2*(1), 25–37. doi:10.100741252-017-0045-1

Atkin, K., & Lorch, M. P. (2014). An ecological method for the sampling of nonverbal signalling behaviors of young children with profound and multiple learning disabilities (PMLD). *Developmental Neurorehabilitation*, 1–15. PMID:25029100

Bellamy, G., Croot, L., Bush, A., Berry, H., & Smith, A. (2010). A study to define: Profound and multiple learning disabilities (PMLD). *Journal of Intellectual Disabilities, 14*(3), 221–235. doi:10.1177/1744629510386290 PMID:21062858

Belva, B. C., Matson, J. L., Sipes, M., & Bamburg, J. W. (2012). An examination of specific communication deficits in adults with profound intellectual disabilities. *Research in Developmental Disabilities, 33*(2), 525–529. doi:10.1016/j.ridd.2011.10.019 PMID:22119701

Bryant, B. R., Bryant, D. P., Shih, M., & Seok, S. (2010). Assistive technology and supports provision: A selective review of the literature and proposed areas of application. *Exceptionality, 18*(4), 203–213. doi:10.1080/09362835.2010.513925

Calculator, S. (1988). Promoting the acquisition and generalization of conversational skills by individuals with severe disabilities. *Augmentative and Alternative Communication, 4*(2), 94–103. doi:10.1080/07434618812331274677

Drasgow, E., Wolery, M., Chezan, L. C., Halle, J., & Hajiaghamohseni, Z. (2017). Systematic instruction of students with significant cognitive disabilities. In *Handbook of special education* (pp. 632–648). Taylor and Francis Inc. doi:10.4324/9781315517698-49

Greathead, S., Yates, R., Hill, V., Kenny, L., Croydon, A., & Pellicano, E. (2016). Supporting children with severe-to-profound learning difficulties and complex communication needs to make their views known. *Topics in Language Disorders, 36*(3), 217–244. doi:10.1097/TLD.0000000000000096

Hutchinson, N., & Bodicoat, A. (2015). The effectiveness of intensive interaction, a systematic literature review. *Journal of Applied Research in Intellectual Disabilities, 28*(6), 437–454. doi:10.1111/jar.12138 PMID:25565017

Johnson, J. J., Rahn, N. L., & Bricker, D. (2015). *An activity-based approach to early intervention* (4th ed.). Paul H. Brookes Publishing Co.

Lancioni, G., Sigafoos, J., O'Reilly, M. F., & Singh, N. N. (2013). *Assistive technology: Interventions for individuals with severe/profound and multiple disabilities.* Springer Science & Business Media. doi:10.1007/978-1-4614-4229-5

Lancioni, G. E., O' Reilly, M. F., Singh, N. N., Sigafoos, J., Didden, R., Oliva, D., & Montironi, G. (2007). Persons with multiple disabilities and minimal motor behavior using small forehead movements and new microswitch technology to control environmental stimuli. *Perceptual and Motor Skills, 104*(3), 870–878. doi:10.2466/pms.104.3.870-878 PMID:17688142

Lancioni, G. E., O'Reilly, M. F., Singh, N. N., Sigafoos, J., Didden, R., Oliva, D., Campodonico, F., de Pace, C., Chiapparino, C., & Groeneweg, J. (2009). Persons with multiple disabilities accessing stimulation and requesting social contact via microswitch and VOCA devices: New research evaluation and social validation. *Research in Developmental Disabilities, 30*(5), 1084–1094. doi:10.1016/j.ridd.2009.03.004 PMID:19361954

Lancioni, G. E., O'Reilly, M. F., Singh, N. N., Sigafoos, J., Oliva, D., & Severini, L. (2008a). Enabling two persons with multiple disabilities to access environmental stimuli and ask for social contact through microswitches and a VOCA. *Research in Developmental Disabilities, 29*(1), 21–28. doi:10.1016/j.ridd.2006.10.001 PMID:17174529

Lancioni, G. E., O'Reilly, M. F., Singh, N. N., Sigafoos, J., Oliva, D., & Severini, L. (2008b). Three persons with multiple disabilities accessing environmental stimuli and asking for social contact through microswitch and VOCA technology. *Journal of Intellectual Disability Research, 52*(4), 327–336. doi:10.1111/j.1365-2788.2007.01024.x PMID:18339095

Lancioni, G. E., O'Reilly, M. F., Singh, N. N., Sigafoos, J., Tota, A., Antonucci, M., & Oliva, D. (2006). Children with multiple disabilities and minimal motor behavior using chin movements to operate microswitches to obtain environmental stimulation. *Research in Developmental Disabilities, 27*(3), 290–298. doi:10.1016/j.ridd.2005.02.003 PMID:16005183

Lancioni, G. E., Olivetti, M., Singh, N. N., O'Reilly, M., Sigafoos, J., & Alberti, G. (2019). Recent technology-aided programs to support adaptive responses, functional activities, and leisure and communication in people with significant disabilities. *Frontiers in Neurology, 10*, 643. doi:10.3389/fneur.2019.00643 PMID:31312169

Maes, B., Lambrechts, G., Hostyn, I., & Petry, K. (2007). Quality-enhancing interventions for people with profound intellectual and multiple disabilities: A review of the empirical research literature. *Journal of Intellectual & Developmental Disability, 32*(3), 163–178. doi:10.1080/13668250701549427 PMID:17885894

Nakken, H., & Vlaskamp, C. (2007). A Need for a Taxonomy for Profound Intellectual and Multiple Disabilities. *Journal of Policy and Practice in Intellectual Disabilities, 4*(2), 83–87. doi:10.1111/j.1741-1130.2007.00104.x

Nind, M., & Hewett, D. (1988). Interaction as curriculum. *British Journal of Special Education, 15*(2), 55–57. doi:10.1111/j.1467-8578.1988.tb00314.x

Nind, M., & Hewett, D. (2012). *Access to communication: Developing the basics of communication with people with severe learning difficulties through intensive interaction*. Routledge. doi:10.4324/9780203462409

Nind, M., & Thomas, G. (2005). Reinstating the value of teachers' tacit knowledge for the benefit of learners: Using 'intensive interaction'. *Journal of Research in Special Educational Needs*, *5*(3), 97–100. doi:10.1111/j.1471-3802.2005.00048.x

O'Reilly, M. F., Renzaglia, A., Hutchins, M., Koterba-Buss, L., Clayton, M., Halle, J. W., & Izen, C. (1992). Teaching systematic instruction competencies to special education student teachers: An applied behavioral supervision model. *Research and Practice for Persons with Severe Disabilities*, *17*, 104–111.

Petry, K., & Maes, B. (2007). Description of the support needs of people with profound multiple disabilities using the 2002 AAMR system: An overview of literature. *Education and Training in Developmental Disabilities*, *42*, 130–143.

Petry, K., Maes, B., & Vlaskamp, C. (2005). Domains of quality of life of people with profound multiple disabilities: The perspective of parents and direct support staff. *Journal of Applied Research in Intellectual Disabilities*, *18*(1), 35–46. doi:10.1111/j.1468-3148.2004.00209.x

Roche, L., Sigafoos, J., Lancioni, G. E., O'Reilly, M. F., & Green, V. (2015). Microswitch technology for enabling self-determined responding in children with profound and multiple disabilities: A systematic review. *Augmentative and Alternative Communication*, *31*(3), 246–258. doi:10.3109/07434618.2015.1024888 PMID:25791421

Schweigert, P., & Rowland, C. (1992). Early communication and microtechnology: Instructional sequence and case studies of children with severe multiple disabilities. *Augmentative and Alternative Communication*, *8*(4), 273–286. doi:10.1080/07434619212331276313

Sigafoos, J., Roche, L., & Tait, K. (2021). Challenges in providing AAC intervention to people with profound intellectual and multiple disabilities. In B. T. Ogletree (Ed.), *Augmentative and Alternative Communication: Challenges and Solutions* (pp. 229–252). Plural Publishing.

Sigafoos, J., Woodyatt, G., Keen, D., Tait, K., Tucker, M., Roberts-Pennell, D., & Pittendreigh, N. (2000). Identifying potential communicative acts in children with developmental and physical disabilities. *Communication Disorders Quarterly*, *21*(2), 77–86. doi:10.1177/152574010002100202

Simacek, J., Pennington, B., Reichle, J., & Parker-McGowan, Q. (2018). Aided AAC for people with severe to profound and multiple disabilities: A systematic review of interventions and treatment intensity. *Advances in Neurodevelopmental Disorders*, *2*(1), 100–115. doi:10.100741252-017-0050-4

Snell, M. E. (1987). *Systematic instruction of people with severe handicaps*. Prentice Hall.

Sparrow, S. S., Balla, D. A., & Cicchetti, D. V. (2005). *Vineland-II Adaptive Behavior Scales* (2nd ed.). Pearson.

Stasolla, F., Caffò, A. O., & Perilli, V. (2018). Assistive Technology-Based Programs and Cognitive-Behavioral Interventions for Helping Adaptive Responding of Children and Adolescents with Rett Syndrome: A Selective Overview. In Y. Kats & F. Stasolla (Eds.), *Education and Technology Support for Children and Young Adults with ASD and Learning Disabilities* (pp. 167–188). IGI Global.

Stasolla, F., Perilli, V., & Boccasini, A. (2019). Assistive Technology for Supporting Communication, Occupation, and Leisure by Children with Severe to Profound Developmental Disabilities. In Advanced Methodologies and Technologies in Artificial Intelligence, Computer Simulation, and Human-Computer Interaction (pp. 237-249). IGI Global.

Chapter 6
New Technologies to Support Adaptive Responding in Children and Adolescents With Neurodevelopmental Disorders

Fabrizio Stasolla
https://orcid.org/0000-0003-1626-9664
University Giustino Fortunato of Benevento, Italy

Donatella Ciarmoli
University Giustino Fortunato of Benevento, Italy

ABSTRACT

The chapter provides the reader with a narrative overview on the newest empirical evidence available on the use of new technologies to help individuals with neurodevelopmental disorders. Three main categories of studies were identified, namely (1) virtual reality, (2) mobile technologies, and (3) wearable technologies. Results were satisfactory although failures occurred. Findings were critically discussed, and different technological solutions were emphasized. Some useful insights for both future and practice were critically discussed.

INTRODUCTION

Individuals with neurodevelopmental disorders (NDD) and severe to profound and multiple disabilities (i.e., intellectual, motor, and communication impairments) may pose serious challenges to daily life contexts, due to their clinical conditions (e.g., medical, breath, postural abnormalities, lack of speech, challenging behaviors, isolation, passivity) and may consequently pose serious problems to parents, staff, teachers, and caregivers (Edwards, Rudaizky, Toner, & Chen, 2021; Gardiner,Miller, & Lach, 2020). Next to physiotherapeutic and pharmacological strategies, those children and adolescents may need specific help to: (a) engage positively and independently with surrounding preferred items, (b) improve favor-

DOI: 10.4018/978-1-7998-7430-0.ch006

able opportunities for communication, occupation and leisure, and (c) redirect challenging behaviors. Furthermore, people with NDD may be unable to develop request and choice responses autonomously, although they are capable of learning skills (Neville, Draper, Cooper, Adullah, & Lakes, 2021; Koly et al., 2021; Pastorino et al., 2021). The aforementioned conditions may have deleterious outcomes on their quality of life (Lopez-Sastre et al., 2021; Remmele et al., 2021; Ueda et al., 2021).

One way to promote self-determination, constructive engagement, and positive participation among children and adolescents with NDD is to resort on the use of assistive technology (AT)-based interventions combined to motivational strategies and learning principles (Manta et al., 2020). Among AT, new technologies (i.e., virtual reality, augmented reality, mobile technologies, and wearable technologies) have been recently and growingly developed (Bailey, Bryant, & Hemsley, 2021; Banta Lavenex & Lavenex, 2021; Valentine et al., 2020). Augmented reality (AR) includes digital environments, people, objects, and materials into the user's real word surroundings. Virtual reality (VR) refers to technologies which generate a three-dimensional environment that incorporates the users, enabling interactions with digital people, objects, and/or materials (Dellazizzo, Potvin, Luigi, & Dumais, 2020; Mesa-Gresa, Gil-Gomez, Lozano-Quillis, & Gil-Gomez, 2018). Mobile technologies (MT) include transportable devices or tools capable of automatically deliver self-directed interventions, foster the access to therapies, entitle the therapies to be distantly administrated, enhance clinical effectiveness, and customize treatment strategies (Hermes, Lyon, Schueller, & Glass, 2019: Kellstedt, Spengler, Foster, Lee, & Maddock, 2021). Wearable technologies (WT) have rapidly been developed in recent years as crucial means of human-computer interaction with the growing complexity of information and communication technology. WT comprise the features of mobility and connectivity ensuring users with the online information and communication while moving (Lee, Kim, Ryoo, & Shin, 2016).

Banta Lavenex and Lavenex (2021) carried out a critical review, through a VR-based setup, on spatial abilities in Down and Williams syndromes and evidenced that most individuals with Down syndrome exhibited low-resolution egocentric and allocentric spatial learning memory abilities similarly to typically developed children. Conversely, children with Down syndrome exhibited impaired high-resolution allocentric spatial and facilitated response learning as compared to typically developed children. Individuals with Williams syndrome also demonstrated facilitated response learning but their low-resolution allocentric spatial learning and memory abilities were significantly compromised, if compared to both Down syndrome and typically developed children.

Colombini, Duradoni, Carpi, Vagnoli, and Guazzini (2021) conducted a systematic mini-review on hand-movements sensing in individuals with NDD and neurodegenerative diseases. Results showed that protocols for attention deficits hyperactivity disorders (ADHD) and autism spectrum disorders (ASD) successfully promoted psychomotor and psychosocial rehabilitation in setting that stimulated learning. VR seemed to be encouraging for assessment and screening of executive functions in individuals with NDD, mild cognitive impairments, and dementia.

Bioulac, Taillard, Philip, and Sagaspe (2020) proposed a narrative review on the excessive daytime sleeping (EDS) in the context of ADHD with first a summary of the objective and subjective tools to evaluate it. Furthermore, perspectives in terms of electroencephalogram (EEG) markers and neurofeedback were suggested. Additionally, the possibilities of new kinds of assessment were critically discussed (i.e., VR and ecological momentary evaluation). Finally, the authors constructively argued on specific clinical conditions with EDS in an ADHD framework as links with narcolepsy and the comorbidity with other psychiatric disorders.

Lau-Zhu, Lau, and McLoughlin (2019) presented a brief overview of recent developments in mobile EEG technologies, and emphasized the proliferation of studies in several neuroscientific domains. Moreover, the authors identified three research opportunities, namely (a) increase in the ease and flexibility of brain data acquisition in NDD population, (b) integration into powerful developmentally-informative research designs, and (c) development of innovative non-stationary paradigm.

Georgescu, Kuzmanovic, Roth, Bente, and Vogeley (2014) elaborated and reviewed the use and the validity of virtual characters (VCs) in non-verbal research in high-functioning autism (HFA). Current relevant paradigms and findings from social-cognitive neuroscience were highlighted. The use of VCs as either agents or avatars in the context of transformed social interactions was considered highly promising. The implementation of real-time social interaction in virtual experimental settings was fostered and represented a more sensitive measure of socio-communicative delays in HFA.

Despite the concise overview on the use of AR, VR, MT, and WT in NDD individuals, a comprehensive review of the literature including new technologies was actually missing. Thus, by using AR, VR, MT, WT, ADHD, ASD, cerebral palsy (CP), rare genetic diseases or syndromes, and NDD no records were found in SCOPUS database.

Accordingly, the first aim of the chapter was to present a narrative and selective overview of the empirical studies published in the last five years (i.e., period from 2015 to 2021) to emphasize the most recent intervention approaches mediated by new technologies in children with NDD, to provide a comprehensive picture of the different options available. Consequently, the second objective of the chapter was to emphasize strengths and weaknesses of the reviewed studies. Finally, the third goal of the chapter was to highlight some useful insights for future research and practice as well as to put forward some helpful options to enhance adaptive skills among NDD individuals. Targeted readers (i.e., caregivers, clinicians, families, professionals, teachers, and users) may find interesting solutions for daily use, added to some helpful insights to improve the quality of life of individuals with NDD.

1. BACKGROUND

New technologies in persons with NDD may be used for a dual purpose such as (a) assessment, and (b) rehabilitation (Simeoli, Milano, Rega, & Marocco, 2021). To evaluate the clinical level of severity in NDD, one may envisage a VR setup (Kayabinar, Alemdaroglu-Gurbuz, & Yilmaz, 2021). To recovery both cognitive and/or motor functions one may design a technology-based program (Aida & Feng, 2021; Bergh & Wennerholm, 2020). For example, Hickie et al. (2019) proposed a highly customized and measurement-based care model to manage youth mental health. A new comprehensive assessment framework to capture biopsychosocial profile of young persons with mental care needs was warranted. A multidimensional measure including five domains (i.e., social and occupational functions, self-harm, suicidal thoughts and behaviors, physical health, and illness type, stage and trajectory) was putted forward.

A further illustrative example was provided by Sgandurra et al. (2018) who detailed a new rehabilitative protocol which included a randomized controlled trial (RCT) aimed to evaluate in a sample of infants at high risk for CP the efficacy of the RCT program compared to the infant message (IM) intervention. Based on assignment, infants performed a 8-week RCT or IM treatment. Dependent measures were the infant motor profile and video-recordings of parent-infant interactions. Finally, parents filled a questionnaire (i.e., the Bayley Social-Emotional, Parents Stress Index). A three-point observation was considered.

Specifically, at the beginning of the study or baseline (T0), at the end of the 8-week program (T1), after two months (T2), and finally at 18 months of age (T3), respectively data were recorded.

Broadly speaking, cognitive and executive functions, communication skills, and emotional competence, posture, gait, and motor movements were adequately targeted in individuals with ADHD and ASD. Conversely, participants with CP and rare genetic diseases (e.g., Angelman, Cornelia de Lange, Down, fragile X, Rett, and/or Williams syndromes) were still uninvestigated as well as request and choice opportunities, leisure options, or challenging behaviors considered as a primary or a secondary outcome. In light of the above, the current narrative overview tentatively summarized some representative studies on the use of AR, VR, MT, and WT to promote adaptive skills and enhance cognitive, communicative, and motor functioning of individuals with NDD.

2. METHOD

A computerized search has been carried out in SCOPUS, ERIC, PubMed, and Psych-Info databases. AR, VR, NDD, ADHD, ASD, CP, rare genetic diseases and syndromes, new technologies, AT, quality of life, developmental disabilities, intellectual disabilities, multiple disabilities, motor impairments, communication deficits, challenging behaviors, and clinical/health conditions were merged as keywords. A manual search on the published literature was added as completion. Eligibility criteria included (a) at least a child, an adolescent or a young adult (i.e., aged within 19 years old), (b) at least an empirical study based on the use of new technologies, (c) English as language of the paper, and (d) publication year comprised between 2015 and 2021, Three main groups of studies were identified, namely (a) AR and VR, (b) MT, and (c) WT. The following section includes a concise overview of the reviewed studies described with the objectives, the participants, the procedures and the results. To summarize the studies synoptic tables were embedded. Irrespective of the number of the study included in each group, three contributions were briefly detailed in each sub-section for practical reasons. The reader may find the reviewed studies summarized in the synoptic tables.

3. LITERATURE OVERVIEW

3.1. Augmented and Virtual Reality

VR, including aug AR, recently emerged as crucial means of effective and suitable intervention in different area of public health, namely (a) assessment, (b) diagnosis, (c) recovery (i.e., rehabilitation), and well-being or quality of life. With regard to rehabilitative program, VR has been widely used to favorably address NDD such as ADHD and ASD. VR ensures individuals with NDD with sensory experiences, computer-mediated in artificial environments, enhancing virtual interactions similarly to the real life. AR, as part of VR, enables an interaction in a physical condition, differently from the artificial context provided by VR. That is, VR usually requires the use of specific headsets, which may not be easily wearable for individuals with NDD. Conversely, AR may be viewed as simpler because it refers to smartphones, tablets, and I-PAD, which might be more adaptable to the real world (Akin & Gokturk, 2019; Berenguer, Baixauli, Gomez, Andres, & De Stasio, 2020; Mesa-Gresa, Gil-Gomez, Lozano-Quilis,

& Gil-Gomez, 2018). Behavioral tracking, ecological validity, and experimental control are commonly acknowledged as main advantages of VR (Birenboim, Bloom, Levit, & Omer, 2021; Parra et al., 2021).

Selander, Strand, Almberg, and Lidestam (2021) evaluated a simulator driving test (SDT) and two neuropsychological tests (i.e., the Useful Field of View or UFV, and the Test of Variable Attention or TOVA) with regard to validity for fitness to drive in 51 young participants with ADHD, 33 of whom had ASD and 38 adolescents without a NDD diagnosis. Results showed a general greater variability and poorer performance in the SDT and the TOVA among participants with ADHD and ASD. Data suggested greater effort and susceptibility to motivational issues, and decline in sustained attention over several tests. In conclusion, the SDT was highly sensitive and had good face validity. The TOVA was sensitive to neuropsychological features of safe driving. The SDT and TOVA were viewed as complimentary one to each other, and discrepancy between test scores required specific considerations.

Wiguna et al. (2020) proposed a four-step mixed-method research design that combined both qualitative and quantitative strategies to reduce bias and collect essential information along a VR-based setup and machine learning technologies such as deep learning application. A perspective ADHD-VR digital game diagnostic tool for children using a deep learning model and its development were proposed. It represented a highly promising assessment tool for individuals with ADHD and an optimal solution because it was designed to improve the completeness and transparency of reports of diagnostic tool accuracy studies. Beside a concise review on ADHD-VR game diagnostic tool prototype with a deep learning model, the study presented a new four-step method for its development in children with ADHD.

Noel, Lakshminarasimhan, Park, and Angelaki (2020) used a naturalistic visual path integration task that encompassed continuous action with active sensing and enabled tracking of participants' dynamics belief states. Thirty-nine participants completed the firefly catching task. Fourteen were individuals aged between 12 and 17 years diagnosed with autism matched with their peers. Both groups showed a previously documented bias pattern by overshooting the radial distance and angular eccentricity of targets. Both groups were driven by misestimating velocity signals due to a non-uniform speed prior rather than imperfect integration. No differences were found in participants' beliefs relatively to the speed prior but there was heightened variability in the ASD group. Both end point variance and trajectory irregularities correlated with ASD symptoms severity. With feedback, variance was reduced and ASD performance was close to their controls. In line with the findings, the contribution highlighted the need for both more naturalistic tasks and a broader computational perspective to define the ASD phenotype and pathology.

3.2. Mobile Technologies

MT are usually used for cellular communication. MT evolved rapidly over last years. Standard MT has recently gone from being more than a simple two-way paper to being a mobile phone, GPS navigation device, an embedded web-browser, or a handheld gaming console. MT have different meanings in different aspects, basically MT in information technology and based on the wireless technology of wireless devices. Laptops, tablets, phones, and equipment information technology integration are commonly included (Brandt, Jensen, Saberg, Andersen, & Sund, 2020; Koumpouros, 2021; Kroesch, Douglas, Jozwik, Uphold, & Chung, 2020).

For instance, Davidson et al. (2019) conducted a pilot evaluation of a tablet-based application to improve quality of care in children with mental health treatment. The application was designed to enhance via technology the quality of delivery of trauma-focused cognitive-behavioral therapy (TF-CBT). Its use was piloted in four community mental health service organizations using a blocked randomized controlled

Table 1. Reviewed studies on AR and VR arranged in alphabetic order

Authors	Participants	Ages	Strategy	Main Outcomes
Ghanouni et al. (2019)	ASD Parents + Clinicians	non specified	Social stories	Validation Acceptance
Liu et al. (2017)	ASD boys	8-9	Digital Aid	Both Positive
Noel et al. (2020)	ASD Adolescents	12-17	Naturalistic path	Mixed Results
Romero-Ayuso et al. (2020)	Non specified NDD	6-11	Naturalistic path	Protocol Study
Selander et al. (2021)	ADHD + ASD adolescents	15-19	Driving simulator	Positive assessment
Simoes et al. (2018)	ASD adolescents	13-19	Serious game	Positive learning
Wiguna et al. (2020)	ADHD children	Non specified	Digital game	Diagnostic tool

trial to examine the feasibility of implementing tablet-assisted TF-CBT versus standard TF-CBT with 13 providers and 27 families. Provider fidelity and child engagement in treatment were observationally measured via session audio recording. Parent and child perceptions of the tablet application were evaluated using structured interviews and mixed-method analysis. Providers actively and appropriately used the tablet-based application as a TF-CBT to enhance treatment activities. Both providers and parents expressed high satisfaction with its use, emphasizing acceptability of the approach. Youth and caregivers reported high alliance with the providers in both conditions. The tablet-based application was helpful and could be integrated into mental health treatment with a minimal training. Further investigations were warranted to evaluate the extent to which technology-based applications may improve the reach, quality, and clinical outcomes of mental health intervention delivered to children and families.

Zamin, Norwawi, Nursyafira, Arshad, & Rambli (2019) enrolled a 9-year-old girl with CP born with an auditory and speech disorder including motor difficulties that affected her mobility in an assisted-technology based program finalized at promoting her communication skills. Her senses and brain did not fully coordinate and this create communication problems with her parents. The study was designed to provide the participant with crucial means of communication without using any sign of communication. An alternative and augmentative tool using mobile technology was developed to help people with CP to positively communicate with people surrounding them. The application was not limited to individuals with CP. It was considered useful for anyone with communication disorders. It was developed in a dual language (i.e., English and Malay) with a customized content. Results demonstrated that the participant successfully managed the application, and her adaptive responding was purposeful. The research corroborated the social innovation initiative for people with developmental disabilities as described in the Eleventh Malaysia Plan (i.e., RMK-11).

Zhang, Vallabhajosyula, & Fung (2020) collated health care professionals' perspectives on the limitation of the existing task, and determined if gamification elements could be incorporated to refine the conventional intervention. A protocol study was presented with an adopted qualitative research approach and focus group interviews among professionals in the field of mental health. During the focus group, participants were requested to comment on the limitations of the existing emotional bias interventions. Next, they were asked to recommend strategies useful to improve the intervention, and provide their perspectives pertaining the use of gamification to enhance the intervention itself. The study was expected to be completed in 12 months.

Table 2. Reviewed studies on MT arranged in alphabetic order

Authors	Participants	Ages	Strategy	Main Outcomes
Davidson et al. (2019)	Providers and families	not applicable	Tablet Application	Users satisfaction
Vrana-Diaz et al. (2020)	Prader-Willy adolescents	13-19	Prospective cohort	Weight reduction
Zamin et al. (2019)	Child with CP	9	Communication application	Improved skills
Zhang et al. (2020)	Professionals	not applicable	Gamification	Users acceptance

3.3. Wearable Technologies

WT include basic options and play a primary role in daily life and in the healthcare industry. Covid-19 pandemic dramatically interrupted the healthcare services and negatively affected national medical systems. Actually, the provision and diffusion of the vaccine progressively improved our health conditions and social interactions. However, WT have the potential to support and provide safety and assistance to both healthcare professionals and users. Communication with distant partners, real-time remote monitoring, symptoms predictions, assessment, and recovery objectives may be easily pursued and acknowledged as primary targets (Clark. Bisi, Duncan, & Stagni, 2021; Irvin et al., 2017).

Gualniera, Singh, Fiori, and Santosh (2021) tackled behavioral, clinical and emotional assessments in individuals with Rett syndrome (RTT) through a web-based technology to measure the phenotype. Furthermore, a non-invasive wearable sensor technology was adopted to evaluate autonomic function through electrodermal activity (EDA) and heart-rate variability (HRV). Ten participants with RTT were recruited. Emotional, behavioral, and autonomic dysregulation (EBAD) was recorded as an outcome measure. Participants were additionally exposed to pharmacological treatment. Results evidenced that three participants improved EBAD and normalized EDA. One participant improved marginally. Moreover, two participants partially increased their performance. Mixed results suggested an association between EDA normalization and symptomatic improvements in RTT. Very high levels of EDA were considered as a biomarker for concurrent serious physical illness in RTT.

Billeci et al. (2018) assessed the feasibility of using WT for characterizing the Autonomic Nervous System (ANS) response in ASD toddlers during the presentation of joint attention (JA) stimuli. Twenty ASD toddlers and 20-age and gender matched typically-developed peers were recorded at baseline and during a JA task through an unobtrusive chest strap for electrocardiography (ECG). Different dependent measures were recorded and applied to ECG (i.e., heart rate, standard deviation of the Normal-to-Normal intervals, Coefficient of Variation, and both low and high frequencies). Data emphasized the feasibility of the WT to characterize the ANS in toddlers with autism. The results of this study indicated the feasibility of characterizing the ANS in ASD toddlers through a minimally intrusive tool. The analysis showed an increased Standard Deviation of the Normal-to-Normal intervals and of the Coefficient of Variation in toddlers with ASD at baseline compared to typically developed children, and lower Low Frequency during the task. Findings suggested the opportunity of using the proposed approach for assessing psychological correlates of JA in young children with ASD.

Di Palma et al. (2017) monitored the physiological response (i.e., autonomic nervous system, ANS) during the engagement of ASD children exposed to socio-cognitive tasks. A variable chest belt for ECG signal recording was used. Socio-cognitive tasks were mediated by serious games (SG) implemented on two tablets. A longitudinal assessment of the ANS response for the children during six months of intervention was performed. Results showed a link between ANS response (i.e., decreased level of physiological response and children's engagement). Data fostered the feasibility of such methodology to be implemented in clinical settings to supervise the ANS response of children with ASD during treatment. A larger sample of participants to confirm preliminary findings was warranted.

Table 3. Reviewed studies on WT arranged in alphabetic order

Authors	Participants	Ages	Strategy	Main Outcomes
Airaksinen et al. (2020)	ASD and CP infants	7 months	Machine learning	Movement tracking
Billeci et al. (2018)	ASD toddlers	2-3	Chest strap ECG	ANS response recording
Di Palma et al. (2017)	ASD children	6-8	Chest belt for ECG	Physiological response
Gualniera et al. (2021)	RTT participants	7-15	Web-based technology	Improved performance
Santosh et al. (2017)	RTT children	11	Longitudinal trial	Protocol study
Sgandurra et al. (2018)	CP infants	6-9 months	Randomized controlled trial	Protocol study

4. DISCUSSION

Empirical data of the reviewed studies on the three technological issues (i.e., AR/VR. MT, and WT) evidenced the affordability, effectiveness, and suitability of the adopted technologies to ensure children and adolescents with NDD with adaptive skills. Results were largely satisfactory although mixed outcomes emerged (Gualniera et al., 2021; Noel et al., 2021). Furthermore, some studies (Ghanouni et al., 2019; Romero-Ayuso et al., 2020; Wiguna et al., 2020) did not clarify NDD characteristics nor the participants' ages. Both assessment and rehabilitative goals were positively pursued. Cognitive and executive functions, behavioral, communication and emotional competences, posture and motor movements were broadly targeted in individuals with ADHD and ASD. Conversely, participants with cerebral palsy and rare genetic diseases (e.g., Rett syndrome) were still uninvestigated as well as request and choice opportunities, leisure options, and challenging behaviors viewed as a primary or a secondary outcome (Lancioni et al., 2007, 2008; Perilli et al., 2019).

Recently, some perspective studies developed new virtual reality-aided solutions to remotely evaluate and recovery cognitive functioning among individuals with neurodegenerative diseases to promote cognitive empowerment (Fabio et al., 2020). Internet access and leisure option were embedded in patients with neurological disorders. Additionally, Bernini et al. (2021) implemented HomeCoRe (i.e., Home Cognitive Rehabilitative software) as an innovative approach and a valid strategy for home-based cognitive rehabilitation in neurodegenerative impairments in clinical settings, specifically useful in the Covid-19 pandemic era. Finally, Bottiroli et al. (2021) developed *Smart Aging*, a serious game platform that generates a 3D VR environment in which users may perform a set of screening tasks finalized at a broadly and global cognition's evaluation. A suitable extension might be proposed for children and adolescents with NDD. For example, one may envisage an adapted version to evaluate request, choice, and leisure opportunities and internet access. Similarly, challenging behaviors and positive participation might be recorded as primary and secondary outcomes, respectively. Alternatively, telerehabilitation strategies can be implemented or combined to remotely supervise and recovery individuals with NDD (Iannizzotto, Nucita, Fabio, Caprì, & Lo Bello, 2020).

5. CONCLUSION

Findings of the current narrative review emphasized the effectiveness and the suitability of the new technologies to support adaptive skills in children and adolescents with NDD. The outcomes of the studies were satisfactory. However, caution was mandatory with concerns to the empiric data reported by different contributions. Thus, some issues seemed relevant such as (a) some of the recordings adopted for determining the effects of the technological-aided programs and some of the evidence available on them, (b) the lack of control over the time (history) variable characterizing some of the studies, and (c) the absence of direct emphasis on the participants' acquisition of a constructive engagement role. Given the aforementioned criticisms and the consequent caution necessary in interpreting part of the available literature, the need of extending the research activity seems necessary. Furthermore, it is indeed critical to analyze the studies reviewed in terms of (a) their size (i.e., the quantitative relevance of the changes observed), and (b) their credibility/reliability based on the methodological conditions underlying the programs (Barlow, Nock, & Hersen, 2009; Kazdin, 2001; Kennedy, 2005).

With regard to the first point, one may argue that there were substantial differences among the studies. Many of them reported statistically and functionally significant modifications in the participants' behavior, which were measured through specific measures or by means of response frequencies (Fabio et al., 2016; Puglia et al., 2020). Other studies (a) reported changes, which were not specifically related to such measures or response frequencies but rather to behavioral ratings expressed by professionals involved in the intervention program and other representative figures (e.g., parents) (Lancioni et et al., 2006) and/or (b) presented partial, inconclusive or negative statistical evidence on formal measures (Siegel & Castellan, 1988). The outcomes of the studies using single-subject designs could be taken as more solid and reliable, because these designs allow for control over the time (history) variable (Kennedy, 2005). The quantitative relevance and credibility are the two important criteria on which to judge the outcomes. A supplementary criterion could be the practical relevance of changes observed in terms of participants' environmental engagement and interaction involvement. With regard to this criterion, it might be noted that not all the studies code this outcome, although that goal was progressively considered within this framework.

6. FUTURE RESEARCH

In line with above, the following perspectives for future research could be considered. A first research effort could be aimed at evaluating the extension to the new technologies such as serious games to other children with developmental disabilities than those involved in the studies reviewed. Those efforts should be made taking into account (a) the extensive literature on the use of this intervention approach in other rehabilitation areas such as acquired or pathology, (b) the ethical considerations related to whether and when the participants' legal representatives have the right to decide the use of such an approach, and (c) the need of methodological sophistication so as to ensure that the contribution of this approach to any performance improvement can be detected with certitude.

A second extension may concern the settings, the generalization and the maintenance over the time. With respect to the first point, one may design intervention programs in different settings, involving school, home, rehabilitative and/or medical center. With respect to the second point, one may consider different tasks or different caregivers or research assistant, parents or teachers concerned in the intervention programs, while with the respect to the third point one may design maintenance and/or post intervention phases systematically within those studies.

A third extension may regard the technologies. One may project new devices and new technological solutions and options responding to participants characteristics on one hand and to contexts' resources on the other. With respect to participants characteristics, one may emphasize new technologies ensuring participants to interact actively to the surrounding world, with minimal effort, developing new behavioral responses. With respect to the second point, one should consider economical resources available to the families and the suitability to rehabilitative centers.

REFERENCES

Aida, T., & Feng, G. (2020). The dawn of non-human primate models for neurodevelopmental disorders. *Current Opinion in Genetics & Development, 65*, 160–168. doi:10.1016/j.gde.2020.05.040 PMID:32693220

Airaksinen, M., Räsänen, O., Ilén, E., Häyrinen, T., Kivi, A., Marchi, V., Gallen, A., Blom, S., Varhe, A., Kaartinen, N., Haataja, L., & Vanhatalo, S. (2020). Automatic posture and movement tracking of infants with wearable movement sensors. *Scientific Reports, 10*(1), 169. Advance online publication. doi:10.103841598-019-56862-5 PMID:31932616

Akin, N. T. A., & Gokturk, M. (2019). *Comparison of theory of mind tests in augmented reality and 2D environments for children with neurodevelopmental disorders.* . doi:10.1007/978-3-319-94334-3_26

Bailey, B., Bryant, L., & Hemsley, B. (2021). Virtual reality and augmented reality for children, adolescents, and adults with communication disability and neurodevelopmental disorders: A systematic review. *Review Journal of Autism and Developmental Disorders*. Advance online publication. doi:10.100740489-020-00230-x

Banta Lavenex, P., & Lavenex, P. (2021). A critical review of spatial abilities in down and williams syndromes: Not all space is created equal. *Frontiers in Psychiatry, 12*, 669320. Advance online publication. doi:10.3389/fpsyt.2021.669320 PMID:34122185

Barlow, D. H., Andrasik, F., & Hersen, M. (2006). *Single-case experimental designs* (3rd ed.). Allyn & Bacon.

Berenguer, C., Baixauli, I., Gómez, S., Andrés, M. E. P., & De Stasio, S. (2020). Exploring the impact of augmented reality in children and adolescents with autism spectrum disorder: A systematic review. *International Journal of Environmental Research and Public Health, 17*(17), 1–15. doi:10.3390/ijerph17176143 PMID:32847074

Bergh, C., & Wennerholm, U. (2020). Long-term health of children conceived after assisted reproductive technology. *Upsala Journal of Medical Sciences, 125*(2), 152–157. doi:10.1080/03009734.2020.1729904 PMID:32101068

Bernini, S., Stasolla, F., Panzarasa, S., Quaglini, S., Sinforiani, E., Sandrini, G., Vecchi, T., Tassorelli, C., & Bottiroli, S. (2021). Cognitive telerehabilitation for older adults with neurodegenerative diseases in the COVID-19 era: A perspective study. *Frontiers in Neurology*, *11*, 623933. Advance online publication. doi:10.3389/fneur.2020.623933 PMID:33519704

Billeci, L., Tonacci, A., Narzisi, A., Manigrasso, Z., Varanini, M., Fulceri, F., Lattarulo, C., Calderoni, S., & Muratori, F. (2018). Heart rate variability during a joint attention task in toddlers with autism spectrum disorders. *Frontiers in Physiology*, *9*(May), 467. Advance online publication. doi:10.3389/fphys.2018.00467 PMID:29765335

Bioulac, S., Taillard, J., Philip, P., & Sagaspe, P. (2020). Excessive daytime sleepiness measurements in children with attention deficit hyperactivity disorder. *Frontiers in Psychiatry*, *11*, 3. Advance online publication. doi:10.3389/fpsyt.2020.00003 PMID:32174847

Birenboim, A., & Bloom, P. B. (2021). The study of walking, walkability and wellbeing in immersive virtual environments. *International Journal of Environmental Research and Public Health*, *18*(2), 1–18. doi:10.3390/ijerph18020364 PMID:33418896

Bottiroli, S., Bernini, S., Cavallini, E., Sinforiani, E., Zucchella, C., Pazzi, S., Cristiani, P., Vecchi, T., Tost, D., Sandrini, G., & Tassorelli, C. (2021). The smart aging platform for assessing early phases of cognitive impairment in patients with neurodegenerative diseases. *Frontiers in Psychology*, *12*, 635410. Advance online publication. doi:10.3389/fpsyg.2021.635410 PMID:33790839

Brandt, Å., Jensen, M. P., Søberg, M. S., Andersen, S. D., & Sund, T. (2020). Information and communication technology-based assistive technology to compensate for impaired cognition in everyday life: A systematic review. *Disability and Rehabilitation. Assistive Technology*, *15*(7), 810–824. doi:10.1080/17483107.2020.1765032 PMID:32407217

Clark, C. C. T., Bisi, M. C., Duncan, M. J., & Stagni, R. (2021). Technology-based methods for the assessment of fine and gross motor skill in children: A systematic overview of available solutions and future steps for effective in-field use. *Journal of Sports Sciences*, *39*(11), 1236–1276. doi:10.1080/02640414.2020.1864984 PMID:33588689

Colombini, G., Duradoni, M., Carpi, F., Vagnoli, L., & Guazzini, A. (2021). LEAP motion technology and psychology: A mini-review on hand movements sensing for neurodevelopmental and neurocognitive disorders. *International Journal of Environmental Research and Public Health*, *18*(8), 4006. Advance online publication. doi:10.3390/ijerph18084006 PMID:33920362

Davidson, T. M., Bunnell, B. E., Saunders, B. E., Hanson, R. F., Danielson, C. K., Cook, D., Chu, B. C., Dorsey, S., Adams, Z. W., Andrews, A. R. III, Walker, J. H., Soltis, K. E., Cohen, J. A., Deblinger, E., & Ruggiero, K. J. (2019). Pilot evaluation of a tablet-based application to improve quality of care in child mental health treatment. *Behavior Therapy*, *50*(2), 367–379. doi:10.1016/j.beth.2018.07.005 PMID:30824252

Dellazizzo, L., Potvin, S., Luigi, M., & Dumais, A. (2020). Evidence on virtual reality-based therapies for psychiatric disorders: Meta-review of meta-analyses. *Journal of Medical Internet Research*, *22*(8), e20889. Advance online publication. doi:10.2196/20889 PMID:32812889

Di Palma, S., Tonacci, A., Narzisi, A., Domenici, C., Pioggia, G., Muratori, F., & Billeci, L.The Michelangelo Study Group. (2017). Monitoring of autonomic response to socio-cognitive tasks during treatment in children with autism spectrum disorders by wearable technologies: A feasibility study. *Computers in Biology and Medicine*, *85*, 143–152. doi:10.1016/j.compbiomed.2016.04.001 PMID:27080078

Edwards, S., Rudaizky, D., Toner, M., & Chen, W. (2021). A qualitative study of factors perceived by parents as promoting personal recovery in children and young people with attention deficit hyperactivity disorder. *Advances in Neurodevelopmental Disorders*, *5*(1), 102–115. doi:10.100741252-020-00187-2

Fabio, R. A., Billeci, L., Crifaci, G., Troise, E., Tortorella, G., & Pioggia, G. (2016). Cognitive training modifies frequency EEG bands and neuropsychological measures in Rett syndrome. *Research in Developmental Disabilities*, *53-54*, 73–85. doi:10.1016/j.ridd.2016.01.009 PMID:26859707

Fabio, R. A., Gangemi, A., Semino, M., Vignoli, A., Canevini, M. P., Priori, A., ... Caprì, T. (2020). Effects of combined transcranial direct current stimulation with cognitive training in girls with Rett syndrome. *Brain Sciences*, *10*(5), 276. Advance online publication. doi:10.3390/brainsci10050276 PMID:32370253

Gardiner, E., Miller, A. R., & Lach, L. M. (2020). Service adequacy and the relation between child behavior problems and negative family impact reported by primary caregivers of children with neurodevelopmental conditions. *Research in Developmental Disabilities*, *104*, 103712. Advance online publication. doi:10.1016/j.ridd.2020.103712 PMID:32554267

Georgescu, A. L., Kuzmanovic, B., Roth, D., Bente, G., & Vogeley, K. (2014). The use of virtual characters to assess and train non-verbal communication in high-functioning autism. *Frontiers in Human Neuroscience*, *8*(Oct). Advance online publication. doi:10.3389/fnhum.2014.00807 PMID:25360098

Ghanouni, P., Jarus, T., Zwicker, J. G., Lucyshyn, J., Mow, K., & Ledingham, A. (2019). Social stories for children with autism spectrum disorder: Validating the content of a virtual reality program. *Journal of Autism and Developmental Disorders*, *49*(2), 660–668. doi:10.100710803-018-3737-0 PMID:30203311

Gualniera, L., Singh, J., Fiori, F., & Santosh, P. (2021). Emotional behavioural and autonomic dysregulation (EBAD) in Rett syndrome – EDA and HRV monitoring using wearable sensor technology. *Journal of Psychiatric Research*, *138*, 186–193. doi:10.1016/j.jpsychires.2021.03.052 PMID:33862302

Hermes, E. D. A., Lyon, A. R., Schueller, S. M., & Glass, J. E. (2019). Measuring the implementation of behavioral intervention technologies: Recharacterization of established outcomes. *Journal of Medical Internet Research*, *21*(1), e11752. Advance online publication. doi:10.2196/11752 PMID:30681966

Hickie, I. B., Scott, E. M., Cross, S. P., Iorfino, F., Davenport, T. A., Guastella, A. J., Naismith, S. L., Carpenter, J. S., Rohleder, C., Crouse, J. J., Hermens, D. F., Koethe, D., Markus Leweke, F., Tickell, A. M., Sawrikar, V., & Scott, J. (2019). Right care, first time: A highly personalized and measurement-based care model to manage youth mental health. *The Medical Journal of Australia*, *211*(S9), S3–S46. doi:10.5694/mja2.50383 PMID:31679171

Iannizzotto, G., Nucita, A., Fabio, R. A., Caprì, T., & Bello, L. L. (2020). Remote eye-tracking for cognitive telerehabilitation and interactive school tasks in times of COVID-19. *Information (Switzerland)*, *11*(6), 296. Advance online publication. doi:10.3390/info11060296

Irvin, D. W., Crutchfield, S. A., Greenwood, C. R., Simpson, R. L., Sangwan, A., & Hansen, J. H. L. (2017). Exploring classroom behavioral imaging: Moving closer to effective and data-based early childhood inclusion planning. *Advances in Neurodevelopmental Disorders, 1*(2), 95–104. doi:10.100741252-017-0014-8

Kayabinar, B., Alemdaroğlu-Gürbüz, İ., & Yilmaz, Ö. (2021). The effects of virtual reality augmented robot-assisted gait training on dual-task performance and functional measures in chronic stroke: A randomized controlled single-blind trial. *European Journal of Physical and Rehabilitation Medicine, 57*(2), 227–237. doi:10.23736/S1973-9087.21.06441-8 PMID:33541040

Kazdin, A. E. (2001). *Behavior modification in applied settings* (6th ed.). Wadsworth.

Kellstedt, D. K., Spengler, J. O., Foster, M., Lee, C., & Maddock, J. E. (2021). A scoping review of bikeability assessment methods. *Journal of Community Health, 46*(1), 211–224. doi:10.100710900-020-00846-4 PMID:32419079

Kennedy, K. (2005). *Single case designs for educational research.* Allyn & Bacon.

Koly, K. N., Martin-Herz, S. P., Islam, M. S., Sharmin, N., Blencowe, H., & Naheed, A. (2021). Parent mediated intervention programmes for children and adolescents with neurodevelopmental disorders in South Asia: A systematic review. *PLoS One, 16*(3). . doi:10.1371/journal.pone.0247432

Koumpouros, Y. (2021). An "all-in-one" wearable application for assisting children with autism spectrum disorder. *Technology and Disability, 33*(1), 65–75. doi:10.3233/TAD-200291

Kroesch, A. M., Douglas, K. H., Jozwik, S., Uphold, N. M., & Chung, Y. (2020). Teaching american government content to students with developmental disabilities using technology and constant time delay. *Journal of Developmental and Physical Disabilities, 32*(6), 925–941. doi:10.100710882-019-09726-9

Lancioni, G. E., Belardinelli, M. O., Chiapparino, C., Angelillo, M. T., Stasolla, F., Singh, N. N., O'Reilly, M. F., Sigafoos, J., & Oliva, D. (2008). Learning in post-coma persons with profound multiple disabilities: Two case evaluations. *Journal of Developmental and Physical Disabilities, 20*(3), 209–216. doi:10.100710882-008-9105-9

Lancioni, G. E., O'Reilly, M. F., Singh, N. N., Groeneweg, J., Bosco, A., Tota, A., Smaldone, A., Stasolla, F., Manfredi, F., Baccani, S., & Pidala, S. (2006). A social validation assessment of microswitch-based programs for persons with multiple disabilities employing teacher trainees and parents as raters. *Journal of Developmental and Physical Disabilities, 18*(4), 383–391. doi:10.100710882-006-9024-6

Lancioni, G. E., Singh, N. N., O'Reilly, M. F., Sigafoos, J., Chiapparino, C., Stasolla, F., Bosco, A., De Pace, C., & Oliva, D. (2007). Enabling a young man with minimal motor behavior to manage independently his leisure television engagement. *Perceptual and Motor Skills, 105*(1), 47–54. doi:10.2466/pms.105.1.47-54 PMID:17918548

Lau-Zhu, A., Lau, M. P. H., & McLoughlin, G. (2019). Mobile EEG in research on neurodevelopmental disorders: Opportunities and challenges. *Developmental Cognitive Neuroscience, 36*, 100635. Advance online publication. doi:10.1016/j.dcn.2019.100635 PMID:30877927

Lee, J., Kim, D., Ryoo, H., & Shin, B.-S. (2016). Sustainable wearables: Wearable technology for enhancing the quality of human life. *Sustainability (Switzerland), 8*(5), 466. Advance online publication. doi:10.3390u8050466

Liu, R., Salisbury, J. P., Vahabzadeh, A., & Sahin, N. T. (2017). Feasibility of an autism-focused augmented reality smart-glasses system for social communication and behavioral coaching. *Frontiers in Pediatrics, 5*, 145. Advance online publication. doi:10.3389/fped.2017.00145 PMID:28695116

López-Sastre, R. J., Baptista-Ríos, M., Acevedo-Rodríguez, F. J., Pacheco-Da-costa, S., Maldonado-Bascón, S., & Lafuente-Arroyo, S. (2021). A low-cost assistive robot for children with neurodevelopmental disorders to aid in daily living activities. *International Journal of Environmental Research and Public Health, 18*(8), 3974. Advance online publication. doi:10.3390/ijerph18083974 PMID:33918839

Manta, O., Androutsou, T., Anastasiou, A., Koumpouros, Y., Matsopoulos, G., & Koutsouris, D. (2020). Innovative technological advancements to improve cognitive and social skills of students with neurodevelopmental disorders. *Technology and Disability, 32*(4), 243–253. doi:10.3233/TAD-200288

Mesa-Gresa, P., Gil-Gómez, H., Lozano-Quilis, J., & Gil-Gómez, J.-A. (2018). Effectiveness of virtual reality for children and adolescents with autism spectrum disorder: An evidence-based systematic review. *Sensors (Switzerland), 18*(8), 2486. Advance online publication. doi:10.339018082486 PMID:30071588

Neville, R. D., Draper, C. E., Cooper, T. J., Abdullah, M. M., & Lakes, K. D. (2021). Association between engagement in physical activity and adaptive behavior in young children with autism spectrum disorder. *Mental Health and Physical Activity, 20*, 100389. Advance online publication. doi:10.1016/j.mhpa.2021.100389

Noel, J., Lakshminarasimhan, K. J., Park, H., & Angelaki, D. E. (2020). Increased variability but intact integration during visual navigation in autism spectrum disorder. *Proceedings of the National Academy of Sciences of the United States of America, 117*(20), 11158-11166. 10.1073/pnas.2000216117

Parra, E., Chicchi Giglioli, I. A., Philip, J., Carrasco-Ribelles, L. A., Marín-Morales, J., & Alcañiz Raya, M. (2021). Combining virtual reality and organizational neuroscience for leadership assessment. *Applied Sciences (Switzerland), 11*(13), 5956. Advance online publication. doi:10.3390/app11135956

Pastorino, G. M. G., Operto, F. F., Padovano, C., Vivenzio, V., Scuoppo, C., Pastorino, N., Roccella, M., Vetri, L., Carotenuto, M., & Coppola, G. (2021). Social cognition in neurodevelopmental disorders and epilepsy. *Frontiers in Neurology, 12*, 658823. Advance online publication. doi:10.3389/fneur.2021.658823 PMID:33935956

Perilli, V., Stasolla, F., Caffò, A. O., Albano, V., & D'Amico, F. (2019). Microswitch-cluster technology for promoting occupation and reducing hand biting of six adolescents with fragile X syndrome: New evidence and social rating. *Journal of Developmental and Physical Disabilities, 31*(1), 115–133. doi:10.100710882-018-9634-9

Puglia, M. H., Krol, K. M., Missana, M., Williams, C. L., Lillard, T. S., Morris, J. P., Connelly, J. J., & Grossmann, T. (2020). Epigenetic tuning of brain signal entropy in emergent human social behavior. *BMC Medicine, 18*(1), 244. Advance online publication. doi:10.118612916-020-01683-x PMID:32799881

Remmele, J., Helm, P. C., Oberhoffer-Fritz, R., Bauer, U. M. M., Pickardt, T., Ewert, P., & Tutarel, O. (2021). A national comparative investigation of twins with congenital heart defects for neurodevelopmental outcomes and quality of life (same same, but different?): Protocol for a prospective observational study. *JMIR Research Protocols*, *10*(5), e26404. Advance online publication. doi:10.2196/26404 PMID:33983133

Romero-Ayuso, D., Alcántara-Vázquez, P., Almenara-García, A., Nuñez-Camarero, I., Triviño-Juárez, J. M., Ariza-Vega, P., Molina, J.-P., & González, P. (2020). Self-regulation in children with neurodevelopmental disorders "SR-MRehab: Un colegio emocionante": A protocol study. *International Journal of Environmental Research and Public Health*, *17*(12), 1–23. doi:10.3390/ijerph17124198 PMID:32545534

Santosh, P., Lievesley, K., Fiori, F., & Singh, J. (2017). Development of the tailored Rett intervention and assessment longitudinal (TRIAL) database and the Rett evaluation of symptoms and treatments (REST) questionnaire. *BMJ Open*, *7*(6), e015342. Advance online publication. doi:10.1136/bmjopen-2016-015342 PMID:28637735

Selander, H., Strand, N., Almberg, M., & Lidestam, B. (2021). Ready for a Learner's permit? clinical neuropsychological off-road tests and driving behaviors in a simulator among adolescents with ADHD and ASD. *Developmental Neurorehabilitation*, *24*(4), 256–265. doi:10.1080/17518423.2020.1869339 PMID:33459571

Sgandurra, G., Beani, E., Giampietri, M., Rizzi, R., Cioni, G., Cecchi, F., & .... (2018). Early intervention at home in infants with congenital brain lesion with CareToy revised: A RCT protocol. *BMC Pediatrics*, *18*(1), 295. Advance online publication. doi:10.118612887-018-1264-y PMID:30185165

Siegel, S., & Castellan, N. J. (1988). *Non parametric statistics* (2nd ed.). Mc Graw Hill.

Simeoli, R., Milano, N., Rega, A., & Marocco, D. (2021). Using technology to identify children with autism through motor abnormalities. *Frontiers in Psychology*, *12*, 635696. Advance online publication. doi:10.3389/fpsyg.2021.635696 PMID:34113283

Simões, M., Bernardes, M., Barros, F., & Castelo-Branco, M. (2018). Virtual travel training for autism spectrum disorder: Proof-of-concept interventional study. *JMIR Serious Games*, *20*(3), e5. Advance online publication. doi:10.2196/games.8428 PMID:29559425

Ueda, R., Okada, T., Kita, Y., Ozawa, Y., Inoue, H., Shioda, M., Kono, Y., Kono, C., Nakamura, Y., Amemiya, K., Ito, A., Sugiura, N., Matsuoka, Y., Kaiga, C., Kubota, M., & Ozawa, H. (2021). The quality of life of children with neurodevelopmental disorders and their parents during the coronavirus disease 19 emergency in japan. *Scientific Reports*, *11*(1), 3042. Advance online publication. doi:10.103841598-021-82743-x PMID:33589663

Valentine, A. Z., Brown, B. J., Groom, M. J., Young, E., Hollis, C., & Hall, C. L. (2020). A systematic review evaluating the implementation of technologies to assess, monitor and treat neurodevelopmental disorders: A map of the current evidence. *Clinical Psychology Review*, *80*, 101870. Advance online publication. doi:10.1016/j.cpr.2020.101870 PMID:32712216

Vrana-Diaz, C. J., Balasubramanian, P., Kayadjanian, N., Bohonowych, J., & Strong, T. V. (2020). Variability and change over time of weight and BMI among adolescents and adults with Prader-Willi syndrome: A 6-month text-based observational study. *Orphanet Journal of Rare Diseases*, *15*(1), 233. Advance online publication. doi:10.118613023-020-01504-7 PMID:32883323

Wiguna, T., Wigantara, N. A., Ismail, R. I., Kaligis, F., Minayati, K., Bahana, R., & Dirgantoro, B. (2020). A four-step method for the development of an ADHD-VR digital game diagnostic tool prototype for children using a DL model. *Frontiers in Psychiatry*, *11*, 829. Advance online publication. doi:10.3389/fpsyt.2020.00829 PMID:32973578

Zamin, N., Norwawi, N. M., Nursyafira, Arshad, N. I., & Rambli, D. R. A. (2019). Make me speak: A mobile app for children with cerebral palsy. *International Journal of Advanced Trends in Computer Science and Engineering, 8*(S1), 368-373. . doi:10.30534/ijatcse/2019/5681.42019

Zhang, M., Vallabhajosyula, R., & Fung, D. (2020). Emotional bias modification for individuals with attention deficit hyperactivity disorder: Protocol for a co-design study. *JMIR Research Protocols*, *9*(12), e24078. Advance online publication. doi:10.2196/24078 PMID:33355536

ADDITIONAL READING

Hosseiniravandi, M., Kahlaee, A. H., Karim, H., Ghamkhar, L., & Safdari, R. (2020). Home-based telerehabilitation software systems for remote supervising: A systematic review. *International Journal of Technology Assessment in Health Care*, *36*(2), 113–125. doi:10.1017/S0266462320000021 PMID:32151291

Jahn, F. S., Skovbye, M., Obenhausen, K., Jespersen, A. E., & Miskowiak, K. W. (2021). Cognitive training with fully immersive virtual reality in patients with neurological and psychiatric disorders: A systematic review of randomized controlled trials. *Psychiatry Research*, *300*, 113928. Advance online publication. doi:10.1016/j.psychres.2021.113928 PMID:33857847

Majidi Fard Vatan, H., Nefti-Meziani, S., Davis, S., Saffari, Z., & El-Hussieny, H. (2021). A review: A comprehensive review of soft and rigid wearable rehabilitation and assistive devices with a focus on the shoulder joint. *Journal of Intelligent and Robotic Systems: Theory and Applications*, *102*(1), 9. Advance online publication. doi:10.100710846-021-01353-x

Pittman, C. A., Ward, B. K., & Nieman, C. L. (2021). A review of adult-onset hearing loss: A primer for neurologists. *Current Treatment Options in Neurology*, *23*(7), 20. Advance online publication. doi:10.100711940-021-00674-4

Pratviel, Y., Deschodt-Arsac, V., Larrue, F., & Arsac, L. M. (2021). Reliability of the dynavision task in virtual reality to explore visuomotor phenotypes. *Scientific Reports*, *11*(1), 587. Advance online publication. doi:10.103841598-020-79885-9 PMID:33436738

Sulzer, J., & Karfeld-Sulzer, L. S. (2021). Our child's TBI: A rehabilitation engineer's personal experience, technological approach, and lessons learned. *Journal of Neuroengineering and Rehabilitation*, *18*(1), 59. Advance online publication. doi:10.118612984-021-00862-y PMID:33827612

Wu, J., Kuruvithadam, K., Schaer, A., Stoneham, R., Chatzipirpiridis, G., Easthope, C. A., Barry, G., Martin, J., Pané, S., Nelson, B. J., Ergeneman, O., & Torun, H. (2021). An intelligent in-shoe system for gait monitoring and analysis with optimized sampling and real-time visualization capabilities. *Sensors (Basel)*, *21*(8), 2869. Advance online publication. doi:10.339021082869 PMID:33921846

KEY TERMS AND DEFINITIONS

Constructive Engagement: Positive participation, active role of an individual exposed to an AT-based program.

Mobile Technologies: Any technological device with internet capability accessible from anywhere the user is.

Neurodevelopmental Disorders: Disabilities primarily associated with the functioning of the brain and the Nervous Central System in children and adolescents, including ADHD, ASD, CP, and rare genetic syndromes.

Quality of Life: Complex psychological construct which includes happiness, pleasure, satisfaction, fulfilment, and well-being.

Virtual Reality: Simulated experience that can be similar or totally different from real world. It is mediated by artificial intelligence.

Wearable Technologies: Category of electronic devices incorporating a microprocessor and an internet access that can be worn by the user as accessories embedded in clothing, implanted in the user's body, or tattooed in the skin.

Chapter 7
Assistive Technology to Promote Adaptive Skills in Children and Adolescents With Rett Syndrome:
A Selective Review

Donatella Ciarmoli
University Giustino Fortunato of Benevento, Italy

ABSTRACT

Rett syndrome is classified within the rare genetic syndromes, characterised by intellectual delays, extensive motor impairments, lack of speech and communication difficulties, sensorial deficits, and problems in adaptive responding. That clinical conditions may be deleterious on their social image, status, and quality of life. A practice for addressing this problem is technology-based interventions. The use of assistive technologies, in particular microswitches, with children with RTT has been shown to effectively change the impact on their quality of life, facilitating access to recreational activities and improving their performance. Through the use of technology-aided programs, a child with RTT and multiple disabilities will be ensured with an independent access to positive stimulation. In this chapter, a selective literature review was carried out considering Rett Syndrome, assistive technologies, quality of life, and rare genetic syndromes. Empirical data demonstrated the effectiveness and suitability of interventions with AT, allowing participants to increase their level of independence.

INTRODUCTION

Rett syndrome (RTT) is a progressive neurodevelopmental disorder, X linked, due to mutations in the methyl-cytosine phosphate guanine binding protein 2 (MECP2) gene, located on Xq28, largely affecting females, first described by Andreas Rett (1966). It is associated with severe to profound intellectual, communicative and motor impairments, beginning between 6 and 18 months old, preceded by a normal

DOI: 10.4018/978-1-7998-7430-0.ch007

birth and an initial regular development (Didden et al., 2010). RTT traditionally follows four stages, namely: (a) stagnation, (b) regression, (c) stationary, and (d) motor deterioration (Stasolla & Caffò, 2013).

Subsequently to an apparent regular birth, the stagnation commonly includes a global arrest of child's development between 5 and 6 months. The regression usually has an onset between 1 and 4 years old. A general loss of adaptive functions occurs. Thus, either a progressive speech or a social interactions' impairments are frequently observed. Nevertheless, eye contact for communicative goals is preserved. During the stationary phase stereotypical hand-related behaviors emerge (e.g., clapping and washing). In addition, respiratory abnormalities (i. e., hyperventilation) and behavioral problems (e. g., night crying and laughing attacks) may be highlighted. Seizures, ataxia, apraxia, motor scoliosis are broadly embedded, between 2 and 8 years. The motor deterioration is described by motor decline, reduced physical activity, decreased stereotyped behaviors, and withdrawal, after 10 years old. Beside the aforementioned clinical conditions, failing locomotion is one of the most common negative functional consequences of RTT (Neul et al., 2010; Rett 1966; Stasolla et al., 2015)

Individuals with RTT usually present a vast array of orthopedic and neurological difficulties. Typical challenges, which may need to be addressed, when treating this population are functional limitations, low cardiovascular capacity, hypotonia, ataxia, apraxia, loss of transitional movements, spasticity, scoliosis and/or kyphosis, loss of ambulation, loss of hand function, foot deformities, and spatial disorientation (Lotan, 2006). Moreover, individuals with RTT are frequently describes as isolated, with minimal opportunities to interact positively with their environment and surrounding objects. Additionally, reduced sensory stimulation, deprivation, and negative consequences on their quality of life may be evidenced (Felce & Perry, 1995). Finally, the latter conditions (i.e., deprivation, isolation, passivity, and withdrawal) may seriously hamper their social image and status (Stasolla et al., 2014).

Interventions for people with RTT may be aimed at compensating and reducing physical impairment and include therapeutic interventions, adaptive techniques, environmental changes and assistive technology-based interventions (AT) (Lancioni, Sigafoos, O'Reilly, & Singh, 2012). That is, by using technological aids such as sensors and personal computers, one may envisage to improve self-determination, with the opportunity of enhancing occupation, constructive engagement, and choice options, almost lacking among children with RTT. The Australian RTT study (Leonard, 2002) has gathered information regarding the use of assistive technology among individuals with RTT. Their findings suggest that the majority of individuals with RTT are using such devices. As detailed in this review, the most commonly used AT for people with RTT are: (a) mobility aids, (b) AT for physiological needs, (c) transport aids, (d) foot supports, (e) communication aids, (f) arm supports, and (g) lifting aids. (see Figure 1).

For instance, Sigafoos et al. (2019) reviewed 38 studies and identified promising approaches that sought to improve adaptive functioning in cases of regression. Thus, 132 participants with RTT were involved in cases where developmental regression was either already occurred or was likely to occur. Interventions targeted a range of variables (e.g., challenging behaviors, communication, motor, and social skills). Multi-component interventions based on learning principles were the norm, suggesting the need for clinical expertise in the application of behavior analytic principles.

Hornof, Whitman, Sutherland, Gerendasy, and McGrenere (2017) exposed a 20-month-old girl who was diagnosed with RTT to a Motivating Music system. The girl presented severe to profound developmental delays, and no specific interactions with her environment. An easy-to-use and engaging music-playing system was designed for motivating her constructive engagement and positive occupation. During the intervention phases, the in-home girl's therapists (i.e., speech, physical, and occupational caregivers) noticed that the girl was highly motivated to use the technological system and incorporated it into their in-home working sessions. The girl consolidated the use of the system along three years and remained strongly engaged when using it.

Recently, Rose, Wass, Jankowski, Feldman, and Djukic (2017) investigated the sustained attention by using an innovative gaze-based task that minimized demands on limited verbal and motor skills of girls with RTT. Thirty-two participants who were aged between 2 and 12 years were involved. They were compared to thirty-two typically developed children, who constituted the control group. The task required the ability of sustained attention on a visual target (i.e., a butterfly) while inhibiting a relevant response to look to moving distractors (i.e., trees and clouds), available in the peripheral visual field. Children with RTT had more difficulty in sustaining attention. Thus, the control group averaged 60% looking at the butterfly versus only 25% for the RTT group. Moreover, RTT participants were closely associated with significant difficulties in three basic features modulating the sustained attention: (a) engagement, (b) distractibility, and (c) re-engagement. That is, RTT group was slower to engage, more distractible, and slower to re-engage. A substantial disruption in sustained attention was identified among RTT girls. The specific characteristics of these impairments have been emphasized and cognitive areas have been outlined that could serve as markers to evaluate the effectiveness of pharmacological and behavioural interventions.

Early research has found that there are few literature reviews based on AT interventions for people with RTT. In light of the above, the chapter included a selective review of the last two decades categorizing the use and effectiveness of AT-based programs for people with RTT. Finally, the implications of the findings have been critically argued and some useful insights for future directions in both research and practice have been highlighted.

1.BACKGROUND

AT refers to any piece, device or equipment enabling people with developmental disabilities independence and self-determination towards their environment. The equipments are commonly used to improve functional capacities of persons with disabilities. They ensure people to perform occupation tasks which were formerly inaccessible, by modifying the methods and enhancing the skills necessary to accomplish the tasks (Reichle, 2001). The term may be used narrowly to include special tools used to profitably complete an activity (e.g., a walker), or orthotics (e.g., braces, splints), as well as some adaptive techniques, which allow the activity' s modifications (Hoening, 2004). By using AT an individual with RTT may enhance his/her independence, self-determination, and active role within home, school and/or rehabilitative settings, significantly reducing caregivers' burden, and fostering his/ her inclusion (Lancioni et al., 2012).

Furthermore, AT-based programs might improve the academic performance and the on-task behavior of participants with RTT. The final objective of an AT-based intervention is to enhance the learning process and to seek for its consolidation, generalization and maintenance over the time (Kazdin, 2001). Based on learning principles (i.e., causal link between behavioral responses and environmental events or consequences), an individual with a rare genetic syndrome and severe to profound neurodevelopmental disorders will be enabled to independently tackle daily life requests. Accordingly, constructive engagement, positive participation, and occupation will be fostered and challenging behaviors added to isolation and passivity should be significantly reduced. Both caregivers and families' burden should be relevantly decreased (Perrilli et al, 2019).

Figure 1. Equipment use in RTT. AT most commonly used in families with a dependent with RTT as shown by Leonard's monitoring in 2002.

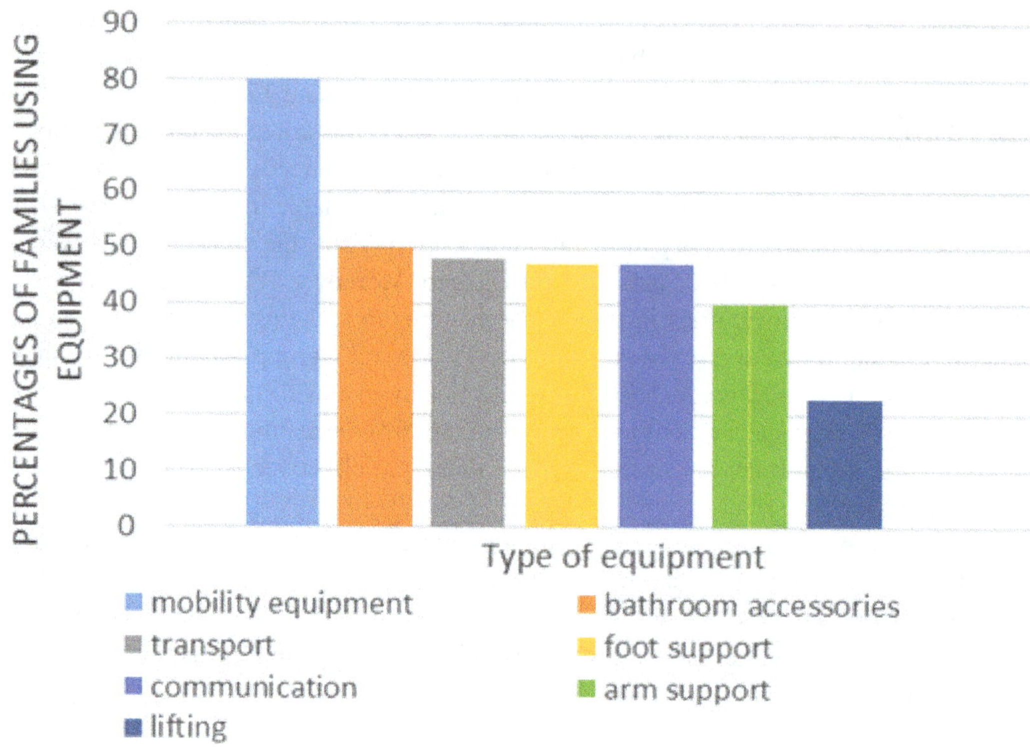

2. METHOD

A computer search was carried out in Scopus, ResearchGate, and PubMed databases. Rare genetic syndromes, RTT, AT, academic performance, ambulation, challenging behavior, communication. constructive engagement, executive functions, locomotion, occupation, and participation were merged as keywords.

The eligibility criteria were (a) an empirical, evidence-based study including an AT-based intervention, (b) children and adolescents as participant, between the ages of 2 and 18; (c) last two decades of publication interval (i.e., 2000-2020), and (d) English as language of the paper. Consequently, twenty-one studies were reviewed with 241 participants included and grouped according to five main categories, namely: (a) adaptive responding, (b) challenging behaviors, (c) communication, (d) executive functions, and (e) locomotion. In the following section, the retained studies were concisely described and a synoptic table summarized the main findings.

3. LITERATURE OVERVIEW

The reviewed studies were arranged in alphabetic order and summarized in Table 1. The reader may note that reviews or theoretical papers were not included because their inclusion would exceed the aim and scope of the current chapter (see above the eligibility criteria in the Method section).

3.1 Adaptive Responding

The first critical issue among individuals with rare genetic syndromes and neurodevelopmental disorders is an adaptive response. Five studies were retained with 21 participants involved. Children with RTT and severe to profound neurodevelopmental and multiple disabilities may experience significant difficulties while dealing with everyday environmental requests. Beside intellectual delays, extensive motor impairments, lack of speech and communication difficulties, they may present sensorial deficits and be unable of an adaptive responding (Stasolla & Ciarmoli, 2020). It is essential that a child or an adolescent with severe to profound multiple disabilities may have an initial minimal response in his/her own behavioral repertoire to be used and optimized during the learning process. Otherwise, an AT-based intervention could not be implemented (Stasolla, Caffò, & Perilli, 2020).

Go (2007) assessed the use of a push-button switch to enable a child with Rett syndrome with the independent access to brief periods of favourite music. A special music keyboard was connected with the pressure switch. The rehabilitative program was designed to recovery neuromuscular disorders and developmental disabilities as a basic mean of adaptive responding. Furthermore, the intervention was planned to improve the participant's quality of life. Results evidenced that the AT-based treatment was effective to ensure a girl with Rett syndrome and severe to profound impairments with play music and actively participate to social life.

Hornof et al. (2017) adapted participatory design techniques to work with five women with RTT, and their families, to design and evaluate new assistive technologies for these women. The process suggested a class of media-playing devices that would be generally useful to women with RTT. Such a system can load multiple audio or video sessions, be activated by many different switches, and respond instantly to switch-hits. Additionally, the system should allow a caregiver to set both the start and the end time of each session. The study also discussed patterns that were observed when collaborating with the families. For example, parents shared longstanding but untried ideas for new assistive technology, and expressed a strong interest in any device that would help their daughters do things for themselves.

Stasolla et al. (2019) evaluated the effectiveness of a microswitch-based intervention on choice making and constructive engagement in a targeted sorting activity, added to indices of happiness (i.e., as an outcome measure of the participants' quality of life), and decreased stereotypic behaviors for six girls with Rett syndrome. Targeted dependent variables were also assessed at a six month post-intervention phase. Following the intervention study, 90 external raters completed a social validation procedure. An ABABAB experimental sequence was implemented for each participant with a cross-over effect. Data emphasized an improved performance for each participant involved (i.e., adaptive responses). Five participants showed a capacity of independent choice. One participant seemed to be closely linked to the behavioral response. Social raters favorably endorsed the use of the program since they positively evaluated the use of the technology on all the investigated dimensions. A microswitch intervention may improve choice making and activity engagement for children with Rett syndrome.

Stasolla et al. (2015) extended the use of assistive technology (i. e. photocells, interface, and personal computers) to support the choice strategies of three girls with Rett syndrome and severe developmental disabilities. A second purpose of the study was to reduce stereotypic behaviors exhibited by the participants involved (i. e. body rocking, hand washing and hand mouthing). Finally, a third goal of the study was to monitor the effects of such program on the participants' indices of happiness. The study was carried out according to a multiple probe design across responses for each participant. Results showed that the three girls increased the adaptive responses and decreased the stereotyped behaviors during intervention phases compared to the baseline. Moreover, during intervention phases, the indices of happiness augmented for each girl as well.

3.2 Challenging Behaviors

This section deals with challenging behavior. Five studies were retained with 106 participants involved. Challenging behavior is broadly defined as a behavior which may be dangerous or deleterious for own or other safety or negatively interfere with a regular learning process (Bowring, Totsika, Hastings, Toogood, & McMahon, 2017). It should be noted that many of the previous reviewed studies addressed their impact on the reduction of stereotypic or challenging behaviors. However, it was considered a secondary outcome. Conversely, in that section, were included studies which addressed the challenging behavior as a primary outcome. Accordingly, the reviewed studies were focused on the microswitch-cluster technology, which pursues the dual simultaneous goal of promoting an adaptive responding and reducing a challenging behavior (Stasolla et al., 2017).

Challenging behaviors (CB) are broadly defined as behaviors that may be dangerous for the own and/or other safety and/or may negatively interfere with the learning process, and/or the normal daily life functioning of individuals with severe to profound developmental disabilities (Noriega & Savelkoul, 2014; Siniscalco, Cirillo, Bradtreet, & Antonucci, 2013). The most common challenging behaviors frequently observed in RTT is represented by hand-related stereotypy and body rocking (Stasolla & Perilli, 2015).

Byiers, Payen, and Symons (2014) enrolled 5 participants with RTT and used direct behavioral observations to quantify and compare their frequency of hand stereotypy and signs of negative affect during presumed periods of high and low stress associated with functional assessment (i.e., negative reinforcement as escape and control as free play respectively). Negative affect was more likely to occur during negative reinforcement (i.e., stress condition) for each participant, whereas hand stereotypy did not differ across conditions for any participant. Although preliminary, the findings suggested that hand stereotypy could not be a valid predictor of behavioral stress-response in girls with RTT. Otherwise, one may argue that the approach used did not adequately evoke a stress response.

Downs et al. (2008) used video-report data provided by parents to describe the gross motor profile of ninety-nine girls with RTT and studied the impact of age, genotype, scoliosis and hand stereotypy. Factor analysis allowed the calculation of general and complex scores of gross motor skills. The majority of the participants were able to sit, slightly less than half were capable of walking, and a minority were able to transfer without assistance. General gross motor skills declined with age, and were poorer in those who had surgically treated scoliosis but not conservatively managed scoliosis. Complex gross motor skills did not decline with age and were higher in those without scoliosis. Motor scores were closely related to the frequency of hand stereotypy.

Lancioni et al. (2014) extended the evidence of microswitch-aided programs in terms of participants involved and responses adopted. One of the two participants in this study was a woman with Rett syndrome. Adults with this syndrome have not been involved in microswitch programs and the possibility of achieving positive effects with her was viewed as relevant for future work with this group of persons. The targeted responses for the two participants consisted respectively of flexible activations of the head and right hand. Flexibility meant that such activations could occur via left or right head movements, or through forward, upward, or downward hand movements. Allowing the participants to use any of several movements (rather than a single/specific one) was thought to make their response easier, given their limited control of their neuro-motor behavior. The possible impact of the program on the participants' mood (happiness) was also assessed. Data showed an increasing in microswitch responses and level of happiness for both participants during the intervention phases of the study.

Mraz et al. (2016) developed a virtual reality (VR)- based therapeutic intervention that (a) decreased upper extremity stereotypies (i.e., repetitive movements that served no function) that interfered with purposeful arm and hand use, (b) promoted purposeful, goal-directed arm function, and (c) improved upper extremity motor skills of a nine-year-old girl with RTT. Using an adapted software and Microsoft Kinect sensor, the participant was exposed to a 12-week VR intervention (i.e., 1 hour/session, 3 sessions/week, 36 total hours). Pre-and post-assessments were administrated to evaluate any modifications in upper extremity function. The VR increased the use of the upper extremities allowing the positive completion of self-care activities, an improvement of reaches completed in a 15-min period, and decreased the stereotypic hand movements.

Perilli et al. (2019) exposed six adolescents with RTT and severe to profound developmental impairments to a microswitch-cluster technology focused on pursuing the dual rehabilitative objective of promoting occupation and reducing hand biting simultaneously. The adaptive responding consisted on inserting three different objects in three different containers within a 4 s time interval. The challenging behavior consisted on hand biting. An ABB^1AB^1 experimental design was implemented. During baselines (i.e., A phases) both behaviors were monitored and recorded. No environmental consequences were delivered by the technological system (i.e., optic sensors and a battery-powered control system unit) even if an adaptive response occurred free of the challenging behavior. During intervention (i.e., B) phase an adaptive response was contingently and positively reinforced irrespective of the simultaneous absence or presence of the challenging behavior. Finally, during the cluster (i.e., B1) phases the adaptive response was contingently reinforced only if occurred totally free of the challenging behavior. Indices of positive participation as sign of constructive engagement and active role were additionally recorded. A social validation assessment with 66 external raters was conducted. A one-year follow-up was carried out. Results demonstrated an improved performance for all the participants who consolidated their learning process over the time (during the follow-up). Indices of positive participation increased as well. Social raters endorsed the use of microswitch-cluster technology.

3.3 Communication

The largest category (i.e., higher number of published studies and participants involved) is represented by communication skills. Four studies were retained with 12 participants involved. Either AT-based programs or cognitive-behavioral interventions, based on learning principles were aimed at promoting communication capacities of individuals with RTT.

Hetzroni et al. (2002) investigated whether the use of AT would support the capacity to recognize symbols by girls with Rett syndrome. Three girls diagnosed at the third clinical stage of the disease were recruited for an individualized educational program. Six types of significant referents (i.e., true name, storybook, food, song, verb, and communication) were used. An individualized multimedia program was created to support the skill to match spoken words to symbols. A multiple probe design across four symbol sets was implemented to evaluate the recognition of graphic and orthographic symbols. Results evidenced a regular learning curve across symbol sets and a partial maintenance of knowledge throughout follow-up probes.

Simacek, Dimian, and Mc Comas (2017) examined the efficacy of parent-implemented communication assessment and intervention with remote coaching via telehealth on the acquisition of early communication skills of three children with RTT (i.e., their age varied between 3 and 5 years). Efficacy of the intervention was evaluated using single-case experimental design. First, functional assessment was adopted to identify idiosyncratic/potentially communicative responses for each child. Next, parents implemented functional communication training (FCT). All of the participants acquired the targeted communication responses. The findings supported the efficacy of telehealth as a service delivered model to coach parents on intervention strategies for enhancing their children's early communication skills.

Stasolla et al. (2014) compared PECS (Picture Exchange Communication System) and VOCA (Vocal Output Communication Aids) intervention strategies to promote communication opportunities for three girls with Rett syndrome and severe to profound developmental disabilities. The first aim of the study was to assess the effectiveness of both aforementioned strategies by enhancing request and choices of preferred items by the participants involved to a caregiver. The second goal of the study was to assess the effects of the intervention program by reducing stereotyped behaviors (i. e. body rocking and hand movements). Finally, the third purpose was to carry out the indices of happiness and monitor quality of life concerning the participants exposed to the intervention program. The study was carried out according to an alternating treatments design with a final preference check phase for each participant. Results showed an increasing of independent requested and chosen items as well as of indices of happiness during intervention phases for all participants. Moreover, two of them chose VOCA strategy during preference checks phase, while the third one equally chose both strategies.

Woodyatt and Ozanne (1992) investigated the intent of the interactive behaviors of six females with Rett syndrome through observation. The authors found that the nonverbal behaviors exhibited by the children in the study were pre-intentional. Caregivers, therefore, should recognize nonverbal behaviors as possible attempts to communicate and seek to determine the intent of these behaviors when responding to them. A 3-year-old child with Rett syndrome was presented with four computer games over the course of 8 months that elicited specific behaviors, including reaching, kicking, visual regard, and vocalization. These games allowed the child to express preference and were intended to improve the child's social interaction skills. The results showed how interactions between the child and computer games increased the ability of preference and intention. Finally, a preschool-age child with Rett syndrome was presented with two switches that could be activated by her head or hand. After pressing the two switches, the child was presented with toys as part of contingent reinforcement regimen. Data revealed that the child quickly mastered the use of the head switch; however, use of the hand switch was less frequent and more variable.

3.4 Executive Functions

Next to other groups, executive functions are usually considered essential for a steady information cognitive processing. Individuals with rare genetic diseases, neurodevelopmental disorders, and intellectual disabilities may systematically fail in executive functions. AT-based protocols and trainings may be relevant to visual attention, procedural or working memory, and speed processing. Three studies were retained with 87 participants involved.

Fabio et al. (2019) explored three cognitive processes in 21 girls with Rett syndrome matched to typically developed peers (i.e., twenty-one girls). The three cognitive functions explored were: (a) the ability to deal with visual stimuli, (b) the ability to identify identical stimuli, and (c) the ability to identify similar stimuli. Through an eye-tracking technology, three different tasks were proposed, namely (a) attention, (b) identification of identical stimuli, and (c) identification of similar stimuli. Results underlined that girls with Rett syndrome had lower performances than their peers in all the cognitive tasks and experimental conditions. Lack of meaningful interactions between groups and the type of task and between groups and contents suggested that the attention behavior in girls with Rett syndrome was significantly impaired and reflected a broad delay in cognitive development.

Rose et al. (2012) examined attention and recognition memory for faces and patterns in Rett syndrome, a severely disabling neurodevelopmental disorder caused by mutations in the X-linked MECP2 gene. Because Rett syndrome impaired speech and hand use, precluding most neuropsychological testing, the visual paired-comparison paradigm (VPC) was used, together with eye tracking. In the VPC, two identical stimuli were presented for familiarization. On test, the familiar stimulus and a new one was paired, and recognition inferred from preferential looking to the novel target. Attention was measured by recording time, gaze dispersion, and number/length of fixations. Twenty-seven females with Rett syndrome (mean age 10 years, age range 2–22 years) from the Rett clinic at a children's hospital were assessed in this study, along with 30 age- and sex-matched typically developing participants (outpatients from the same hospital). Although patients with Rett syndrome showed recognition of both faces and patterns, with novelty scores greater than chance (50%), their performance was significantly poorer compared to the typically developing comparison group. Their attention to both was less mature and marked by a more narrowly focused gaze, with fewer and longer fixations. When inspecting faces, attention to the eyes was similar in both groups. However, patients with Rett syndrome tended to ignore the nose and mouth.

Wandin et al. (2020) carried out a two-phases study focused on developing a tool finalized at assessing visual attention in individuals with Rett syndrome using an aided-alternative and augmentative strategy (AAC) with a communication partner during naturalistic interactions in clinical settings. Moreover, the tool's reliability, validity, and usability were evaluated. The assessment of visual attention in interaction (AVAI) tool was developed to visual attention operationalized at the communication partner, a symbol or an object. Along the study six video-recorded interactions of 9 girls with Rett syndrome were analyzed. Intra- and inter-rater agreements were additionally considered. A strong difference emerged in the AVAI between conditions (i.e., with or without aided-language modeling). Results suggested that AVAI differentiated the participants. The AVAI was reliable, valid and socially accepted by the participants.

3.5 Locomotion

Beside cognitive processes and communication skills, motor abilities with balance, posture, gait, ambulation, and locomotion may be seriously compromised among individuals with RTT and neurodevelopmental disorders. Accordingly, AT-based programs based on learning principles may be supportive and motivating in executing single step responses and/or locomotion fluency (Stasolla, Caffò, et al., 2019). Four studies were retained with 10 participants involved.

Pizzamiglio et al. (2008), explored the possibility of rehabilitating purposeful use of the hands and hand-eye coordination in individuals with RTT. A child affected by RTT, received experimental, computerized visual-motor coordination training and a sensory-motor rehabilitative program specifically designed and based on Piaget's (1937) theory of cognitive development. After 3 years of therapy, the participant partially regained the use of her hands as an instrument of object knowledge and as a means of communicating with people.

Schafer and Norah (2015), described the process of selecting an assistive device for a child with RTT to promote ambulation. A 5-year-old girl with RTT was enrolled. The child was able to perform the farthest distances with a metal toy shopping cart and with an anterior facing four-wheeled walker. The result suggested that physiotherapists and health professionals caring for young children with RTT should consider using a shopping trolley. of a metal toy to establish and practise walking before choosing a longer-term adjustable front walker, such as the one in this case.

Stasolla and Caffò (2017), assessed a microswitch-based program to improve self-determination to access to preferred stimuli and to foster locomotor behavior by two girls with Rett syndrome and multiple disabilities. To enhance the first behavior (access to preferred stimuli) a wobble microswitch (sensitive touch sensor) was used while for the second behavior (step responses) optic sensors were applied. A second aim of the study was to monitor indices of happiness as consequence of the use of assistive technology. Finally, a third objective of the study was the reduction of hand washing and body rocking related stereotypies. The study was carried out according to a multiple probe design across behaviors for both participants, where the two behaviors were first learned independently, then combined together. Results showed an increasing of performance and of indices of happiness and a decreasing of stereotyped behaviors for both participants during intervention phases.

Stasolla et al. (2017), extended the use of a microswitch-based program for assessing contingency awareness and promoting locomotion fluency of five adolescents with Rett syndrome. A second goal was to evaluate the effectiveness and the suitability of the rehabilitative intervention on participants' indices of happiness as outcome measure of their quality of life and on the reduction of their stereotypic behaviors. Finally, a social validation procedure involving 40 parents of children with severe developmental disabilities and 40 caregivers was carried out. The study was conducted according to an ABABCBCB experimental sequence for each participant, with A representing baselines, B indicating the contingent intervention closely linked to the adaptive responding, and C reporting a non-contingent control phase with positive stimulation occurring throughout the session, irrespective of the adaptive behavior. Results showed an improved performance for all the participants during contingent intervention phases. The control phases revealed that all participants acquired the contingency awareness. The indices of happiness increased as sign of an enhanced quality of life. Both groups of raters favorably scored the use of such technology.

4.DISCUSSION

This review demonstrated the validity, suitability, and effectiveness of using AT-based programs for children with RTT to enable self-determined pleasurable stimuli and increase their independence by addressing problems in locomotion, communication, executive functions, adaptive responses and reduction of challenging behaviors. Whenever available, social validation procedures, preference checks, maintenance or follow-up phases confirmed social and clinical validities of the adopted programs, which were consolidated over the time. Essentially, AT-based programs functionally filled the existing gap between the individual skills and the environmental requests. Individuals with RTT and multiple disabilities will be ensured with an independent access to positive stimulation. A beneficial coping will be outlined with positive outcomes on the participants' quality of life (Amoako & Hare, 2020). The findings suggested the following considerations.

First, AT-based programs have been helpful in improving the independence and self-determination in daily life of individuals with RTT. Thus, by using AT devices or setups the gap between behavioural and cognitive abilities and environmental demands was favorably bridged. An active role was promoted and the centrality of the individual was emphasised. The participants enrolled in the retained studies successfully performed the required responses and tasks and their behaviour seemed to be purposeful.

Consequently, it could be argued that the fulfilment and motivation were adequately reinforced and positively satisfied (Alquraini & Rao, 2020; Cook, Adams, Encarnacao, & Alvarez, 2012).

Second, challenging behaviours through microswitch-cluster technology were significantly reduced. That is, although challenging behaviour has been targeted in many studies, interventions with microswitch-clusters have targeted the simultaneous dual goals of promoting an adaptive response and decreasing challenging behaviour as a primary outcome, ensuring through the use of technology a positive reinforcement contingency or feedback on the contingency itself (Lancioni et al., 2007, 2009).

Third, communication skills were promoted through the use of technological equipment, fostering social interactions and enhancing participants' constructive engagement. Consequently, both caregivers and teachers' burden were reduced. The participants' constructive engagement was enhanced accordingly. Their positive participation to social life was additionally consolidated (Townend, Bartolotta, Urbanowicz, Wandin, & Curfs, 2020).

Fourth, executive functions were supported. In this way, attention, procedural and working memory were encouraged through AT-mediated cognitive training. It can be argued that AT-based programs and computer-based systems were effective in assessing and recovering cognitive functions with beneficial results on participants' involvement in academic life (Arthanat, Curtin, & Knotak, 2013).

Fifth, gait, appropriate posture, gait responses and locomotion fluency improved by relying on basic forms of AT such as microswitches and contingent positive stimulation were useful to highly motivate and reward individuals with rare genetic diseases while performing one-step responses or locomotion fluency (Lancioni et al., 2003, 2004). Gait and posture were fostered accordingly.

5. CONCLUSION

Assistive technologies provide people with RTT with the ability to self-determine their favourite stimuli and increase their independence by avoiding social isolation. Various categories of assistive technologies have been examined to help and manage some of the symptoms of RTT.

The current chapter identified five different groups of studies (adaptive responses, challenging behaviors, communication, executive functions and mobility) for patients with RTT. There were few studies on AT in RTT and more specifically on the use of AT in executive functions and challenging behaviors. New technological and sophisticated options should be designed and implemented to meet both human expertise and financial resources. Both qualitative and quantitative analyses should be considered in the future. In addition, further experimental phases of follow-up, generalisation, maintenance and preference control can be envisaged to assess participants' choices combined with consolidation of learning over time and in different settings.

6. FUTURE RESEARCH

In the light of the above, future research should extend the number of samples examined in empirical contributions, include additional technological and individualised solutions to meet more complex needs of the participants involved by considering (where possible) more sophisticated targeted behaviors. Whenever available, virtual reality technologies (e. g., serious games) could be used. Wearable technologies focused on promoting locomotion, posture, and gait might additionally be adopted. Telerehabilitation should be widely implemented to allow patients to remain in a highly comfortable and safe environment. Communication with distant partners could also have a positive impact on people with RTT, who could easily communicate in the Covid-19 pandemic era.

REFERENCES

Amoako, A. N., & Hare, D. J. (2020). Non-medical interventions for individuals with Rett syndrome: A systematic review. *Journal of Applied Research in Intellectual Disabilities*, *33*(5), 808–827. doi:10.1111/jar.12694 PMID:31833197

Bowring, D. L., Totsika, V., Hastings, R. P., Toogood, S., & McMahon, M. (2017). Prevalence of psychotropic medication use and association with challenging behavior in adults with an intellectual disability. A total population Study. *Journal of Intellectual Disability Research*, *61*(6), 604–617. doi:10.1111/jir.12359 PMID:28090687

Downs, J. A., Bebbington, A., Jacoby, P., Msall, M. E., Mcllroy, O., Fyfe, S., ... Leonard, H. (2008). Gross motor profile in Rett syndrome as determined by video analysis. *Neuropediatrics*, *39*(04), 205–210. doi:10.1055-0028-1104575 PMID:19165708

Fabio, R. A., Giannatiempo, S., & Caprì, T. (2019). Attention and identification of the same and the similar visual stimuli in Rett syndrome. *Life Span and Disability*, *22*, 113–127.

Felce, D., & Perry, J. (1995). Quality of life: Its definition and measurement. *Research in Developmental Disabilities*, *16*(1), 51–74. doi:10.1016/0891-4222(94)00028-8 PMID:7701092

Giesbers, S., Didden, R., Radstaake, M., Korzilius, H., Gontard, A., & Lang, R. (2012). Incontinence in individuals with Rett syndrome: A comparative study. *Journal of Developmental and Physical Disabilities*, *24*(3), 287–300. doi:10.100710882-012-9271-7 PMID:22639525

Goo, T. (2007). Medical music therapy based on baby science (baby-science-based music therapy) and assistive technology for children. *Current Pediatric Reviews*, *3*(3), 198–206. doi:10.2174/157339607781369573

Hetzroni, O., Rubin, C., & Konkol, O. (2002). The use of assistive technology for symbol identification by children with Rett syndrome. *Journal of Intellectual & Developmental Disability*, *27*(1), 57–71. doi:10.1080/13668250120119626-1

Hoenig, H. (2004). Assistive technology and mobility aids for the older patient with disability. *The Annals of Long-Term Care: the Official Journal of the American Medical Directors Association*, *12*, 12–13.

Hornof, A., Whitman, H., Sutherland, M., Gerendasy, S., & McGrenere, J. (2017). Designing for the "universe of one": Personalized interactive media systems for people with the severe cognitive impairment associated with Rett syndrome. *Conference on Human Factors in Computing Systems - Proceedings*, 2137-2148. 10.1145/3025453.3025904

Hornof, A., Whitman, H., Sutherland, M., Gerendasy, S., & McGrenere, J. (2017). Designing for the "Universe of One": Personalized Interactive Media Systems for People with the Severe Cognitive Impairment Associated with Rett Syndrome. *Perspectives on Cognitive Impairment*, *8*, 546–558. doi:10.1145/3025453.3025904

Kazdin, A. E. (2001). *Behavior modification in applied settings*. Wadsworth: Thomson Learning.

Lancioni, G. E., Sigafoos, J., O'Reilly, M. F., & Singh, N. N. (2012). *Assistive technology: Interventions for individuals with severe/profound and multiple disabilities*. Springer.

Lotan, M. (2006). Management of Rett Syndrome in the Controlled Multisensory (Snoezelen) Environment. A Review with Three Case Stories. *The Scientific World Journal*, *6*, 791–807. doi:10.1100/tsw.2006.159 PMID:16830051

Marz, K., Eisenberg, G., Diener, P., Amadio, G., Foreman, M. H., & Engsberg, J. R. (2016). The effects of virtual reality on the upper extremity skills of girls with Rett syndrome: A single case study. *Journal of Intellectual Disability - Diagnosis and Treatment, 4,* 152-159.

Neul, J. L., Kaufmann, W. E., Glaze, D. G., Christodoulou, J., Clarke, A. J., Bahi-Buisson, N., ... Percy, A. K. (2010). Rett syndrome: Revised diagnostic criteria and nomenclature. *Annals of Neurology*, *68*(6), 944–950. doi:10.1002/ana.22124 PMID:21154482

Noriega, D. B., & Savelkoul, H. F. J. (2014). Immune dysregulation in autism spectrum disorder. *European Journal of Pediatrics*, *173*(1), 33–43. doi:10.100700431-013-2183-4 PMID:24297668

Perilli, V., Stasolla, F., Caffò, A. O., Albano, V., & D'Amico, F. (2019). Microswitch-cluster technology for promoting occupation and reducing hand biting of six adolescents with fragile X syndrome: New evidence and social rating. *Journal of Developmental and Physical Disabilities*, *31*(1), 115–133. doi:10.100710882-018-9634-9

Pizzamiglio, M. R., Vitturini, C., Piccardi, L., & Spitoni, G. (2008). Sensor-Motor Rehabilitation in Rett Syndrome: A Case Report. *Focus on Autism and Other Developmental Disabilities*, *23*(1), 49–62. doi:10.1177/1088357607311446

Reichle, J. (2011). Evaluating assistive technology in the education of persons with severe disabilities. *Journal of Behavioral Education*, *20*(1), 77–85. doi:10.100710864-011-9121-1

Rett, A. (1966). Uber ein eigenartigers himatrophisches syndrom bei hyperamonaemie im kinsalter. *Wiener Medizinische Wochenschrift*, *116*, 723–728. PMID:5300597

Rose, A. S., Djukic, A., Janjowski, J., Feldman, J. F., Fishman, I., & McDermott, M. V. (2012). Rett syndrome: An eye-tracking study of attention and recognition memory. *Developmental Medicine and Child Neurology*, *8*, 301–302. PMID:23488948

Rose, S. A., Wass, S., Jankowski, J. J., Feldman, J. F., & Djukic, A. (2017). Sustained attention in the face of distractors: A study of children with Rett syndrome. *Neuropsychology*, *31*(4), 403–410. doi:10.1037/neu0000369 PMID:28383972

Schaefer, C., & Norah, L. J. (2014). Fostering Ambulation for a Preschool Child with Rett Syndrome: A Case Report. *College of Nursing Faculty Research and Publications*, *323*, 1–12.

Sigafoos, J., O'Reilly, M. F., Ledbetter-Cho, K., Lim, N., Lancioni, G. E., & Marschik, P. B. (2019). Addressing sequelae of developmental regression associated with developmental disabilities: A systematic review of behavioral and educational intervention studies. *Neuroscience and Biobehavioral Reviews*, *96*, 56–71. doi:10.1016/j.neubiorev.2018.11.014 PMID:30481529

Simacek, J., Dimian, A. F., & McComas, J. J. (2017). Communication intervention for young children with severe neurodevelopmental disabilities via telehealth. *Journal of Autism and Developmental Disorders*, *47*(3), 744–767. doi:10.100710803-016-3006-z PMID:28093677

Siniscalco, D., Cirillo, A., Bradstreet, J. J., & Antonucci, N. (2013). Epigenetic findings in autism: New perspectives for therapy. *International Journal of Environmental Research and Public Health*, *10*(9), 4261–4273. doi:10.3390/ijerph10094261 PMID:24030655

Stasolla, F., & Caffò, A. O. (2013). Promoting adaptive behaviors by two girls with Rett syndrome through a microswitch-based program. *Research in Autism Spectrum Disorders*, *7*(10), 1265–1272. doi:10.1016/j.rasd.2013.07.010

Stasolla, F., Caffò, A. O., & Perilli, V. (2020). Fostering inclusion of children and adolescents with autism spectrum disorders in daily settings through technological supports: A selective overview. In Y. Kats & F. Stasolla (Eds.), *Education and technology support for children and young adults with ASD and learning disabilities* (pp. 224–245). IGI Global.

Stasolla, F., Caffò, A. O., Perilli, V., & Albano, V. (2019). Experimental Examination and Social Validation of a Microswitch Intervention to Improve Choice-Making and Activity Engagement for Six Girls with Rett Syndrome. *Developmental Neurorehabilitation*, *22*(8), 527–541. doi:10.1080/17518423.2019.1624655 PMID:31169045

Stasolla, F., Caffò, A. O., Perilli, V., Boccasini, A., Damiani, R., & D'Amico, F. (2019). Assistive technology for promoting adaptive skills of children with cerebral palsy: Ten cases evaluation. *Disability and Rehabilitation. Assistive Technology*, *14*(5), 489–502. doi:10.1080/17483107.2018.1467972 PMID:29732901

Stasolla, F., Caffò, A. O., Perilli, V., Boccasini, A., Stella, A., Damiani, R., & Damato, C. (2017). A microswitch-based program for promoting initial ambulation responses: An evaluation with two girls with multiple disabilities. *Journal of Applied Behavior Analysis*, *50*(2), 345–356. doi:10.1002/jaba.374 PMID:28128442

Stasolla, F., Caffò, A. O., Perrilli, V., Boccasini, A., Damiani, R., & D'Amico, F. (2017). Fostering Locomotion Fluency of Five Adolescents with Rett Syndrome through a Microswitch-Based Program: Contingency Awareness and Social Rating. *Journal of Developmental and Physical Disabilities*, *30*(2), 239–258. doi:10.100710882-017-9582-9

Stasolla, F., & Ciarmoli, D. (2020). Supporting Adaptive Responding and Reducing Challenging Behaviors of Children with Rare Genetic Syndromes and Severe to Profound Developmental Disabilities Through Assistive Technology-Based Programs. *International Journal of Behavioral Research & Psychology*, *8*, 1–3. doi:10.19070/2332-3000-2000010e

Stasolla, F., Damiani, R., Perilli, V., Di Leone, A., Albano, V., Stella, A., & Damato, C. (2014). Technological supports to promote choice opportunities by two boys with fragile X syndrome and severe to profound developmental disabilities. *Research in Developmental Disabilities*, *35*(11), 2993–3000. doi:10.1016/j.ridd.2014.07.045 PMID:25118066

Stasolla, F., De Pace, C., Damiani, R., Di Leone, A., Albano, V., & Perrilli, V. (2014). Comparing PECS and VOCA to promote communication opportunities and to reduce stereotyped behaviors by three girls with Rett syndrome. *Research in Autism Spectrum Disorders*, *8*(10), 1269–1278. doi:10.1016/j.rasd.2014.06.009

Stasolla, F., & Perilli, V. (2015). Assistive technology to promote communication, leisure, occupation skills by children with Rett syndrome and severe to profound developmental disabilities: A literature overview. In D. Kolby (Ed.), *Rett syndrome and other communication disorders: Symptoms, treatments and Prognosis* (pp. 32–48). Nova Publisher.

Stasolla, F., & Perilli, V. (2015). Microswitch-based programs (MBP) to promote communication, occupation, and leisure skills for children with multiple disabilities: a literature overview. In N. R. Silton (Ed.), *Recent advances in assistive technologies to support children with developmental disorders* (pp. 195–216). Nova Science Publishers. doi:10.4018/978-1-4666-8395-2.ch009

Stasolla, F., Perrilli, V., Di Leone, A., Damiani, R., Albano, V., Stella, A., & Damato, C. (2015). Technological aids to support choice strategies by three girls with Rett syndrome. *Research in Developmental Disabilities*, *36*, 36–44. doi:10.1016/j.ridd.2014.09.017 PMID:25310833

Wandin, H., Lindberg, P., & Sonnander, K. (2020). Development of a tool to assess visual attention in Rett syndrome: A pilot study. *AAC: Augmentative and Alternative Communication*, *36*, 118–127. PMID:32791851

Woodyatt, G., & Ozanne, C. (1992). Breaking the silence in Rett Syndrome. *Nature Genetics*, *23*, 127–128. PMID:10508498

ADDITIONAL READING

Huisman, S., Mulder, P., Kuijk, J., Kerstholt, M., van Eeghen, A., Leenders, A., van Balkom, I., Oliver, C., Piening, S., & Hennekam, R. (2018). Self-injurious behavior. *Neuroscience and Biobehavioral Reviews*, *84*, 483–491. doi:10.1016/j.neubiorev.2017.02.027 PMID:28694012

Kouroupetroglou, G. (2014). *Assistive technologies and computer access for motor disabilities*. IGI Global. doi:10.4018/978-1-4666-4438-0

Lancioni, G. E., & Singh, N. N. (2014). *Assistive technologies for people with diverse abilities*. Springer. doi:10.1007/978-1-4899-8029-8

Sigafoos, J., Kagohara, D., Van Der Meer, L., Green, V. A., O'Reilly, M. F., Lancioni, G. E., Lang, R., Rispoli, M., & Zisimopoulos, D. (2011). Communication assessment for individuals with Rett syndrome: A systematic review. *Research in Autism Spectrum Disorders*, *5*(2), 692–700. doi:10.1016/j.rasd.2010.10.006

Stasolla, F. (2020). *Understanding children with cerebral palsy*. Nova Publisher.

Wadhera, T., & Kakkar, D. (2020). *Interdisciplinary Approaches to Altering Neurodevelopmental Disorders*. IGI Global. doi:10.4018/978-1-7998-3069-6

KEY TERMS AND DEFINITIONS

Assistive Technology: Umbrella term including any piece, device, tool, or equipment enabling self-determination and independence in individuals with developmental disorders.

Quality of Life: Complex psychological construct which includes pleasure, satisfaction, fulfilment, well-being, and happiness.

Rare Genetic Syndromes: Medical conditions caused by inherited gene mutations. These can be passed down from parents to children and run along families.

Rett Syndrome: Progressive neuro-developmental disorder, X-linked, caused by mutations of MECP2 gene, located on Xq28 chromosome.

Chapter 8
Family-Centered Telehealth Supporting Motor Skills and Activity in Individuals With Rett Syndrome

Meir Lotan
Ariel University, Israel

Michelle Stahlhut
https://orcid.org/0000-0002-4551-5265
Rigshospitalet, Denmark

Alberto Romano
https://orcid.org/0000-0001-9774-2964
Italian Rett Association (AIRett), Italy

Jenny Downs
https://orcid.org/0000-0001-7358-9037
Telethon Kids Institute, Australia

Cochavit Elefant
University of Haifa, Israel

ABSTRACT

Rett syndrome is a rare genetically caused condition associated with severe disability and impaired motor functions. Local therapists typically see small numbers of affected individuals, and this limits their capacity to gain experience. Telehealth is being used increasingly to counter poor access to rehabilitation services. Moreover, there is a need to develop management plans that support individuals with Rett syndrome over their lifespan. Three projects in which telehealth support was provided by therapists experienced in Rett syndrome and supported by available local resources are presented in this chapter. The three projects responded to locally identified needs in a cost-efficient way and empowered those working with people with Rett syndrome to maintain and improve their clients' physical function and activity. This chapter will discuss the conceptual underpinnings of delivering a service using a telehealth approach and describe the results and the strategies implemented in the projects mentioned above.

DOI: 10.4018/978-1-7998-7430-0.ch008

INTRODUCTION

Remote Telehealth Services

Telehealth services (THS) are the goal-oriented use of various remote technology applications, such as mobile phone, computer, computer sharing, and television applications, to access individuals who need rehabilitation services. Telehealth services are managed by professionals and have explicit goals as with other rehabilitation (Salminen et al., 2016). The development of THS has responded to the need to reduce medical costs, to provide professional expertise with rare syndromes from a central location, and to counter long distances to access health services, especially for those living in rural areas (Patel et al., 2012). These challenges have challenged the development of cost-effective and technology-based solutions to provide remote health care and rehabilitation. Telehealth services might help to solve the problems related to patient access to rehabilitation, therapies, or physician expertise. Such technology could extend or replace some outpatient care or rehabilitation processes (Calouro et al., 2014) There are many areas where THS have been found useful in evaluation (Mani et al., 2017) and therapeutic settings, including for cardiac patients (Anttila et al., 2019), neurological rehabilitation (Jagos et al., 2015), orthopedics (Bell et al., 2019), improvement of adaptive skills (Caprì et al., 2021) and physiotherapy (Gal et al., 2015). Most of these intervention projects have been implemented with individuals with less severe disability. The question is, can individuals with severe disability, such as those diagnosed with Rett syndrome (RTT), benefit from technologically advanced medical and therapy services, such as THS?

Rett Syndrome (RTT)

RTT is a neurological disorder mostly found in females and is caused by a mutation in the MECP2 gene (Amir et al., 1999). The child with RTT has apparently initial normal psychomotor development during the first 6-18 months but then presents with regression in language, gross motor, and manual skills. The hallmark of the disease includes the onset of repetitive stereotypical hand movements which appear during the regression period (Neul et al., 2010). Comorbidities associated with RTT usually include the development of scoliosis by approximately 80% of those diagnosed (Downs et al., 2016) and seizures occurring in 50%-85% of individuals (Glaze et al., 2010). Many females with RTT will survive into adulthood (Anderson et al., 2014). Therefore, setting achievable long-term therapeutic goals for these individuals over the lifespan is vital (Cass et al., 2003). Therapies for RTT have had some success when delivered in clinic (Budden, 1995) or school settings (Elefant, 2001). Several studies have investigated the application of an enriched therapeutic environment to small samples of individuals with RTT. Although evidence is limited, these examples suggest that programs can maintain and even increase gross motor function and wellbeing (Downs et al., 2018; Lotan et al., 2012). Recent reviews on rehabilitation interventions show that individuals with RTT can achieve functional improvements in gross motor, fine motor, and communication skills (Amoako & Hare, 2020; Fonzo et al., 2020; Lim et al., 2020). Cumulative evidence suggests that intensive, high-quality, ecologically focused interventions at a young age can yield significant positive results. Therefore, most research projects, including those targeting people with RTT are aimed at participants at younger ages (Ramey & Ramey, 1998).

Telehealth Services and Rett Syndrome

As with other rare disorders, those affected by RTT are scattered geographically, and individual medical practitioners and therapists typically see small numbers of individuals. This limits the capacity of local therapists working hands-on with this population to develop specific expertise to provide the very best care. However, some practitioners and therapists who, often because of particular research interest in the condition, have developed specialist expertise, but their geographical location is distant from many families. There is a need to develop and test cost-effective mechanisms by which therapists with expertise in a rare disorder can provide support to families or caregivers over long distances. This service delivery model to local home and community settings could support optimal functioning in individuals with RTT. Recently, an interactive school program have been provided to children and young adults with RTT during the COVID-19 pandemic (Dovigo et al., 2021). This program promoted social and cognitive interactions. As such Telehealth services in RTT could be a promising opportunity within several areas of health care.

This chapter will describe the conceptual underpinnings for three Telehealth projects within the field of physical therapy which have been implemented in different regions of Europe for individuals with RTT. These projects involved individuals with RTT in Ireland, the second in Sicily, and the third in northern Italy. We present models for planning and evaluation, using a Participatory Action Research (PAR) within the Family-Centered Care (FCC) approach and the Goal Attainment Scale (GAS) as an outcome measure, suitable for a research population presenting a broad functional range. The here presented projects proposed a combination of a direct (in vivo) functional and environmental assessment of the participants with a remote-conducted supervision of a therapeutic activities program implementation by local resources. Therefore, a strict combination of the remote practice with direct intervention is proposed as a model to cope with the difficulties that occurred when telehealth is applied to physical therapy for people with developmental disorders such as RTT.

CONCEPTUAL UNDERPINNINGS TO APPLICATION OF TELEHEALTH SERVICES FOR RTT

Planning Individually-Adapted Physical Therapy Programs for Telehealth Delivery

At initial contact with each family, we evaluated the availability of the family and participant to be involved in a physical intervention program. Our decision-making process was then based on the framework of the Rehab-CYCLE developed by Stucki and Sangha (Stucki & Sangha, 1998) and the "Rehabilitation Problem Solving Form" which are based on the ICF model (World Health Organization, 2007), used to identify specific and relevant target problems, discern factors that cause or contribute to these problems, and after that plan the most appropriate interventions (Steiner et al., 2002). The Rehab-CYCLE is an ICF-based tool characterized with a problem-solving approach that can facilitate the structuring, organization and documentation of the rehabilitation process including the coordination and a multidisciplinary team. It comprises four key elements integrated in an iterative process aimed to comprehensively describe the functioning of persons experiencing disability, to guide the planning of functioning-oriented rehabilitation services and evaluate changes in the functioning status over a certain time period. The four key elements in the Rehab-CYCLE are the following: assessment (aimed at understanding a person functioning and identifying the needs to be addressed with a rehabilitative intervention), assignment (of identified relevant therapeutic objectives to specific interventions and appropriate healthcare professionals), intervention (the individual team member selects a suitable intervention and appropriate instruments to pursue the identified objective using an evidence-based and hypothesis-driven approach), and evaluation (each team member conducts an evaluation of the impact of the intervention using a previously selected evaluation tools, this element comprises the tam discussion on how the Rehab-CYCLE proceeded) (Rauch et al., 2008). In the ICF model, non-problematic aspects of health are summarized under the umbrella term "functioning," whereas "disability" serves as an umbrella term for impairments, activity limitations, or participation restrictions. The ICF model describes ingredients related to human functioning and disability and serves as a framework to organize information.

By using such definitions, statements specifying the influence of different aspects such as functioning or disability as well as environmental factors as facilitators or barriers on gross motor function were evaluated using the following elements:

1. **Body structures/functions:** Relates to the health condition of the participants (e.g., what are the child's health issues and abilities?).
2. **Coping strategies:** Measures the level of child and family's readiness to participate (e.g., what is the reaction of the child and family to the performed exercise?).
3. **Mediators:** Elements that influence the individual with RTT either directly or indirectly. They are divided into supportive mediators or resources, and adverse mediators or barriers.
    a. Resources: Elements that can support the program implementation (e.g., are there adult children who can provide assistance to the parents, a socio-economic situation with relevant resources, or supportive grandparents living close by).
    b. Barriers - Elements that can prevent the program implementation (e.g., how many small children are in the family and at what ages? How many jobs are held by the parents? Are there any background health limitations of the parents\other children or a poor socio-economic situation?).
    c. Availability: Hourly availability of the individual with RTT and the people involved in carrying out the program (e.g., how many hours is the individual with RTT at home every day? How many hours a day are other family members who can contribute at home with the participant?).
4. **Environmental factors:** Characteristics of the environment in which the family lives (e.g., does the family live in a rural area, by the sea, near a mountain or a forest? What environmental settings are available in the surroundings?).
5. **Motivational factors/facilitators:** Elements that positively modify the motivation of the individual with RTT. (e.g., What does she like? What motivates her to initiate and complete an action?).

Therefore, a 4-point scale that codes all the elements mentioned above according to the ICF model's coding structure was developed (see Table 1).

Although personal factors or resources are essential in the rehabilitation process (Lorish et al., 1991), they are not classified within the ICF model due to the significant social and cultural variance associated with them (World Health Organization, 2007). Yet, this is a crucial part affecting adherence to the program by most girls with RTT. Therefore, personal factors relevant to each participant were included within the scoring system to guide the development of a specific, individually tailored intervention

Table 1. Consideration of personal characteristics of participants

Term / Level	0	1	3	4	Score
Body structures / Functions	There are many limitations and few functions.	There are few limitations and some functions.	There are very few limitations and moderate functions.	There are no limitations.	
Coping strategies	Both child and parents negate the presented exercises.	The child or parents present some personal restrictions.	There are but few personal restrictions presented by the child or parents.	The family is willing and excited to participate.	
Positive mediators - Resources	There is no support for the program.	Some aspects are supporting the program, and some are negating the implementation of the program.	Most aspects are supporting the program, and some are negating the implementation of the program.	The family's situation highly supports all aspects of the program.	
Negative mediators - Barriers	Many aspects are preventing this program from happening.	Some aspects are supporting, and some are negating the implementation of the program.	Most aspects support the program, and few negate the implementation of the program.	There are no factors negatively influencing the performance of the activity program.	
Availability	The child and parents have no time to perform the program.	The family has a restricted timetable to implement the program.	The child and parents have a fluent timetable enabling program implementation	Both child and parents have unlimited time to implement the program.	
Environmental factors	The environmental factors do not support the implementation of the program.	The environmental factors have few advantages and mostly disadvantages in implementing the program.	The environmental factors have some advantages and few disadvantages in program implementation.	The environmental factors fully support the implementation of the program (live close to appropriate social attractors).	
Motivational factors	The child does not seem to be interested in anything	The child has a but limited number of motivational factors	The child has some motivational factors	The child has many motivational factors (food, music, dance, social interaction)	
Total score for the participant					

program. Participants and families receiving a score less than 14 are considered paerticipants with less resources to perform the program and adhere to it. Therefore, they should only be asked to participate if resources can be improved, or barriers removed (an example: if the mother is pregnant for instance then starting the program after the birth could be more suitable).

The researchers would like to emphasize that this should not be a one-sided decision-making process by the researchers but an ongoing discussion between the researchers and the parents. For example, discussions could indicate motivational factors that are overlooked or suggest simple resources within the household appliances to enable rehabilitation. This process improved communication between the researchers and the participating families and enabled the construction of an intervention program specifically tailored to each participant and her family.

The programs were performed using Skype or Zoom technologies. However, the authors emphasize that any direct video-based technology enabling real-time observation of the participants [Skype, WhatsApp video, Zoom and others] are all likely to achieve similar outcomes. Similar to others (Steiner et al., 2002), we recommend routine checks and revision of goals in rehabilitation programs for complex conditions such as RTT. During the calls the researchers were guided by the Rehab-CYCLE model (Stucki & Sangha, 1998) to revise the program and adapt it in relation to problems or success mentioned by the family members during program implementation. Such decisions should be taken to meet the individual's expectations or needs while always considering the researchers' practical, clinical, and evidence-based knowledge regarding RTT.

Due to phenotypic variability, individuals with RTT present a variety of clinical presentations and family needs. When implementing programs within such a population, the program's effectiveness may depend on the personal characteristics of each client and their family. For a heterogenic population such as this, no 'one type fits all' therapy can be defined. Therefore, the therapist should seek to understand the participants and be able to adapt intervention techniques to each individual and family, focusing on their specific needs. When evaluating the child and family's abilities and needs, the therapist should work within the ICF model suggested by Steiner and associates (Steiner et al., 2002) and take into account all elements which might have negative (barriers) and positive (resources) effect on the suggested program including the client and family physical and emotional capabilities and limitations. In the words of Yalom (2002), "inspire yourself to create a new treatment for each client".

Content of the Program

When a program is initiated, it should be implemented as any exercise or training program. Due to the fact that the family members are considered as "un-trained personnel" We observed that the activities should be implemented for shorter durations and intensities at the beginning of the program, with progressive building of the activities within daily routines. Activities within routines were expanded further with time, guided by evaluations as to their value. The activities should always include an adequate motivational factor that supports the program's execution (e.g., enabling the individual to view a favorite cartoon, receive praise from parents, family members, and friends, or go for a walk in the park or mall). The program should be flexible in order to adapt to any sudden change in comorbidity status, sleep habits, or changes in medication, including changes of dosage. The activities should be carried out daily to create a stable regular structure that is easy to follow. The program should also take advantage of the moments in which the client carries out activities similar to those of the program, e.g., take advantage of the times when they have to go out and return home to go up and down the stairs (instead of using the elevator), walk during indoor transitions instead of using a wheelchair, etc. Moreover, during all three programs described in this chapter, it was clear that the attitudes of parents and therapists can positively or negatively affect the program outcomes. Therefore, the therapist in charge must consider the attitudes of the participants and, through THS access (in these projects such as the Skype and Zoom calls), to adapt the program (updating the program constantly sometimes by reducing the load and in other cases enhancing the program intensity or difficulty level) and maintain adherence of all involved. The remote supervisions are suggested here as an integral part of any THS program allowing the program manager to accompany family members and therapists in carrying it out, intercepting needs as soon as they arise.

Settings

Some settings may have limited rehabilitative support for individuals with a disability, yet many families want to engage with programs for their children. Hence, the locations for the programs described in this chapter were extremely accepting of this type of intervention and the parents embraced it wholeheartedly. In a different setting, a slightly changed program might be required. Yet, it is the responsibility of the therapist in charge to adapt the program to entail factors that will positively influence the acceptance of the program and the adherence to it, to maximize the positive effects. Individual circumstances (such as divorce, changing residence, etc.) can influence intervention outcomes as well. It is challenging to master personal events, but some can be predicted and therefore prevented. For example, if the family is planning to move to a new apartment, the program's initiation should be postponed as the involvement of the parents in the event will not allow them to start the program. Moreover, the new house might be built differently from the old one, presenting new difficulties, thereby needing reconstruction of the rehabilitation program. If a family is due to have a new baby, the mother's pregnancy might prevent the program's full implementation, and the planned exercise program may need adjustment.

Participatory Action Research and Family-Centered Care

The principles of participatory action research (PAR) and family-centered care (FCC) guided the designs of the three THS projects described in this chapter. PAR is defined as "a participatory, democratic process concerned with developing practical knowing to pursue worthwhile human purposes" (Reason & Bradbury, 2001). Action research involves clients (in this case, families, and support staff for the individual with RTT) throughout the research process through problem identification and disentangling. The steps representing the progression of a PAR process involves numerous cycles of: Assessment (of each participant's therapeutic needs by the first author), Mutual goal attainment (joint goals are constructed for each client together with the family regarding their feasibility and availability within the family's framework), Action (the families implement the program), Reflection (the program is discussed/presented over Skype meetings and re-evaluated by supervisor and parents), and Evaluation (the program is modified if necessary and re-implemented). Action research assumes that the participant's involvement is empowering for them with the final results of achieving greater welfare for the person with RTT and her family. Action researchers seek change and develop solutions in collaboration with the client while maintaining sensitivity to the family's needs and desires (Ozanne & Saatcioglu, 2008). PAR design has a weaker level of evidence than randomized controlled trial designs but is well suited to developing an evolving program that includes highly personal collaborations.

FCC can be defined as placing the clients' needs, within the context of their family and community, at the center of care and planning an individualized and dynamic model of care in collaboration with the client and family that will best meet these needs (Siebes et al., 2007). More precisely, the Institute for Family-Centered Care stated that FCC is an innovative approach to planning, delivering, and evaluating health care grounded in a mutually beneficial partnership among patients, families, and providers. It applies to patients of all ages and may be practiced in any health care setting (Institute for Patient- and Family-Centered Care, 2011). FCC puts the intervention emphasis on the needs of the child and family to support the patterns of living and be supported by the family's strengths and resources (Dunst et al., 1988; King et al., 2004). Within FCC practice, the family is recognized as the constant in the child's life and his primary source of strength and support. Family members are involved in their child's care and learn more about their child and their child's treatment. In turn, they can share their knowledge with professionals, and this provides a more holistic picture of the child and a way to heighten awareness of the child as part of the family (Siebes et al., 2007). Families are not referred to or treated as dependent clients, with professionals and policymakers viewing families as equals, citizens with whom they collaborate and empower. Thus, the family plays a fundamental role in the decision-making process concerning services for their child (Bamm & Rosenbaum, 2008). With the family unit as the primary and principal context for promoting child health and well-being, FCC has been shown to contribute to developmental progress and skill development (Caro & Derevensky, 1991; Law et al., 1998; Moxley-Haegert & Serbin, 1983). Therefore, the healthcare professional must involve family members in all areas of assessment, planning, and delivery of health-related services.

SOLUTIONS AND RECOMMENDATIONS

Three Example Projects

Participants (In All Three Projects)

Overall, 58 individuals with RTT participated in all three projects. Five individuals living in Ireland participated in project I, 13 individuals living in Sicily participated in project II, and 40 individuals living in northern Italy participated in project III. Their characteristics are specified within each project description.

Intervention Procedure for All Three Programs

All participants underwent four assessment sessions at approximately three-month intervals (±1month). These sessions were performed with physical attendance of the researchers who examined the participant and discussed the program with the parents. During the first meeting, relevant information was collected on medical and clinical conditions (e.g., epilepsy, osteoporosis, sleep disturbances associated with RTT), current motor skills and activities, and any ongoing therapeutic interventions (e.g., physiotherapy, psychomotor, hydrotherapy) and other environmental enablers or barriers. Information was collected for each of the ICF domains. During the meetings, parents' expectations and wishes regarding the improvement of motor function for their daughters were discussed together with the researcher and referred professionals. A draft of the individualized rehabilitation goals for the intervention phase was compiled and discussed with parents and available local rehabilitation professionals (if present) to address the availability of resources to implement these programs.

In the second assessment session, the rehabilitation goals were again discussed with each family and available local rehabilitation professional and revised as necessary. Categories for Goal Attainment Scaling (GAS) were then compiled for each goal. The therapeutic objectives referred to five different areas: increments in joint mobility of the limbs; improvements of spinal asymmetries; enhancements of gross motor function; increased functional use of the hands; improvements of general physical health.

After constructing the program, the family and available local rehabilitation professionals were provided with an individualized program of simple therapeutic activities. The aims were to achieve therapeutic objectives by practicing simple daily physical activities incorporated into the girl's everyday life for a total time of about one non-continuous hour a day for five days a week. Each family was able to organize the activities during the week according to their routines and habits. The rehabilitation activities foreseen in the programs included but were not limited to maintaining passive postures to prevent the onset or worsening of musculoskeletal problems secondary to RTT; maintaining active symmetrical and asymmetrical postures to rebalance the trunk muscles and improve balance; exercise of functional skills (e.g., sitting position, standing position, walking, climbing or descending stairs); and functional use of hands. The goals and activities identified were different for each individual with RTT in content, difficulty, and intensity. After two weeks to develop familiarity with the program, the family was contacted remotely every two weeks for approximately one hour each through a videoconference platform (Skype/Zoom) until the end of the intervention period. The first remote-supervision meeting was mainly used to clarify questions relating to the practical implementation of the activities proposed in the program. The subsequent supervision meetings were aimed at supporting the execution of the programs by answering the parents' questions, adapting them to emerging needs, solving problems, rearranging the timetable, adapting the proposed exercises, evaluating, and sharing the achievement of objectives, and, if necessary, setting new goals.

At the end of the intervention phase, the third evaluation session identified the level of achievement of the objectives established in the GAS, and the parents' considerations relating to the intervention phase were collected.

The telehealth supervision meetings were suspended between the third and fourth (follow-up) evaluation sessions (wash-out phase). The fourth evaluation was performed as a repetition of the last three evaluations, assessing the participant's functional level (see Figure 1).

Outcome Measures

As the participants presented different functional abilities (from girls showing minimal functional difficulties to people who have been wheelchair users throughout their life), the selected outcome measure which was able to collect all outcomes into one scale was the GAS.

The GAS was administered to assess the degree of achievement of the rehabilitation objectives identified for each participant. This scaling system represents a mathematical technique used to quantify the achievement (or not) of the identified rehabilitation goals and can be used in rehabilitation (Turner-Stokes, 2009). The GAS represents a sensitive measure of patient changes after intervention in relation to a specific therapeutic objective. It has been identified as the most sensitive tool to reflect and measure small changes in patients' functioning and conditions that otherwise would not be found using standardized or physiological measures (Mailloux et al., 2007). Goals (between 3-5 for each participant) set should follow the SMART principle. To best suit the individual's potential, they should be specific, measurable, attainable, realistic, and timely (Bovend'Eerdt et al., 2009). Each identified rehabilitation goal received a weight of significance from 1 (a little – such as joint range of motion) to 3 (very – such as elements related to participation) to take account of the relative importance of the goal to the individual and the difficulty that the rehabilitation team anticipates in achieving it. Higher weight represents higher importance or difficulty of goal achievement (Rushton & Miller, 2002). The degree of achievement of each objective is assessed on a 5-points scale: if the patient reaches the expected level, this is assigned the value 0. If obtained results are better than expected, these are given the values +1 (a little more than expected) or +2 (much more than expected). If results are lower than expected, these are assigned the values -1 (a little less than expected) or -2 (no change from baseline). In our investigation, a score of -1 represents the maintenance of the pre-intervention situation, and a score of -2 means worsening with respect to pre-intervention assessment. Each level of each goal is defined by the team or the experimenter and should be objective and observable.

Figure 1. Flow chart of the three protocols – all meetings depicted in gray were performed with physical attendance of the researchers

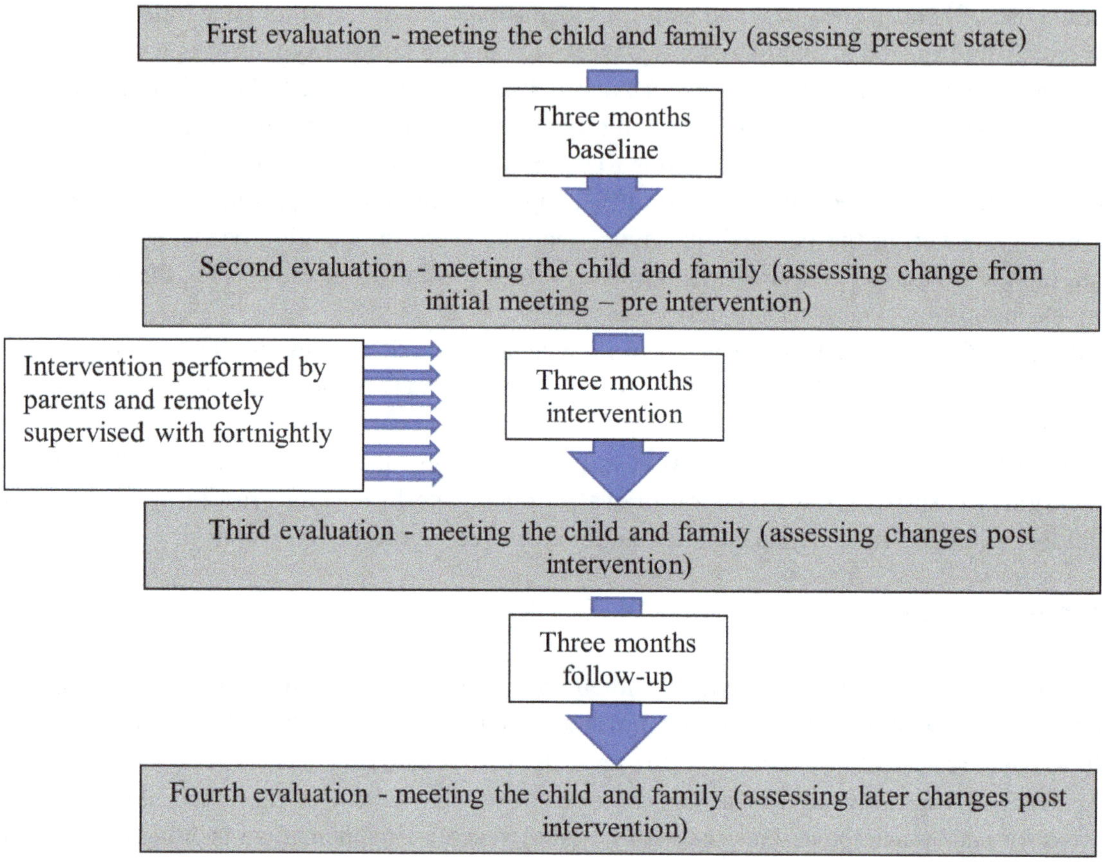

The outcome score and weight of each goal were incorporated into a single aggregated T-score to obtain one numerical score for each patient regarding the rehabilitation goal achievement by applying the following formula (Turner-Stokes, 2009):

$$T-score = 50 + \frac{10 \cdot \Sigma(w_i x_i)}{\sqrt{\left[(1-\rho)\cdot \Sigma w_i^2 + \rho \cdot (\Sigma w_i)^2\right]}}$$

Where wi = the weight assigned to each goal, xi = the numerical value achieved for each goal (between -2 and +2), and ρ (rho) = the expected correlation of the goal scales, for practical purposes, ρ most commonly approximates to 0.3 (Kiresuk & Sherman, 1968). Therefore, the composite goal score (the sum of the attainment levels × the relative weights for each goal) is transformed into a standardized measure or T-score with a mean of 50 and a standard deviation of 10. T-score represents an overall measure of the adequacy of the proposed objectives. A T-score of 50 ± 10 indicates that overall, the goals set were adequate to the intervention's potential. A T-score > 60 indicates that the rehabilitation team has underestimated the treatment potential, and a T-score < 40 indicates that the objectives were overestimated for the intervention (Turner-Stokes, 2009).

Study I: Ireland

The Setting

As reported by the participants' parents, there were no regular physical therapy services in many of the special education facilities in their local area. Therefore, implementing such a program in such an environment empowered both the parents and educational teams and was accepted by the individuals with RTT and their families.

Participants

Nine individuals were invited to participate in the project. All agreed to participate, yet two families did not return the signed informed consent form and two other families did not have internet services to enable Skype calls. Therefore, five families participated in the telehealth intervention program. The participants' age ranged from 5 - 18 (Mean: 9; SD ± 5.6) years, and functional abilities were variable (see Table 2).

Table 2. Functional abilities of participants

Child	Age (years)	Sitting on floor	Standing	Walking	Going down-stairs	Running	Jumping	Stand on one leg
1	6	I	I	I	I	I	N	N
2	5	I	I	I	A	N	N	N
3	18	I	A	A	A	N	N	N
4	11	I	I	I	A	N	N	N
5	5	N	N	N	N	N	N	N

Abbreviations list: N = Not able; A = Assisted; I = Independent.

Evaluation and Intervention

All participants were assessed, and a home-based exercise program was developed in adherence to functional goals. Participants' parents and local therapists (when available) participated in the evaluation meetings and in the goal definition process. Families then participated in fortnightly Skype sessions over a three-month period, guided by a researcher physiotherapist to monitor progress and adjust the program as necessary. These remote supervision meetings concerned a discussion of the program implementation with parents and other involved people (when available). If needed the execution of the activities were remotely observed by the researcher to better understand the difficulties and find a solution. The intervention was performed by the available local resources. The participants' parents were the main active party in carrying out the program activities but also other family members, caregivers, teachers, and local rehabilitation professionals participation were included in the program when they gave their availability. GAS was used to evaluate progress, and a parental satisfaction questionnaire was administered following the program.

Results

All participants presented improvements in functional abilities (see Table 3).

A Case Study

The most severe child (#5) was five years old. She was presenting shortening of knee flexors (Hamstrings), the beginning of right C-shaped scoliosis, was unable to sit on the floor independently and was constantly showing significant dislike from any movement or exercise (expressed by frown face and shouting when being moved. Her exercise program included: sitting against the wall with extended knees to elongate hamstrings muscles, exercises to counter the development of scoliosis, standing in a standing frame, and supported walking with the mother holding her by the pelvic for short distances. Later on, when she improved, independent sitting was exercised for longer durations, and walking was exercised for longer distances with a gradual reduction of support. At the end of the program, she sat unsupported for an unlimited duration and stood between two sofas independently for extended durations (up to an hour) (see Figure 2). She could also sit alone on the horse for half an hour during an entire hippotherapy session. But the most significant change was her attitude which was completely altered. Instead of rejecting any form of exercise and movement (as she behaved during the initial assessment), she was now calling her mother repeatedly asking to stand up, walk, and move.

Study 2: Sicily

Setting

The place where the Sicily investigation took place showed little support to adults with disabilities. Therefore, many family members were keen for a program for their daughter (mainly adults) with RTT. The setting was extremely accepting of this type of intervention, and the parents embraced it wholeheartedly.

Participants

Thirteen participants with genetically confirmed classic RTT and their families were involved in this study. (mean age: 17y 9m ± 7y 9m; range: 3y 4m – 34y 4m). Five subjects (at school age) attended regular school with typically developed peers for at least four our per day, and one subject attended an educational center for more than an hour a day (other participants were not enrolled in any educational/ rehabilitation facility). The level of severity of RTT and gross motor functional ability level varied between participants.

Table 3. Goals, post-intervention skills, and GAS score following the six-month Telehealth intervention

Participant	Baseline skill (GAS score -2)	Goal (GAS score 0)	Post-intervention skills	Post-intervention GAS score
1	Unable to jump independently	To jump two consecutive jumps independently	Can jump five consecutive jumps independently	2
	Unable to throw lightweight pillow	To be able to throw a lightweight pillow forward	Able to hit a lightweight pillow to a basket 5/5	2
	Unable to stand with one leg on a therapeutic peanut roll	To stand with one leg on a peanut for 5 second	Able to stand with one leg on a peanut for 10 seconds	2
	Unable to stand on one leg following assistance to lift one leg	To be able to stand on one leg for 2 seconds when assisted into the position	Able to stand on one leg for 4 seconds when assisted into the position	1
	Median GAS score: 2			
2	Falls almost every 5 minutes when walking independently outdoors	Fall twice when walking for 20 minutes outdoors	Falls once when walking for 20 minutes outdoors	1
	Can walk quickly outdoors	Will be able to take 5 running steps when walking outdoors	She takes 20 running steps when walking outdoors	2
	Can stand on balance board for only 1 second and falls down	Will be able to stand on balance board for 30 seconds	She was able to stand on the balance board for 30 minutes	+2
	Able to go down 1 stair with intense support only	Will be able to go down 1 stair with slight parental support	Able to go down 1 stair with intense support only	-1
Median GAS score: 1.5				
3	Able to walk with support for 10 minutes indoors	Will be able to walk with support for 15 minutes indoors	Able to walk for 25 minutes indoors	2
	Able to walk with support for 5 minutes outdoors	Will be able to walk with support for 10 minutes outdoors	Able to walk with support for 20 minutes outdoors	2
	Able to walk with support for 10 steps outdoors	Will be able to walk 3 steps indoors unaided	Able to walk more than 50 steps indoors unaided	2
	Able to dance to slow music for 10 minutes with support	Will be able to dance to fast rhythmic music for 10 minutes with support	Able to dance to slow music for 10 minutes with support	-1
Median GAS score: 2				
4	Can walk unaided indoors	Will be able to negotiate a two-meter obstacle course unaided within five minutes	Negotiates a two-meter obstacle course for 1 minute (achieved in 23 seconds)	2
	She dislikes dancing with her parents	Will dance with parents while held in a support belt for 1 minute[1] (footnote)	Dances with parents while held in a support belt for five minutes	1
	Picking up medium-sized objects (ring/ball) from the table when sitting on a chair	Will be able to pick up medium-sized objects from the floor when sitting on a chair	Able to pick up medium-sized objects (ring/ball) from the floor when sitting on a therapeutic peanut roll and when standing	1
	Usually afraid of movement on a trampoline	Will walk aided across the trampoline	Walks aided across the trampoline	0
	[1]The use of a support belt prevents the child from leaning on the hands of the parents/caregivers (an external stability point) and makes her rely on his core muscles (internal stability), thereby enhances her own stability towards independent mobility			
	Median GAS score: 1			
5	Unable to sit independently on the floor with knees flexed	Will be able to sit independently on the floor with knees flexed for 5 second	Able to sit independently on the floor with knees flexed no time restriction	2+
	She can sit with her back to the wall with four towels supporting (elevating) her pelvis	Will be able to sit on the floor with her back to the wall with one towel under (elevating) her pelvis[2]	Able to sit on the floor with her back to the wall without towels and a rolled towel under (elevating) her heels	2+
	Dislikes movement, able to be move slowly for a maximum of one minute with significant support	Will be able to move to slow music for five minutes with assistance	Able to dance fast rhythmic music for 15 minutes with minimal assistance to move – appears to enjoy movement	2+
	Cannot sit independently on a horse	Will be able to sit independently on a horse for 5 minutes	Able to sit independently on a horse for 30 minutes	2+
	[2]Due to hamstrings shortening, straightening the knees was only possible with pelvic elevated from the floor at program initiation.			
Median GAS score: 2				

Abbreviation list: GAS = Goal Attainment Scaling

Figure 2. Standing between two sofas

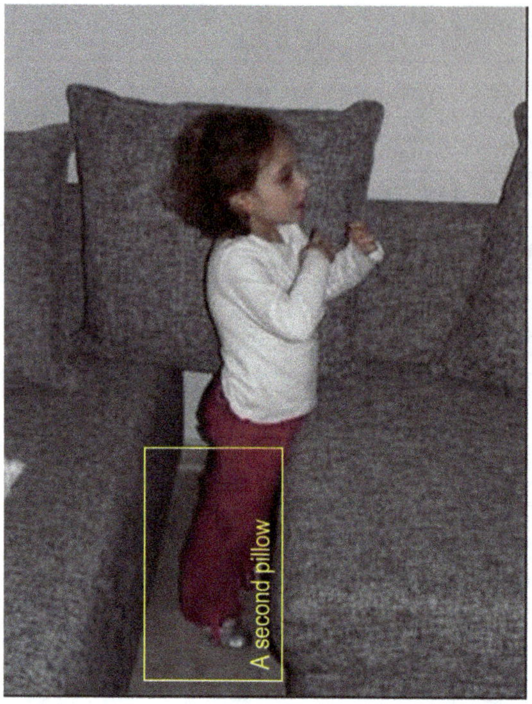

Evaluation and Intervention

The evaluation sessions were carried out by two physiotherapists experienced in treating people with RTT at the participants' homes. Participants' parents and reference local physical therapists (when available) participated in the evaluation meetings. Participants' parents carried out the intervention phase at their houses, and if local therapists of the participants offered their participation in the project, they were happily recruited. Intervention settings and materials were different between participants and individually adapted to each client.

Results

The following table (Table 4) presents a summary of the pre- and post-intervention situation and the outcome measure for each objective, for each participant with the relative weight and score obtained at the GAS (GAS Score). The weight of each goal is classified according to the rehabilitation relevance on a scale from 1 (unimportant goal) to 3 (very important goal).

A Case Study

During the evaluation stage of the project (which included the gathering of medical information from the parents and a functional evaluation), one of the young women participating (21 years of age) was carried into the room by both her parents, each holding her under her armpit. Her functional abilities at that point were similar to the ones of a person who was wheelchair-bound. Yet, by challenging her to

Table 4. Sicily project; GAS Goals with T-scores for each participant

Pt.	Pre-Intervention Situation	Expected outcome (GAS score 0)	Post-Intervention Situation	Weight	GAS Score	T-Score
1	Can walk independently for <10 steps	Can walk independently for 20-30 steps	Can walk independently for more than 150 steps	3	2	70,2
	Can stand for <1 minute independently	Can stand for 2-3 minutes independently	Can stand for more than 3 minutes independently	2	1	
	While lying on the back with one knee flexed at the stomach other knee rise 20 cm from the mattress	While lying on the back with one knee flexed at the stomach other knee rise 10 cm from the mattress	While lying on the back with one knee flexed at the stomach, the other knee rises 6 cm from the mattress	1	1	
	Can climb the stairs with strong trunk support	Can climb the stairs with slight unilateral arm support	Can climb the stairs with slight unilateral palm support	2	1	
	Can descend the stairs with strong trunk support	Can descend the stairs with slight unilateral arm support	Can descend the stairs with slight unilateral palm support	2	1	
	Resting pulse is at 75bpm	Resting pulse is at 70-71bpm	Resting pulse was at 71bpm	1	0	
2	Can walk for a maximum of 90 seconds before fall	Can walk for a maximum of 3 minutes before fall	Can walk for more than 5 minutes before fall	3	2	51,6
	Can maintain all four position for 20 seconds	Can maintain all four position for at least 1 minute	Can maintain all four position for 1 minute	2	0	
	Cannot stand up from a chair	Try to get up from a chair with strong support given to one hand (make the helping movement)	Try to get up from a chair with strong support given to both hands (make the helping movement)	3	-1	
	Never activate hand reaching	She activates initial reaching movement of the hands to interesting objects	She activates body part to initiate hand reaching movement	2	-1	
3	Can walk independently for <10 steps	Can walk independently for 15-20 steps	Can walk independently for more than 70 steps	3	2	77,4
	Can stand for <1 minute with support to one hand	Can stand for 1,5-2 minutes with support given to one hand	Can stand for >3 minutes with support given to one hand	2	2	
	Severe PRoM reduction at both knees' extension and ankles dorsiflexion	Improve for 10° in at least one knee extension or improve for 10° in at least one ankle dorsiflexion	Improve for 10° in at least one knee extension or improve for 10° in at least one ankle dorsiflexion	1	0	
	Can sit on a stool with feet on the floor for 1 minute	Can sit on a stool with feet on the floor for 2-2,5 minutes	Can sit on a stool with feet on the floor for >3 minutes	2	2	
4	Her weight is at 28 kg	Her weight is at 29 ± 0.5 kg	Her weight is at 27kg	2	-2	39,1
	Likert parent satisfaction for stomach bloating (1 = very unhappy about situation and frequency)	Stomach bloating it's reduced a little but nothing special = 3 on (0-5 Likert scale)	Stomach bloating it's reduced a little but nothing special = 3 on (0-5 Likert scale)	1	0	
	Grabbing big objects and holding them for more than two seconds	Grabbing small objects and holding them for 1 second	Grabbing small objects and holding them for 1 second	1	1	
5	HR at rest 92bpm	HR at rest 87-88bpm	HR at rest 78bpm	2	2	72,4
	Need to be pulled up with two hands to stand from a chair	Can stand up from a chair with slight unilateral palm support	Need to be pulled up with one hand to stand from a chair	2	-1	
	Can stand for <45 seconds with support to one hand	Can stand for 60-75 seconds with support to one hand	Can stand for more than 60 seconds independently	3	2	
	Can walk with one support (held to the hand/wrist) for <10 steps	Can walk with one support (held to the hand/wrist) for 10-15 steps	Can walk for >10 steps independently	3	2	
6	Never activate hand reaching	Activate initial reaching movement of the hands to interesting objects	Reach the object and touch it	1	1	54,8
	Can stand for less than 10 seconds independently	Can stand for 30-45 seconds independently	Can stand for less than 10 seconds independently	2	-1	
	Can walk with one support (held to the hand/wrist) for less than 10 steps	Can walk with one support (held to the hand/wrist) for 20-30 steps	Can walk with one support (held to the hand/wrist) for more than 30 steps	3	1	
7	Can stand independently for <30 seconds	Can stand independently for 45-60 seconds	Can stand independently for more than 75 seconds	3	2	75,6
	Can walk independently for <10 steps	Can walk independently for 10-15 steps	Can walk independently for more than 20 steps	3	2	
	Can stand up from a chair (and vice versa) with little help to one hand	Can stand up from a chair (and vice versa) independently (with a verbal cue) at least 1 time on 5 tries	Can stand up from a chair (and vice versa) independently (no verbal cue) at least 3 times on 5 tries	2	2	
	HR at rest 98bpm	HR at rest 93-94bpm	HR at rest 92bpm	2	0	
8	HR at rest 135bpm	HR at rest 125bpm	HR at rest 130bpm	3	-1	50,0
	Can walk on a treadmill at initial speed (0.5 km/h)	Can walk on a treadmill at initial speed + 1 km/h	Can walk on a treadmill at initial speed + 1 km/h	1	0	
	Her BMI is 30	Her BMI is 29	Her BMI is 28,5	3	1	

continued on following page

Table 4. Continued

Pt.	Pre-Intervention Situation	Expected outcome (GAS score 0)	Post-Intervention Situation	Weight	GAS Score	T-Score
	Can climb the stairs with strong unilateral arm support	Can climb the stairs with slight unilateral palm support	Can climb the stairs independently using the handrail	2	1	
9	Can descend the stairs with strong unilateral arm support	Can descend the stairs with slight unilateral palm support	Can descend the stairs independently using the handrail	2	1	67,7
	HR at rest 110bpm	HR at rest 100bpm	HR at rest 74bpm	1	2	
	Can sit on a stool with feet on the floor for <10 seconds	Can sit on a stool with feet on the floor for 30-60 seconds	Can sit on a stool with feet on the floor for 2 minutes	3	2	
10	Range of motion of Elbows R -10/L-20	Improvement of 10° of range of motion in at least one of the elbows	Worsening occurs in at least one elbow	1	-2	58,3
	Range of motion of knees R -45/L-45	Improvement of 10° of range of motion in at least one of the knees	Range of motion of knees R -45/L-45	1	-1	
11	Can sit on the floor at the end of a wedge with crossed legs for <10 seconds	Can sit on the floor at the end of a wedge with crossed legs for 15-20 seconds	Can seat at the end of a wedge on the floor for >25 seconds	2	2	76,4
	Lose >10° Knees extension (in at least one knee)	Actual ROM (-40° Knees extension bilaterally)	Improve >10° Knees extension (in at least one knee)	3	2	
	Right knee is at -25 degrees	Improvement of 10° of extension range of motion in the right knee	Right knee is at -25 degrees	2	-1	
12	Can sit on a stool without feet support for <1 minute	Can sit on a stool without feet support for 1.5-2 minutes	Can sit on a stool without feet support for >3 minutes	3	2	59,8
	When lying supine with the hands over the head, the elbow is 25cm far from the mattress	When lying supine with the hands over the head, the elbow is 10cm far from the mattress	One elbow touches the table with slight pressure, and the other is at less than 10cm far from the mattress	1	1	
	Can sit on a stool with feet on the floor for <30 seconds	Can sit on a stool with feet on the floor for 1-1,5 minute	Can sit on a stool with feet on the floor for >2 minutes	3	2	
	Range of motion of hips R-20/L-20	Improvement of 10° of extension range of motion in at least one hip	Improvement <10° of extension range of motion in at least one hip	2	-1	
13	Range of motion of knees R-40/L-40	Improvement of 10° of extension range of motion in the left knee	Improvement of 10° of extension range of motion in the left knee	2	0	66,6
	Heart rate at rest 80bpm	Heart rate at rest 75-76bpm	Heart rate at rest 76bpm	1	0	
	Can't actively rotate the head to the right	Can actively rotate the head 30° to the right from midline	Can actively rotate the head to the right for the full range of motion	2	2	
					Mean	63,1
					SD	11,9

Abbreviation list: Pt. = Participants; GAS = Goal Attainment Scaling; bpm = Beats Per Minute; HR = Heart Rate; PRoM = Passive Range of Motion; BMI = Body Mass Index; R = Right; L = Left; SD = Standard Deviation.

stand and walk without assistance (despite the terrified look in her parents' eyes), it was soon evident that her abilities were higher than as first observed. Her therapist was instructed to work with her on independent walking and stair climbing (not the parents who could not bring themself to challenge their daughter). At the end of the three months, she walked independently, including walking over obstacles, and overcoming an obstacle course alone. She needed but little help (held by one hand) to ascend and descend the stairs. Her new abilities were a significant improvement in her quality of life and health state, as well as a considerable relief to her parents.

Study 3: Northern Italy

Setting

The project was implemented within Veneto and Lombardia counties in the northeastern part of Italy. This location was chosen by the Italian Rett syndrome Association (AIRett), the leading RTT parents' organization in Italy.

Participants

Participants involved in this study were 40 girls and women with genetically confirmed classic RTT and their families, members of the Italian Rett syndrome association (AIRett). This study included girls and women with ages ranging from 2.8 – 40.3 (mean 15.7 ± 9.7) years. The clinical severity varied substantially within our sample. All participants lived at home with their parents.

Results

This project involved 40 girls and women and summary data for the overall goals for the specific goal areas and related levels of achievement are presented in Table 5.

Table 5. Descriptive statistics of goals distribution and level of achievement for each area

Goal area		Amount (%)	GAS score at T3, median (range)	T-score at T3, mean (SD)	GAS score at T4, median (range)	T-score at T4, mean (SD)
Functional goals	Sitting	10 (4.9%)	64,7 (5,4)	1 (0,5 – 2)	2 (0,5 – 2)	67,3 (6,7)
	Standing	21 (10.2%)	56,3 (12,4)	1 (-2 – 2)	0,25 (-2 – 2)	51,4 (13,7)
	Transitional change	17 (8.3%)	53,0 (8,9)	0 (-0,5 – 2)	0 (-1 – 2)	52,5 (9,5)
	Walking	35 (17.1%)	59,7 (10,2)	1 (-2 – 2)	1 (-2 – 2)	59,9 (12,5)
	Challenging	38 (18.5%)	54,2 (10,2)	0 (-1 – 2)	0,5 (-1,5 – 1,5)	53,7 (10,1)
	Balance	5 (2.4%)	51,1 (8,8)	0,25 (-1 – 1)	0,25 (0 – 1)	53,7 (5,0)
	Hand function	15 (7.3%)	57,1 (14,3)	0 (-1 – 2)	0,5 (-1 – 2)	59,3 (14,3)
General physical health*		7 (3.4%)	-0,5 (-2 – 1)	45,2 (11,3)	-0,75 (-2 – 1)	41,6 (12,2)
Range of joint motion		28 (13.7%)	1 (-1 – 1)	54,9 (10,0)	0 (-2 – 2)	51,7 (13,7)
Spine asymmetries		29 (14.2%)	\	\	-1 (-2 – 1)	40,7 (10,4)
Total		205 (100%)	\	\	0,25 (-2 – 2)	55,9 (10,7)

Abbreviation list: GAS = Goal Attainment Scale; SD = Standard Deviation; T3 = Post-intervention evaluation, T4 = Follow-up evaluation.

*General physical health: Activities include treadmill training, taking long walks, and others to increase the participant's daily physical activity level. Success can be determined by a reduction of heart rate at rest or weight loss.

A Case Study

When first evaluating this three-year-old child, we found a scared young child with a significant fear of movement. Every time she woke up from bed, she needed her parents to hold her firmly in their arms for about 20-30 minutes while she was vigorously screaming (The researchers suspected that the screaming episodes were due to an extreme case of fear of movement). Therefore, her program included daily use of a "splint- standing- frame" (a splint standing frame is the use of old splints intended to be used by adults, bolted into a piece of wood, and used as a standing frame with minimal support - see Figure 3).

Figure 3. The use of a splint standing frame and "dance parties" with her parents to her favorite tunes. At the end of the program, she was no longer screaming each time she woke up, which was a huge relief to her parents; she enjoyed moving independently around the living room while holding to furniture and was even able to complete 26 steps independently.

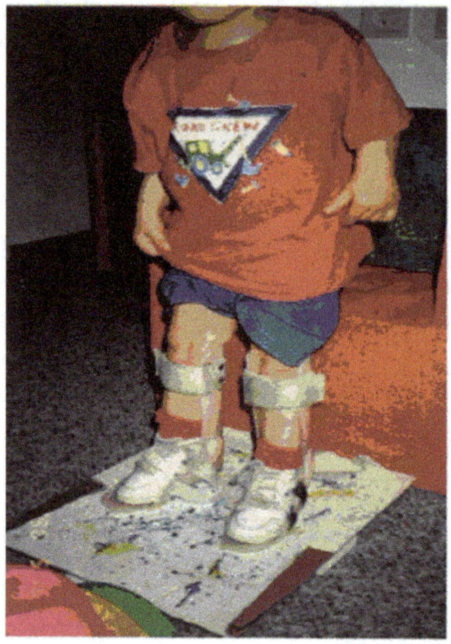

Parental Satisfaction

For the three projects, the parent caregivers reported a high level of satisfaction (during the skype calls and satisfaction questionnaires) and a good level of adherence to the proposed activities. This finding suggests that creating and supervising a home-based, family-centered individualized rehabilitation program focused on the person and adapted to her and family needs motivates family members who mostly report a positive attitude towards the program. The identification of functional activities that could lead to visible results in everyday life led to better adherence to the program by the family, contributing to a good level of parental satisfaction and positive functional outcomes. This information suggests that when building programs such as the ones presented within this chapter, the therapist should consider the family members' motivation to carry out the activities and the possibility of integrating them into the daily routine. Comparable results have also been found in other populations of individuals with disabilities when considering the parents' predisposition, availability, and previous experiences (Lee et al., 2016; Lee et al., 2018). The participants' parents reported a high level of satisfaction regarding the habilitation program suggested by the researchers. This result is attributed to the relationship of trust that the rehabilitation team established with families by following them remotely via Skype, addressing their concerns and suggestions. Therefore, the authors suggest the need for remote supervision to similar programs at regular and frequent intervals to support the family in overcoming obstacles and maintaining a positive attitude towards the proposed activities.

As several activities included in the programs were functional exercises that could facilitate visible outcomes, their execution was easily integrated into the participants' and families' daily routines. They began to use the suggested methods for the exercises during everyday activities. The above-described projects support the fact that identifying the functional activities which concern the parents of children with RTT (and probably to others with severe disabilities) was of immense importance. Therefore, prescribing those specific activities as part of the home exercise program caused improved adherence to the program, leading to the exercise integration in the daily routine, thereby increasing parental satisfaction and positive functional outcomes.

FUTURE RESEARCH DIRECTIONS

This chapter described the concept and the results of a three-month, Skype-supervised, home-based, family-centered, individualized rehabilitation program for individuals with RTT. The authors identified motorically oriented rehabilitation objectives for all participants and barriers preventing improvement in this group of participants, and then constructed individualized, home rehabilitation programs which yielded positive outcomes. The findings suggest that Skype-supervised family-centered rehabilitation interventions are effective for individuals with RTT for achieving functional rehabilitation goals when support is provided to participants, their family members, and local professionals. Similar results were found in all three projects presented in this chapter coherently with those observed in other populations with family members' involvement (Randström et al., 2013). These findings coincide with Kerr's statement that the exercises performed by caregivers are highly recommended for the physical and functional state of the individual with RTT, stressing the significance of regular daily activity for the long-term health of this population (Kerr, 2007). THS hold the potential to support the achievement and generalization of therapeutic goals in the clients' daily living environment in cost-effective and low-technological ways. The authors believe that similar projects involving supervised, home-based, family-centered, individualized rehabilitation programs can be generalized for other individuals presenting an array of diagnosis and disabilities.

CONCLUSION

The results presented within the present chapter suggest that an individually adapted, Skype supervised, client-centered, home-based exercise program is an efficient way to improve the motor and functional abilities of individuals with RTT. The findings of the current research projects are of particular importance when considering the participants' age. Our three projects included a wide age range from age 3 to 40 years. The implemented programs led to improvements in participants from childhood to adulthood, suggesting that people with RTT and possibly others with disabilities across all ages can benefit from such home-based interventions. According to existing literature, deterioration in health and function is expected during adulthood in RTT (Hagberg et al. 1993), as well as in other disabilities (Tse et al., 2018) but, at the same time, despite such deterioration, a reduction in health services is registered for this population (Leonard et al. 2001). Since there is more support to young children (by educational facilities) where their weight and size do not hinder supported movements (as is the case in adults), and the parents are younger, we suspect that, if such a program had been implemented at a younger age, it might have produced even better outcomes.

Moreover, the involved parents supported the implementation of the program and presented a high level of satisfaction. The results also reveal that implementing such a project within the PAR concept, which requires working with and being guided by the participants (and their families in these cases), is highly recommended. Our qualitative findings reveal that the participants' parents' satisfaction with the program might have facilitated them to experience the therapeutic effects of the exercise, and this might have promoted their involvement and resolve in continuation of the prescribed exercises, integrating the exercise program as a part of their daily activities. Many of the activities in the programs were functional exercises, and their execution was easily integrated into the participants' daily routines. Families began to use the suggested methods for the exercises during everyday activities.

We can affirm that identifying the functional activities that concern the parents of children with disabilities and prescribing those specific activities as part of the home exercise program caused improved adherence to the program, leading to exercise integration in the daily routine, increasing parental satisfaction, and positive functional outcomes. Therefore, our findings suggest that a THS program can support and advance the physical abilities of individuals with RTT at all ages and functional abilities. Most likely, it can improve the lives of all individuals with severe disabilities and their families.

ACKNOWLEDGMENT

The International Rett Syndrome Foundation partially funded this project within the HeART Grant [grant number 3610].

We would like to thank the International Rett syndrome Foundation for supporting this research project. We would also like to thank the Italian Rett Association (AIRett) and the head of the organization Lucia Dovigo for supporting this project connecting researchers and involved families, and constantly supporting the experimentation of therapeutic strategies based on telerehabilitation. Last but not least, we would also like to thank the parents and individuals with RTT involved in this project.

REFERENCES

Amir, R. E., Van den Veyver, I. B., Wan, M., Tran, C. Q., Francke, U., & Zoghbi, H. Y. (1999). Rett syndrome is caused by mutations in X-linked MECP2, encoding methyl-CpG-binding protein 2. *Nature Genetics*, *23*(2), 185–188. doi:10.1038/13810 PMID:10508514

Amoako, A. N., & Hare, D. J. (2020). Non-medical interventions for individuals with Rett syndrome: A systematic review. In Journal of Applied Research in Intellectual Disabilities (Vol. 33, Issue 5, pp. 808–827). Blackwell Publishing Ltd. doi:10.1111/jar.12694

Anderson, A., Wong, K., Jacoby, P., Downs, J., & Leonard, H. (2014). Twenty years of surveillance in Rett syndrome: What does this tell us? *Orphanet Journal of Rare Diseases*, *9*(1), 87. doi:10.1186/1750-1172-9-87 PMID:24942262

Anttila, M. R., Kivistö, H., Piirainen, A., Kokko, K., Malinen, A., Pekkonen, M., & Sjögren, T. (2019). Cardiac rehabilitees' technology experiences before remote rehabilitation: Qualitative study using a grounded theory approach. *Journal of Medical Internet Research*, *21*(2), e10985. doi:10.2196/10985 PMID:30730298

Bamm, E. L., & Rosenbaum, P. (2008). Family-centered theory: Origins, development, barriers, and supports to implementation in rehabilitation medicine. *Archives of Physical Medicine and Rehabilitation*, *89*(8), 1618–1624. doi:10.1016/j.apmr.2007.12.034 PMID:18586223

Bell, K. M., Onyeukwu, C., McClincy, M. P., Allen, M., Bechard, L., Mukherjee, A., Hartman, R. A., Smith, C., Lynch, A. D., & Irrgang, J. J. (2019). Verification of a portable motion tracking system for remote management of physical rehabilitation of the knee. *Sensors (Switzerland)*, *19*(5), 1021. doi:10.339019051021 PMID:30823373

Bovend'Eerdt, T. J. H., Botell, R. E., & Wade, D. T. (2009). Writing SMART rehabilitation goals and achieving goal attainment scaling: A practical guide. *Clinical Rehabilitation*, *23*(4), 352–361. doi:10.1177/0269215508101741 PMID:19237435

Budden, S. (1995). Management of Rett Syndrome: A Ten Year Experience. *Neuropediatrics*, *26*(02), 75–77. doi:10.1055-2007-979727 PMID:7566457

Calouro, C., Kwong, M. W., & Gutierrez, M. (2014). An Analysis of State Telehealth Laws and Regulations for Occupational Therapy and Physical Therapy. *International Journal of Telerehabilitation*, *6*(1), 17–24. doi:10.5195/ijt.2014.6141 PMID:25945218

Caprì, T., Nucita, A., Iannizzotto, G., Stasolla, F., Romano, A., Semino, M., Giannatiempo, S., Canegallo, V., & Fabio, R. A. (2021). Telerehabilitation for Improving Adaptive Skills of Children and Young Adults with Multiple Disabilities: A Systematic Review. *Review Journal of Autism and Developmental Disorders*, *8*(2), 244–252. doi:10.100740489-020-00214-x

Caro, P., & Derevensky, J. L. (1991). Family-Focused Intervention Model: Implementation and Research Findings. *Topics in Early Childhood Special Education*, *11*(3), 66–91. doi:10.1177/027112149101100307

Cass, H., Reilly, S., Owen, L., Wisbeach, A., Weekes, L., Slonims, V., Wigram, T., & Charman, T. (2003). Findings from a multidisciplinary clinical case series of females with Rett syndrome. *Developmental Medicine and Child Neurology*, *45*(5), 325–337. doi:10.1111/j.1469-8749.2003.tb00404.x PMID:12729147

Dovigo, L., Caprì, T., Iannizzotto, G., Nucita, A., Semino, M., Giannatiempo, S., Zocca, L., & Fabio, R. A. (2021). Social and Cognitive Interactions Through an Interactive School Service for RTT Patients at the COVID-19 Time. *Frontiers in Psychology*, *12*, 2417. doi:10.3389/fpsyg.2021.676238 PMID:34248774

Downs, J., Rodger, J., Li, C., Tan, X., Hu, N., Wong, K., de Klerk, N., & Leonard, H. (2018). Environmental enrichment intervention for Rett syndrome: An individually randomised stepped wedge trial. *Orphanet Journal of Rare Diseases*, *13*(1), 3. doi:10.118613023-017-0752-8 PMID:29321033

Downs, J., Torode, I., Wong, K., Ellaway, C., Elliott, E. J., Christodoulou, J., Jacoby, P., Thomson, M. R., Izatt, M. T., Askin, G. N., McPhee, B. I., Bridge, C., Cundy, P., & Leonard, H. (2016). The natural history of scoliosis in females with rett syndrome. *Spine*, *41*(10), 856–863. doi:10.1097/BRS.0000000000001399 PMID:26679887

Dunst, C. J., Trivette, C. M., Davis, M., & Cornwell, J. (1988). Enabling and Empowering Families of Children With Health Impairments. *Children's Health Care*, *17*(2), 71–81. doi:10.120715326888chc1702_2

Elefant, C. (2001). Speechless yet communcative: revealing the person behind the disablity of Rett syndrome through clinical research on songs in music therapy. In D. Aldridge, G. Di Franco, E. Ruud, & T. Wigram (Eds.), *Music Therapy in Europe. The 5th European Music Therapy Congress (Napoli, April 2001)* (pp. 113–128). Ismez.

Epstein, L. G. (1995). Rett Syndrome--Clinical and Biological Aspects: Studies on 130 Swedish Females. In Archives of Neurology (Vol. 52, Issue 4). Cambridge University Press. doi:10.1001/archneur.1995.00540280025011

Fonzo, M., Sirico, F., & Corrado, B. (2020). Evidence-based physical therapy for individuals with rett syndrome: A systematic review. In Brain Sciences (Vol. 10, Issue 7, pp. 1–20). MDPI AG. doi:10.3390/brainsci10070410

Gal, N., Andrei, D., Nemeş, D. I., Nədəşan, E., & Stoicu-Tivadar, V. (2015). A Kinect based intelligent e-rehabilitation system in physical therapy. *Studies in Health Technology and Informatics*, *210*, 489–493. doi:10.3233/978-1-61499-512-8-489 PMID:25991195

Glaze, D. G., Percy, A. K., Skinner, S., Motil, K. J., Neul, J. L., Barrish, J. O., Lane, J. B., Geerts, S. P., Annese, F., Graham, J., McNair, L., & Lee, H. S. (2010). Epilepsy and the natural history of Rett syndrome. *Neurology*, *74*(11), 909–912. doi:10.1212/WNL.0b013e3181d6b852 PMID:20231667

Institute for Patient- and Family-Centered Care. (2011). *Advancing the practice of patient- and family-centered care in hospitals - how to get started* (Vol. 20814, Issue 301). Author.

Jagos, H., David, V., Haller, M., Kotzian, S., Hofmann, M., Schlossarek, S., Eichholzer, K., Winkler, M., Frohner, M., Reichel, M., Mayr, W., & Rafolt, D. (2015). A framework for (tele-) monitoring of the rehabilitation progress in stroke patients. *Applied Clinical Informatics*, *6*(4), 757–768. doi:10.4338/ACI-2015-03-RA-0034 PMID:26767068

Kerr, A. (2007). *Understanding Rett Disorder: A Guide for Professionals*. University of Glasgow.

King, S., Teplicky, R., King, G., & Rosenbaum, P. (2004). Family-Centered Service for Children with Cerebral Palsy and Their Families: A Review of the Literature. In Seminars in Pediatric Neurology (Vol. 11, Issue 1, pp. 78–86). W.B. Saunders. doi:10.1016/j.spen.2004.01.009

Kiresuk, T. J., & Sherman, R. E. (1968). Goal attainment scaling: A general method for evaluating comprehensive community mental health programs. *Community Mental Health Journal*, *4*(6), 443–453. doi:10.1007/BF01530764 PMID:24185570

Law, M., Darrah, J., Pollock, N., King, G., Rosenbaum, P., Russell, D., Palisano, R., Harris, S., Armstrong, R., & Watt, J. (1998). Family-centred functional therapy for children with cerebral palsy: An emerging practice model. *Physical & Occupational Therapy in Pediatrics*, *18*(1), 83–102. doi:10.1080/J006v18n01_06

Lee, F. K. I., Lee, T. F. D., & So, W. K. W. (2016). Effects of a tailor-made exercise program on exercise adherence and health outcomes in patients with knee osteoarthritis: A mixed-methods pilot study. *Clinical Interventions in Aging*, *11*, 1391–1402. doi:10.2147/CIA.S111002 PMID:27785001

Lee, I. F. K., Yau, F. N., Yim, S. S. H., & Lee, D. T. F. (2018). Evaluating the impact of a home-based rehabilitation service on older people and their caregivers: A matched-control quasi-experimental study. *Clinical Interventions in Aging*, *13*, 1727–1737. doi:10.2147/CIA.S172871 PMID:30254432

Leonard, H., Fyfe, S., Leonard, S., & Msall, M. (2001). Functional status, medical impairments, and rehabilitation resources in 84 females with Rett syndrome: A snapshot across the world from the parental perspective. *Disability and Rehabilitation*, *23*(3–4), 107–117. doi:10.1080/09638280150504180 PMID:11247006

Lim, J., Greenspoon, D., Hunt, A., & McAdam, L. (2020). Rehabilitation interventions in Rett syndrome: a scoping review. In Developmental Medicine and Child Neurology (Vol. 62, Issue 8, pp. 906–916). Blackwell Publishing Ltd. doi:10.1111/dmcn.14565

Lorish, C. D., Abraham, N., Austin, J., Bradley, L. A., & Alarcon, G. S. (1991). Disease and psychosocial factors related to physical functioning in rheumatoid arthritis. *The Journal of Rheumatology*, *18*(8), 1150–1157. PMID:1834844

Lotan, M., Schenker, R., Wine, J., & Downs, J. (2012). The conductive environment enhances gross motor function of girls with Rett syndrome. A pilot study. *Developmental Neurorehabilitation*, *15*(1), 19–25. doi:10.3109/17518423.2011.629374 PMID:22256830

Mailloux, Z., May-Benson, T. A., Summers, C. A., Miller, L. J., Brett-Green, B., Burke, J. P., Cohn, E. S., Koomar, J. A., Parham, L. D., Roley, S. S., Schaaf, R. C., & Schoen, S. A. (2007). Goal attainment scaling as a measure of meaningful outcomes for children with sensory integration disorders. *The American Journal of Occupational Therapy*, *61*(2), 254–259. doi:10.5014/ajot.61.2.254 PMID:17436848

Mani, S., Sharma, S., Omar, B., Paungmali, A., & Joseph, L. (2017). Validity and reliability of Internet-based physiotherapy assessment for musculoskeletal disorders: A systematic review. *Journal of Telemedicine and Telecare*, *23*(3), 379–391. doi:10.1177/1357633X16642369 PMID:27036879

Moxley-Haegert, L., & Serbin, L. A. (1983). Developmental education for parents of delayed infants: Effects on parental motivation and children's development. *Child Development*, *54*(5), 1324–1331. doi:10.2307/1129685 PMID:6194944

Neul, J. L., Kaufmann, W. E., Glaze, D. G., Christodoulou, J., Clarke, A. J., Bahi-Buisson, N., Leonard, H., Bailey, M. E. S., Schanen, N. C., Zappella, M., Renieri, A., Huppke, P., & Percy, A. K. (2010). Rett syndrome: Revised diagnostic criteria and nomenclature. *Annals of Neurology*, *68*(6), 944–950. doi:10.1002/ana.22124 PMID:21154482

Ozanne, J. L., & Saatcioglu, B. (2008). Participatory action research. *The Journal of Consumer Research*, *35*(3), 423–439. doi:10.1086/586911

Patel, S., Park, H., Bonato, P., Chan, L., & Rodgers, M. (2012). A review of wearable sensors and systems with application in rehabilitation. *Journal of Neuroengineering and Rehabilitation*, *9*(1), 1–17. doi:10.1186/1743-0003-9-21 PMID:22520559

Ramey, C. T., & Ramey, S. L. (1998). Early Intervention and Early Experience. *The American Psychologist, 53*(2), 109–120. doi:10.1037/0003-066X.53.2.109 PMID:9491742

Randström, K. B., Asplund, K., Svedlund, M., & Paulson, M. (2013). Activity and participation in home rehabilitation: Older people's and family members' perspectives. In Journal of Rehabilitation Medicine (Vol. 45, Issue 2, pp. 211–216). doi:10.2340/16501977-1085

Rauch, A., Cieza, A., & Stucki, G. (2008). How to apply the international classification of functioning, disability and health (ICF) for rehabilitation management in clinical practice. *European Journal of Physical and Rehabilitation Medicine, 44*(3), 329–342. PMID:18762742

Reason, P., & Bradbury, H. (2001). *Handbook of action research: Participative inquiry and practice*. Sage.

Rushton, P. W., & Miller, W. C. (2002). Goal Attainment Scaling in the rehabilitation of patients with lower-extremity amputations: A pilot study. *Archives of Physical Medicine and Rehabilitation, 83*(6), 771–775. doi:10.1053/apmr.2002.32636 PMID:12048654

Salminen, A.-L., Hiekkala, S., & Stenberg, J.-H. (2016). *Remote rehabilitation. Research of the Social Insurance Institution of Finland*. KELA.

Siebes, R. C., Wijnroks, L., Ketelaar, M., van Schie, P. E. M., Gorter, J. W., & Vermeer, A. (2007). Parent participation in paediatric rehabilitation treatment centres in the Netherlands: A parents' viewpoint. *Child: Care, Health and Development, 33*(2), 196–205. doi:10.1111/j.1365-2214.2006.00636.x PMID:17291324

Steiner, W. A., Ryser, L., Huber, E., Uebelhart, D., Aeschlimann, A., & Stucki, G. (2002). Use of the ICF model as a clinical problem-solving tool in physical therapy and rehabilitation medicine. *Physical Therapy, 82*(11), 1098–1107. doi:10.1093/ptj/82.11.1098 PMID:12405874

Stucki, G., & Sangha, O. (1998). Principles of rehabilitation. *Rheumatology, 1*, 517–530.

Tse, M. M. Y., Kwan, R. Y. C., & Lau, J. L. (2018). Ageing in individuals with intellectual disability: Issues and concerns in Hong Kong. *Hong Kong Medical Journal, 24*(1), 68–72. doi:10.12809/hkmj166302 PMID:29326402

Turner-Stokes, L. (2009). Goal attainment scaling (GAS) in rehabilitation: A practical guide. *Clinical Rehabilitation, 23*(4), 362–370. doi:10.1177/0269215508101742 PMID:19179355

World Health Organization. (2007). *International Classification of Functioning, Disability, and Health: Children & Youth Version: ICF-CY*. World Health Organization.

Yalom, I. D. (2002). *The gift of therapy : reflections on being a therapist*. Piatkus London.

ADDITIONAL READING

Barnsteiner, J., Disch, J., & Walton, M. (2014). *Person and family centered care, 2014 AJN award recipient*. Sigma Theta Tau.

Effgen, S., & LaForme Fiss, A. (2021). *Meeting the Physical Therapy Needs of Children*. F.A. Davis Company.

Elefant, C. (2002). *Enhancing Communication in Girls with Rett Syndrome through Songs in Music Therapy*. Aalborg Universitet.

Fabio, R. A., Caprì, T., & Martino, G. (2019). *Understanding Rett Syndrome: A guide to symptoms, management and treatment*. Routledge. doi:10.4324/9780429470851

Hagberg, B., Anvret, M., Wahlstrom, J., & Wahlström, J. (1993). Rett syndrome-Clinical and biological aspects: Studies on 130 Swedish females (Issue 127). Cambridge University Press.

Lotan, M., & Merrick, J. (2011). *Rett Syndrome: Therapeutic Interventions*. Nova Science Publishers Inc.

Murphy, K. P., McMahon, M. A., & Houtrow, A. J. (2020). *Pediatric rehabilitation: principles and practice*. Springer Publishing Company. doi:10.1891/9780826147073

Reason, P., & Bradbury, H. (2001). *Handbook of action research: Participative inquiry and practice*. Sage.

Smith, L. (2009). *Child and family-centred healthcare: Concept, theory and practice*. Macmillan International Higher Education.

KEY TERMS AND DEFINITIONS

Family-Centered Care: Innovative approach to planning, delivering, and evaluating health care grounded in a mutually beneficial partnership among patients, families, and providers.

Habilitation: Process by which a person acquires new skills previously denied due to a disorder or impairment that had prevented their development. The term habilitation usually refers to the development of cognitive, social, fine motor, gross motor, or other skills that contribute to mobility, communication, and performance of activities of daily living and enhance the individual's quality of life.

Individualized Treatment: The concept for which each person's rehabilitation treatment must be planned based on his unique and peculiar characteristics and needs.

Motor Skill: The ability to perform a voluntary complex motor act.

Participatory Action Research: A shared, democratic process of research concerned with developing practical knowing to pursue worthwhile human purposes.

Rett Syndrome: A neurodevelopmental X-linked disorder characterized by apparently normal development until the age of 6-25 months when progressive loss of voluntary control of hand movements and communication skills; ataxia; seizures; autistic behavior; intermittent hyperventilation; hyperammonemia; and other comorbidities appear.

Telerehabilitation: Delivery of therapeutic rehabilitation at a distance or offsite using telecommunication technologies.

Section 3
Neurodegenerative Diseases

Chapter 9
Assistive Technology for Promoting the Independence and the Quality of Life in Persons With Alzheimer's Disease:
A Selective Review

Donatella Ciarmoli
University Giustino Fortunato of Benevento, Italy

ABSTRACT

Persons with Alzheimer's disease (AD) may present a loss of cognitive functioning, memory impairments, communication difficulties, obstacles to perform daily activities, disorientation, and challenging behaviours. Currently, there is no cure for AD. However, there are valid treatments to alleviate AD-related symptoms and to reduce the burden on carers; for example, the effectiveness of the use of assistive technology (AT) has been seen. The aim was to provide, in this chapter, an overview of the newest empirical evidences available on the use of AT-based programs to improve the independence and the quality of life of patients with Alzheimer's disease and their caregivers. A selective literature review was carried out considering Alzheimer's, assistive technologies, dementia, quality of life, and caregivers. Empirical data demonstrated the effectiveness and the suitability of the AT interventions allowing participants to improve their quality of life, as well as to mitigate the mental and physical burden of their caregivers.

INTRODUCTION

Alzheimer's disease (AD) is the most common form of dementia and accounts for 50–80% of dementia cases. It is characterized by memory loss and rapidly progresses to symptoms such as personality modifications and language difficulties, leading to a loss of the ability to perform routine activities and

DOI: 10.4018/978-1-7998-7430-0.ch009

eventual death for AD. Less than 1% of AD cases are related to genetic mutations; these cases generally occur in younger adults (approximately 45 years old) (Stoccoro & Coppedè, 2018). Alzheimer's disease is characterized by a progressive loss of cognitive functions. It is considered that neuroinflammation plays a fundamental role in its onset and progression (Carrillo-Avila, Melgar-Rodriguez, Díaz-Zuñiga & Martínez-Aguilar, 2020). The development and progression of AD are linked to the dysfunction and death of neurons, which generally appear to originate in the hippocampus, frontal, temporal lobes, and the limbic system, extending to neocortex regions as the disease progresses (Li et al., 2004). Currently, AD can be diagnosed in living patients by positron emission tomography (PET) and cerebrospinal fluid (CSF) techniques (Stoccoro & Coppedè, 2018). Additionally, AD may have social-emotional negative outcomes such as depression, withdrawal, and passivity (i.e., physical inactivity) (Ciro, Park, Burkhard, Yan & Geula, 2013). Accordingly, persons with AD may experience a growing negative impact on their quality of life (LoPresti, Bodine, & Lewis, 2008; Westphal, Dingjan, & Attoe, 2010).

Actually, there is no cure for AD, but some medication and therapies have been shown to reduce the behavioural and psychological symptoms, alleviating pressures and improving quality of life for individuals as well as their caregivers. Two basic categories of interventions have been up to date assessed for reducing the decline deterioration of AD, namely (a) pharmacological treatments, and (b) behavioral strategies (LoPresti, et al., 2008).

Five medications are currently used to treat the cognitive problems of AD: four are acetylcholinesterase inhibitors (tacrine, rivastigmine, galantamine and donepezil) and the other (memantine) is an NMDA receptor antagonist. The benefit from their use is small (Birks & Harvey, 2018). Any medication has been clearly shown to delay or halt the progression of the disease. Psychosocial interventions are used as an adjunct to pharmaceutical treatment and can be classified within behaviour, emotion, cognition, or stimulation-oriented approaches (Rabins, Blacker, & Rovner, 2007). The behavioral strategies or psychosocial interventions used for AD are: (a) Behavioural interventions attempt to identify and reduce the antecedents and consequences of target behaviors, to help reduce some specific problem behaviors, such as incontinence (Doody, Stevens, & Beck, 2001); (b) Stimulation-oriented treatments include art, music and pet therapies, exercise, and any other kind of recreational activities; (c) Emotion-oriented interventions include reminiscence therapy, validation therapy, supportive psychotherapy and sensory integration, and (d) cognition-oriented treatments, which include reality orientation and cognitive re-training, is the reduction of cognitive deficits ((Bottino, Carvalho, & Alvarez, 2005; Doody, Stevens, & Beck, 2001, Rabins, Blacker, & Rovner, 2007; Chung, Lai, Chung, & French, 2002; Spector et al., 2003).

The number of older affected by Alzheimer disease and related dementias will triple to 13 million persons by 2050, consequently increasing healthcare is needed. An approach to this emerging crisis is the development and deployment of intelligent assistive technologies that compensate for the specific physical and cognitive deficits of older adults with dementia, and thereby also reduce caregiver burden (Ashok et al., 2009).

Assistive Technology (AT) has been suggested as means by which people with dementia can be helped to live independently, while also leading to greater efficiencies in care. However, little is known about how AT is being used by people with dementia and their caregivers in their daily routines (Gibson, Dickinson, & Brittain, 2015). Assistive technology (AT) has been identified as one area in which both improvements and possible cost savings, in care delivery can be made (Duff & Dolphin, 2007). The term assistive technology incorporates a wide range of devices, ranging from simple, low-cost devices to complex home monitoring systems using electronic information and communication technology (ICT). In addition, technology use in everyday dementia care also includes the use of a range of everyday or household devices and objects, which will not be defined as 'AT' or even as 'technology' but which are routinely used to assist with care functions and household tasks (Astell, Malone, Williams, Hwang, & Ellis, 2014). Even the simplest technology tools offer Alzheimer's patients a great degree of help. To begin with, reminders in the form of messages can be recorded on a device at home and then played back out loud at the appropriate time. Some devices can even play messages based on the person's activity. Medication management technology can be as simple as a pillbox marked with days of the week or as high-tech as automated pill dispensers which beep and open to remind caregivers and those with dementia to take their medication (Grindrod & Gates, 2014).

Diaz-Orueta et al. (2014) clarified how some cognitive function (i.e., attention and verbal memory) may determine the interaction of cognitively impaired elderly people with technology. Twenty persons ranging between the mild and moderate level of AD were assessed by a means of neuropsychological and functional battery and were asked to follow simple commands from an avatar appearing on a TV by means of remote control, such as asking the participants to confirm their presence or to respond YES/NO to a proposal to see a TV program. The number of correct answers and command repetitions required for the user to respond were recorded. The results showed an improved performance in the TV task by the participants who were less impaired. Accordingly, neuropsychological assessment was considered a useful complementary tool for AT developers in the adaptation and the implementation to the elderly with different cognitive and functional profiles.

Carrasco et al. (2008) proposed a natural human computer interaction paradigm for persons with cognitive impairments such as Alzheimer's Disease. The paradigm consisted of using a realistic virtual character, rendered on a common television set, to play the role of a virtual personal assistant that shows reminders, notifications and performs short dialogues with the user. In this paradigm, the television remote control is used as a return channel to capture the user's responses. To test this concept, a functional prototype was built and then validated by a group of 21 persons with Alzheimer's Disease ranging from mild to moderate level. For this validation two simple dialogues were developed that consisted of simple Yes/No type questions. The test results showed that with both dialogues all users engaged naturally with the avatar. All of the users understood the information conveyed by the avatar and answered successfully by means of the TV remote control.

Recently, there has been a growing interest in employing serious games (SGs) for the assessment and rehabilitation of elderly people with mild cognitive impairment (MCI), Alzheimer's disease (AD), and related disorders. Manera et al. (2015) examined the acceptability of 'Kitchen and cooking' – a SG developed in the context of the EU project VERVE in these populations. In this game a cooking plot is employed to assess and stimulate executive functions (such as planning abilities) and praxis. The game is installed on a tablet, to be flexibly employed at home and in nursing homes. Twenty-one elderly participants (9 MCI and 12 AD, including 14 outpatients and 7 patients living in nursing homes, as well as 11 apathetic and 10 non-apathetic) took part in a 1-month trail, including a clinical and neuropsychological assessment, and 4-week training where the participants were free to play as long as they wanted on a personal tablet. During the training, participants met once a week with a clinician in order to fill in self-report questionnaires assessing their overall game experience (including acceptability, motivation, and perceived emotions). The results of the self-report and of the data concerning game performance (e.g., time spent playing or number of errors) confirmed the overall acceptability of Kitchen and cooking for both patients with MCI and patients with AD and related disorders, and the utility to employ it for training purposes. Interestingly, the results confirm that the game is suitable also to apathetic patients. Technological solutions are divided into different groups according to their using. Four main groups of ambient assisted living (AAL): daily task facilitation, mobility assistance, healthcare and rehabilitation, and social inclusion and communication have been introduced (Li, Lu & McDonald-Maier, 2015). Ranasinghe et al., (2020) have differentiated the application of motion systems, health monitoring, and activity recognition.

Chan et al. (2016) proposed grouping technology solutions into four categories: invasive wearable, non-invasive wearable, combined and others. This approach is important from the technology point of view because wearable or other invasive sensors have bigger concerns regarding their reception by patients (battery issues, technology acceptance). There is a whole range of categorizing options that usually take into account either the nature of the technology or the needs of senior citizens (Maresova, Tomsone, & Lameski, 2018).

The current chapter aims to present a selective review of the last two decades, categorizing the use and effectiveness of AT to support people with AD and their caregivers. In order to gain a deep understanding of the current state of assistive technology research and development in this domain, and to guide future research, a selective review was carried out. This focussed on the types of technology reported to have been designed, developed and evaluated across a broad sample of research literature. The implications of the findings were critically discussed. Some useful guidelines for future research and practice were detailed.

1. BACKGROUND

Assistive technology can be defined as "any device or system that allows an individual to perform a task that they would otherwise be unable to do or increases the ease and safety with which the task can be performed." This includes a wide range of devices that can grouped according to their purpose. People with AD experience very different symptoms that require different responses. Additionally, the most appropriate assistive technology will depend on an individual's lifestyle and circumstances which change over time.

2. METHODS

A computerized search was conducted in Scopus and PubMed databases. Alzheimer disease, dementia, assistive technologies and quality of life were merged as keywords.

The eligibility criteria were (a) an evidence-based study including an AT-based intervention, (b) old adults as participants (i.e., 70-95 years of age), (c) last two decades of publication interval (i.e., 2000-2020), and (d) English as language of the paper. Consequently, twenty-eight studies were reviewed with 818 participants included and grouped according to eight main categories, namely (a) aid to careers, (b) communication, (c) daily activities, (d) executive functions, (e) urinary incontinence, (f) spatial orientation, (g) physical activity and (h) positive participation (see Table 1). As introduced above, twenty-eight records were found. In the following section, the retained studies were concisely described and the synoptic table (i.e., Table 1) summarized the main findings.

3. LITERATURE OVERVIEW

The reviewed studies were arranged in alphabetic order and summarized in Table 1. The reader may note that review or theoretical papers were not included because their inclusion would exceed the aim and scope of the current chapter (see above the eligibility criteria in the Method section).

3.1 Aid to Careers

The first critical issue to resolve among individuals with AD is aids to caregivers. A range of interventions have been introduced to alleviate the adverse outcomes of dementia caregiving (Matthews et al., 2019). These interventions include programs to provide training in the management of dementia-related symptoms, bolstering resources through social support coordination, and respite designed to help caregivers maximize time free from care responsibilities (Brodaty, Green, & Koschera, 2003). There is growing recognition of the need for assistive technology for caregivers of persons with dementia as well (Sriram, Jenkinson, & Peters, 2019). Two studies with a total of 529 participants are reviewed in this group.

Peterson et al. (2020) aimed to evaluate Personal Health Record for Persons with Dementia and Their Family Caregivers (PHR-ADRD), a free web-based information exchange tool, using a multiphase mixed methods approach. Dementia caregivers (N=34) were surveyed for their well-being and perceptions of PHR-ADRD feasibility and utility at 6 and 12 months using close- and open-ended questions as well as a semi-structured interview (n=8). Exploratory analyses compared participants' characteristics as well as PHR-ADRD use and experiences based on overall favorable status. Feasibility and utility scores decreased over time, but a subset of participants indicated that the system was helpful. Quantitative comparisons could not explain why some participants indicated favorable, neutral, or negative views of the system overall or had not engaged with PHR-ADRD. Qualitative findings suggested that technology literacy and primary care provider buy-in were barriers. Both qualitative and qualitative findings indicated that time constraints to learn and use the system affected most participants. Development and dissemination of PHRs for family caregivers of persons with ADRD should aim to make systems user-friendly for persons with limited time and technological literacy. Establishing health care provider buy-in may be essential to the future success of any PHR system.

Davies et al. (2020) assessed the impact of AT on informal caregivers' burden and psychological well-being. Individuals with dementia and their informal caregivers were recruited to a randomized-controlled trial assessing effectiveness of AT. Caregivers were allocated to two groups according to their cared-for person's randomization to a full or basic package of AT and were assessed on caregiver burden, state anxiety, and depression. Caregivers' data from three assessments over 6 months of the trial were analyzed. No significant between- or within-group differences at any time point on caregivers' burden, anxiety, and depression levels were found. Full AT for people with dementia did not impact caregivers' psychological outcomes compared to basic AT. The length of follow up was restricted to 6 months.

3.2 Communication

A second crucial issue commonly addressed by AT-based programs is the individual's communication skills, because AD is a neurodegenerative disorder that progressively undermines the intellectual and physical functioning of the persons affected, with an increasing deterioration of their general performance including communication skills. Four studies with a total of 35 participants are reviewed in this group.

Lancioni et al. (2014) assessed a simple computer-aided program for helping patients with moderate Alzheimer's disease engage in verbal reminiscence. Practically, the program was aimed at fostering the patient's verbal engagement on a number of life experiences/topics previously selected for him or her and introduced in the sessions through a friendly female, who appeared on the computer screen. The female asked the patient about the aforementioned experiences/topics, and provided him or her with positive attention, and possibly verbal guidance (i.e., prompts/encouragements). Eight patients were involved in the study, which was carried out according to non-concurrent multiple baseline designs across participants. Seven of them showed clear improvement during the intervention phase (i.e., with the program). Their mean percentages of intervals with verbal engagement/reminiscence ranged from close to zero to about 15 during the baseline and from above 50 to above 75 during the intervention. The results were discussed in relation to previous literature on reminiscence therapy, with specific emphasis on the need for (a) replication studies and (b) the development of new versions of the technology-aided program to improve its impact and reach a wider number of patients.

Lancioni et al. (2012) developed a technology-aided intervention strategy relying on pictorial cues alone or in combination with verbal instructions and assessed these two versions of the strategy with three persons with moderate Alzheimer's disease. In Section I of the study, the strategy version with pictorial cues plus verbal instructions was compared with an existing technology-based strategy with verbal instructions. Each strategy was used with one specific activity. In Section II of the study, the strategy version with pictorial cues alone was compared with the aforementioned strategy with verbal instructions. Again, each strategy was used with one activity. Both strategy versions were effective with all three participants. The percentages of correct activity performance observed with those versions increased to above 90 and were comparable with those obtained with the existing verbal instructions strategy. A social validation assessment of the version with pictorial cues alone and the existing strategy with verbal instructions (employing university psychology students as raters) showed differences in the latter strategy in terms of practicality and in the former in terms of respect of participants' dignity.

Lancioni et al (2015) focused on the assessment of a program recently developed for helping patients with moderate Alzheimer's disease engage in computer-mediated verbal reminiscence (Lancioni et al., 2014a). Sixteen participants were involved in the study. Six of them used the original program version with the computer showing a virtual partner posing questions and providing attention and guidance. The other 10 used a slightly modified program version with the computer presenting photos and videos and providing encouragements to talk as well as attention and guidance. Participants were exposed to brief program sessions individually. The results showed that 15 participants (five of those using the first version and all of those using the second version) had a clear and lasting increase in verbal engagement/reminiscence during the intervention sessions with the program. Those 15 participants had mean percentages of intervals with verbal engagement/reminiscence below 10 during baseline and between about 45 and 75 during the intervention.

Lancioni et al. (2016) implemented a program for verbal reminiscence and assessed it with eight new participants. Have monitored the participants' verbal production during the intervention in which photos and brief videos were used to foster verbal reminiscence. Monitoring allowed computer approval and reminders to be consistent with the participants' behavior. The results showed that the participants' mean percentages of intervals with verbal engagement/reminiscence were below 10 during baseline and control sessions and between above 50 and nearly 80 during the intervention.

3.3 Daily Activities

Next to communication skills, daily activities are considered essential, because persons affected by AD experience a progressive decline of their condition with a gradual loss of their independence in daily functioning (Ambrose, 2012). Indeed, they are less autonomous in important areas involving, among others, (1) managing medication and finances, (2) using typical communication means to interact with family and friends (e.g., using the telephone), (3) performing daily activities such as preparing food, (4) managing orientation and travel within circumscribed and familiar places, such as home or daily centers and (5) engaging in recreation activities such as listening to music (Lancioni et al. 2014). In this group, five studies with a total of 19 participants are reviewed.

Lancioni et al. (2014) proposed two studies that aimed to evaluating standard technology resources for supporting activity and travel among patients with moderate Alzheimer's disease. Specifically, Study I assessed a pictorial instruction program relying on the use of a portable computer and a commercially available and inexpensive video editing software for supporting the performance of daily activities with three patients. Study II assessed the indoor travel performance of four patients (i.e., the three involved in Study I and a fourth patient with no previous research exposure) using a commercially available, basic doorbell system with sound and light cues. The percentages of correct activity steps obtained with the instruction program used in Study I were relatively high and largely like the percentages reported in previous studies using more sophisticated technology. During Study II, the percentages of correct travels of two patients matched the data of the most successful patients involved in previous studies with more sophisticated technology. The percentages of the other two patients tended to be lower than those obtained previously but were still practically relevant.

Lancioni et al. (2014) assessed technology-aided programs to support performance of daily activities and selection/activation of music items with patients with moderate AD. A four patients, during the intervention, were presented with activity-related pictorial instructions via a computer fitted with inexpensive, commercial software. At the same time as a second group of four patients were (a) presented with different music options and (b) allowed to select and activate the preferred option via a microswitch response. The first group showed that each patient learned to perform the two activities available with percentages of correct responses exceeding 85 by the end of the intervention. The second group showed that all patients learned to choose and activate music options. Psychology students, involved in a social validation procedure, scored the patients' behavior within the program better than their behavior in a control moment.

Lancioni et al. (2018) evaluated technology-based behavioral interventions for promoting daily activities in people with mild-to-moderate AD. Eight participants who were taught to start and carry out daily activities on their own using a tablet or a smartphone device, which provided activity reminders, step instructions, and praise were enrolled. The participants succeeded in starting the activities independently and carrying them out accurately; concluding that aforementioned technology-based interventions may represent practical means for supporting people with Alzheimer's disease.

Lancioni et al. (2014) conducted a study to assess technology-aided programs to promote leisure engagement in persons with AD. Specifically, a program aimed at enabling three patients with mild or moderate AD to choose among different music options and favorite stimuli was assessed. The study was carried out according to a nonconcurrent multiple baseline design across patients. Results were very encouraging. The patients learned to choose and activate their preferred music pieces.

Gobeil et al. (2019) conduced a qualitative, descriptive single-case study with an older woman with mild AD and her caregiver to document the acceptability of AMELIS. Ten learning sessions were performed (1989), errorless learning and multi-layer approach. Data collection comprised pre- and post-intervention interviews with the participant and her caregiver, logbooks, and experimenter's summaries. A thematic analysis was conducted, and Technology Acceptance Model (TAM) was used to structure the presentation of the results. This study revealed that the acceptability of AMELIS was positive mainly because the tool was reported as useful by the participant and her caregiver. The large touchscreen and the personalized learning method also influenced their attitude towards the use of the tool. Thus, AMELIS is an innovative technology that has the potential to be accepted by older people with AD and their families.

3.4 Executive Functions

Assistive technology has been recognized as a promising tool to improve the lives of persons living with memory loss and their caregivers. The use of assistive technology in dementia care is expanding, although it is most often intended to manage care and promote safety. There is a lack of assistive technology designed to aid persons with memory loss in participating in meaningful activities. Four studies with a total of 148 participants are reviewed in this group.

McCarron (2019) used a pilot randomized controlled trial (RCT) design to evaluate the Social Support Aid (SSA). The SSA is a mobile phone-based app that employs facial recognition software. It was designed to assist persons with memory loss remember the names and relationships of the people they interact with to promote social engagement. The objectives were to ascertain (1) the feasibility and utility of the SSA, (2) whether the outcomes of SSA use suggested potential benefits for persons living with memory loss and their care partners, and (3) how study design components could inform subsequent RCTs. Persons with memory loss were randomized to the SSA (n=20) or the usual care control group (n=28). Quantitative data were collected at three timepoints (baseline, 3 months, and 6 months). Participants in the intervention group participated in qualitative interviews following completion of their 6-month survey. Participant eligibility, willingness to be randomized, and retention were not barriers to conducting a full scale RCT; however, recruitment strategies should be addressed before. Feasibility and utility scores indicated that participants felt neutral about the technology. Use of the SSA was not significantly associated with changes in quality of social interactions or quality of life measures over the 6 months of follow-up (P>.05). The qualitative analysis revealed three themes that described how and why the SSA worked or not: (1) outcomes, (2) reasons why it was or was not useful, and (3) recommendations. There is a need to develop effective assistive technology that improves the quality of life of persons with memory loss. Assistive technology for memory loss should be a priority for future research.

Recently, virtual reality memory training demonstrated effectiveness in improving memory functions in older people with MCI. In fact, Optale et al. (2010) evaluated in a 6-month randomized controlled trial (n = 36), an intervention group which received immersive computer-generated virtual reality memory training through a head-mounted display using a combination of auditory (music) and visual stimuli to create a virtual environment and participants navigated the virtual surroundings using a joystick. The control group received a musical therapy intervention. The primary outcome measure in the study was the Mini-Mental State Examination (MMSE) a commonly used screening tool for cognitive impairment. Other aspects of cognition function were also assessed including attention, and verbal fluency through navigating the environment, learning routes, and remembering objects. After a period of 36 sessions over a 3-month training period, the intervention group showed improvements in the MMSE ($p = 0.014$), with maintenance of the benefits following a 3-month booster phase of 24 sessions ($p = 0.044$), while the control group MMSE scores decreased ($p = 0.001$ and $p = 0.003$, respectively) compared to baseline. Other improvements were also observed, particularly in digit span forward and verbal story recall (all $p < 0.05$). Depressive symptoms measured using the Geriatric Depression Scale decreased after the initial 3-month training period ($p = 0.025$) but not after the booster period. Higher depressive symptoms were observed in the control group after 3 months but not after the booster.

Similarly, Man et al. (2012) have reported in another randomized controlled trial (n = 44) of participants with questionable dementia (indicated by the CDR scale as consistent with MCI) using non-immersive scenario-based virtual reality memory training, while participants in the control groups underwent therapy-led non-virtual reality sessions of memory training using similar procedures The computer-generated virtual reality experience presented 2 scenarios: firstly, a home setting with 2 bedrooms, a living room, a dining room, a kitchen, and a bathroom, and, secondly, a convenience store with several products, refrigerators, and a cashier. Participants were given verbal and written instructions and timed while navigating the scenarios using a joystick and carrying out specific tasks. Practice effects were observed in both groups; however, the intervention group performed better in total encoding, total recall and delayed recall in the Fuld Object Memory Evaluation and the Multifactorial Memory Questionnaire (strategy) (all $p < 0.001$). However, only the non-virtual reality group reported improvements in the Multifactorial Memory Questionnaire (contentment).

A study by Siriaraya and Ang (2014) conducted intriguing virtual reality mixed-method investigations (n = 20) using different prototypes to recreating memories and social engagement in People Living with Dementia (PLWD) in long-term aged care. Over 9 visits, 3 different virtual reality settings ("reminiscence room," "virtual tool," and "gardening") were tested in 2 aged care facilities, followed by semi-structured interviews with care staff regarding the efficacy of the interventions. Results showed that virtual reality activities triggered reminiscence. Reminiscence also occurred through their interaction with virtual objects, particularly with objects of personal relevance. A sense of escapism was reported among participants, with reports of "being slipped into an alternate reality" along with positive feelings. However, in 1 participant, reminiscence led to feelings of sadness while reflecting on past experiences, prompting care staff to redirect the participant back into the virtual garden. More studies are needed to assess the ability of virtual reality to facilitate reminiscence in PLWD, including studies of reminiscence therapy which provides structure and support for the participant during and after the virtual experience.

3.5. Uninary Incontinence

Urinary incontinence and toileting problems in general are quite frequent among older people, particularly those affected by Alzheimer's disease and other dementias (Adkins & Mathews, 1997). Cognitively competent older people are expected to benefit from combinations of habit training, bladder and pelvic muscle exercise, and biofeedback (Goode, Burgio, Richter, & Markland, 2010). Only one study with three participants is reviewed in this group.

Lancioni et al (2011) assessed whether three patients with Alzheimer's disease could learn to use urine alarms and caregivers' prompts to eliminate large urinary accidents. As soon as the patient began to release urine, the alarm system presented auditory and vibratory signals. In relation to those signals, the caregiver would prompt/encourage the patient to stop urinating and accompany him or her to the toilet to void. After urination, the caregiver provided the patient positive social attention. The results of the intervention showed that the use of the alarm system and caregivers' prompts was effective in helping the three patients to reduce their large urinary accidents to zero or near zero levels. Self-initiated toileting, which was minimal during baseline, accounted for nearly 35%, 50% and 75% of the patients' toileting occasions during the intervention. Fifty-two caregivers, who participated in a social validation assessment of toileting approaches relying on alarm systems or timed toileting, seemed to find the former preferable for the patients, for the context, as well as for themselves.

3.6 Orientation

The persons affected by AD gradually lose their abilities to, among others, find the way within familiar contexts and even indoor areas, such as the home. Behavioral interventions have traditionally involved strategies such as reality orientation training, memory training and stimulation enrichment (Arkin, 2007). Three studies with a total of 11 participants are reviewed in this group.

Lancioni et al (2014) proposed two studies extended the assessment of programs recently developed for promoting activity and orientation in persons with moderate AD. Specifically, Study I pursued a new evaluation of a program, in which pictorial instructions of activity steps are presented on a computer screen at intervals. Study II pursued a new evaluation of a program using music and strobe lights (emitted at the destinations) as spatial cues to support indoor orientation and travel. Six participants were included, three per study. The results of Study I showed that the participants reached high percentages of correct steps in each of the two activities targeted. The results of Study II showed that the participants had high percentages of correct orientation and travel within their day care context. The results of both studies were in line with the data of previous studies in these areas.

Lancioni et al. (2013) extended the assessment of an orientation program involving auditory cues (i.e., verbal messages automatically presented from the destinations) with five patients with AD; compared the effects of this program with those of a program with light cues (i.e., a program in which strobe lights were used instead of the verbal messages) with the same five patients, and (b) conducted a social validation assessment of the two programs with 70 university psychology students employed as social raters. Results confirmed the effectiveness of the program with auditory cues and showed an equally strong impact of the program with light cues with all five patients. The psychology students involved in the social validation assessment provided significantly higher scores for the program involving light cues on a six-item questionnaire. Those scores suggested that this program was perceived as a practically and socially preferable choice.

Lancioni et al (2011) assessed whether three patients with Alzheimer's disease could learn to use a basic orientation technology to reach different rooms within a medical center. At each travel instance, the technology provided verbal messages (cues) from the room to reach. For the first two patients, the messages were presented at intervals of about 15 s. For the third patient (who had more extensive orientation problems), shorter intervals combined with the voice of the research assistant were initially used. Results showed that all three patients were successful in using the technology to orient their travel and find the rooms correctly. A social validation assessment, in which university psychology students were asked to rate the patients' travel performance with the technology and with the help of a caregiver, provided generally higher (more positive) scores for the technology-assisted performance.

3.7 Positive Participation

For patients who are in the severe and lower end of the moderate stage of the disease, intervention programs may be more simply directed at promoting participation in (i.e., attention/orientation to and possible physical involvement with) positive environmental events (Gerdner, 2000). Four studies with a total of 30 participants are reviewed in this group.

Lancioni et al. (2012), extended the comparison of active (self-regulated) music stimulation versus passive (outer-regulated) music stimulation with seven new patients in the severe or low moderate stage of Alzheimer's disease. In the active condition, the patients used a simple hand response and a microswitch to self-regulate music stimulation inputs. In the passive condition, music stimulation was automatically presented throughout the sessions (i.e., continuously). Data showed an increase in the patients' indices of positive participation (e.g., singing or music-related movements, and smiles) during both music conditions. The increase in the active condition was greater than that in the passive condition for five of the seven patients. The other two patients showed comparable data across conditions and a smaller increase in the active condition, respectively.

Pino, Granata, Legouverneur, and Rigaud (2012) developed a robot (i.e., graphical user interface; GUI) aimed at providing cognitive and social support, through a suite of applications (i.e., task reminder, navigation support, and communication). The GUI delivered these services for eleven elderly patients with MCI. A user-centered design for the GUI was adopted. First, the moderator described the purpose of the research, introduced the robot, and explained the evaluation procedure. Then participants were asked to complete a series of tasks using the main menu of the GUI and navigate through its different applications. Performance and satisfaction measures were collected (i.e., time to complete each task, number of errors due to manipulation, and number of help requests). Test were carried out individually. Findings confirmed that most of the features of the GUI were adapted to the needs and capacities of older adults with cognitive impairments. However, individual factors (e.g., age, education level, and computer experience) were found to affect task performances. Finally, some specific characteristics of the interfaces (i.e., icons and navigation system) had to be modified to make the application usable by the largest number of patients suffering from cognitive deficits.

Lancioni et al. (2013), assessed the impact and social rating of an active and a passive music condition implemented with six patients with Alzheimer's disease. In the active condition, the patients used a simple hand response and a microswitch to self-regulate music stimulation inputs. In the passive condition, music stimulation was automatically presented throughout the sessions. Active and passive stimulation sessions were preceded and followed by control (non-stimulation) sessions. The active condition sessions showed an increase in the patients' indices of positive participation (e.g., singing or music-related movements, and smiles) greater than that observed in the passive condition sessions for five of the six patients. Positive intervention effects could also spread to the post-intervention sessions. Social raters (42 care and rehabilitation staff members working with persons with multiple disabilities) positively scored the active condition on a six-item questionnaire dealing with, among others, conditions' suitability, respect of patients' dignity and independence, and practicality.

Nijhof, van Hoof, van Rijn, and van Gemert-Pijnen (2013) planned a technology-supported leisure game for people with dementia in relation to the stimulation of social behavior. Its impact on behavioral outcomes of persons with dementia was explored in a nursing home and day care setting in comparison to a traditional leisure activity. The technology was aimed to stimulate social behavior and interaction among 10 participants with AD, via its design features, including a TV, radio, telephone, and treasure box. A mixed-method research design was applied. The observations were conducted using the Oshkosh Social Behavior Coding scale. Results showed that social behavior was found to occur more often than non-social behavior. Specifically, participants with a low Mini-Mental State Evaluation Score, scored higher for non-social and non-verbal behavior. Females scored higher for social behavior than males. The interviewed activities facilitators claimed that the technology-supported leisure game helped them with their professional tasks.

3.8 Physical Activity

Behavioral interventions available for persons in the mild or early moderate stages of the disease may include technology-aided programs aimed at supporting different types of functional engagement concerning, among others, daily activities, leisure/entertainment, communication, reminiscence, and physical activity. Four studies with a total of 43 participants are reviewed in this group.

Lancioni et al. (2019) assessed a smartphone-based program to promote practical and mildly demanding arm responses and personal satisfaction and increase physical exertion (heart rates) in people with advanced Alzheimer's disease. The program relied on a Samsung Galaxy A3 smartphone with Android 6.0 operating system. Two groups of 10 and 11 participants, respectively, were assigned different responses (i.e., placing cards into an elevated box and moving bottles with water from a table into a container). Responses activated the smartphone, which produced brief periods of preferred stimulation. Lack of responding led the smartphone to produce a verbal prompt. All participants significantly increased the independent response frequencies, level of personal satisfaction, and heart rates during program sessions as opposed to baseline or control sessions. A smartphone-based program may help people with advanced Alzheimer's disease increase independent occupation with possible benefits in terms of satisfaction and physical condition.

Lancioni et al. (2018) evaluated technology-based interventions for promoting daily activities and supported ambulation in people with mild-to-moderate and moderate-to-severe Alzheimer's disease, respectively. This study included 9 participants who were taught to engage in brief periods of ambulation using a walker combined with a tilt microswitch and a notebook computer, which monitored step responses and provided stimulation and prompts. The participants largely increased their ambulation levels and also showed signs of positive involvement (e.g., smiles and verbalizations).

Lancioni et al (2016) used technology-aided programs to promote mild physical activity (i.e., positive forms of engagement) in persons with moderate or severe Alzheimer's disease have provided promising results. This study extended the assessment of the program for promoting mild physical activity with 10 new participants for whom arm-raising responses were targeted. The results showed that the mean frequencies of arm-raising responses were about or below four and between about 10 and 19 per session during the baseline and the intervention, respectively.

Lancioni et al. (2014) conducted two studies to assess technology-aided programs to promote mild physical activity, directed at patients in the low moderate or severe stages of the Alzheimer's disease who were no longer capable of ambulating and spent their time generally inactive, sitting in their wheelchairs. In particular, Study I used a program to help three patients exercise an arm-raising movement. Study II used a program to help three patients exercise a leg-foot movement. Each study was carried out according to a non-concurrent multiple baseline design across patients. Results were very encouraging. The patients enhanced their performance of the target movements and increased their indices of positive participation (e.g., smiles and verbalizations) during the sessions.

Table 1. Reviewed studies arranged in alphabetic order

Authors	Participants	Mean ages	Groups
Davies et al (2020)	495	-	aid to carers
Gobeil (2019)	1	78	daily activities
Lancioni et al. (2011)	3	78	orientation
Lancioni et al. (2011)	3	84.5	incontinence
Lancioni et al. (2012)	3	-	positive partecipation
Lancioni et al. (2012)	3	76.3	comunication
Lancioni et al. (2013)	5	77	orientation
Lancioni et al. (2013)	6	81	positive partecipation
Lancioni et al. (2014)	4	80	daily activities
Lancioni et al. (2014)	3	74.6	orientation
Lancioni et al. (2014)	8	83	comunication
Lancioni et al. (2014)	3	82.3	daily activities
Lancioni et al. (2014)	3	72.3	daily activities
Lancioni et al. (2014)	3	89.66	physical activity
Lancioni et al. (2015)	16	81.5	comunication
Lancioni et al. (2016)	8	82	comunication
Lancioni et al. (2016)	10	82	physical activity
Lancioni et al. (2018)	8	82.5	daily activities
Lancioni et al. (2018)	9	81	physical activity
Lancioni et al. (2019)	21	84.5	physical activity
Man et al. (2012)	44		executive function
Mc Carron et al. (2019)	48	74.9	executive function
Nijhof et al. (2013)	10	80	positive partecipation
Optale et al. (2010)	36	80	executive function
Peterson et al. (2020)	34	-	aid to carers
Pino et al. (2012)	11	78	positive partecipation
Siriaraya and Ang ()	20	86	executive function

4. DISCUSSION

Data of the reviewed studies evidenced an overall effectiveness, suitability, and validity of the AT-based interventions to enable patients with AD to orient themselves in space, perform physical activities while combating sedentariness, perform daily activities, have positive participation, avoid incontinence, improve executive functions, and help careers. Results observed in the reviewed studies were satisfactory. Whenever available, social validation procedures, maintenance or follow-up phases confirmed social and clinical validities of the adopted programs, which were consolidated over the time.

AT-based interventions may be viewed as great educational, psychological, and rehabilitative resources. In fact, they prevent isolation, withdrawal, and passivity. The AT-based programs were helpful for promoting the independence and an active role of the participants involved in the selected studies. The patients with AD were positively occupied and constructively engaged. Thus, the participants of the reviewed studies profitably learned the use of the technology. Their physical exercises were supported, their daily activities profitably managed, their communication skills promoted, their leisure and occupation opportunities significantly increased. Furthermore, their challenging behaviors were relevantly reduced. One may argue that the AT-based strategies may have beneficial effects on the participants' quality of life (Span et al., 2018; Zellefrow et al., 2017). Furthermore, the caregivers' burden may be decreased because independent adaptive responding of the participants with AD was improved. Accordingly, AD patients no more relied on caregivers' assistance, with reciprocal positive outcomes. The participants restored the loosed skills and were rewarded and motivated through an individualized selection of the positive stimulation. Similarly, the technological solutions were personalized for fostering their adaptation to each participant. One may argue that by designing a customer-tailored solution, the user may largely benefit of the learning process, with significant outcomes in daily contexts (Billis, Mantziari, Zilidou, & Bamidis, 2018; Rosenberg & Nygard, 2017). On many occasions, AT-based programmes have also been favourably evaluated by external evaluators and their own families.

As to the social aspect of this topic, research suggested that senior patients and their caregivers are willing to accept technological solutions and, after overcoming the initial hesitation, are ready to actively use them. In this respect, it was essential for the technological solutions to be easy to operate and easy to carry around. Surveys investigating the attitudes of elderly patients to new technologies showed that they appreciated the benefits of the technology and comparatively easily accepted non-intrusive devices and tools. Intrusive gadgets and wearables are not universally popular. The target group, however, values the increased autonomy, independence, safety, as well as the social connectivity that these devices bring (Ozturk et al., 2018).

For the individual AT-groups reviewed, the data suggest the following considerations: 1) First of all, we can say that AT is useful in order to alleviate the adverse outcomes that are reflected on the people who help Alzheimer's patients, and therefore on their carers (Davies et al., 2020; Peterson et al., 2012); 2) the communication skills of people with AD are found to be greatly improved through the use of assistive technology to promote verbal reminiscence (Lancioni et al, 2014;2015); 3) Daily activities are easy to perform thanks to the implementation of programs based on AT, integrating equipment capable of improving autonomy in the performance of simple daily activities (Gobeil et al., 2019; Lancioni et al., 2018); 4) Equipping people with Alzheimer's with assistive technology that can improve executive functions such as memory allows you to help the patient with memories but also their caregivers (Man et al., 2012); 5) Although incontinence problems in patients with Alzheimer's disease are quite frequent, to date few studies have focused on this problem. However, this problem is critical for both patients and their carers. The use of "urinary alarms" could be one of the possible solutions to this problem (Lancioni et al., 2011); 6) Programs based on the use of AT are found to give positive performance on orientation ability in people with AD (Lancioni et al., 2013); 7) Little is being done for people with severe-to-moderate stages of Alzheimer's, however, the importance of designing technology-based interventions to promote positive participation has been seen (Lancioni et al., 2013; Pino et al., 2012); and 8) Technological aid programs to promote functional engagement (such as physical activities) appear to be valuable for people with AD (Lancioni et al., 2014).

5. CONCLUSION

Assistive technologies, as we have seen, offer the opportunity for Alzheimer's patients to live in a safe and controlled environment, avoid social isolation and perform simple daily activities. Moreover, assistive technologies in some cases allowed carers to lower their level of responsibility with aids that allow tracking of people with AD. Various types of assistive technologies have been examined to help to manage some of the symptoms of Alzheimer. Although there are obvious ethical and practical difficulties, more research needs to be done in the specified targeted population in order to develop interventions which offer more appropriate care. The symptoms and effects of dementia presented above can be used to suggest that there is both high potential for assistive technologies to have a positive impact in this area, but also a need for these technologies to be designed with an in-depth understanding of constraints on interaction caused by the disease. The majority of AT currently available support day-to-day living activities, safety monitoring and can assist in health care. However, these devices merely address the 'ease of living' rather than focus on 'quality of life'. One potential area for development is recreational devices to encourage individuals with dementia to participate in hobbies which they once enjoyed. There are already a number of technologies in use, including digital devices, smart sensors, and intelligent applications, that assist elderly people with their everyday needs in their own homes. Developing a strategy for an integrated technological solution would resolve many issues faced by elderly patients and would lead to improving their quality of life, health, and safety.

6. FUTURE RESEARCH

New research should deal with the following topics (a) new extension of the AT-based programs with new patients with AD, (b) the assessment of maintenance, generalization, and/or follow-up phases for evaluating the learning process, (c) new preference check assessment phases for the participants involved, and (d) the recruitment of new groups of external raters for further social validation procedures.

In light of the above, the future research should consider the following features. A first research effort should deal with samples extension. Further empirical contributions should evaluate the use of AT-based interventions on a larger and representative sample of patients with AD. In addition, few studies have focused on problems of incontinence and executive functions. Therefore, research effort should include further technological and individualized solutions for incontinence and executive functions.

Lastly, more consideration should be given to telerehabilitation services, remote technologies should be adopted. For instance, telerehabilitation could be useful for both assessment and recovery purposes. Because telemedicine can provide follow-up care to help people with dementia to maintain their independence and continue living in their own homes, improve their safety, ameliorate clinical outcomes, and reduce access to health services. Ecological validity, experimental control, and tracking of behavioral responses may be easily managed.

REFERENCES

Adkins, V. K., & Mathews, R. M. (1997). Prompted voiding to reduce incontinence in community-dwelling older adults. *Journal of Applied Behavior Analysis*, *30*(1), 153–156. doi:10.1901/jaba.1997.30-153 PMID:9103990

Ambrose, C. T. (2012). Neuroangiogenesis: A vascular basis for Alzheimer's disease and cognitive decline during aging. *Journal of Alzheimer's Disease*, *32*(3), 773–778. doi:10.3233/JAD-2012-120067 PMID:22850316

Arkin, S. (2007). Language-enriched exercise plus socialization slows cognitive decline in Alzheimer's disease. *American Journal of Alzheimer's Disease and Other Dementias*, *22*(1), 62–77. doi:10.1177/1533317506295377 PMID:17534004

Ashok, J., Bharucha, C., Anand, V., Forlizzi, J., Dew, M. A., & Charles, F. (2009). Reynolds, Scott Stevens, Howard Wactlar, Intelligent Assistive Technology Applications to Dementia Care: Current Capabilities, Limitations, and Future Challenges. *The American Journal of Geriatric Psychiatry*, *17*, 84–88.

Astell, A., Malone, B., Williams, G., Hwang, F., & Ellis, M. (2014). Leveraging everyday technology for people living with dementia: A case study. *Journal of Assistive Technologies*, *8*(4), 164–176. doi:10.1108/JAT-01-2014-0004

Bankole, A., Anderson, M., Smith-Jackson, T., Knight, A., Oh, K., Brantley, J., Barth, A., & Lach, J. (2012). Validation of noninvasive body sensor network technology in the detection of agitation in dementia. *American Journal of Alzheimer's Disease and Other Dementias*, *27*(5), 346–354. doi:10.1177/1533317512452036 PMID:22815084

Billis, A., Mantziari, D., Zilidou, V., & Bamidis, P. D. (2018). Co-Creation of an Innovative Vocational Training Platform to Improve Autonomy in the Context of Alzheimer's Disease. *The American Journal of Geriatric Psychiatry*, 309–323. PMID:29968665

Birks, J. S., & Harvey, R. J. (2018). Donepezil for dementia due to Alzheimer's disease. *Cochrane Database of Systematic Reviews*, *8*, 12–13. doi:10.1002/14651858.CD001190.pub3 PMID:29923184

Bottino, C. M., Carvalho, I. A., Alvarez, A. M., Avila, R., Zukauskas, P. R., Bustamante, S. E. Z., Andrade, F. C., Hototian, S. R., Saffi, F., & Camargo, C. H. P. (2005, December). Cognitive rehabilitation combined with drug treatment in Alzheimer's disease patients: A pilot study. *Clinical Rehabilitation*, *19*(8), 861–864. doi:10.1191/0269215505cr911oa PMID:16323385

Brodaty, H., Green, A., & Koschera, A. (2003). Meta-analysis of psychosocial interventions for caregivers of people with dementia. *Journal of the American Geriatrics Society*, *51*(5), 657–664. doi:10.1034/j.1600-0579.2003.00210.x PMID:12752841

Camilo, M. C. (2009). *Tecnologie quotidiane per la cura della malattia di Alzheimer: risultati della ricerca, direzioni e sfide*. Elsevier.

Carrasco, E., Epelde, G., Moreno, A., Ortiz, A., Garcia, I., Buiza, C., Urdaneta, E., Etxaniz, A., Gonz'alez, M. F., & Arruti, A. (2008). *Natural Interaction between Virtual Characters and Persons with Alzheimer's Disease*. University of the Basque Country.

Carrillo-Avila, A., Melgar-Rodriguez, S., Díaz-Zuñiga, J., & Martínez-Aguilar, V. (2020). Periodontitis and alzheimer´s disease. *Medicina Oral Patología Oral y Cirugia.*

Chan, D., Gallaher, L. M., Moodley, K., Minati, L., Burgess, N., & Hartley, T. (2016). The 4 Mountains Test: A Short Test of Spatial Memory with High Sensitivity for the Diagnosis of Pre-dementia Alzheimer's Disease. *Journal of Visualized Experiments, 116*(116), 54–55. doi:10.3791/54454 PMID:27768046

Cheong, C. K., Lim, K. H., Jang, J. W., & Jhoo, J. H. (2015). The effect of telemedicine on the duration of treatment in dementia patients. *Journal of Telemedicine and Telecare, 21*(4), 214–218. doi:10.1177/1357633X14566571 PMID:25586813

Chung, J. C., Lai, C. K., Chung, P. M., & French, H. P. (2002). Snoezelen for dementia. *Cochrane Database of Systematic Reviews, 4*, 15–18. PMID:12519587

Ciro, A., Park, J., Burkhard, G., Yan, N., & Geula, C. (2012). Biochemical differentiation of cholinesterases from normal and Alzheimer's disease cortex. *Current Alzheimer Research, 9*(1), 138–143. doi:10.2174/156720512799015127 PMID:21244353

Davies, A., Brini, S., Hirani, S., Gathercole, R., Forsyth, K., Henderson, C., Bradley, R., & Davies, L. (2020). The impact of assistive technology on burden and psychological well-being in informal caregivers of people with dementia (ATTILA Study). *Translational Research & Clinical Interventions,* 1-10.

Diaz-Orueta, U., Etxaniz, A., Gonzalez, M. F., Buiza, C., Urdaneta, E., & Yanguas, J. (2014). Role of cognitive and functional performance in interactions between older people with cognitive decline and an avatar on TV. *Universal Access in the Information Society, 13*(1), 89–97. doi:10.100710209-013-0288-1

Doody, R. S., Stevens, J. C., Beck, C., Dubinsky, R. M., Kaye, J. A., Gwyther, L., Mohs, R. C., Thal, L. J., Whitehouse, P. J., DeKosky, S. T., & Cummings, J. L. (2001). Practice parameter: Management of dementia (an evidence-based review). Report of the Quality Standards Subcommittee of the American Academy of Neurology. *Neurology, 56*(9), 1154–1166. doi:10.1212/WNL.56.9.1154 PMID:11342679

Duff, P., & Dolphin, C. (2007). Cost-benefit analysis of assistive technology to support independence for people with dementia – part 2. Results from employing the ENABLE cost-benefit model in practice. *Technology and Disability, 19*(2-3), 79–90. doi:10.3233/TAD-2007-192-305

Gibson, G., Dickinson, C., & Brittain, K. (2015). The everyday use of assistive technology by people with dementia and their family carers: A qualitative study. *BMC Geriatrics, 15*, 89.

Gobeil, G., Pigot, H., Laliberté, C., Dépelteau, A., Laverdière, O., Grégoire, M.A.D., Laprise, N., Beauchamp, I., Couture, M., Adelise, Y., & Bier, N. (n.d.). Facilitating day-to-day life management of older people with Alzheimer's disease: A revelatory single-case study on the acceptability. *AMELIS Interactive Calendar, 18*, 241-257.

Goode, P. S., Burgio, K. L., Richter, H. E., & Markland, A. D. (2010). Incontinence in older women. *Journal of the American Medical Association, 303*(21), 2172–2181. doi:10.1001/jama.2010.749 PMID:20516418

Gregg, L., & Tarrier, N. (2007). Virtual reality in mental health: A review of the literature. *Social Psychiatry and Psychiatric Epidemiology, 42*(5), 343–354. doi:10.100700127-007-0173-4 PMID:17431528

Grindrod, K. A., Li, M., & Gates, A. (2014). Evaluating user perceptions of mobile medication management applications with older adults: A usability study. *JMIR mHealth and uHealth*, *2*(1), 11. doi:10.2196/mhealth.3048 PMID:25099993

Kalová, E., Vlcek, K., Jarolímová, E., & Bures, J. (2005). Allothetic orientation and sequential ordering of places is impaired in early stages of Alzheimer's disease: Corresponding results in real space tests and computer tests. *Behavioural Brain Research*, *159*(2), 175–186. doi:10.1016/j.bbr.2004.10.016 PMID:15817181

Khanuja, K., Joki, J., Bachmann, G., & Cuccurullo, S. (2018). Gait and balance in the aging population: Fall prevention using innovation and technology. *Maturitas*, *110*, 51–56. doi:10.1016/j.maturitas.2018.01.021 PMID:29563035

Lancini, G., Singh, N.N., O'Reilly, M.F., Sigafoos, J., Bosco, A., Zonno, N., & Badagliacca, F. (2011). Persons with mild or moderate Alzheimer's disease learn to use urine alarms and prompts to avoid large urinary accidents. *Research in Developmental Disabilities, 32,* 1998-2004.

Lancioni, G., De Caro, M.F., Singh, N.N., O'Reilly, M.F., Sigafoos, J., & Buono, S. (2014). Further evaluation of programs for promoting daily activities and indoor orientation and travel in persons with moderate Alzheimer's disease. *Life Span and Disability, 2,* 245-263..

Lancioni, G., Nirbhay, N. S., O'Reilly, M. F., Sigafoos, J., D'Amico, F., Ferlisi, G., Denitto, F., De Vanna, F., & Belardinelli, M. O. (2015). Patients with moderate Alzheimer's disease engage in verbal reminiscence with the support of a computer-aided program: A pilot study. *Frontiers in Aging Neuroscience*, *7*, 1–9. doi:10.3389/fnagi.2015.00109 PMID:26089797

Lancioni, G., Nirbhay, N. S., O'Reilly, M. F., Sigafoos, J., D'Amico, F., Sasanellli, G., De Vanna, F., & Signorino, M. (2015). Persons with Alzheimer's disease engage in leisure and mild physical activity with the support of technology-aided programs. *Research in Developmental Disabilities*, *37*, 55–63. doi:10.1016/j.ridd.2014.11.004 PMID:25460220

Lancioni, G., Nirbhay, N. S., O'Reilly, M. F., Sigafoos, J., Renna, C., Ventrella, M., Pinto, K., & Minervini, M. G. (2014). Supporting daily activities and indoor travel of persons with moderate Alzheimer's disease through standard technology resources. *Research in Developmental Disabilities*, *34*(8), 2351–2359. doi:10.1016/j.ridd.2013.04.020 PMID:23711628

Lancioni, G., O'Reilly, M. F., Nirbhay, N., Singh, C., Sigafoos, J., Grumo, G., Pinto, K., Stasolla, F., Signorino, M., & Groeneweg, J. (2013). Assessing the impact and social perception of self-regulated music stimulation with patients with Alzheimer's disease. *Research in Developmental Disabilities*, *34*(1), 139–146. doi:10.1016/j.ridd.2012.07.026 PMID:22944256

Lancioni, G., O'Reilly, M. F., Singh, N. N., Sigafoos, J., Rigante, V., De Franciscis, L., Stasolla, F., Perilli, V., & Lang, R. (2013). A Further Evaluation of the Impact of Self-regulated Music Stimulation on Positive Participation of Patients with Alzheimer's Disease. *Journal of Developmental and Physical Disabilities*, *25*(3), 273–283. doi:10.100710882-012-9301-5

Lancioni, G., Perilli, V., O'Reilly, M. F., Nirbhay, N., Singh, C., Sigafoos, J., Bosco, A., Caffò, A., Picucci, L., Cassano, G., & Groeneweg, J. (2013). Technology-based orientation programs to support indoor travel by persons with moderate Alzheimer's disease: Impact assessment and social validation. *Research in Developmental Disabilities*, *34*(1), 286–293. doi:10.1016/j.ridd.2012.08.016 PMID:22982468

Lancioni, G., Perilli, V., Singh, N. N., O'Reilly, M. F., & Sigafoos, J. (2016). Technology-Aided Programs to Support Positive Verbal and Physical Engagement in Persons with Moderate or Severe Alzheimer's Diseas. *Frontiers in Aging Neuroscience*, *8*, 1–8. doi:10.3389/fnagi.2016.00087 PMID:27148050

Lancioni, G., Perilli, V., Singh, N. N., O'Reilly, M. F., Sigafoos, J., Cassano, G., Pinto, K., Minervini, M. G., & Oliva, D. (2012). Technology-aided pictorial cues to support the performance of daily activities by persons with moderate Alzheimer's disease. *Research in Developmental Disabilities*, *33*(1), 265–273. doi:10.1016/j.ridd.2011.09.017 PMID:22093673

Lancioni, G., Perilli, V., Singh, N. N., O'Reilly, M. F., Sigafoos, J., D'Amico, F., Laporta, D., Cattaneo, M. G., Scordamaglia, A., & Pinto, K. (2018). Technology-Based Behavioral Interventions for Daily Activities and Supported Ambulation in People With Alzheimer's Disease. *American Journal of Alzheimer's Disease and Other Dementias*, *33*(5), 318–326. doi:10.1177/1533317518775038 PMID:29742903

Lancioni, G., Perilli, V., Singh, N. N., O'Reilly, M. F., Sigafoos, J., D'Amico, F., Turnone, B., Laporta, D., Scordamaglia, A., & Pinto, K. (2019). Smartphone-Based Interventions to Foster Simple Activity and Personal Satisfaction in People With Advanced Alzheimer's Disease. *American Journal of Alzheimer's Disease and Other Dementias*, *34*(7-8), 478–485. doi:10.1177/1533317519844144 PMID:31014071

Lancioni, G., Perrilli, V., Singh, N.N., O'Reilly, M.F., Sigafoos, J., Bosco, A., De Caro, M.F., Cassano, G., Pinto, K., & Minervini, M. (2011). *Persons with mild or moderate Alzheimer's disease use a basic orientation technology to travel to different rooms within a day center*. Academic Press.

Lancioni, G., Singh, N., O'Reilly, M. F., Renna, C., Pinto, K., De Vanna, F., Caffò, A., & Stasolla, F. (2014). Persons with moderate Alzheimer's disease use simple technology aids to manage daily activities and leisure occupation. *Research in Developmental Disabilities*, *35*(9), 2117–2128. doi:10.1016/j.ridd.2014.05.002 PMID:24881006

Lancioni, G., Singh, N., O'Reilly, M. F., Sigafoos, J., Ferlisi, G., Zullo, V., Schirone, S., Prisco, R., & Denitto, F. (2014). A computer-aided program for helping patients with moderate Alzheimer's disease engage in verbal reminiscence. *Research in Developmental Disabilities*, *35*(11), 3026–3033. doi:10.1016/j.ridd.2014.07.047 PMID:25124700

Landau, R., Werner, S., Auslander, G. K., Shoval, N., & Heinik, J. (2009). Attitudes of family members and care professionals towards the use of GPS for monitoring patients with dementia: An exploratory study. *British Journal of Social Work*, *39*, 670–692. doi:10.1093/bjsw/bcp037

Lauriks, S., Reinersmann, A., Van der Roest, H. G., Meiland, F. J., Davies, R. J., Moelaert, F., Mulvenna, M. D., Nugent, C. D., & Dröes, R. M. (2007). Review of ICT-based services for identified unmet needs in people with dementia. *Ageing Research Reviews*, *6*(3), 223–246. doi:10.1016/j.arr.2007.07.002 PMID:17869590

Lee, J. H., Kim, J. H., Jhoo, J. H., Lee, K. U., Kim, K. W., Lee, D. Y., & Woo, J. I. (2008). A telemedicine system as a care modality for dementia patients in Korea. *Alzheimer Disease and Associated Disorders, 14*(2), 94–101. doi:10.1097/00002093-200004000-00007 PMID:10850748

Li, R., Lindholm, K., Yang, L. B., Yue, X., Citron, M., Yan, R., Beach, T., Sue, L., Sabbagh, M., Cai, H., Wong, P., Price, D., & Shen, Y. (2004). Amyloid beta peptide load is correlated with increased beta-secretase activity in sporadic Alzheimer's disease patients. *Proceedings of the National Academy of Sciences*, 101.

Li, R., Lu, B., & McDonald-Maier, K.D. (2015). Cognitive assisted living ambient system: a survey. *The Digital Competence Framework 2.0, 1*, 229-252.

LoPresti, E., Bodine, C., & Lewis, C. (2008). Assistive technology for cognition: Understanding the needs of persons with disabilities. *IEEE Engineering in Medicine and Biology Magazine, 27*(2), 29–39. doi:10.1109/EMB.2007.907396 PMID:18463019

Man, D. W., Chung, J. C., & Lee, G. Y. (2012). Evaluation of a virtual reality-based memory training programme for Hong Kong Chinese older adults with questionable dementia: A pilot study. *International Journal of Geriatric Psychiatry, 27*(5), 513–520. doi:10.1002/gps.2746 PMID:21681818

Manera, V., Petit, P. D., Derreumaux, A., Orvieto, I., Romagnoli, M., Lyttle, G., David, R., & Robert, P. H. (2015). 'Kitchen and cooking,' a serious game for mild cognitive impairment and Alzheimer's disease: A pilot study. *Frontiers in Aging Neuroscience, 7*, 24. doi:10.3389/fnagi.2015.00024 PMID:25852542

Maresova, P., Tomsone, S., Lameski, P., Madureira, J., Mendes, A., Zdravevski, E., Chorbev, I., Trajkovik, V., Ellen, M., & Rodile, K. (2018). Technological Solutions for Older People with Alzheimer's Disease [Review]. *Current Alzheimer Research, 15*(10), 975–983. doi:10.2174/1567205015666180427124547 PMID:29701154

Matthews, K. A., Xu, W., Gaglioti, A. H., Holt, J. B., Croft, J. B., Mack, D., & McGuire, L. C. (2019). Racial and ethnic estimates of Alzheimer's disease and related dementias in the United States (2015-2060) in adults aged ³65 years. *Alzheimer's & Dementia, 15*(1), 17–24. doi:10.1016/j.jalz.2018.06.3063 PMID:30243772

McCarron, H., Zmora, R., & Gaugler, J.E. (n.d.). A Web-Based Mobile App With a Smartwatch to Support Social Engagement in Persons With Memory Loss: Pilot Randomized Controlled Trial. *JIMIR Aging, 2*, 1-15.

Meiland, F. (2007). COGKNOW: Development of an ICT device to support people with dementia. *The Journal on Information Technology in Healthcare, 5*, 324–334.

Melander, C., Martinsson, J., & Gustafsson, S. (2017). Measuring electrodermal activity to improve the identification of agitation in individuals with dementia. *Dementia and Geriatric Cognitive Disorders, 7*(3), 430–409. doi:10.1159/000484890 PMID:29430245

Miskelly, F. (2005). Tracciamento elettronico di pazienti con demenza e vagabondi utilizzando la tecnologia dei telefoni cellulari. *Age and Ageing, 34*, 497–499. doi:10.1093/ageing/afi145 PMID:16107453

Morris, M., Lundell, J., & Dishman, E. (2004). Catalyzing social interaction with ubiquitous computing: a needs assessment of elders coping with cognitive decline. *Human Factors in Computing Systems*, 5-6.

Newell, A. F., Carmichael, A., Gregor, P., & Alm, N. (2007). *Information technology for the cognitive support*. Lawrence Erlbaum Associates.

Nijhof, N., Van Hoof, J., Van Rijn, H., & Van Gemert-Pijnen, J. E. (2013). The behavioral outcomes of a technology-supported leisure activity in people with dementia. *Technology and Disability*, *25*(4), 263–273. doi:10.3233/TAD-140398

Optale, G., Urgesi, C., Busato, V., Marin, S., Piron, L., Priftis, K., Gamberini, L., Capodieci, S., & Bordin, A. (2010). Controlling memory impairment in elderly adults using virtual reality memory training: A randomized controlled pilot study. *Neurorehabilitation and Neural Repair*, *24*(4), 348–357. doi:10.1177/1545968309353328 PMID:19934445

Ozturk, E., van Iersel, M., van Loon, K., den Rooijen, C., van Dongen, E., & van Wijngaarden, R. D. (2018). Interactive online learning on perioperative management of elderly patients. *Frontiers in Aging Neuroscience*, *5*, 45–48. PMID:29502855

Peterson, C. M., Mikal, J. P., McCarron, H. R., Finlay, J. M., Mitchell, L. L., & Gaugler, J. E. (2020). The Feasibility and Utility of a Personal Health Record for Persons With Dementia and Their Family Caregivers for Web-Based Care Coordination: Mixed Methods Study. *JMIRI Aging*, *3*(1), 1–16. doi:10.2196/17769 PMID:32589158

Pino, M., Granata, C., Legouverneur, G., & Rigaud, A. S. (2012). Assessing design features of a graphical user interface for a social assistive robot for older adults with cognitive impairment. *International Symposium of Automation and Robotics in Construction*, *7*, 55-86. 10.22260/ISARC2012/0085

Rabins, P. V., Blacker, D., & Rovner, B. W. (2007). (Steering Committee on Practice Guidelines) "American Psychiatric Association practice guideline for the treatment of patients with Alzheimer's disease and other dementias. *The American Journal of Psychiatry*, *164*, 5–56. PMID:18340692

Ranasinghe, K. G., Cha, J., Iaccarino, L., Hinkley, L. B., Beagle, A. J., Pham, J., Jagust, W. J., Miller, B. L., Rankin, K. B., Rabinovici, G. D., Vossel, K. A., & Nagarajan, N. N. (2020). Neurophysiological signatures in Alzheimer's disease are distinctly associated with TAU, amyloid-β accumulation, and cognitive decline. *Journal of Translational Medicine*, 12. PMID:32161102

Robinson, H. (2012). *Suitability of healthcare robots for a dementia unit and suggested improvements*. Elsevier.

Rosenberg, L., & Nygård, L. (2017). Learning and knowing technology as lived experience in people with Alzheimer's disease: A phenomenological study. *Aging & Mental Health*, *21*(12), 1272–1279. doi:10.1080/13607863.2016.1222347 PMID:27592720

Schwickert, L., Becker, C., Lindemann, U., Maréchal, C., Bourke, A., Chiari, L., Helbostad, J. L., Zijlstra, W., Aminian, K., Todd, C., Bandinelli, S., & Klenk, J. (2013). Fall detection with body-worn sensors: A systematic review. *Zeitschrift für Gerontologie und Geriatrie*, *46*(8), 706–719. doi:10.100700391-013-0559-8 PMID:24271251

Sherzai, A., & Sherzai, D. (2017). *The Alzheimer's Solution: A Breakthrough Program to Prevent and Reverse the Symptoms of Cognitive Decline at Every Age*. HarperOne.

Siriaraya, P., & Ang, C. S. (2014). Recreating living experiences from past memories through virtual worlds for people with dementia. *Proceedings of the SIGCHI Conference on Human Factors in Computing Systems*. 10.1145/2556288.2557035

Span, M., Hettinga, M., Groen-van de Ven, L., Jukema, J., Janssen, R., Vernooij-Dassen, M., Eefsting, J., & Smits, C. (2018). Involving people with dementia in developing an interactive web tool for shared decision-making: Experiences with a participatory design approach. *Disability and Rehabilitation*, *40*(12), 1410–1412. doi:10.1080/09638288.2017.1298162 PMID:28286969

Spector, A., Thorgrimsen, L., Woods, B., Royan, L., Davies, S., Butterworth, M., & Orrell, M. (2003). Efficacy of an evidence-based cognitive stimulation therapy programme for people with dementia: Randomised controlled trial. *The British Journal of Psychiatry*, *183*(3), 248–254. doi:10.1192/bjp.183.3.248 PMID:12948999

Sriram, V., Jenkinson, C., & Peters, M. (2019). Informal carers' experience of assistive technology use in dementia care at home: A systematic review. *BMC Geriatrics*, *14*(1), 160. doi:10.118612877-019-1169-0 PMID:31196003

Stoccoro, A., & Coppedè, F. (2018). Role of epigenetics in Alzheimer's disease pathogenesis. *Neurodegenerative Disease Management*, *8*(3), 181–193. doi:10.2217/nmt-2018-0004 PMID:29888987

Westphal, A., Dingjan, P., & Attoe, R. (2010). What can low and high technologies do for late life mental disorders? *Current Opinion in Psychiatry*, *23*(6), 510–505. doi:10.1097/YCO.0b013e32833d74d4 PMID:20717039

Wherton, J.P. (2007). Technological opportunities for supporting people with dementia who are living at home. *International Journal of Human-Computer Studies, 56*, 65-66.

Zellefrow, B., Shanaei, S., Salam, R., El Nasan, A., & Elzabadani, H. (2017). Halcyon – Assistive technology for Alzheimer's patients. *The British Journal of Psychiatry*, 375.

ADDITIONAL READING

Arkin, S. (2007). Language-enriched exercise plus socialization slows cognitive decline in Alzheimer's disease. *American Journal of Alzheimer's Disease and Other Dementias*, *22*(1), 62–77. doi:10.1177/1533317506295377 PMID:17534004

Astell, A., Smith, S. K., & Joddrell, P. (2018). Using Technology in Dementia Care. Londra: Jessica Kingsley Publishers.

Bucciarelli, A. (2015). *Alzheimer's Diseas*. Bridge: Mercury Learning & Information.

Lancioni, G. E., Perilli, V., Singh, N. N., O'Reilly, M. F., Sigafoos, J., & Cassano, G. (2012). Technology-aided pictorial cues to support the performance of daily activities by persons with mild or moderate Alzheimer's disease. *Research in Developmental Disabilities*, *33*(1), 265–273. doi:10.1016/j.ridd.2011.09.017 PMID:22093673

Mulvenna, M. D., & Nugent, C. D. (2010). *Supporting People with Dementia Using Pervasive Health Technologies*. Springer. doi:10.1007/978-1-84882-551-2

KEY TERMS AND DEFINITIONS

Alzheimer's Disease: Degenerative neurological disease affecting the brain, progressively leading the sufferer to a state of total dependency.

Assistive Technology: Umbrella term including any piece, device, tool or equipment enabling self-determination and independence in individuals with developmental disorders.

Caregiver: Caregiver and naturally refers to all family members caring for a sick and/or disabled relative.

Communication: The process and manner of transmitting information from one individual to another, through the exchange of a message processed according to the rules of a given common code.

Quality of Life: Complex psychological construct which includes pleasure, satisfaction, fulfilment, well-being, and happiness.

Review: Categorization of empirical studies available in the literature along a determined time interval on a specific topic.

Chapter 10
Assistive Technology-Based Programs and Telerehabilitation Strategies to Support Adaptive Responding of Individuals With Neurodegenerative Diseases

Fabrizio Stasolla
https://orcid.org/0000-0003-1626-9664
University Giustino Fortunato of Benevento, Italy

Donatella Ciarmoli
University Giustino Fortunato of Benevento, Italy

ABSTRACT

Individuals with neurodegenerative diseases (NDD) may pose serious challenges to daily life medical contexts. In fact, they commonly fail while dealing with environmental requests. To overcome this issue, one may rely on assistive technology-based programs. The COVID-19 pandemic suddenly exacerbated their clinical conditions. Telerehabilitation may be useful to profitably tackle the latter issue. A concise survey on the newest empirical contributions available was proposed. Five main categories of studies were identified. Results were satisfactory, although failures occurred. Findings were critically discussed and some useful insights for both research and practice were highlighted.

INTRODUCTION

Young and older adults with neurodegenerative diseases (e.g., Alzheimer disease, Parkinson disease, amyotrophic lateral sclerosis and multiple sclerosis) may pose serious challenges to daily contexts such as families, caregivers, professionals, and medical or rehabilitative centers. Thus, they commonly exhibit communicative, emotional, intellectual, motor, and social impairments while tackling day life requests.

DOI: 10.4018/978-1-7998-7430-0.ch010

Because of their significantly compromised clinical conditions, individuals with severe disabilities frequently experience isolation, passivity, and detachment with negative consequences on their quality of life. That situation may be meaningfully deleterious for their social image, desirability, and status. In fact, they constantly rely on caregivers' assistance (Bassi et al., 2020; Gil-Gonzales, Perez-San-Gregorio, Conrad, & Martin-Rodriguez, 2021; Schischlevskij et al., 2021). To positively address this issue, one may rely on assistive technology-based programs (AT). Such approach includes basic aids to support people with relevant disorders within daily settings. AT-based interventions are implemented to fill the existing gap between the individual's capacities and the environmental' s requests. Moreover, AT may build a functional bridge enabling self-determination of persons with different levels of disabilities and decreasing caregivers' burden accordingly (Behera, Condell. Dora, Gibson. And Leavy, 2021; Gongora Alonso et al., 2019). Thus, an active role, constructive engagement, and functional occupation of individuals with neurodegenerative disorders may be enhanced (Leuty, Boger, Young, Hoey, & Mihaillidis, 2013; Savvidis et al., 2018).

Recently, Covid-19 pandemic drastically exacerbated the precarious conditions of persons with neurodegenerative diseases (NDD) due to quarantine and social distancing preventive measures. Additionally, the unavailability of National Medical Services reduced the opportunity in NDD people to receive adequate medical care. The diffusion of the vaccine partially improved that situation. To overcome this latter issue, one may use telerehabilitation strategies (TR) (Akbas & Mummolo, 2021; Caprì et al., 2021).

For example, Hung and Fong (2019) reviewed the current literature on the application of TR in occupational therapy practice and its clinical outcomes over last decade. Studies retrieved from seven electronic databases were assessed and findings evidenced positive therapeutic effects although data were considered insufficient to demonstrate the validity of TR compared to face – to – face interventions. Caprì et al. (2021) systematically reviewed the literature on the use of TR in individuals with multiple disabilities, and examined the effects of TR on adaptive skills of individuals with severe to profound and multiple delays. Furthermore, the different types of devices and families' satisfaction were assessed. Nevertheless, by including AT, NDD, and TR in Scopus, no records were found.

In light of the above, the first goal of the chapter was to provide the readers with an update and concise survey on the use of AT-based programs and TR to promote cognitive, communicative, and motor functions in persons with NDD. Positive participation and leisure opportunities were additionally examined. The second objective of the chapter was to emphasize advantages and limitations of the adopted technological solutions. Finally, some useful insights for both future research and practice were critically discussed.

1. BACKGROUND

AT-based strategies may provide persons diagnosed with different neurodegenerative diseases and various levels of disabilities with a valid aid in basic problem domains. For instance, independent access to positive stimulation, functional activities, physical exercise, reminiscence, communication skills, leisure and recreation, request and choice processes are frequently included (De Pace & Stasolla, 2014; Stasolla, Perilli, & Boccasini, 2016). Furthermore, the area of detachment and passivity encompasses the difficulty of being favorably committed in adaptive behaviors and/or physical activities with beneficial consequences. Functional activities may be considered as crucial for occupational purposes. Communication skills and reminiscence are essential for social interaction and recovery of personal events. Leisure and recreation domains include the inability of manage leisure or recreation opportunities independently. Request and choice processes refer to the awareness and the capacity to select and ask for desired items, and satisfy personal needs (Lancioni & Singh, 2014). AT-based interventions are designed to provide devices, instruments, or tools aimed at reducing the distance between the individual's skills and the requested environmental skills to achieve specific objectives. It is critical that an AT-based option is customer tailored and strictly individualized (Lancioni, Sigafoos, O'Reilly, & Singh, 2012).

Beside the aforementioned approach, telerehabilitation (TR) may be considered for assessment and rehabilitative purposes. In fact, TR offers advantages in terms of both synchronous or asynchronous data recording, assessment, and recovery processes. Thus, persons with neurodegenerative diseases may be assessed and recovered for cognitive, communicative, and motor functions through TR strategies (Asano et al., 2021; Kim et al., 2021). Moreover, TR may be viewed as a valid strategy to overcome Covid-19 pandemic negative consequences (Langer et al., 2021).

Although a substantial body of literature exists for both practical and clinical areas of investigation (AT and TR; Belic et al., 2019; Koumakis, Chatzaki, Kazantzaki, Maniadi, & Tsiknakis, 2019; Stamford, Schmidt, & Friedl, 2015), none of the available review papers presents a combination of both domains. Additionally, the published reviews are exclusively focused on a specific disease (e.g., Parkinson or sclerosis) rather than provide the reader with a comprehensive review targeted on different neurodegenerative diseases.

2. METHOD

A computerized search was performed in Scopus database. Neurodegenerative diseases, Alzheimer disease, Parkinson disease, amyotrophic lateral sclerosis, multiple sclerosis, young and older adults, assessment, rehabilitation, AT, TR, neurological disorders, intellectual disabilities, motor impairments, communication disorders, isolation, passivity, active role, constructive engagement, positive participation, quality of life, pain, reminiscence, functional activities, leisure, occupation, physical exercise, and detachment were merged as keywords. A manual search was added as completion. Including criteria were: (a) empirical studies with an AT-based intervention or a TR-based program, (b) a participant with a neurodegenerative disease with an age of 20 years or older, (c) English language of the paper, and (d) 2011-2021 as time interval publication year. Excluding criteria were: (a) review papers, (b) theoretical papers, (c) book chapters, (d) conference papers, and (e) only children or adolescents as participants (i.e., 19 years old or younger). Five main categories of studies were identified, namely (a) recovering of functional and physical activities, (b) communication abilities, (c) positive participation, (d) leisure and recreation, and (e) telerehabilitation. The following section (i.e., literature overview) includes a concise description of the reviewed studies. Synoptic tables were additionally included to improve the readability and the clarity of the overview. The authors of the studies, the recruited participants, their ages, the setups used, and the outcomes were presented. Irrespective of the number of the studies retained in each section, three contributions were concisely detailed along each category for practical reasons.

3. LITERATURE OVERVIEW

3.1. Functional and Physical Activities

To prevent isolation and passivity, the recovery of daily functional and physical activities may be considered essential. Thus, AT-based programs are commonly focused on reactivate occupational tasks among persons with mild to moderate Alzheimer Disease or to promote basic physical exercises of patients with moderate to severe Alzheimer Disease. The completion of daily functional activities may be pursued through a task analysis and either visual or verbal prompts, which may eventually be combined in a unique solution. Otherwise, one can use reminders, step instructions, and praise provision. Backward or Forward chaining may be additionally acknowledged. Different technological devices may be used such as microswitches, laptops, tablets, and/or smart-phones and mobile technologies equipped with an adapted software (Mancioppi, Fiorini, Timpano, Sportiello, & Cavallo, 2019). Physical exercise may be supported by microswitches, contingent positive stimulation, walkers, and both physical and verbal prompts as reminders in case of no responding (Klimova, Valis, & Kuca, 2018; Stasolla, Caffò, et al., 2017). Otherwise, persons with Parkinson disease may be helped along walking process because they may be affected by motor blocks known as freezing of gait (Stamford, Schmidt, & Friedl, 2015). Ten studies were selected along this section with 144 participants included (Imbeault, Langlois, Bocti, Gagnon, & Bier, 2018; Lancioni, Singh, O'Reilly, et al., 2017, 2018, 2019; Lazarou et al., 2019; Oksnebjerg, Woods, & Waldermar, 2019; Rohrbach et al., 2019; Stummer et al., 2015; Wang, Sudhama, Begum, Huq, & Mihailidis, 2017; Zhao et al., 2016; see Table 1).

For instance, Oksnebjerg et al. (2019) evaluated four steps of an interactive user including a rehabilitation program based on cognitive support technology, through an app design process. In the first step, a pilot investigation was carried out to explore beneficial outcomes and challenges of adopting existing off-the-shelf app to support self-management with living with the early stages of dementia. The second step included focus-group interviews conducted in-depth comprehension of the needs and perspectives of potential end-users of the app. The third step consisted of a product benchmarking process, which was useful to further evaluate the design process. The final step considered an iterative co-design process, which encompassed the three previous steps. Twenty-eight participants with dementia who were aged between 53 and 82 years, seventeen family caregivers (i.e., mean age 60 years), and 10 professional caregivers (i.e., mean age 49 years) were enrolled. Results evidenced the effectiveness and the suitability of the app for helping people with dementia in the self-management of everyday life functional activities. Memory support and structure in daily living were recognized as basic needs and the adopted technology was identified as a suitable solution with a tailor-made calendar as key-feature.

Rohrbach et al. (2019) conducted a crossover study with 10 patients who were aged between 51 and 84 years and suffered from mild to moderate Alzheimer Disease using an augmented reality approach based on a Microsoft HoloLens to support participants in a tea making task. The participants were tested and post-hoc semi-structured interviews were carried out to assess the usability. The study took place in a qualified medical center for cognitive disorders. Two experimental conditions were implemented, namely (a) natural or control condition and (b) trials (i.e., experimental condition) guided by an augmented reality, which consisted of an application developed within a user centered strategy including four iterative cycles though mutual collaboration between researchers, clinicians, and family members. A step-by-step guidance system for a multi-step activity daily living task (i.e., preparation of a cup of tea) with embedded audio-visual cues was assessed. Results demonstrated that participants failed when they executed the task with or without holographic assistance. No statistical differences emerged in success rates or error frequencies. However, data showed participants' prolonged trial durations when equipped with the augmented reality headset. Moreover, a multiple linear regression revealed an influence of the errors in the control condition and a moderation of the errors in the experimental condition. Participants who presented more severe problems in the natural condition emphasized lower improvements in trials duration once provided with the technology (i.e., augmented reality).

Zhao et al. (2016) exposed twelve participants aged between 53 and 78 years and diagnosed with Parkinson disease to a rehabilitative program focused on the improvement of their gait through the use of new mobiles like smart-glasses. The technology was used to deliver external cues that could enhance ambulation process in a natural environment. Specifically, the study analyzed rhythmic visual and auditory cueing in a laboratory with a customer-made application for the Google Glass. Different gait parameters were compared (i.e., walking speed, cadence, stride length, and its variability). Freezing of gait was additionally recorded. Three types of external cues were evaluated, namely (a) metronome, (b) flashing light, and (c) optic flow. A fourth control condition (i.e., no cue) was included. Participants completed several walking tasks with various complexities. Seven inertial sensors attached to the feet, legs, and pelvis monitored and coded motion data for gait analysis. Two professional raters scored gait freezing severity through video-recording. User experience was evaluated with a semi-open interview. During cueing, a more stable gait pattern emerged, specifically on complicated walking courses. Nevertheless, freezing of gait did not decrease. The metronome was more effective compared to the visual cues and more preferred by the participants. The technology was successfully adopted and suitable for fostering gait fluency.

Table 1. Reviewed studies on Physical and functional activities

Studies	Participants	Ages	Technology	Disease	Outcomes
Imbeault et al. (2018)	1	65	Tablet and App	Alzheimer	One positive
Lancioni et al. (2017)	21	72-93	Microswitches	Alzheimer	One negative
Lancioni et al. (2018)	17	70-92	Microswitches	Alzheimer	Two negative
Lancioni et al. (2019)	21	73-96	Smartphone and App	Alzheimer	All positive
Lazarou et al. (2019)	6	69-84	Smart system	Alzheimer	Six positive
Oksnebjerg et al. (2019)	28	53-82	Interactive program	Dementia	All positive
Rohrbach et al. (2019)	10	51-84	Augmented Reality	Alzheimer	Ten positive
Stummer et al. (2015)	18	55-71	Walk-bicycle	Parkinson	Two negative
Wang et al. (2017)	10	59-88	Robot	Alzheimer	Ten positive
Zhao et al. (2016)	12	53-78	Smart-glasses	Parkinson	Twelve positive

3.2. Communication Abilities

Communication skills are considered crucial for social interactions, inclusion, participation and societal affiliation. Additionally, interdependence is embedded based on the principle of give-and-take (Koldrack, Luplow, Kirste, & Teipel, 2013). Being related with other individuals may be viewed as a basic feature of quality of life. Social relations ensure emotional support and positively involve people in daily activities, being constructively engaged (Holthe & Wulff-Jacobsen, 2016). Due to either intellectual disabilities or extensive motor impairments, young and older adults with neurodegenerative disease may systematically fail to communicate with other people (Kotipalli, Praveen Kumar, Mohan Raju, & Murali Krishna, 2019). AT-based programs and aided-alternative and augmentative communication strategies may be useful to enable people with neurodegenerative disease to profitably cope with their environment (Asghar, Cang, & Yu, 2018; Brownlee & Bruening, 2012; Fried-Oken, Mooney, & Peters, 2015). Thus, computerized systems, tablets, I-PAD, I-POD, Smartphone with adapted software and specific sensors capable of adequately detect even small behavioral response are commonly used (Sigafoos et al., 2019; van der Meer et al., 2017). Ten studies were reviewed with 75 participants involved (Caligari, Godi, Giardini, & Colombo, 2019; Lancioni, Simone, et al., 2015; Lancioni, Singh, O'Reilly, Sigafoos, D'Amico, et al., 2015a, b, 2016, 2017; Lancioni, Singh, O'Reilly, Sigafoos, D'Amico, Sasanelli, et al., 2016; Santos, Licursi, Amaral, Cavalcanti, & Silveira, 2019, see Table 2).

For example, Caligari et al. (2019) designed a new sensor (i.e., the Lever Magnetic-spring Mechanical Switch, LeMMS), ensuring repeated activation and/or releasing cycles requiring a very small action force. Twenty participants, mean aged of 59 years and diagnosed with advanced amyotrophic lateral sclerosis (ALS) were enrolled and exposed to the new technology focused on the enhancement of their communication skills. All the participants regularly used other sensors but they were unable manage the technology due to their clinical conditions, except for the new LeMMS. Observations occurred at the baseline (T0), and after one (T1), six (T2), and twelve months (T3). At baseline, participants were evaluated through standardized clinical scales. The click-Test-30 considered the maximum number of the LeMMS activations along 30 s and thumb/fingers strength evaluation was monitored through the Kendall scale. The QUEST 2.0 Dev questionnaire was administrated at T1. Some use-related information added to the Click-Test-30 were collected at T1, T2, and T3. Results demonstrated that after one training session, all the participants were capable of use the LeMMS with a minimal effort (i.e., minimal residual movement of one finger). The mean score of QUEST 2.0 Dev questionnaire suggested a strong satisfaction with the LeMMS. No significant differences emerged at Click-Test-30 between T0 and T1. However, at T2 and T3 the performance significantly decreased. At T3 half of the participants were able to use their communication device.

Jarosiewicz et al. (2016) exposed a 52-years old man diagnosed with ASL to the use of brain computer interface (BCI) and a kinematic decoder (i.e., a decoder that controlled cursor movements) to demonstrate its calibration using collected data during practical point-and-click control of the BCI. A retrospective inference of the user's intended movement directions was adopted, based on subsequent selections. An extension of such method was investigated to allow the click decoder to also be recalibrated using acquired data during practical BCI use. Neural data patterns were retrospectively labeled as equivalent to click during all time bins in which the click log-likelihood was above the click threshold that was adopted during real-time neural control. The click decoder using standard supervised classifier training method was labeled as "non-click". The participant was enabled to freely type across 11 research sessions spanning 29 days, maintaining high performance neural control over cursor movement and click without needing to interrupt virtual keyboard use for explicit calibration task through a combined real-time bias correction and baseline firing rate tracking. That approach successfully corroborated the clinical validity of intra-cortical BCI for individuals with extensive motor impairments by eliminating the need for calibration task with prescribed targets and click times.

Santos et al. (2019) presented the design process of an AT device for people with Parkinson disease and some tremor in the hands. A user-center design approach was proposed based on the integration of the tools House of Quality (QFD) and TRIZ, seeking for a feasible innovative technical solution focused on meeting users' requirements. Additionally, a 3D printing was adopted as a tool to enhance and refine the design, through the manufacture of mock-ups and prototypes used in interaction and testing with users. Four main features were relevantly fostered, namely (a) the communication among members of multidisciplinary team, (b) a clearer identification of the design demands and users' needs, (c) a development time reduction, and (d) creation of feasible and innovative solution. Preliminary test involved a 60-years old man with Parkinson disease, who followed a regular medication treatment and a single-case experimental design was applied to demonstrate the impact on the quality of the feeding task with regard to both performance and satisfaction.

Table 2. Reviewed studies on communication skills

Studies	Participants	Ages	Technology	Disease	Outcomes
Caligari et al. (2019)	20	42-84	Mechanical switch	ASL	Twenty Positive
Jarosiewicz et al. (2016)	1	52	BCI	ASL	One Positive
Lancioni, Simone et al. (2015)	5	54-67	Computer + Microswitch	ASL	Five Positive
Lancioni et al. (2015a)	3	65-85	Computer + Microswitch	Alzheimer	Three Positive
Lancioni et al. (2015b)	16	72-93	Computer + Microswitch	Alzheimer	One Negative
Lancioni et al. (2016)	8	73-96	Computer + Microswitch	Alzheimer	Eight Positive
Lancioni et al. (2017)	4	52-68	Computer + Microswitch	ASL	Four Positive
Lancioni, Sasanelli et al. (2016)	3	71-80	Computer + Microswitch	Parkinson	One Negative
Mc Cane et al. (2015)	14	41-72	BCI	ASL	Four Negative
Santos et al. (2019)	1	60	Design Approach	Parkinson	One Positive

3.3. Positive Participation

A further feature that represents a critical basis of constructive engagement, active role, and quality of life is positive participation. Because persons with neurodegenerative diseases commonly experience isolation and passivity, to promote positive participation may be viewed as a primary rehabilitative goal among researchers and clinicians. Thus, AT-based interventions may be helpful to enhance it by fostering social interactions. Accordingly, the technological supports ensure individuals with neurodegenerative disease with the independent access to positive stimulation. That is, participants with neurodegenerative disease will be capable of independently interact with the surrounding environment and positively participate to the daily social life (Klimova, Valis, & Kuca, 2018; Savvidis et al., 2018). Four studies were retained with 34 participants recruited (Lancioni, Bosco, et al., 2015; Lancioni, O'Reilly, Singh, et al., 2013a, b; Lancioni, Singh, O'Reilly, Green, et al., 2013, see Table 3).

Table 3. Reviewed studies on positive participation

Studies	Participants	Ages	Technology	Disease	Outcomes
Lancioni, Bosco et al.(2015)	11	71-94	Computer + Microswitch	Alzheimer	Five Negative
Lancioni et al. (2013a)	6	76-89	Computer + Microswitch	Alzheimer	One Negative
Lancioni et al. (2013b)	7	75-90	Computer + Microswitch	Alzheimer	Two negative
Lancioni, Singh, et al. (2013)	10	72-92	Computer + Microswitch	Alzheimer	Ten Positive

Lancioni, Bosco, et al. (2015) assessed the outcomes of response-related music stimulation versus unrelated-response (i.e., general) music stimulation on positive participation of 11 participants with severe and low-moderate levels Alzheimer disease, who were aged between 71 and 94 years. Positive participation encompassed behavioral signs of singing and/or rhythmic movements and smiles. Both experimental conditions were delivered through a computerized system which provided the participants with preferred music/song and amusing videos. In the experimental condition (i.e., related music stimulation), the participants were requested to activate a pressure circular button to receive brief periods of pleasant events. In the control condition (i.e., general) music stimulation was automatically determined throughout the sessions (i.e., continuously). Six participants evidenced higher intervals of positive participation in the experimental condition, conversely to five participants who emphasized no significant differences between conditions.

Lancioni et al. (2013a) evaluated the impact on positive participation added to social rating of an AT-based program which included six participants diagnosed within the severe range of the Alzheimer disease and who were aged between 76 and 89 years. Two conditions were implemented, namely (a) an active condition, and (b) a passive condition. During the active conditions the participants were equipped with the technology (i.e., computer and microswitch) ensuring them with brief periods of positive stimulation contingent to an active responding (i.e., simple hand response). In the passive condition, the stimulation was automatically provided by the system, irrespective of the participants' responding. The active condition revealed higher levels of intervals with positive participation for five of the six participants. The learning process was consolidated during the post-intervention checks. Social raters favorably endorsed the use of the technology.

Lancioni et al. (2013b) extended the comparison between active (i.e., self-regulated) and passive (i.e., outer-regulated) music stimulation with seven participants who were aged between 75 and 90 years and diagnosed between the severe and low-moderate range of Alzheimer's disease. In the active condition, the participants used a simple hand response and a related pressure microswitch to activate music inputs independently. In the passive condition, music stimulation was delivered through the sessions. Results demonstrated an increased levels of intervals with positive participation during both conditions. The improved performance was higher in the active condition for five of the seven participants. No relevant differences were evidenced for two participants.

3.4. Leisure and Recreation

A supplementary feature significantly enhanced by the AT-based programs may be leisure and recreation activities. Thus, individuals with neurodegenerative disease may greatly benefit from technological aids and computerized systems because they may be profitably involved in recreation opportunities, which may be favorably fostered through different technological solutions. Essentially, constructive engagement and positive roles may be improved with beneficial effects on participants' quality of life with a contingent reduction of both caregivers and families' burden (Asghar, Cang, & Yu, 2017). Six studies were reviewed along the section with 102 participants involved (Lancioni, Perilli, et al., 2011; Lancioni, Singh, O'Reilly, 2014; Lim, Wallace, Luszcz, & Reynolds, 2013; Neven et al., 2013; Nijhof, Van Hoof, Van Rijn, & Van Gemert-Pijnen, 2013; Plow & Finlayson, 2013, see Table 4).

For instance, Lancioni et al. (2014) exposed four patients diagnosed with moderate Alzheimer's disease aged between 75 and 89 years to a computerized hierarchical program combined with a microswitch enabling the participants to select desired leisure options. The technology additionally included an amplifier, an interface and adapted software. The participants were requested to choose among four different music styles (i.e., classical, opera, pop male singers, and pop female singers). Each option was automatically scanned and identified with a double (i.e., verbal and visual) cue. Once the participants selected the category, they were asked to choose among the singers of the selected category. Finally, they were asked to select a specific song of the selected singer. Once completed the selection with three different responses useful to minimize unintentional choices, they could listen 2-3 min of the desired song. Results showed that all the participants learned to profitably use the technology for leisure purposes. External raters (i.e., forty-four psychology students) favorably endorsed the use of such technology.

Lim et al. (2013) investigated the usability of tablet computers as part everyday living in people with dementia. Twenty-one participants with an early stage of dementia and career-dyads were recruited for a seven-day in home setting. Sessions were collected to determine whether patients with early stage of dementia were capable of using a tablet-based program independently and reduce caregivers' burden accordingly. Feedbacks were returned through questionnaires from both patients and personnel enrolled. Results evidenced that half of the participants were able to constructively engage with and use the tablet computer independently and demonstrated to be useful to their caregivers. No significant traits were recorded to uniquely identified who were the patients less likely to use the tablet computer. Caregivers' relief was measured by the amount of time participants with dementia spent adopting the device without supervision.

Nijhof et al. (2013) examined the effectiveness and suitability of a technology-supported leisure game for people with dementia in relation to the stimulation of social behavior. Specifically, the additional impact of the technological equipment was assessed in a nursing home and daycare setting compared with a traditional leisure activity. The technology-supported game pursued the stimulation of social behavior and interaction among participants via its design features, which included a TV, radio, telephone, and treasure box. A mixed-method research design was implemented. Ten participants diagnosed with a moderate range of dementia were recruited. Data demonstrated that social behaviors occurred more frequently than non-social behavior during the sessions. Females scored higher than males in social behavior. Caregivers were significantly facilitated and their work was easier with the use of the technology. The activities resulted more person-centered.

Table 4. Reviewed studies on leisure and Recreation.

Studies	Participants	Ages	Technology	Disease	Outcomes
Lancioni, Perilli, et al. (2011)	1	85	Technological equipment	Alzheimer	One Positive
Lancioni et al. (2014)	4	75-89	Computer + Microswitch	Alzheimer	Four Positive
Lim et al. (2013)	21	55-70	Tablet Computer	Dementia	Eleven Negative
Neven et al. (2013)	36	27-63	GPS tracking device	Multiple Sclerosis	Fifteen Negative
Nijhof et al. (2013)	10	61-78	Technological equipment	Dementia	Ten Positive
Plow and Finlayson (2013)	30	52-68	Technological equipment	Multiple Sclerosis	Thirty Positive

3.5. Telerehabilitation

TR as part of telemedicine, is currently adopted to remotely supervise and evaluate users in a synchronous or asynchronous way (Brunner, Hemsley, Togher, & Palmer, 2017). During Covid-19 pandemic both strategies may be helpful to promote participants' active role, constructive engagement, and functional occupation, next to assessment and diagnosis objectives. Thus, users' s quality of life (QoL) might be enhanced with families and professionals' burden reduction. Although both approaches were documented in the literature, no records were found on both combined approaches in NDD. Five studies were included in the current section (Albiol-Perez et al., 2017; Bernini et al., 2021; Cikajlo & Potisk, 2019; Mantovani et al., 2020; Matamala-Gomez etal., 2021).

Bernini et al. (2021) conducted a perspective study and proposed a home-care rehabilitation equipment to recovery cognitive functions in young and older patients with neurodegenerative diseases. A usable and safe cognitive rehabilitation tool was assessed. Its use was demonstrated in clinical settings with evidence-based data and several advantages for both patients and professionals. It provided users, families, professionals, and caregivers with a valid instrument to be remotely monitored and supervised.

Cikajlo and Potisk (2019) designed a randomized study with 97 patients diagnosed with Parkinson diseases with only 20 eligible participants randomized in two groups. A first group used a 3D technological system and a second group used a traditional laptop. Both groups participated to a 10-session 3 weeks training with a pick and a place task in the virtual world requiring precise hand movement to manipulate virtual cubes. Results showed a higher performance of participants in the experimental group. The 3D immersive, remotely controlled, technology was helpful to enhance users' motor performance.

Albiol-Perez et al. (2017) exposed 10 participants with Parkinson disease to 15 rehabilitation sessions. A groundbreaking system based on a virtual motor rehabilitation was implemented. Two points observations (i.e., baseline and end of the intervention) were recorded. A customizable intervention was performed. A low-cost telerehabilitation system was used. Postural control was examined as an outcome measure. Results demonstrated the effectiveness and the suitability of the technological system to improve motor performance and postural control.

Table 5. Reviewed studies on TR

Studies	Participants	Ages	Technology	Disease	Outcomes
Albiol-Perez et al. (2017)	10	not specified	virtual reality	Parkinson	Ten positive
Bernini et al. (2021)	not applicable		Intelligent System	NDD not specified	Cognitive Rehabilitation
Cikajlo and Potisk (2019)	20	not specified	virtual reality	Parkinson	Twenty Positive
Mantovani et al. (2020)	not applicable		Virtual reality +TR	Neurological diseases	Cognitive Rehabilitation
Matamala-Gomez et al. (2021)	not applicable		Flow healthcare	Neurological diseases	Remote Supervision

4. DISCUSSION

Data of the reviewed studies demonstrated that AT-based interventions were suitable and effective to promote daily life skills of persons with neurodegenerative diseases. Results were largely positive although soma failures occurred (i.e., 3.75%). The recruited participants were progressively capable of independent responding and enabled with profitably cope with their environment. Their self-determination was fostered and positive participation relevantly improved. Both caregivers and families' burden were significantly reduced. External raters involved in social validation procedures favorably corroborated the clinical validity of the implemented programs. TR and new technologies were helpful to assess and recover individuals with neurodegenerative disease through remote supervision. The findings were largely supported by the existing literature (Gongora Alonso et al., 2019; Stasmford, Schmidt, & Friedl, 2015; Stasolla, Boccasini, et al., 2014) and suggested the following the following considerations.

First, AT-based programs may be considered a great practical and rehabilitative resource helping young and older adults with neurodegenerative diseases to promote daily adaptive skills and enhance self-determination. Thus, patients with neurodegenerative enrolled in the retained studies diseases were capable of achieving both functional and physical activities. The participants' communication skills were relevantly promoted and leisure opportunities were fostered. Accordingly, caregivers and families' burden were meaningfully reduced. The management of daily life was improved (Lancioni et al., 2004; 2007a; Stasolla & De Pace, 2014).

Second, positive participation and functional occupation were supported. Thus, the recruited participants were constructively engaged in the proposed activities and/or tasks with beneficial outcomes on their quality of life. Consequently, isolation, passivity, and detachment were practically prevented. The participants improved their active role and were profitably included in the implemented programs. Their positive mood, whenever recorded, was inceased accordingly. One may reasonably argue that AT-based interventions had a beneficial impact on the participants' wellbeing, pleasure, and fulfillment (Lancioni et al., 2007b; Stasolla, Damiani, et al., 2014).

Third, the participants consolidated the learning process over the time. Thus, the performances were encouraged over the time and across settings along the studies in which both features were recorded. One may argue that the learning process was significantly enhanced and strengthened. Thus, the assiduity and regularity of the collected sessions allowed the acquisition of the participants' adaptive behaviors. Moreover, data indicated that their adaptive responding was purposeful (Catania, 2012).

Fourth, external raters included in social validation assessments, either professionals (e.g., caregivers, neurologists, psychologists, and physiotherapists), or families' members (i.e., parents) favorably scored the use of the technology. Traditionally, they evaluated the dimensions of (a) participant's comfort, (b) program's rehabilitative and/or practical impact, (c) participant's independence and/or self-determination, (d) suitability in home and medical centers care settings, and (e) rater's involvement as researcher in that implemented program (Lancioni, O'Reilly, et al., 2006).

Fifth, TR and new technologies seemed to be a valid way for both clinicians and researchers to assess and recover adaptive behaviors and cognitive skills of individuals with neurodegenerative diseases remotely. Researchers could either track behavioral responses or evaluate brain activities though virtual environments. Furthermore, TR included experimental controlled settings and/or ecological contexts. One may argue that differences between younger and older adults emerged with regard to the acquired confidence with the technology itself. That differences might influence their performance (Caffò et al., 2016, 2020).

Sixth, despite the aforementioned positive outcomes some failures occurred. By reading the synoptic tables included along the chapter, one may emphasize that that TR approach seemed to be an encouraging and promising strategy as a future perspective. Data on AT-based interventions were mixed. Although extensively encouraging and promising, some participants failed, as above reported. Two considerations can be emphasized with this regard. Next to the technological solutions adopted to be further customized, one may argue that the selected behavioral responses required an excessive effort. A further explanation might be that the collected sessions were not systematically conducted over the time to corroborate the learning process (Chalmers, Hurst, Mackay, & Fergus, 2019; Tang, Wang, Ramhumar, & Nair, 2020).

5. CONCLUSION

The current overview emphasized five categories of studies on the use of AT and TR to support adaptive responding of individuals with NDD. Technological aids enhanced the participants' active role, self-determination, positive participation. The users were enabled in communication skills, physical activities, leisure and occupation opportunities. Moreover, they were easily monitored and supervised remotely through TR strategies. During Covid-19 pandemic it was very useful because the pandemic event suddenly interrupted medical assistance and rehabilitation care. With virtual reality setups and telerehabilitation, professionals could easily assess the users' daily performances and provided feedback on learning process. Technological supports were effective and reliable to help persons with neurodegenerative diseases even if physically distanced. Thus, through TR professionals were capable to provide timely feedback on daily use, with beneficial outcomes on both users and families. Their constructive engagement and positive occupation were fostered accordingly. Assessment and rehabilitative objectives were successfully achieved.

6. FUTURE RESEARCH

New research within this framework should deal with the following features and topics: (a) extension to a larger sample including further pathologies (e.g., stroke and/or post-coma), (b) design new technological solutions and/or options to adequately satisfy both behavioral minimal responses, and more complex environmental requests, (c) a systematic inclusion along the conducted studies of maintenance and/or generalization phases, added to social validation procedures, and (d) differentiate between single-subject and between groups experimental designs.

For example, one could rely on robots-assisted programs to enhance positive, physical, and social participation of patients with stroke. Otherwise, a combination of microswitches and VOCA could be implemented in post-coma persons in a minimally conscious state to enable the participant with self-administration of positive stimulation and/or asking for social contact with a caregiver. Finally, systematic comparisons of virtual reality setups, mobile technologies, and wearable technologies might be envisaged (Stasolla, 2021; Stasolla et al., 2021).

REFERENCES

Akbas, K., & Mummolo, C. (2021). A computational framework towards the tele-rehabilitation of balance control skills. *Frontiers in Robotics and AI*, *8*, 648485. Advance online publication. doi:10.3389/frobt.2021.648485 PMID:34179106

Asano, M., Koh, G. C., Madhukumar, P., Teng, G. Y. H., Liew, P. L. L., Nagalingam, S., Tan, M. L. M., Ng, Y. S., & Tan, B. K. T. (2021). Study protocol: A pilot quasi-experimental trial of tele-rehabilitation and tele-drain care post-mastectomy. *Pilot and Feasibility Studies*, *7*(1), 39. Advance online publication. doi:10.118640814-021-00776-5 PMID:33522962

Asghar, I., Cang, S., & Yu, H. (2018). Usability evaluation of assistive technologies through qualitative research focusing on people with mild dementia. *Computers in Human Behavior*, *79*, 192–201. doi:10.1016/j.chb.2017.08.034

Bassi, M., Cilia, S., Falautano, M., Grobberio, M., Negri, L., Niccolai, C., Pattini, M., Pietrolongo, E., Quartuccio, M. E., Viterbo, R. G., Allegri, B., Amato, M. P., Benin, M., De Luca, G., Gasperini, C., Minacapelli, E., Patti, F., Trojano, M., & Delle Fave, A. (2020). The caring experience in multiple sclerosis: Caregiving tasks, coping strategies and psychological well-being. *Health & Social Care in the Community*, *28*(1), 236–246. doi:10.1111/hsc.12858 PMID:31524966

Behera, C. K., Condell, J., Dora, S., Gibson, D. S., & Leavey, G. (2021). State-of-the-art sensors for remote care of people with dementia during a pandemic: A systematic review. *Sensors (Basel)*, *21*(14), 4688. Advance online publication. doi:10.339021144688 PMID:34300428

Belić, M., Bobić, V., Badža, M., Šolaja, N., Đurić-Jovičić, M., & Kostić, V. S. (2019). Artificial intelligence for assisting diagnostics and assessment of Parkinson's disease—A review. *Clinical Neurology and Neurosurgery*, *184*, 105442. Advance online publication. doi:10.1016/j.clineuro.2019.105442 PMID:31351213

Bernini, S., Stasolla, F., Panzarasa, S., Quaglini, S., Sinforiani, E., Sandrini, G., Vecchi, T., Tassorelli, C., & Bottiroli, S. (2021). Cognitive telerehabilitation for older adults with neurodegenerative diseases in the COVID-19 era: A perspective study. *Frontiers in Neurology*, *11*, 623933. Advance online publication. doi:10.3389/fneur.2020.623933 PMID:33519704

Brownlee, A., & Bruening, L. M. (2012). Methods of communication at end of life for the person with amyotrophic lateral sclerosis. *Topics in Language Disorders*, *32*(2), 168–185. doi:10.1097/TLD.0b013e31825616ef

Brunner, M., Hemsley, B., Togher, L., & Palmer, S. (2017). Technology and its role in rehabilitation for people with cognitive-communication disability following a traumatic brain injury (TBI). *Brain Injury: [BI]*, *31*(8), 1028–1043. doi:10.1080/02699052.2017.1292429 PMID:28471267

Caffò, A. O., Lopez, A., Spano, G., Saracino, G., Stasolla, F., Ciriello, G., Grattagliano, I., Lancioni, G. E., & Bosco, A. (2016). The role of pre-morbid intelligence and cognitive reserve in predicting cognitive efficiency in a sample of italian elderly. *Aging Clinical and Experimental Research*, *28*(6), 1203–1210. doi:10.100740520-016-0580-z PMID:27149863

Caffò, A. O., Lopez, A., Spano, G., Stasolla, F., Serino, S., Cipresso, P., Riva, G., & Bosco, A. (2020). The differential effect of normal and pathological aging on egocentric and allocentric spatial memory in navigational and reaching space. *Neurological Sciences*, *41*(7), 1741–1749. doi:10.100710072-020-04261-4 PMID:32002741

Caligari, M., Godi, M., Giardini, M., & Colombo, R. (2019). Development of a new high sensitivity mechanical switch for augmentative and alternative communication access in people with amyotrophic lateral sclerosis. *Journal of Neuroengineering and Rehabilitation*, *16*(1), 152. Advance online publication. doi:10.118612984-019-0626-5 PMID:31783763

Caprì, T., Nucita, A., Iannizzotto, G., Stasolla, F., Romano, A., Semino, M., Giannatiempo, S., Canegallo, V., & Fabio, R. A. (2021). Telerehabilitation for improving adaptive skills of children and young adults with multiple disabilities: A systematic review. *Review Journal of Autism and Developmental Disorders*, *8*(2), 244–252. doi:10.100740489-020-00214-x

Catania, A. C. (2012). *Learning* (5th ed.). Sloan.

Chalmers, C., Hurst, W., Mackay, M., & Fergus, P. (2019). Identifying behavioral changes for health monitoring applications using the advanced metering infrastructure. *Behaviour & Information Technology*, *38*(11), 1154–1166. doi:10.1080/0144929X.2019.1574900

Cikajlo, I., & Peterlin Potisk, K. (2019). Advantages of using 3D virtual reality-based training in persons with parkinson's disease: A parallel study. *Journal of Neuroengineering and Rehabilitation*, *16*(1), 119. Advance online publication. doi:10.118612984-019-0601-1 PMID:31623622

De Pace, C., & Stasolla, F. (2014). Promoting Environmental Control, Social Interaction, and Leisure/Academy Engagement Among People with Severe/Profound Multiple Disabilities Through Assistive Technology. In G. Kouroupetroglou (Ed.), *Assistive Technologies and Computer Access for Motor Disabilities* (pp. 285–319). doi:10.4018/978-1-4666-4438-0.ch010

Dockx, K., Van Remoortel, H., De Buck, E., Schelstraete, C., Vanderheyden, A., Lievens, T., Kinyagu, J. T., Mamuya, S., & Vandekerckhove, P. (2019). Effect of contextualized versus non-contextualized interventions for improving hand washing, sanitation, and health in rural tanzania: Study design of a cluster randomized controlled trial. *International Journal of Environmental Research and Public Health, 16*(14), 2529. Advance online publication. doi:10.3390/ijerph16142529 PMID:31311186

Fried-Oken, M., Mooney, A., & Peters, B. (2015). Supporting communication for patients with neurodegenerative disease. *NeuroRehabilitation, 37*(1), 69–87. doi:10.3233/NRE-151241 PMID:26409694

Gil-González, I., Pérez-San-Gregorio, M. Á., Conrad, R., & Martín-Rodríguez, A. (2021). Predicting improvement of quality of life and mental health over 18-months in multiple sclerosis patients. *Multiple Sclerosis and Related Disorders, 53*, 103093. Advance online publication. doi:10.1016/j.msard.2021.103093 PMID:34175814

Góngora Alonso, S., Hamrioui, S., De La Torre Díez, I., Motta Cruz, E., López-Coronado, M., & Franco, M. (2019). Social robots for people with aging and dementia: A systematic review of literature. *Telemedicine Journal and e-Health, 25*(7), 533–540. doi:10.1089/tmj.2018.0051 PMID:30136901

Holthe, T., & Wulff-Jacobsen, I. (2016). Matching user needs to technology in dementia care: Experiences with the alma supervisor educational program. *Family Medicine and Primary Care Review, 18*, 492–496. doi:10.5114/fmpcr.2016.63710

Hung, K. N. G., & Fong, K. N. K. (2019). Effects of telerehabilitation in occupational therapy practice: A systematic review. *Hong Kong Journal of Occupational Therapy, 32*(1), 3–21. doi:10.1177/1569186119849119 PMID:31217758

Imbeault, H., Langlois, F., Bocti, C., Gagnon, L., & Bier, N. (2018). Can people with Alzheimer's disease improve their day-to-day functioning with a tablet computer? *Neuropsychological Rehabilitation, 28*(5), 779–796. doi:10.1080/09602011.2015.1133431 PMID:28278593

Kim, E. S., Laird, L., Wilson, C., Bieg, T., Mildner, P., Möller, S., Schatz, R., Schwarz, S., Spang, R., Voigt-Antons, J.-N., & Rochon, E. (2021). Implementation and effects of an information technology-based intervention to support speech and language therapy among stroke patients with aphasia: Protocol for a virtual randomized controlled trial. *JMIR Research Protocols, 10*(7), e30621. Advance online publication. doi:10.2196/30621 PMID:34255727

Klimova, B., Valis, M., & Kuca, K. (2018). Exploring assistive technology as a potential beneficial intervention tool for people with Alzheimer's disease – a systematic review. *Neuropsychiatric Disease and Treatment, 14*, 3151–3158. doi:10.2147/NDT.S181849 PMID:30532546

Koldrack, P., Luplow, M., Kirste, T., & Teipel, S. (2013). Cognitive assistance to support social integration in Alzheimer's disease. *Geriatric Mental Health Care, 1*(2), 39–45. doi:10.1016/j.gmhc.2013.04.005

Kotipalli, P., Praveen Kumar, E. R., Mohan Raju, M. A. S., & Murali Krishna, D. (2019). *Supportive communication system for the elderly disabled people.* . doi:10.1007/978-981-13-1921-1_45

Koumakis, L., Chatzaki, C., Kazantzaki, E., Maniadi, E., & Tsiknakis, M. (2019). Dementia care frameworks and assistive technologies for their implementation: A review. *IEEE Reviews in Biomedical Engineering, 12*, 4–18. doi:10.1109/RBME.2019.2892614 PMID:30640629

Lancioni, G. E., Bosco, A., De Caro, M. F., Singh, N. N., O'reilly, M. F., Green, V. A., Ferlisi, G., Zullo, V., D'Amico, F., Addante, L. M., Denitto, F., & Zonno, N. (2015). Effects of response-related music stimulation versus general music stimulation on positive participation of patients with Alzheimer's disease. *Developmental Neurorehabilitation, 18*(3), 169–176. doi:10.3109/17518423.2013.802388 PMID:23869934

Lancioni, G. E., O'Reilly, M. F., Singh, N. N., Groeneweg, J., Bosco, A., Tota, A., Smaldone, A., Stasolla, F., Manfredi, F., Baccani, S., & Pidala, S. (2006). A social validation assessment of microswitch-based programs for persons with multiple disabilities employing teacher trainees and parents as raters. *Journal of Developmental and Physical Disabilities, 18*(4), 383–391. doi:10.100710882-006-9024-6

Lancioni, G. E., O'Reilly, M. F., Singh, N. N., Sigafoos, J., Grumo, G., Pinto, K., Stasolla, F., Signorino, M., & Groeneweg, J. (2013a). Assessing the impact and social perception of self-regulated music stimulation with patients with Alzheimer's disease. *Research in Developmental Disabilities, 34*(1), 139–146. doi:10.1016/j.ridd.2012.07.026 PMID:22944256

Lancioni, G. E., O'Reilly, M. F., Singh, N. N., Sigafoos, J., Rigante, V., de Franciscis, L., Stasolla, F., Perilli, V., & Lang, R. (2013b). A further evaluation of the impact of self-regulated music stimulation on positive participation of patients with Alzheimer's disease. *Journal of Developmental and Physical Disabilities, 25*(3), 273–283. doi:10.100710882-012-9301-5

Lancioni, G. E., O'Reilly, M. F., Singh, N. N., Stasolla, F., Manfredi, F., & Oliva, D. (2004). Adapting a grid into a microswitch to suit simple hand movements of a child with profound multiple disabilities. *Perceptual and Motor Skills, 99*(2), 724–728. doi:10.2466/pms.99.2.724-728 PMID:15560365

Lancioni, G. E., Perilli, V., Singh, N. N., O'Reilly, M. F., & Cassano, G. (2011). A man with severe Alzheimer's disease stops wandering during a picture coloring activity. *Developmental Neurorehabilitation, 14*(4), 242–246. doi:10.3109/17518423.2011.575439 PMID:21732808

Lancioni, G. E., Sigafoos, J., O'Reilly, M. F., & Singh, N. N. (2012). *Assistive technology: Interventions for individuals with severe/profound and multiple disabilities.* Springer.

Lancioni, G. E., Simone, I. L., De Caro, M. F., Singh, N. N., O'Reilly, M. F., Sigafoos, J., Ferlisi, G., Zullo, V., Schirone, S., Denitto, F., & Zonno, N. (2015). Assisting persons with advanced amyotrophic lateral sclerosis in their leisure engagement and communication needs with a basic technology-aided program. *NeuroRehabilitation, 36*(3), 355–365. doi:10.3233/NRE-151224 PMID:26409339

Lancioni, G. E., & Singh, N. N. (2014). *Assistive technologies for people with diverse abilities.* Springer. doi:10.1007/978-1-4899-8029-8

Lancioni, G. E., Singh, N. N., O'Reilly, M. F., Green, V. A., Ferlisi, G., Ferrarese, G., Zullo, V., Perilli, V., Cassano, G., Cordiano, N., Pinto, K., & Zonno, N. (2013). Self-regulated music stimulation for persons with Alzheimer's disease: Impact assessment and social validation. *Developmental Neurorehabilitation, 16*(1), 17–26. doi:10.3109/17518423.2012.707693 PMID:23030807

Lancioni, G. E., Singh, N. N., O'Reilly, M. F., Sigafoos, J., Chiapparino, C., Stasolla, F., Bosco, A., De Pace, C., & Oliva, D. (2007a). Enabling a young man with minimal motor behavior to manage independently his leisure television engagement. *Perceptual and Motor Skills*, *105*(1), 47–54. doi:10.2466/pms.105.1.47-54 PMID:17918548

Lancioni, G. E., Singh, N. N., O'Reilly, M. F., Sigafoos, J., Chiapparino, C., Stasolla, F., & Oliva, D. (2007b). Using an optic sensor and a scanning keyboard emulator to facilitate writing by persons with pervasive motor disabilities. *Journal of Developmental and Physical Disabilities*, *19*(6), 593–603. doi:10.100710882-007-9073-5

Lancioni, G. E., Singh, N. N., O'Reilly, M. F., Sigafoos, J., D'Amico, F., Ferlisi, G., ... Belardinelli, M. O. (2015b). Patients with moderate Alzheimer's disease engage in verbal reminiscence with the support of a computer-aided program: A pilot study. *Frontiers in Aging Neuroscience*, *7*(JUN). Advance online publication. doi:10.3389/fnagi.2015.00109 PMID:26089797

Lancioni, G. E., Singh, N. N., O'Reilly, M. F., Sigafoos, J., D'Amico, F., Laporta, D., Cattaneo, M. G., Scordamaglia, A., & Pinto, K. (2018). Technology-based behavioral interventions for daily activities and supported ambulation in people with Alzheimer's disease. *American Journal of Alzheimer's Disease and Other Dementias*, *33*(5), 318–326. doi:10.1177/1533317518775038 PMID:29742903

Lancioni, G. E., Singh, N. N., O'Reilly, M. F., Sigafoos, J., D'Amico, F., Pinto, K., & Chiapparino, C. (2017). Supporting simple activity engagement in persons with moderate to severe Alzheimer's disease through a technology-aided program. *American Journal of Alzheimer's Disease and Other Dementias*, *32*(3), 137–144. doi:10.1177/1533317517698793 PMID:28423935

Lancioni, G. E., Singh, N. N., O'Reilly, M. F., Sigafoos, J., D'Amico, F., Renna, C., & Pinto, K. (2016). Technology-aided programs to support positive verbal and physical engagement in persons with moderate or severe Alzheimer's disease. *Frontiers in Aging Neuroscience*, *8*(APR). Advance online publication. doi:10.3389/fnagi.2016.00087 PMID:27148050

Lancioni, G. E., Singh, N. N., O'Reilly, M. F., Sigafoos, J., D'Amico, F., Sasanelli, G., De Vanna, F., & Signorino, M. (2015a). Persons with Alzheimer's disease engage in leisure and mild physical activity with the support of technology-aided programs. *Research in Developmental Disabilities*, *37*, 55–63. doi:10.1016/j.ridd.2014.11.004 PMID:25460220

Lancioni, G. E., Singh, N. N., O'Reilly, M. F., Sigafoos, J., D'Amico, F., Turnone, B., Laporta, D., Scordamaglia, A., & Pinto, K. (2019). Smartphone-based interventions to foster simple activity and personal satisfaction in people with advanced Alzheimer's disease. *American Journal of Alzheimer's Disease and Other Dementias*, *34*(7-8), 478–485. doi:10.1177/1533317519844144 PMID:31014071

Lancioni, G. E., Singh, N. N., O'Reilly, M. F., Sigafoos, J., Renna, C., Pinto, K., De Vanna, F., Caffò, A. O., & Stasolla, F. (2014). Persons with moderate Alzheimer's disease use simple technology aids to manage daily activities and leisure occupation. *Research in Developmental Disabilities*, *35*(9), 2117–2128. doi:10.1016/j.ridd.2014.05.002 PMID:24881006

Langer, A., Gassner, L., Flotz, A., Hasenauer, S., Gruber, J., Wizany, L., Pokan, R., Maetzler, W., & Zach, H. (2021). How COVID-19 will boost remote exercise-based treatment in Parkinson's disease: A narrative review. *NPJ Parkinson's Disease*, *7*(1), 25. Advance online publication. doi:10.103841531-021-00160-3 PMID:33686074

Lazarou, I., Parastatidis, T., Tsolaki, A., Gkioka, M., Karakostas, A., Douka, S., & Tsolaki, M. (2017). International ballroom dancing against neurodegeneration: A randomized controlled trial in Greek community-dwelling elders with mild cognitive impairment. *American Journal of Alzheimer's Disease and Other Dementias*, *32*(8), 489–499. doi:10.1177/1533317517725813 PMID:28840742

Leuty, V., Boger, J., Young, L., Hoey, J., & Mihailidis, A. (2013). Engaging older adults with dementia in creative occupations using artificially intelligent assistive technology. *Assistive Technology*, *25*(2), 72–79. doi:10.1080/10400435.2012.715113 PMID:23923689

Lim, F. S., Wallace, T., Luszcz, M. A., & Reynolds, K. J. (2013). Usability of tablet computers by people with early-stage dementia. *Gerontology*, *59*(2), 174–182. doi:10.1159/000343986 PMID:23257664

Mancioppi, G., Fiorini, L., Timpano Sportiello, M., & Cavallo, F. (2019). Novel technological solutions for assessment, treatment, and assistance in mild cognitive impairment. *Frontiers in Neuroinformatics*, *13*, 58. Advance online publication. doi:10.3389/fninf.2019.00058 PMID:31456679

Mantovani, E., Zucchella, C., Bottiroli, S., Federico, A., Giugno, R., Sandrini, G., Chiamulera, C., & Tamburin, S. (2020). Telemedicine and virtual reality for cognitive rehabilitation: A roadmap for the COVID-19 pandemic. *Frontiers in Neurology*, *11*, 926. Advance online publication. doi:10.3389/fneur.2020.00926 PMID:33041963

Matamala-Gomez, M., Bottiroli, S., Realdon, O., Riva, G., Galvagni, L., Platz, T., Sandrini, G., De Icco, R., & Tassorelli, C. (2021). Telemedicine and virtual reality at time of COVID-19 pandemic: An overview for future perspectives in neurorehabilitation. *Frontiers in Neurology*, *12*, 646902. Advance online publication. doi:10.3389/fneur.2021.646902 PMID:33841313

Matamala-Gomez, M., Donegan, T., Bottiroli, S., Sandrini, G., Sanchez-Vives, M. V., & Tassorelli, C. (2019). Immersive virtual reality and virtual embodiment for pain relief. *Frontiers in Human Neuroscience*, *13*, 279. Advance online publication. doi:10.3389/fnhum.2019.00279 PMID:31551731

Neven, A., Janssens, D., Alders, G., Wets, G., Wijmeersch, B. V., & Feys, P. (2013). Documenting outdoor activity and travel behaviour in persons with neurological conditions using travel diaries and GPS tracking technology: A pilot study in multiple sclerosis. *Disability and Rehabilitation*, *35*(20), 1718–1725. doi:10.3109/09638288.2012.751137 PMID:23343357

Nijhof, N., Van Hoof, J., Van Rijn, H., & Van Gemert-Pijnen, J. E. W. C. (2013). The behavioral outcomes of a technology-supported leisure activity in people with dementia. *Technology and Disability*, *25*(4), 263–273. doi:10.3233/TAD-140398

Oksnebjerg, L., Woods, B., & Waldemar, G. (2019). Designing the ReACT app to support self-management of people with dementia: An iterative user-involving process. *Gerontology*, *65*(6), 673–685. doi:10.1159/000500445 PMID:31266031

Plow, M., & Finlayson, M. (2013). Potential benefits of nintendo wii fit among people with multiple sclerosis: A longitudinal pilot study. *International Journal of MS Care, 15*(S1, SUPPL.1), 13–23. doi:10.7224/1537-2073-15.S1.13 PMID:24453702

Rohrbach, N., Gulde, P., Armstrong, A. R., Hartig, L., Abdelrazeq, A., Schröder, S., Neuse, J., Grimmer, T., Diehl-Schmid, J., & Hermsdörfer, J. (2019). An augmented reality approach for ADL support in Alzheimer's disease: A crossover trial. *Journal of Neuroengineering and Rehabilitation, 16*(1), 66. Advance online publication. doi:10.118612984-019-0530-z PMID:31159816

Santos, A. V. F., Licursi, L. A., Amaral, M. F., Cavalcanti, A., & Silveira, Z. C. (2019). User-centered design of a customized assistive device to support feeding. *Procedia CIRP, 84,* 743-748.

Savvidis, T. P., Konstantinidis, E. I., Dias, S. B., Diniz, J. A., Hadjileontiadis, L. J., & Bamidis, P. D. (2018). *Exergames for Parkinson's disease patients: How participatory design led to technology adaptation.* doi:10.3233/978-1-61499-880-8-78

Schischlevskij, P., Cordts, I., Günther, R., Stolte, B., Zeller, D., Schröter, C., Weyen, U., Regensburger, M., Wolf, J., Schneider, I., Hermann, A., Metelmann, M., Kohl, Z., Linker, R. A., Koch, J. C., Stendel, C., Müschen, L. H., Osmanovic, A., Binz, C., ... Schreiber-Katz, O. (2021). Informal caregiving in amyotrophic lateral sclerosis (als): A high caregiver burden and drastic consequences on caregivers' lives. *Brain Sciences, 11*(6), 748. Advance online publication. doi:10.3390/brainsci11060748 PMID:34200087

Seitz, R. J., & Donnan, G. A. (2015). Recovery potential after acute stroke. *Frontiers in Neurology, 6.* Advance online publication. doi:10.3389/fneur.2015.00238 PMID:26617568

Sigafoos, J., O'Reilly, M. F., Ledbetter-Cho, K., Lim, N., Lancioni, G. E., & Marschik, P. B. (2019). Addressing sequelae of developmental regression associated with developmental disabilities: A systematic review of behavioral and educational intervention studies. *Neuroscience and Biobehavioral Reviews, 96,* 56–71. doi:10.1016/j.neubiorev.2018.11.014 PMID:30481529

Stamford, J. A., Schmidt, P. N., & Friedl, K. E. (2015). What engineering technology could do for quality of life in Parkinson's disease: A review of current needs and opportunities. *IEEE Journal of Biomedical and Health Informatics, 19*(6), 1862–1872. doi:10.1109/JBHI.2015.2464354 PMID:26259205

Stamford, J. A., Schmidt, P. N., & Friedl, K. E. (2015). What engineering technology could do for quality of life in Parkinson's disease: A review of current needs and opportunities. *IEEE Journal of Biomedical and Health Informatics, 19*(6), 1862–1872. doi:10.1109/JBHI.2015.2464354 PMID:26259205

Stasolla, F. (2021). Virtual reality and wearable technologies to support adaptive responding of children and adolescents with neurodevelopmental disorders: A critical comment and new perspectives. *Frontiers in Psychology, 12,* 720626. Advance online publication. doi:10.3389/fpsyg.2021.720626 PMID:34322073

Stasolla, F., Boccasini, A., Perilli, V., Caffò, A. O., Damiani, R., & Albano, V. (2014). A selective overview of microswitch-based programs for promoting adaptive behaviors of children with developmental disabilities. *International Journal of Ambient Computing and Intelligence, 6*(2), 56–74. doi:10.4018/IJACI.2014070104

Stasolla, F., Caffò, A. O., Perilli, V., Boccasini, A., Stella, A., Damiani, R., Albano, V., & Damato, C. (2017). a microswitch-based program for promoting initial ambulation responses: An evaluation with two girls with multiple disabilities. *Journal of Applied Behavior Analysis, 50*(2), 345–356. doi:10.1002/jaba.374 PMID:28128442

Stasolla, F., Damiani, R., Perilli, V., Di Leone, A., Albano, V., Stella, A., & Damato, C. (2014). Technological supports to promote choice opportunities by two children with fragile X syndrome and severe to profound developmental disabilities. *Research in Developmental Disabilities, 35*(11), 2993–3000. doi:10.1016/j.ridd.2014.07.045 PMID:25118066

Stasolla, F., & De Pace, C. (2014). Assistive technology to promote leisure and constructive engagement by two boys emerged from a minimal conscious state. *NeuroRehabilitation, 35*(2), 253–259. doi:10.3233/NRE-141112 PMID:24990021

Stasolla, F., Matamala-Gomez, M., Bernini, S., Caffò, A. O., & Bottiroli, S. (2021). Virtual reality as a technological-aided solution to support communication in persons with neurodegenerative diseases and acquired brain injury during COVID-19 pandemic. *Frontiers in Public Health, 8*, 635426. Advance online publication. doi:10.3389/fpubh.2020.635426 PMID:33665181

Stasolla, F., Perilli, V., & Boccasini, A. (2016). Assistive Technologies for Persons with Multiple Disabilities. In J. Luiselli & A. J. Fisher (Eds.), *Computer-Assisted and Web-Based Innovations in Psychology, Special Education, and Health* (pp. 287–310). Elsevier. doi:10.1016/B978-0-12-802075-3.00011-5

Stummer, C., Dibilio, V., Overeem, S., Weerdesteyn, V., Bloem, B. R., & Nonnekes, J. (2015). The walk-bicycle: A new assistive device for Parkinson's patients with freezing of gait? *Parkinsonism & Related Disorders, 21*(7), 755–757. doi:10.1016/j.parkreldis.2015.04.025 PMID:25983112

Tang, W., Wang, A., Ramkumar, S., & Nair, R. K. R. (2020). Signal identification system for developing rehabilitative device using deep learning algorithms. *Artificial Intelligence in Medicine, 102.* doi:10.1016/j.artmed.2019.101755

van der Meer, L., Matthews, T., Ogilvie, E., Berry, A., Waddington, H., Balandin, S., ... Sigafoos, J. (2017). Training direct-care staff to provide communication intervention to adults with intellectual disability: A systematic review. *American Journal of Speech-Language Pathology, 26*, 1279–1295.

Wang, R. H., Sudhama, A., Begum, M., Huq, R., & Mihailidis, A. (2017). Robots to assist daily activities: Views of older adults with Alzheimer's disease and their caregivers. *International Psychogeriatrics, 29*(1), 67–79. doi:10.1017/S1041610216001435 PMID:27660047

Zhao, Y., Nonnekes, J., Storcken, E. J. M., Janssen, S., van Wegen, E. E. H., Bloem, B. R., Dorresteijn, L. D. A., van Vugt, J. P. P., Heida, T., & van Wezel, R. J. A. (2016). Feasibility of external rhythmic cueing with the Google glass for improving gait in people with Parkinson's disease. *Journal of Neurology, 263*(6), 1156–1165. doi:10.100700415-016-8115-2 PMID:27113598

ADDITIONAL READING

Asghar, I., Cang, S., & Yu, H. (2020). The impact of assistive software application to facilitate people with dementia through participatory research. *International Journal of Human-Computer Studies*, *143*, 102471. Advance online publication. doi:10.1016/j.ijhcs.2020.102471

Cardillo, E., Sapienza, G., Li, C., & Caddemi, A. (2021). Head motion and eyes blinking detection: A mm-wave radar for assisting people with neurodegenerative disorders. *2020 50th European Microwave Conference, EuMC 2020,* 925-928. 10.23919/EuMC48046.2021.9338116

Cortellessa, G., Fracasso, F., Umbrico, A., Cesta, A., Dionisio, P., Ciucci, L., Di Guardo, F., Tamburini, E., Pérez, M. Á., Herrero, J., Triantafyllidou, V., Dewarrat, R., Boghiu, F., Barnestein-Fonseca, P., Goodman-Casanova, J. M., & Mayoral, F. (2021). Co-design of a TV-based home support for early stage of dementia. *Journal of Ambient Intelligence and Humanized Computing*, *12*(4), 4541–4558. doi:10.100712652-020-01823-4

Hamdoun, S., Michael, K., Monteleone, R., & Bookman, T. (2021). Assistive technologies for greatly improved quality of life for people living with MND/ALS. *IEEE Consumer Electronics Magazine*, *10*(3), 76–81. doi:10.1109/MCE.2020.3035523

Pousada, T., Garabal-Barbeira, J., Martínez, C., Groba, B., Nieto-Riveiro, L., & Pereira, J. (2021). How loan bank of assistive technology impacts on life of persons with amyotrophic lateral sclerosis and neuromuscular diseases: A collaborative initiative. *International Journal of Environmental Research and Public Health*, *18*(2), 1–14. doi:10.3390/ijerph18020763 PMID:33477437

Spalla, G., Gouin-Vallerand, C., Yaddaden, A., & Bier, N. (2020). Towards an augmented reality cognitive orthosis to assist people with alzheimer's disease: Preliminary design. *ACM International Conference Proceeding Series*, 60-65. 10.1145/3411170.3411234

KEY TERMS AND DEFINITIONS

Assistive Technology: Umbrella term which includes any device, piece, tool, or equipment ensuring individuals with neurodegenerative diseases with self-determination and independence.

Constructive Engagement: Participant' active role and positive occupation to daily activities.

Neurodegenerative Diseases: Neurological disorders caused by progressive loss of structure or function of neurons, which may ultimately involve cell death.

Quality of Life: Complex psychological construct which includes happiness, pleasure, satisfaction, and fulfillment.

Telerehabilitation: Part of telemedicine with professionals who are able to remotely assess, monitor and supervise users in a synchronous or asynchronous way.

Chapter 11
Using Virtual Reality for Assessment and Rehabilitation of AD and MCI Patients:
A Selective Overview

Giulia Binaghi
Catholic University of Sacred Heart, Milan, Italy

ABSTRACT

Alzheimer's disease (AD) is a primary cause of dementia in the ageing population affecting more than 35 million people around the globe. Acquisition of information in everyday life requires memorization in complex three-dimensional environments. Emerging ICT (information and computer technology) applications based on virtual reality (VR) environments can lead to a behavior modification as they provide a photorealistic virtual environment (VE). This chapter provides a selective overview of the empirical evidence available along last five years on the use of virtual reality (VR) to promote everyday life skills and cognitive impairment mitigation of AD patients. Virtual reality allows us to identify and treat deficits in memory that are relevant to everyday life yet not detectable with list learning. Articles related to virtual reality have been divided in two categories according to their use: whether for assessment and diagnostic or rehabilitative purposes. Clinical implications were critically discussed. Suggestions for future research and practice will also be provided.

1. INTRODUCTION

Alzheimer disease (AD) is the primary cause of dementia worldwide (Ritchie & Lovestone, 2002). AD is defined by the National Institute on Aging-Alzheimer's Association (NIAA; McKhann et al., 2011) as "evidence of progressive cognitive decline on subsequent evaluations based on information from informants and cognitive testing in the context of either formal neuropsychological evaluation or standardized mental status examinations."

DOI: 10.4018/978-1-7998-7430-0.ch011

Currently, more than 35 million people are suffering from this disease around the globe (Brookmeyer, Johnson, Ziegler-Graham, & Arrighi, 2007). The basic pathological hallmarks of AD include widespread neuronal synaptic loss, excessive presence of astrocytes, aggregation of multiple proteinaceous deposits for instance β-amyloid plaques and neurofibrillary tangles (NFT) (Murph & LeVine, 2010).

People suffering from dementia are compromised in several cognitive domain (e.g., executive functions), to impede functioning in everyday life and social and occupational functioning. Impairment in the sense of orientation, and memory difficulties are related to the reduction of the temporal cortex volume, especially concerning the hippocampus, as well as the atrophy of the retro-splenial cortex. Serino and Riva (2013) claim that the translation between egocentric and allocentric frames, supported by the retro-splenial cortex, can be the basis of the spatial disorientation deficits. These deficits compromise the ability to link information between two landmarks (egocentric strategy) (Cushman, Stein, & Duffy, 2008). Patients with AD experience difficulties also when using an allocentric strategy (i.e., mental maps) or changing point of view between egocentric and allocentric views (Morganti, Stefanini, & Riva, 2015). These deficits are followed by a progressive decline in basic Activities of Daily Living (Millán-Calenti, Tubío,Pita-Fernández, Rochette, Lorenzo, & Maseda 2012).

Recently, several AD medical rehabilitation studies have shifted the focus to the field of virtual reality (VR) due to the rapid development of such technologies. To investigate everyday activities, virtual-reality offers the opportunity to bridge the gap between in situ approaches and laboratory settings. VR also demonstrates advantages in the treatment of dementia and reminiscence activities allowing experiences to be shared with family. These applications have an intuitive appeal but it remains unclear whether immersive virtual reality (IVR) can support the diagnosis or treatment of AD dementia (Johnson, 2018).

Until now, VR has been more employed in motor neurological disorders or in the treatment of mental health conditions, such as anxiety disorders or psychosis (Cogné et al., 2017). Researchers feared that patients would not tolerate the VR procedure (Flynn et al., 2003), but recently any danger was excluded (Laver et al., 2015). IVR has been utilized in public awareness campaigns allowing users to take reminiscence activities allowing experiences to be shared with family (Johnson, 2018). However, it remains unclear whether IVR can enhance the diagnosis or treatment of AD dementia. Moreover, VR applications are employed today as relevant experimental models of the real world to study how cognitive processes are embodied in complex and more natural behaviors (Rizzo, Schultheis, Kerns, & Mateer, 2004). Thus, immersive environment can easily stimulate the brain based on quantitative electroencephalogram (QEEG) analysis (Anopas & Wongsawat, 2014).

Few studies have analyzed the effects of topographical disorientation, that is one of the main hallmark of AD, (Aguirre & D'Esposito, 1999), because the lack of available behavioral measures of navigational capacity prevents researchers to detect early AD. Some studies hypothesize that a computer-based virtual reality (VR) test environment might yield comparable measures of broad applicability to the early detection of navigational impairment in mild cognitive impairment (MCI) and AD, identifying task and variables that influence navigational strategies and navigational success (Cushamn & Duffy, 2007; Monacelli, Cushman, Kavcic, & Duffy, 2003). Previous studies also focused on the ability to translate environmental- centered spatial information (allocentric) into body-centered ones (egocentric) in order to perform an efficient wayfinding during the active interaction in a complex virtual environment (Morganti, Carassa & Germiniani, 2007). Additionally, spatial memory difficulties in normal ageing and AD are extensively studied in large-scale environments using VR-based applications with 3D adaptations of both laboratory tests (Laczo et al., 2010) and naturalistic environments, evidencing encouraging results (Widmann, Beinhoff, & Riepe, 2012).

Accordingly, the first aim of this chapter was to provide the reader with an overview of the empirical evidences available between 2010-2020, regarding virtual reality-based programs for both assessment and treatment of Alzheimer's disease. Immersive virtual reality (IVR) tools, virtual brain neuroinformatic platform, Smart Aging Serious Game (SASG), computerized virtual cognitive test, mixed Reality-based Cognitive Training System and augmented reality methods have been systematically reviewed. This review was intended to examine the results from feasibility studies and controlled trials of virtual and augmented reality on AD and MCI rehabilitation and quality of life.

The second aim of the chapter was to illustrate the advantages of VR for diagnosis, dealing with the following topics: (a) visual spatial processes (i.e., navigational abilities, spatial memory and orientation), (b) memory (working, semantic, episodic), (c) functional abilities and (d) neurobiological status.

The third purpose was to emphasize the effectiveness of VR treatment in cognitive functions (i.e., wayfinding, attention, memory) even related to everyday activities, neurobiology (i.e., cerebral blood flow), and general mood (i.e., higher mood, less anxiety and frustration). Safety and efficacy of the current state of VR tools were discussed, providing suggestions for future research in this topic area.

2. BACKGROUND

The use of computers in psychological testing began over a quarter of a century ago (Riva, 1998). Few computer-based exploratory programs have been carried out aimed at older adults who have dementia (Cipriani, Bianchetti, & Trabucchi, 2006; Smith, Housen, Yaffeet, et al., 2009). These devices were effective both for diagnosis and to improve cognitive tasks such as face–name association, memory, attention, and list recall (Belleville et al., 2006).

VR is a novel branch of Information Computer Technology (ICT) that has been recently suggested for use in the area of neuropsychology. 'Immersive' virtual reality is defined as a system that encompasses the user's visual field and where virtual movement replicates actual head or bodily movement (Clay et al., 2020). Virtual reality uses computer simulation to replace an individual's external sensory world with an artificial environment that allows individual's orientation and physical movement. IVR was first presented by Ivan Sutherland (1965), and was intended to make that (virtual) world in the window looks real, sounds real, feels real, and responds realistically to the viewer's actions (Mazuryk & Gervautz,1992). IVR uses head mounted displays (HMD) which adjust the input to each eye to create a true sense of perspective in 3D. Interaction is more naturalistic using head/hand movements or walking within a monitored field. Virtual reality is defined 'immersive' as it encompasses the user's visual field and virtual movement replicates actual head or bodily movement. These sensory cues enable a more accurate representation of position (Clay et al., 2020) and contribute to an experience that is not only immersive but intuitive: participants do not need to be shown how to move, they just move (McNaughton, Battaglia, Jensen, & Moser, 2006). Excluding external visual input and updating the simulated visual environment in relation to head movements, it is possible to integrate vestibular, proprioceptive, and visual information.

The use of VR systems for disease treatment has been already explored in several areas, such as brain damage (Tost et al., 2009). The design and development of cognitive rehabilitation training activities in the framework of VR technology should be carried out for neuropsychological assessment of the following domains: attention, executive functions, memory (Optale et al., 2010), motor rehabilitation (Tost et al., 2009), and spatial orientation (Kober, Wood, Hofer, Kreuzig, & Kiefer, 2013). The design result should be a VR training system that is easy to use by AD patients and that is capable of providing effective feedback of the progress of their rehabilitation. In summary, the use of VR-based cognitive training systems would offer effective support to patients with MCI, early stage of AD, and caregivers. It would, also, place a particular focus on appropriate therapeutic interventions for the pre-dementia phase of AD to slow down its progression and provide effective training interventions to mitigate the symptoms (Garcıa-Betances, Jimenez-Mixco, Arredondo, & Cabrera-Umpierrez, 2015).

Several contributions indicated that patients feel a sense of control and enjoyment while interacting with the VR (Flynn et al., 2003). Moreover, modern IVR technology overcomes mismatch between visual perception and vestibular feedback (e.g., head rotation or walking) that commonly induced nausea in participants (Freeman et al., 2017) through a one-to-one correspondence of movement to visual perception. However, this has not yet been systematically appraised in a patient population. IVR has the advantage to simulate world which could potentially offer accurate discrimination of AD pathology on spatial cognitive tasks (Slobounov, Ray, Johnson, Slobounov & Newell, 2015), as well as the acquired level of spatial mental representations, which involved hippocampal and para-hippocampal gyri in navigation tasks (Burgess, Maguire, & O'Keefe, 2002; Chrastil, 2013; Spiers & Maguire, 2007). Tasks of spatial cognition may therefore offer earlier detection of AD ahead of current gold standard episodic memory measures. The implementation of VR-based tools opens up enormous possibilities for several operational features of cognitive rehabilitation. First, accessibility to a high level of experimental control, allows the study of diverse brain-stimulation activities within different areas (e.g., memory, language, executive functions). Second, researchers' access to real-time feedback allows together performance information during the course of the training and to evaluate its effectiveness (Garcı´a-Betances, Jime´nez-Mixco, Arredondo, & Cabrera-Umpie´rrez, 2015). Third, IVR allows to point out cognitive and functional deficits through use of large landscapes that would not be possible with other techniques (Vlcˇek & Laczo´, 2014).

2. METHOD

A computerized search was carried out within Scopus, PubMed, and Psych-Info databases for journal articles written in English and published in the last decade (i.e., 2010-2020) using combinations of the following keywords: Alzheimer disease, virtual reality, technology-based programs. The adopted including criteria were (a) only virtual reality for cognitive assessment and treatment, (b) AD and MCI patients involved as participant (i.e., ranging age 68-87 years old), and (c) empirical studies with control/clinical group comparison considered. The excluding criteria were: (a) review and book chapters, (b) technological tools not including virtual reality, (c) the absence of a rehabilitative program (i.e., theoretical contribution), (d) participants with intellectual disability not including Alzheimer disease.

Accordingly, 23 studies were retained, with a total of 836 participants enrolled. For practical reasons, they were grouped following the purpose for which virtual reality was used. Thus, two main categories were targeted, namely: 'assessment' and 'rehabilitation'. A synoptic table was added as completion, including the authors of the reviewed studies, participants involved, their ages, the virtual reality tool used, and the outcomes. It should be noticed that the number of studies presented for the two groups are not homogeneous., because currently most virtual reality studies are focused on assessment purposes.

3. LITERATURE OVERVIEW

The selected studies were arranged according to the use of Virtual Reality (i.e., assessment or rehabilitation), as listed in Table 1.

Table 1. Reviewed studies grouped according to the use of Virtual Reality

Authors	Categories	Participants	Mean Ages	Strategies	Main Outcomes
Allain et al., 2014	Assessment	24	75	Preparing a cup of coffee in both real and non-immersive virtual reality allows to assess IADL (instrumental activities of daily living) in AD patients	Were found significant relations ($p \leq .05$; $p \leq .01$, $p \leq .005$) between virtual and real coffee-making scores
Allison et al., 2016	Assessment	79	78.5	VR tasks of wayfinding and route learning assessed spatial navigation performance	AD showed significant ($p=0.001$) deficits in the use of a wayfinding strategy, but not in route learning strategy
Byrns et al., 2020	Rehabilitation	19	72.26	Virtual reality environment consisting of a music theatre as music therapy has to improve emotions and memory performance	Results showed a decrease of negative emotions (from M= 0.69 to M= 0.45). Improvement in memory performances ranged from 1.91% to 36.84%.
Cabinio et al., 2020	Assessment	139	73.59	VR serious game (SASG) platform assessed the cognitive profile of aMCI population and cognitive differences between aMCI and HC	Validity of SASG in discriminating aMCI from HC (AUC: 0.879)
Cogné et al., 2018	Assessment	38	68.25	In a 3D virtual environment were introduced three cueing conditions: salient landmarks, directional arrows and a map to enhance navigational skills in AD patients.	The recognition of landmarks increased significantly ($p=.04$) with directional arrows and with salient landmarks ($p.= 0002$)
Cushman et al., 2008	Assessment	26	74	Real-world and virtual environment assessed navigational deficit in MCI and AD patients	Were found correlations ($r= 0.73$; $p < .001$) between real-world and virtual navigational deficits
Davis & Ohman, 2016	Rehabilitation	40	62	Participants will try to find their way to a location within a virtual reality simulation of senior residence in two environemnts: standard and salient.	A VR environment full of cues is useful to assess wayfinding but also to improve this competence. patients $p < .05$
Doniger et al., 2018	Rehabilitation	70	52,5	How VR cognitive training could improve cognition and cerebral blood flow (CBF) in preclinical AD.	increase of up to 12% in CBF; a reduction of 48% risk of AD
Fasilis et al., 2018	Rehabilitation	10	73.6	Was examined the effect of CCR* and VR on the cognitive enhancement and rehabilitation, in patients with mild AD.	Emerged a statistical significant difference in Memory Retention ($p=0.009$); Working Memory ($p=0.039$); Executive Functions ($p=0.007$)
Foloppe et al., 2020	Rehabilitation	1	79	Cooking activities using interventions based on errorless learning, vanishing-cue, and virtual reality techniques.	Positive results: 15.4% from the virtual; 11.3% from the real condition.
Howett et al., 2019	Assessment	45	71.7	VR path integration test was combined with MRI measures of entorhinal cortex volume	VR task was able to assess biomarker related to AD (area under the curve = 0.90)
Lecouvey et al., 2019	Assessment	17	79.29	Virtual Reality for assessing PM (prospective memory) and RM (retrospective memory)	AD recalled the prospective component better than the retrospective one ($z =3.18$;$p < 0.01$, $r = 0.63$)
Manera et al., 2016	Rehabilitation	57	75.65	Was tested feasibility of both virtual and paper attentional task to train selective and sustained attention	Were identified more target in paper condition (M= 28.5) than in the virtual one (M= 20.6). 70% preferred VR condition
Morganti et al., 2015	Assessment	26	80.96	Two virtual reality tasks (VR-Maze and VR-Road Map tasks) assessed allo- to egocentric translation of spatial knowledge in AD and control group (CG)	The AD group reached significantly ($p < .001$) fewer target points than the CG in both VR task.
Moyle et al., 2006	Rehabilitation	10	89	Testing the effectiveness of a Virtual Reality Forest (VRF) on engagement, apathy, and mood states of people with dementia.	During the VRF experience, residents experienced more pleasure ($p = .008$) but also a greater level of alertness ($p <.001$).
Park et al., 2019	Rehabilitation	21	71.5	Mixed reality MR (augmented and virtual reality) was implemented to assess visuospatial working memory	Significant improvement in visuospatial working memory in the MR group compared with the control group ($t=-2.612$, $p=0.017$)
Plancher et al., 2012	Assessment	30	76.5	Two VR environments (active and passive exploration) assessed episodic memory level.	AD patients showed fewer recognition and allocentric spatial information than older adults ($p < .001$)
Sauzeon et al., 2016	Assessment	16	78.63	VR assessed verbal (objective and subjective) memory	AD showed poor objective memory, learning semantic clustery, and false recognition ($p<.0001$)
Stefanovski et al., 2019	Assessment	18	68.6	The Virtual Brain (TVB) neuroinformatics platform, combined with PET score, was used to assess hyperexcitability in AD related to the protein amyloid beta (Abeta)	It was found a strong inverse dependency for AD ($R2= 0.625$) and lower levels of Abeta
Tarnanas et al., 2014	Assessment	134	71.3	Participants were assessed 2 times with VR-DOT***, magnetic resonance imaging (MRI), event-related potentials (ERPs) and neuropsychological tests.	In AD were found significant correlations ($P <.01$) between VR-DOT scores, ERPs, MRI and neuropsychological tests
White & Moussavi, 2016	Rehabilitation	1	74	How VR navigation (VRN) could enhance navigating and also bring real-life cognitive benefits.	VRN environment led to an improvement in navigating ($R2=4634$).
Widmann et al, 2012	Assessment	15	72.6	A mixed design (CVLT** x VE) was used to assess Everyday- life memory deficits	AD recalled only 40% of items in list learning and 20% in VE (Virtual Environement)

AD= Alzheimer Disease; MCI= mild cognitive impairment;

*CCR= Computerized Cognitive Rehabilitation; **CVLT= California Verbal Learning Test; ***VR-DOT= virtual reality day-out task

3.1 VR for Assessment of AD

Virtual reality allows to evaluate impaired cognitive functions in AD's patients. In this section 13 articles were detailed with 607 participants specifically related to the assessment of Alzheimer's Disease (see Table 1). Since Alzheimer's disease causes impairments affecting instrumental activities of daily living (IADL), some authors (Allain, Foloppe, Besnard, & Yamagouchi, 2014) evaluated its impact through an-immersive virtual coffee task (NI-VCT). Performance on the virtual task was compared to an identical daily living task involving the actual preparation of a cup of coffee. Results showed that AD patients performed worse than control group on all tasks, providing utility of NI-VCT in predicting AD cognitive performance.

The first study focused on navigational abilities in preclinical AD (Allison, Fagan, Morris & Head, 2016) showed that pre-clinical AD is associated with decline in acquiring the spatial information relevant for wayfinding performance. Wayfinding performance was very powerful in discriminating between preclinical AD and healthy group. As the learning phase required the ability to learn the locations of objects in the environment in relation to each other, these results suggested that preclinical AD- deficits are related to the formation of cognitive maps. Early-stage symptomatic AD-related deficits were observed for all of the wayfinding and route learning tasks relative to control group, and for all but the wayfinding learning task relative to control group. Thus, virtual environment allowed to differentiate the visual-spatial processing performance between preclinical AD and healthy group. These findings were consistent with previous works comparing symptomatic AD to normal group (Cherrier, Mendez & Perryman, 2001; Laczó et al., 2010; Lithfous, Dufour, & Després, 2013).

A further study focused on detecting navigational deficits (Cushman, Stein, & Duffy, 2018) described real-world navigation test with a virtual reality (VR) version in aging and AD patients. Three participant groups (young normal controls, older normal controls, patients with MCI) have been exposed to a navigation test. They were randomly assigned to real-world or virtual environment test (Quake3, ID Software). Eight navigation sub-tests were: route learning, free recall, self-orientation, route drawing, landmark recall, photograph recognition, photograph location, and video location. Results showed strong correlations between navigational capacities in real-world and virtual environments. Data supported the use of virtual environment testing to detect impaired navigational capacities (Richardson, Montello, & Hegarty, 1999). The learning of navigational landmarks is equivalent in real-world and virtual environments, suggesting that cognitive mechanisms are similar (Gillner & Mallot, 1998). Unfortunately, the combination of visual and verbal losses in AD included both strategies involved in navigation: self-movement perception and identification of named places (Golledge, 1999).

Virtual reality allows to explore navigational difficulties of patients, as well as the acquired level of spatial mental representations. Virtual reality technology could also be used to assess whether there was a decline in performing the allo-to egocentric translation of spatial knowledge. Morganti, Stefanini and Riva (2015) used VR-Maze spatial task (VRMT) and VR-Road Map task (VR-RMT) to assess AD participants' abilities in exploring a complex environment in an both egocentric and allocentric manner. The strength point of this study was that VR-MT and VR-RMT were actively navigable from an egocentric perspective, so that participants could choose their own path within the environment. That was due to the combination of physical activity (moving in the environment without the possibility of deciding the path) and psychological activity (deciding the route without physically moving). In the VR-Maze spatial task (VR-MT), in order to assess allocentric spatial knowledge in the PP-MT (paper-and-pencil versions of five different complex mazes), participants were requested to draw the path from start to exit, trying to find the most efficient way between the two points. In the VR-Road Map task (VR-RMT), in order to assess egocentric mental rotation, the PP-RMT consisted of a stylized city map in which participants had to indicate the direction in order to follow a designated route. The main purpose of this task was to evaluate if the allo-to egocentric translation of spatial knowledge required for the navigation in the virtual environment could differ from the one required from a mental imagery simulation of the same environment based on a sketched map. The results emphasized that there was a specific reduction in performing allo- to egocentric spatial tasks in AD, whereas this reduction was not as evident in equivalent allocentric spatial tasks. These findings supported the use of VR based spatial tasks as useful tools for the easiest assessment of allo- to egocentric reference frame correspondence and translation, as well as a the efficacy of a more ecological evaluation of the navigational impairment in AD patients. These data confirmed previous results (Hort et al., 2007; Laczo et al., 2009) that emphasized wayfinding impairment based on survey maps in AD patients.

A group of researchers examined how visual cues could be helpful to improve spatial memory of patients with AD and MCI (Cognè et al., 2018). In this study, during virtual intersections within a virtual landmark, three visual cueing conditions for navigation were offered: salient landmarks, directional arrows, and a map. The number of trajectory mistakes did not differ significantly between patients with AD and patients with MCI on all three kind of path (salient landmarks, directional arrows, and map). Conversely, significant correlations emerged between the number of trajectory mistakes under the arrow condition and executive tests, and between the number of trajectory mistakes under the salient landmark condition and memory tests. In summary, visual cueing such as directional arrows and salient landmarks appeared helpful for spatial navigation and memory tasks in AD and MCI patients.

One of the main purposes of using virtual reality is to characterize episodic memory profiles in amnestic mild cognitive impairment (aMCI) and AD patients. Plancher, Tirard, Gyselinck, Nicolas, and Piolino (2011) conducted a study on three different types of population: healthy older adults, MCI and moderate AD patients. The research had to determine whether environmental factors linked to encoding information (active or passive exploration) could influence memory performance. Participants were immersed in two virtual environments characterized by active exploration (driver of a virtual car) and passive exploration (passenger of that car). Recall and recognition of environment's elements, contextual information (temporal, egocentric and allocentric spatial information), and the quality of binding were assessed. In summary, results revealed that AD patients were impaired compared to the healthy older group and also to MCI patients in all recalls, which included central information, its multi-component context, and binding. Only familiarity judgment was preserved. However, the MCI and AD patients were impaired in comparison with the control population for both the immediate and delayed recall of egocentric memory and allocentric spatial information. That was in line with a previous virtual reality study which identified the reduced volume of the hippocampus, the precuneus and parietal regions as the causes of memory impairment (Weniger, Ruhlede, Lange, Wolf, & Irle, 2011). A remarkable point was that all participants benefited from active virtual exploration. AD patients improved the recall of elements, spatial allocentric information and binding, confirming previous study about the utility of an ecological test of memory, such as virtual reality (Chetelat, Desgranges, & Eustache, 2006; Perri, Serra, Carlesimo, & Caltagirone, 2007). Moreover, comparing memory virtual test to classical memory test, emerged correlations in performances on the recall of elements, temporal and spatial information, binding and spatial recognition.

Tarnanas, Tsolaki, Nef, Muria, and Mosimann (2014) used a virtual reality day-out task (VR-DOT) environment to examine executive functions, prospective memory, and reasoning in a complex emergency routine (fire evacuation) that required multitasking. In that sense, VR-DOT was a complex instrumental activity of daily living. In this study, VR-DOT performance was compared to markers of neuro-degeneration and electrophysiologic correlates (ERPs) over different time intervals. Significant correlations were found among these variables, so that this study confirmed that impaired executive functions, as measured with VR-DOT, were predictors of greater cognitive decline. Furthermore, it confirmed usefulness of P3b latencies for assessing declining progression (Bennys, Rondouin, Benattar, Gabelle, & Touchon, 2011).

Likewise, Cabinio et al. (2020) assessed the cognitive profile of an amnestic mild cognitive impairment (aMCI) population through smart aging serious game (SASG), a virtual reality platform. SAGS was an ecological serious game based on a virtual house, in which participants are asked to interact with the different parts of the scenario and to perform specific tasks. SAGS belonged to the so-called 'serious games' (SGs), defined as << *digital applications specialized for purposes other than entertaining*>> (Dubois et al., 2014; Robert et al., 2014), which were able to implement virtual 3D real environments. All the actions performed by the participants within the SAGS were recorded and measured, allowing the assessment of memory, executive functions, working memory, and visual spatial processes (Bottiroli et al., 2017). Results showed the validity of the SASG in discriminating preclinical population with aMCI from health aging individuals. A greater diagnostic efficacy for SASG emerged compared to gold standard tests, so that SASG can be considered a digital biomarker providing objective and clinically meaningful data about the cognitive profile of aMCI participants, in particular for the detection of the reduction in the hippocampal volume. Moreover, SASG interface was specifically implemented for non-expert users and proved a good usability, as it wasalready been demonstrated (Zucchella e al., 2014).

With regard to episodic and semantic memory, Widmann, Beinhoffa, and Riepea (2012) investigated verbal learning in a virtual environment. The primary goal of their study was to assess learning of verbal material in situations imitating naturalistic conditions. In their mixed 2x2 research design each patient was randomly assigned to the first condition (California Verbal Learning Test) and later to the second condition (virtual environment). Results showed that patients with AD only achieved about 40% in list learning (standard condition) and 20% in virtual environment (naturalistic condition), unlike the control group that achieved about 90% of presented items in both conditions. This proved that testing of explicit declarative memory content within a three-dimensional environment was better suited to portray the memory deficits in AD patients. Moreover, recognition of items seemed to be facilitated by learning in a naturalistic environment. In fact, recognition of virtual shop names approached 100% in patients with AD.

To investigate everyday memory, Sauzeon et al. (2016) assessed everyday-like memory in ageing and in AD patients from the virtual reality-based Human Object Memory for Everyday Scenes (HOMES) test (Sauzeon et al., 2012). In this study, memory processes were assessed for multiple objects in a more naturalistic testing situation in both ageing and AD. Secondly, the relationship between self-reported memory complaints and the HOMES (Human Object Memory for Everyday Scenes) measures was examined. The procedure consisted of a learning phase and a retrieval phase. The learning phase consisted of two study-test trials where the presentation of the two versions of targeted apartments was counterbalanced across the participants. This computer-guided 'passive' exploration of the apartment in each version lasted 50 s. After a 10-min delay, a verbal yes/no recognition task was administered. Compared to older adults, AD patients exhibited a poor clustering, learning, and recognition performance, and also a high amount of false recognition. AD related deficits on the HOMES test were mediated by both memory and executive functioning (EF) measures, while those observed on false memory indices were only mediated by episodic memory (EM) measure. Overall, the results supported the fact that the VR-based memory test bridged the gap between in situ approaches and laboratory settings for AD patients and it was an appropriate device to capture age-related differences.

An important feature of memory to investigate is Prospective memory (PM). AD patients reported prospective and retrospective failures in everyday life which are liable to household accidents (Ryu et al., 2016). Prospective memory is defined as the memory for intentions, which enables us to remember to carry out planned actions, while performing a concurrent activity named 'ongoing task'. Lecouvey et al. (2019) studied AD-related PM impairment, comparing cognitively normal older individuals and patients with mild AD on a VR task in which they were asked to retrieve the prospective and retrospective components of EB (event-based) and TB (time-based) intentions. In fact, virtual reality, as immersed individuals in everyday-life situations, may enhance the sensitivity of PM tasks and improve the detection of inconspicuous impairments (Knight & Titov, 2009). In this study, the virtual environment was a virtual town created with an original software (EditoMem and SimulaMem), using VR tools Dev 3.0 (Plancher et al., 2012). Participants navigated in the environment in a virtual car and were asked to recall seven intentions. Results indicated that AD participants had higher difficulties in retrospective component and encoding phase, especially when the link between the prospective cue and the retrospective component was weaker. Thus, VR not only allowed the assessment of cognitive impairments, but also provided insighted into their functional repercussions in real life (Déjos, Sauzéon & N'kaoua, 2012).

Virtual reality could be also applied to neurobiological assessment. Howett et al. (2019) demonstrated that an entorhinal cortex-based virtual reality navigation task could differentiate patients at different level of cognitive impairment with classification accuracy superior to cognitive tests. The path integration task was administered using the HTC Vive IVR kit and was undertaken within virtual open arena environments. Results evidenced that performance on a novel immersive virtual reality path integration paradigm, based on the central role of the entorhinal cortex in navigation, was impaired in MCI patients compared to healthy controls, as previously found (Hort et al., 2007; Laczo´ et al., 2014). Finally, path integration performance differentiated MCI biomarker-positive patients from biomarker-negative patients with markedly higher sensitivity and specificity than a battery of 'gold standard' cognitive tests.

Likewise, Stefanovski, et al. (2019) focused on molecular pathways and computational models, such as TVB (The Virtual Brain), in order to assess Alzheimer's Disease. The Virtual Brain (TVB) neuroinformatics platform allowed standardized large-scale structural connectivity-based simulations of whole brain dynamics. Results derived from the combination of positron emission tomography (PET) with neural function in TVB addressing the phenomenon of hyperexcitability in AD related to the protein amyloid beta (Abeta). Local Abeta-mediated disinhibition and hyperexcitation, analyzed though electroencephalograms (EEG), were considered candidate mechanisms of AD pathogenesis. In TVB simulations, the molecular candidate mechanism has led to macro-scale slowing in EEG and neural signal with a particular shift form alpha to theta previously observed in AD patients (Babiloni et al., 2016; Loewenstein et al., 1989). In summary, this study demonstrated how TVB enabled the simulation of systems effects caused by pathogenetic molecular candidate mechanisms in human virtual brains.

3.2 VR for Rehabilitation of Alzheimer's Disease

While no pharmacological treatment has yet proven to be efficient, it was explored how technology can be integrated into non-pharmacological intervention to enhance its benefits. One alternative for improving the efficiency of Alzheimer's treatment is to use virtual reality cognitive training. In this section will be listed 10 articles with 229 participants related to this topic.

Several empirical studies suggested that virtual reality can be effective, despite the possible production of errors (Dunn & Clare, 2007; Metzler-Baddeley & Snowden, 2005). Foloppe's et al. (2018) implemented VR techniques during a virtual experiment based on cooking activities. Their research questions were: how beneficial the virtual intervention was at experiment time and 6 months later, and if virtual learning context could affect learning progression. Unexpectedly, the real condition was more efficient than the virtual condition in increasing autonomous performance. The results from the real condition suggested that strategies to reduce errors and specific cueing instructions were efficient at improving the assisted autonomy of patients with mild AD, even for 6 months after stopping the intervention, as already emerged previously (Van der Linden et al., 2006). However, it was important to point out that the virtual condition reduced her needs for written instructions and visuospatial indications of the target objects.

Since cues were necessary for effective wayfinding as they provided a reference point to remember one's location (Caduff & Timpf 2008), Davis and Ohman (2017) examined whether salient cues could help AD patients to find their way within a virtual reality simulation of senior residence. Wayfinding problems in AD have been linked to modifications within the hippocampus and related structures, including senile plaques, neurofibrillary tangles and neuron loss. They were causes of compromised learning routes (Rainville, Passini, & Marchand, 2001), recalling landmarks, and remembering of the sequence of landmarks in a route (Jheng & Pai, 2009; Kavcic & Duffy, 2003). In senior living residences, a lack of salient features is common and contributes to wayfinding problems (Passini, Rainville, & Marchand, 1998). The Virtual Senior Living (VSL) was a recently developed, computerized, 3-dimensional computer simulation of a continuing care retirement home. Participants could virtually move about the VSL using a joystick. Visual attention to cues was measured by the use of eye tracking glasses, which tracked eye movements using pupil-corneal reflection. Experiment implied two environments: standard (no cues) and salient (multiple cues) and demonstrated the greater effectiveness of the second one. Thus, the two novel methods, VR and eye tracking, were able to give important information about how older adults with and without AD use cues to find their way in environments. The results provided evidence for ways to make the environment more supportive for wayfinding for older adults with Alzheimer's disease, such that individuals know where they are and can more easily find their way to desired locations.

With regard to neurocognitive training of spatial skills, White and Moussavi (2016) conducted a research program, over a period of approximately 7 weeks, based upon spatial navigation with targets in a symmetric and landmark-less virtual building. Authors evaluated whether an individual with AD could learn to navigate in a simple VR navigation (VRN) environment and whether that training could also bring real-life cognitive benefits. Participant's performance was evaluated by means of the MoCA and by studying the trajectories recorded during the navigation in VRN environment. Comparing the baseline assessment with the end of the training program, a substantial improvement emerged in navigating skills in the VRN assessment. The overall results suggested that immersive VR system could allowed MCI patients to rehabilitate their spatial skills and translate them to overall real-world spatial navigation, such as orientation.

With regard to attentive problems, very common symptoms in early AD patients Manera et al. (2016) conducted an attentional task based on a fully immersive VR system. The attentional task was inspired from the classical cancellation tasks (Zazzo, 1972) to train selective and sustained attention, and was administered in both a VR version and a paper version in a within-subjects design. Results showed that both participants with MCI and dementia were satisfied and reported feelings of security, and low anxiety and fatigue, suggesting that VR task may be employed in patients with different levels of cognitive and functional impairment. Additionally, almost 70% of the participants, reported to be more satisfied in the

VR condition compared to the paper condition, because it was more immersive, engaging and motivating. Apathetic participants reported to be more interested in the VR version compared to the paper version, suggesting that VR can be successfully employed to make a task more interesting for older people with cognitive decline, resulting in a higher adhesion to rehabilitative training.

Also mixed reality (MR)-based technology can be designed to improve cognitive functions related to day-to-day activities (Jak, 2012). In fact, it provided familiar virtual environments situations so that participants can transfer skills learned in the clinical setting to the real world using multimodal feedback (Krasovsky et al., 2018). In the Park, Jung and Jun (2019) pilot study, effects of a mixed reality-based cognitive training system with these from conventional computer-assisted cognitive training system were compared. MR-based cognitive training system was based on vital daily tasks designed to target multiple cognitive domains such as selective attention, visual/verbal working memory, problem solving, executive functions, sequencing, planning, and calculation. Moreover, MR interface (unlike assisted computer-assisted training system) augmented a sense of being in and interacting with a virtual environment. MR-based cognitive training system could enable the transfer of cognitive skills learned in the clinical setting to real-world situations, as already found (Klingberg, 2010). In particular, MR training's participants showed significantly improved performance in visuospatial working memory compared to those involved in the conventional training.

Similarly, Fasilis et al. (2018) designed an interactive cognitive rehabilitation training SG (Serious Game) based on the "Decomposition Hypothesis" (Anderson, 2002), according to which the daily tasks can be decomposed into equally fundamental actions, and through training in those actions/operations, it's possible to achieve an improved performance. Repetition of procedures lead to specialization, generalization of learned skills and the maintenance of a clear mind. Based on this theory, six 'decomposed' categories (functional memory, memory retention, attention, problem solving, executive functions and cognitive flexibility) were tested through Computerized Cognitive Rehabilitation (CCR), Virtual Environments and ICT (Interactive Computer-based Training) in patients with mild dementia. Positive results revealed beneficial effects of SGs computer games, which combined enjoyment with learning, due to the so called "intrinsic transference" (Fabricatore, 2002).

Virtual reality has also been used for the rehabilitation of neurobiological functions. Here it was presented a randomized control trial (Doniger et al., 2018) which examined the ability of *Advanced Cognitive Training for Independent and Vital Elderly* (ACTIVE) to improve cognition and cerebral blood flow (CBF). This intensive VR cognitive training consisted of lifelike cognitive tasks (set of "real-world" VR cognitive tasks) with simultaneous treadmill walking. A variety of long-term benefits, including everyday functional abilities (Rebok et al., 2014), depression onset, quality of life (Wolinsky et al., 2010), and protection against dementia emerged. In fact, these participants were 33% less likely than controls to develop dementia over 10 years. The results of the present trial substantiated the efficacy of a VR-based cognitive-motor training program and its potential to become a standard of care. In particular, CBF showed sensitivity to cognitive training in healthy seniors, who showed a great improvement in memory connected to a CBF improvement.

The effectiveness of Virtual Reality was assessed also on emotions rehabilitation in a Mixed Methods Pilot Study (Moyle, Jones, Dwan, & Petrovich, 2016). In this study, emotions were assessed through *Observed Emotion Rating Scale* (Lawton, Van Haitsma, & Klapper, 1999), an observational tool for rating two positive emotions (pleasure and general alertness), and three negative emotions (anger, anxiety/fear, and sadness). Results showed that Virtual Reality Forest had an overall positive impact on participants, in particular, on those with mid stage dementia. However, the results of the OERS also indicated that residents living with dementia experienced a greater level of fear/anxiety during the forest experience than the normative sample in an activity context. Findings supported the positive perception of Virtual Reality Forest which created a stimulating environment and helped to immerse participants in the experience, which in turn reduced their apathy and improved cognitive abilities.

Recently, a group of researchers (Byrns et al., 2020) proposed a new version of Music Therapy (MT), suitable for the treatment of AD. Music therapy has been shown to be beneficial because improved cognitive, psychological and behavioral impairments induced by Alzheimer's disease (Gallego & Garcia, 2017; Ray & Mittelmann, 2017). In the aforementioned study, a virtual reality environment consisting of a music theatre created using Unity 3D software in which participants were immersed among the audience and whose emotions are assessed by an electroencephalogram device (EEG) was designed. A series of eight 30 second song excerpts are sequentially presented, accompanied by visual scenes designed with specific color shades and lightings in order to achieve the emotional purpose (relaxation, engagement) of the song (Valdez & Mehrabian, 1994). In order to analyze the impact of the Music Therapy environment on memory and attention performances, 6 attention and memory exercises were created. Results showed a reduction of frustration and negative emotions through virtual music therapy and a prolongation of positive effect after the MT. With regard to cognitive functions, results showed a large increase in memory performance but only a small improvement in attention abilities. In summary, reducing negative emotions through MT could improve memory performances.

4. DISCUSSION

Data of this selective overview emphasized the effectiveness and the suitability of Virtual Reality based programs for promoting early diagnosis and effective treatments. In this review, VR advantages and ecological validity were illustrated. As regard, VR assessment, it emerged that VR testing could point out instrumental activities of daily living (IADL) deficits, often not detected using traditional neuropsychological tests (Allain et al., 2014). For example, Sauzeon et al., (2016) found an effective VR tool (VR based *Human Object Memory for Everyday Scenes* test) for screening any early memory hallmark of the Alzheimer disease, notably for MCI people. Through their evaluation in a more ecological context, HOMES test, may tend to diminish age-related differences (i.e., false recognition susceptibility), but without altering the capture of a specific memory profile in the early stages of AD unlike traditional memory tests. Widmann et al. (2012) showed VR efficacy in assessing everyday-life memory deficit (i. e., verbal learning). Since learning in a virtual environment is more difficult, VR highlighted the impairment of recognition more than classical list learning paradigms because they could underestimate memory capacity in day-to-day situations. Virtual reality performances, in terms of VR day-out task (VR-DOT) were found to be correlated with markers of neurodegeneration, assessed by functional MRI (Tarnanas et al., 2014). VR-DOT had the advantage of not being as invasive as MRI, so it could optimize the early diagnosis of AD and could provide the greatest benefit in terms of cost and risk compared with other techniques. Notably, only AD patients' performance in VR test, unlike their scores on the verbal test, correlated with their CDS (daily memory complaints) scores. This result confirmed previous studies (Farias, Harrell, Neumann & Houtz, 2003) about poor correlations between standard neuropsychological memory assessments and behavior-based measures of daily living skills (e.g., dialing a telephone).

As regard memory skills, Lecouvey et al. (2019) study suggested new insights into the nature of PM (prospective memory) and RM (retrospective memory) impairment in mild AD thanks to virtual real assessment. AD patients reported difficulties in retrospective component and the encoding phase, especially for actions and intentions related to short-term memory. Encoding of spatial information through a virtual action appeared to enhance spatial retrieval of the participants. This study confirmed the reliability of VR for assessing complex cognitive functions such as PM. From a clinical point of view, it will be important to incorporate active encoding into episodic memory training in order to encourage patients to use their own actions to encode information in their daily life.

VR has proven its efficacy also in assessing spatial skills. In Morganti et al. (2016) study, virtual reality spatial tasks showed efficiently AD decline in performing the allo- to egocentric translation of spatial knowledge during different types of wayfinding. Main advantage of this study consisted in easy-to-use computerized tools that did not require any sophisticated setting up. Authors stressed on difference between maintaining a spatial perspective in a classical Road Map test (as in the M-RMT) or in a simulated world (as in the VR-RMT). These two methods provided different embodied schemas (the first based on imaginative ability, the second on active performance), which resulted in different allocentric-to-egocentric outcomes. Specifically, the VR-MRT, by providing an external representation of the route perspective, could influence perspective taking and provided different performance in spatial orientation than the Money's Road Map Test. As consequence, an allo-to-egocentric translation task emphasized the differences between a non-pathological cognitive decline in older adults and impairments in this ability connected to Alzheimer's disease. Importance of active exploration in a VR environment was argued also by Plancher et al. (2012), imprinting memory traces of the spatial environment, which facilitated related information retrieval. The data were widely supported by previous literature (Brooks, Attree, Rose, Clifford, & Leadbetter, 1999; Carassa, Geminiani, Morganti, & Varotto, 2002). VR active exploration increased participants' recall of central information and the relationship between pieces of information. In fact, active exploration was based on procedural skills, which have been documented to be one of the most preserved in AD patients (Lipinska & Backman, 1997; Van Halteren-van Tilborget al., 2007). Procedural memory tended to be more pronounced in VR studies using active exploration than in typical laboratory conditions. Also Park et al. (2019) found that VR training system was also more promising to improve visuospatial working memory because it was the only one to allow to actually see own actual body position in the simulated environment.

Moreover, VR environment allowed us to identify valid support for spatial navigation and memory tasks in AD and MCI patients: in particular salient cues such as directional arrows and salient landmarks (Cognè et al., 2018). Likewise, virtual navigational tasks designed to assess a wayfinding strategy could represent a powerful tool for detecting the earliest AD-related deficit (Allison et al., 2016; Cushman et al., 2008).

VR navigation could be useful also for an assessment of neurobiological structures, such as entorhinal cortex (Howett et al., 2019). In that study, through a novel VR path integration paradigm, it was demonstrated that navigation performance based on the entorhinal cortex was impaired in MCI patients compared to healthy controls. In particular, virtual path integration performance differentiated MCI biomarker-positive patients from biomarker-negative patients with markedly higher sensitivity and specificity than a battery of gold standard cognitive tests used in clinical and research practice. Moreover, VR was the only tool capable of simulating of systems effects caused by pathogenetic molecular candidate mechanisms at a multi-scale level in human virtual brains (Stefanovski et al., 2019). Results represented the first proof of concept for linking molecular changes as detected by PET to large-scale brain modeling, using the VR simulation framework. Virtual reality, also in terms of serious games (SGs), proved to be effective in the ability to detect the reduction in the hippocampal volume (Cabinio et al., 2020).

This datum was very important since pre-morbid hippocampal volume was considered a biomarker of Alzheimer disease (Devanand et al., 2007).

As regard the second and last macro-category, 'rehabilitation', virtual reality-based training proved to be a valid support to enhance the functional autonomy and daily-like activities in AD patients. For example, in the single-case by Foloppe et al. (2018), cooking activities learned in virtual training, were transferred to real life and was consolidated over the time in everyday life. In particular, the virtual condition reduced needs for written instructions and visuospatial indications of the target objects. The results from the virtual condition compared to the real condition were consistent with the idea that virtual reality provided ecological contexts and was more sensitive than traditional tests.

VR has proven its efficacy also on a neurobiological level: i.e., improving cerebral blood flow, linked to selective attention, working memory and executive functions (Doniger et al., 2018). These functions underlined the actions of daily life. Thus, the tasks implemented in a daily functional virtual environment improved the ability to plan, organize, problem solve, and multitask. As consequence, an ecologically cognitive-motor VR setting that simulated complex daily activities could promote transfer of trained skills in real conditions. Accordingly, VR trial could be a prophylactic regimen for AD, adaptable for home-based application in high-risk individuals. VR also offered unique advantages, such as adaptability/personalization, ability to synchronously train motor and cognitive processes, multisensory feedback, real-time rewards, and enhanced motivation. Greater engagement coupled with ecological validity emphasized VR training as a prime candidate for transfer training gains to daily activities, as already found (Coyle, Traynor & Solowij, 2015).

Virtual reality environment training also proved to be effective in increasing spatial skills (White & Moussavi, 2016). The overall results suggested that people at the early stages of AD could learn to navigate paths in a suitably immersive VR system, and the learned paths could be translated to overall real-world spatial navigation skills. Thus, cognitive training based on interactive rehabilitation, such as smart aging serious game (SASG), provided benefit for AD rehabilitation (Fasilis et al., 2018).

VR-based training could be a valid tool to train selective and sustained attention (Manera et al., 2016) thanks to its power to engage participants. In fact, MCI and dementia patients reported to be highly satisfied and interested in the virtual version of the attentional task, compared to the paper version. In fact, VR showed its efficacy also in emotions rehabilitation, increasing the level of involvement and positive emotions (Moyle et al., 2006). VR was able to create a stimulating environment and this could help to immerse participants in the experience, which in turn reduced their apathy and improved quality of life. Emotional impact was assessed also in a virtual musical theater (Byrns et al., 2020) where a reduction of negative emotions, most notably frustration, and an improvement of positive emotions over time emerged. Music therapy could be also useful to improve attention and memory performance.

Overall, this review demonstrated the feasibility of using VR technology to study cognitive deficits and daily impairments of patients with aMCI and AD. Its portability, low cost, easy accessibility (it can be implemented at home), its usability, and good user tolerance allowed VR to be integrated successfully into clinical practice. The effectiveness of VR was strengthened by the active use of the participants.

In summary, the strength of this review was to focus on virtual reality as an elective assistive technology for Alzheimer's disease. The choice to focus on the categories of assessment and rehabilitation of cognitive and emotional skills is both a strength and a weakness. It is a strong point as it allows to know the most recent contributions, which could be useful in clinical practice. The limit consisted in excluding other possible applications of virtual reality, for example to improve motor and postural abilities, as examined in previous studies (Bourellier et al., 2016). The application of virtual reality to daily activities has been analyzed (Foloppe et al., 2018) but mainly as a secondary effect of the underlying executive and cognitive functions. Finally, even if virtual reality has already been applied to everyday activities, for example cooking skills (Davis, Ohman, & Weisbeck, 2017), augmented reality (AR) and mixed reality technology (MR) are two kind of assistive technologies which will need to be further explored because could allow more seamless integration.

5. CONCLUSION

The reviewed studies pointed out two main categories based on different use of virtual reality technology in order to evaluate its usefulness in the diagnosis and rehabilitation of AD patients. The outcomes of the studies were largely positive. Many of the studies highlighted VR ecological validity for assessing AD and reported a statistically improvement in cognitive rehabilitation. Studies enrolled in this review had a good methodological structure. For example, the majority used a control group to compare the effectiveness of the empirical data evidenced between virtual reality and real situations. Moreover, some studies showed a good reliability, maintaining positive results obtained with virtual training over the time. Finally, cognitive functions were measured with objective neuronal tools (e.g., PET, EEG), as in Stefanovski et al. (2019) or validated scales with good statistical validity and reliability. For example, Lawton's Spatial Anxiety Scale (Lawton, 1994) for anxiety related to wayfinding (Davis & Ohman, 2016). However, readers should interpret with caution some of these findings. Indeed, questions emerged about (a) size of sample, (b) difficulty in differentiating AD from MCI patients in the sample, (c) emotional problems in fragile patients if special precautions were not taken, (d) absence of follow-up in some studies, and (e) not always representative sample of individuals with MCI or AD. Few limitations in the use of virtual reality for AD patients need to be considered. For instance, VR could lead to difficulties in wearing the 3D glasses and using the mouse. Furthermore, in some studies the participants were unable to familiarize themselves with the VR technology (Byrns et al., 2020). Overall, if outcomes were evaluated on the basis of the criteria of ecological validity and clinical relevance, it should be noticed that all studies met these criteria.

6. IMPLICATIONS FOR FUTURE RESEARCH

In light of the above, the future research perspectives should try to disentangle which aspects of the VR task made it more interesting (e.g., the character's animation, the 3D visualization, the big screen), to allow the replication of the current results in different trainings. Future studies should also test whether security feelings can be further improved by employing a more naturalistic user interface.

The lack of widely accepted paradigms for the diagnosis and therapy is the reason why most of the studies could not be validated and used in clinical practice. Multi-center discussion with creating study guidelines is highly needed. In fact, if such patterns were designed, VR could probably be easily implemented as a valuable diagnostic and therapeutic option (Słyk, Zarzycki, Kocwa-Karnaś, & Domitrz, 2019).

Further empirical testing should be orientated to investigate the different effects of virtual and augmented reality on different aspects of dementia, not only for reminiscence but also for relaxation and enjoyment. In fact, given the prevalence of challenging behaviors and anxiety among these patients, virtual reality could assist by reducing stress levels because participants can potentially experience the same anxiety-provoking scenarios in a safer and more controlled setting. This is applicable if the use of the technology is relatively simple and safety screening is done prior its use (D'Cunha et al., 2019). It is important to ensure that future use of this technology is theoretically grounded and controlled to avoid potential harm to vulnerable patient groups. As consequence, collaboration between clinicians, researchers, and software engineering teams is crucial to build on the early potential demonstrated.

REFERENCES

Aguirre, G. K., & D'Esposito, M. (1999). Topographical disorientation: A synthesis and taxonomy. *Brain*, *122*(9), 1613–1628. doi:10.1093/brain/122.9.1613 PMID:10468502

Allain, P., Foloppe, D. A., Besnard, J., Yamaguchi, T., Etcharry-Bouyx, F., Le Gall, D., Nolin, P., & Richard, P. (2014). Detecting Everyday Action Deficits in Alzheimer's Disease Using a Nonimmersive Virtual Reality Kitchen. *Journal of the International Neuropsychological Society*, *20*(5), 468–477. doi:10.1017/S1355617714000344 PMID:24785240

Allison, S. L., Fagan, A. M., Morris, J. C., & Heada, D. (2016). Spatial Navigation in Preclinical Alzheimer's Disease. *Journal of Alzheimer's Disease*, *52*(1), 77–90. doi:10.3233/JAD-150855 PMID:26967209

Anopas, D., & Wongsawat, Y. (2014). Virtual reality game for memory skills enhancement based on QEEG. *BMEiCON 2014–7th Biomedical Engineering International Conference.*

Babiloni, C., Del Percio, C., Caroli, A., Salvatore, E., Nicolai, E., Marzano, N., Lizio, R., Cavedo, E., Landau, S., Chen, K., Jagust, W., Reiman, E., Tedeschi, G., Montella, P., De Stefano, M., Gesualdo, L., Frisoni, G. B., & Soricelli, A. (2016). Cortical sources of resting state EEG rhythms are related to brain hypometabolismin subjects with Alzheimer's disease: An EEG-PET study. *Neurobiology Aging Journal*, *48*, 122–134. doi:10.1016/j.neurobiolaging.2016.08.021 PMID:27668356

Belleville, S., Gilbert, B., Fontaine, F., Gagnon, L., Menard, E., & Gauthier, S. (2006). Improvement of episodic memory in persons with mild cognitive impairment and healthy older adults: Evidence from a cognitive intervention program. *Dementia and Geriatric Cognitive Disorders*, *22*(5-6), 486–499. doi:10.1159/000096316 PMID:17050952

Bennys, K., Rondouin, G., Benattar, E., Gabelle, A., & Touchon, J. (2011). Can event-related potential predict the progression of mild cognitive impairment? *Journal of Clinical Neurophysiology*, *28*(6), 625–632. doi:10.1097/WNP.0b013e31823cc2d3 PMID:22146349

Bottiroli, S., Tassorelli, C., Lamonica, M., Zucchella, C., Cavallini, E., Bernini, S., Sinforiani, E., Pazzi, S., Cristiani, P., Vecchi, T., Tost, D., & Sandrini, G. (2017). Smart aging platform for evaluating cognitive functions in aging: A comparison with the MoCA in a normal population. *Frontiers in Aging Neuroscience*, *21*(9), 1–14. doi:10.3389/fnagi.2017.00379 PMID:29209200

Bourrelier, J., Ryard, J., Dion, M., Merienne, F., Manckoundia, P., & Mourey, F. (2016). Use of a virtual environment to engage motor and postural abilities in elderly subjects with and without mild cognitive impairment (MAAMI Project). *IRBM*, *37*(2), 75–80. doi:10.1016/j.irbm.2016.02.007

Brookmeyer, R., Johnson, E., Ziegler-Graham, K., & Arrighi, H. M. (2007). Forecasting the global burden of Alzheimer's disease. *Alzheimer's & Dementia Journal*, *3*(3), 186–191. doi:10.1016/j.jalz.2007.04.381 PMID:19595937

Byrns, A., Abdessalem, H. B., Cuesta, M., Bruneau, M. A., Belleville, S., & Frasson, C. (2020). Adaptive Music Therapy for Alzheimer's Disease Using Virtual Reality. In V. Kumar & C. Troussas (Eds.), *Intelligent Tutoring Systems*. Springer International Publishing. doi:10.1007/978-3-030-49663-0_25

Cabinio, M., Rossetto, F., Isernia, S., Saibene, F. L., Di Cesare, M., Borgnis, F., Pazzi, S., Migliazza, T., Alberoni, M., Blasi, V., & Baglio, F. (2020). The Use of a Virtual Reality Platform for the Assessment of the Memory Decline and the Hippocampal Neural Injury in Subjects with Mild Cognitive Impairment: The Validity of Smart Aging Serious Game (SASG). *Journal of Clinical Medicine*, *9*(1355), 1–13. doi:10.3390/jcm9051355 PMID:32384591

Caduff, D., & Timpf, S. (2008). On the assessment of landmark salience for human navigation. *Cognitive Processing*, *9*(4), 249–267. doi:10.100710339-007-0199-2 PMID:17999102

Chai, X. J., & Jacobs, L. F. (2009). Sex differences in directional cue use in a virtual landscape. *Behavioral Neuroscience*, *123*(3), 276–283. doi:10.1037/a0014722 PMID:19331451

Cherrier, M. M., Mendez, M., & Perryman, K. (2001). Route learning performance in Alzheimer disease patients. *Neuropsychiatry, Neuropsychology, and Behavioral Neurology*, *14*(3), 159–168. PMID:11513099

Chetelat, G., Desgranges, B., & Eustache, F. (2006). Brain profile of hypometabolism in early Alzheimer's disease: Relationships with cognitive deficits and atrophy. *Revista de Neurología*, *162*(10), 945–951. PMID:17028562

Cipriani, G., Bianchetti, A., & Trabucchi, M. (2006). Outcomes of a computer based cognitive rehabilitation program on Alzheimer's disease patients compared with those on patients affected by mild cognitive impairment. *Archives of Gerontology and Geriatrics*, *43*(3), 327–335. doi:10.1016/j.archger.2005.12.003 PMID:16451811

Clay, B., Howett, D., FitzGerald, J., Fletcher, P., Chan, D., & Price, A. (2020). Use of Immersive Virtual Reality in the Assessment and Treatment of Alzheimer's Disease: A Systematic Review. *Journal of Alzheimer's Disease*, *75*(1), 23–43. doi:10.3233/JAD-191218 PMID:32280091

Cogné, M., Auriacombe, S., Vasa, L., Tison, F., Klinger, E., Sauzeon, H., Joseph, P.-A., & N'Kaoua, B. (2018). Are Visual Cues Helpful for Virtual Spatial Navigation and Spatial Memory in Patients With Mild Cognitive Impairment or Alzheimer's Disease? *Neuropsychology*, *4*(32), 385–400. doi:10.1037/neu0000435 PMID:29809030

Cogné, M., Taillade, M., N'Kaoua, B., Tarruella, A., Klinger, E., Larrue, F., Sauze'on, H., Joseph, P. A., & Sorita, E. (2017). The contribution of virtual reality to the diagnosis of spatial navigation disorders and to the study of the role of navigational aids: A systematic literature review. *Annals of Physical and Rehabilitation Medicine*, *60*(3), 164–176. doi:10.1016/j.rehab.2015.12.004 PMID:27017533

Coyle, H., Traynor, V., & Solowij, N. (2015). Computerized and virtual reality cognitive training for individuals at high risk of cognitive decline: Systematic review of the literature. *The American Journal of Geriatric Psychiatry*, *4*(23), 335–359. doi:10.1016/j.jagp.2014.04.009 PMID:24998488

Cushman, L. A., & Duffy, C. J. (2007). The sex specificity of navigational strategies in Alzheimer disease. *Alzheimer Disease and Associated Disorders*, *21*(2), 122–129. doi:10.1097/WAD.0b013e318047df2f PMID:17545737

Cushman, L. A., Stein, K., & Duffy, C. J. (2008). Detecting navigational deficits in cognitive aging and Alzheimer disease using virtual reality. *Neuorology*, *71*(12), 888–895. doi:10.1212/01.wnl.0000326262.67613.fe PMID:18794491

D'Cunha, N. M., Nguyen, D., Naumovski, N., McKune, A. J., Kellett, J., Georgousopoulou, E. N., Frost, J., & Isbel, S. (2019). A mini-review of virtual reality-based interventions to promote well-being for people living with dementia and mild cognitive impairment. *Gerontology*, *65*(4), 430–440. doi:10.1159/000500040 PMID:31108489

Davis, O., & Ohman, J. (2017). Wayfinding in Aging and Alzheimer's Disease within a Virtual Senior Residence: Study Protocol. *Journal of Advanced Nursing*, *72*(7), 1677–1688. doi:10.1111/jan.12945 PMID:26915997

Davis, R., Ohman, J. M., & Weisbeck, C. (2017). Salient cues and wayfinding in Alzheimer's disease within a virtual senior residence. *Environment and Behavior*, *49*(9), 1038–1065. doi:10.1177/0013916516677341 PMID:29230067

Déjos, M., Sauzéon, H., & N'kaoua, B. (2012). Virtual reality for clinical assessment of elderly people: Early screening for dementia. *Revue Neurologique*, *168*(5), 404–414. doi:10.1016/j.neurol.2011.09.005 PMID:22137150

Devanand, D. P., Pradhaban, G., Liu, X., Khandji, A., De Santi, S., Segal, S., Rusinek, H., Pelton, G. H., Honig, L. S., Mayeux, R., Stern, Y., Tabert, M. H., & de Leon, M. J. (2007). Hippocampal and entorhinal atrophy in mild cognitive impairment: Prediction of Alzheimer disease. *Neurology*, *68*(11), 828–836. doi:10.1212/01.wnl.0000256697.20968.d7 PMID:17353470

Doeller, C. F., King, J. A., & Burgess, N. (2008). Parallel striatal and hippocampal systems for landmarks and boundaries in spatial memory. *Proceedings of the National Academy of Sciences of the United States of America*, *105*(15), 5915–5920. doi:10.1073/pnas.0801489105 PMID:18408152

Doniger, G. M., Schnaider Beeri, A., Bahar-Fuchs, A., Gottlieb, A., Tkachov, A., & … . (2018). Virtual reality-based cognitive-motor training for middle-aged adults at high Alzheimer's disease risk: A randomized controlled trial. *Alzheimer's & Dementia: Translational Research & Clinical Interventions*, *4*(4), 118–129. doi:10.1016/j.trci.2018.02.005 PMID:29955655

Dubois, B., Feldman, H. H., Jacova, C., Hampel, H., Molinuevo, J. L., Blennow, K., DeKosky, S. T., Gauthier, S., Selkoe, D., Bateman, R., Cappa, S., Crutch, S., Engelborghs, S., Frisoni, G. B., Fox, N. C., Galasko, D., Habert, M.-O., Jicha, G. A., Nordberg, A., ... Cummings, J. L. (2014). Advancing research diagnostic criteria for Alzheimer's disease: The IWG-2 criteria. *Lancet Neurology*, *13*(6), 614–629. doi:10.1016/S1474-4422(14)70090-0 PMID:24849862

Dunn, J., & Clare, L. (2007). Learning face–name associations in early-stage dementia: Comparing the effects of errorless learning and effortful processing. *Neuropsychological Rehabilitation*, *17*(6), 735–754. doi:10.1080/09602010701218317 PMID:17852759

Fabricatore, C. (2002). *Learning and Videogames: An Unexploited Synergy*. Springer Science & Business Media.

Farias, S. T., Harrell, E., Neumann, C., & Houtz, A. (2003). The relationship between neuropsychological performance and daily functioning in individuals with Alzheimer's disease: Ecological validity of neuropsychological tests. *Archives of Clinical Neuropsychology*, *18*(6), 655–672. doi:10.1093/arclin/18.6.655 PMID:14591439

Fasilis, T., Patrikelis, P., Siatouni, A., Alexoudi, A., Veretzioti, A., Zachou, L., & Gatzonis, S.-S. (2018). A pilot study and brief overview of rehabilitation via virtual environment in patients suffering from dementia. *Psychiatriki*, *29*(1), 42–51. doi:10.22365/jpsych.2018.291.42 PMID:29754119

Flynn, D., van Schaik, P., Blackman, T., Femcott, C., Hobbs, B., & Calderon, C. (2003). Developing a virtual reality-based methodology for people with dementia: A feasibility study. *Cyberpsychology Behavior Journal*, *6*(6), 591–611. doi:10.1089/109493103322725379 PMID:14756925

Foloppe, D., Richard, P., Yamaguchi, T., Etcharry-Bouyx, F., & Allain, P. (2018). The potential of virtual reality-based training to enhance the functional autonomy of Alzheimer's disease patients in cooking activities: A single case study. *Neuropsychological Rehabilitation*, *28*(5), 709–733. doi:10.1080/09602011.2015.1094394 PMID:26480838

Freeman, D., Reeve, S., Robinson, A., Ehlers, A., Clark, D., Spanlang, B., & Slater, M. (2017). Virtual reality in the assessment, understanding, and treatment of mental health disorders. *Psychological Medicine*, *47*(14), 2393–2400. doi:10.1017/S003329171700040X PMID:28325167

Gallego, M. G., & García, J. G. (2017). Music therapy and Alzheimer's disease: Cognitive, psy-chological, and behavioural effects. *Neurologia (Barcelona, Spain)*, *32*(5), 300–308. PMID:26896913

Garcı'a-Betances, R. I., Jime'nez-Mixco, V., Arredondo, M. T., & Cabrera-Umpie'rrez, M. F. (2015). Using Virtual Reality for Cognitive Training of the Elderly. *American Journal of Alzheimer's Disease and Other Dementias*, *30*(1), 49–54. doi:10.1177/1533317514545866 PMID:25107931

Gillner, S., & Mallot, H. A. (1998). Navigation and acquisition of spatial knowledge in a virtual maze. *Journal of Cognitive Neuroscience*, *10*(4), 445–463. doi:10.1162/089892998562861 PMID:9712675

Golledge, R. G. (1999). *Wayfinding Behavior: Cognitive Mapping and Other Spatial Processes*. The Johns Hopkins University Press.

Hill, N. T., Mowszowski, L., Naismith, S. L., Chadwick, V. L., Valenzuela, M., & Lampit, A. (2017). Computerized cognitive training in older adults with mild cognitive impairment or dementia: A systematic review and meta-analysis. *The American Journal of Psychiatry*, *174*(4), 329–340. doi:10.1176/appi.ajp.2016.16030360 PMID:27838936

Hort, J., Laczo, J., Vyhnalek, M., Bojar, M., Bures, J., & Vlcek, K. (2007). Spatial navigation deficit in amnestic mild cognitive impairment. *Proceedings of the National Academy of Sciences of the United States of America*, *104*(10), 4042–4047. doi:10.1073/pnas.0611314104 PMID:17360474

Howett, D., Castegnaro, A., Krzywicka, K., Hagman, J., Marchment, D., Henson, R., Rio, M., King, J. A., Burgess, N., & Chan, D. (2019). Differentiation of mild cognitive impairment using an entorhinal cortex-based test of virtual reality navigation. *Brain*, *142*(6), 1751–1766. doi:10.1093/brain/awz116 PMID:31121601

Jak, A. J. (2012). The impact of physical and mental activity on cognitive aging. *Current Topics in Behavioral Neurosciences*, *10*, 273–291. doi:10.1007/7854_2011_141 PMID:21818703

Jheng, S. S., & Pai, M. C. (2009). Cognitive map in patients with mild Alzheimer's disease: A computer-generated arena study. *Behavioural Brain Research*, *200*(1), 42–47. doi:10.1016/j.bbr.2008.12.029 PMID:19162077

Johnson, L. (2018). For people with dementia, virtual reality can be life-changing. *Wired*. https://www.wired.co.uk/article/virtual-reality-dementia-technology

Kavcic, V., & Duffy, C. (2003). Attentional dynamics and visual perception: Mechanisms of spatial disorientation in Alzheimer's disease. *Brain*, *126*(5), 1173–1181. doi:10.1093/brain/awg105 PMID:12690056

Klingberg, T. (2010). Training and plasticity of working memory. *Trends in Cognitive Sciences*, *14*(7), 317–324. doi:10.1016/j.tics.2010.05.002 PMID:20630350

Kober, S. E., Wood, G., Hofer, D., Kreuzig, W., Kiefer, M., & Neuper, C. (2013). Virtual reality in neurologic rehabilitation of spatial disorientation. *Journal of Neuroengineering and Rehabilitation*, *10*(1), 1–13. doi:10.1186/1743-0003-10-17 PMID:23394289

Laczó, J., Andel, R., Vyhnálek, M., Vlcek, K., Magerova, H., Varjassyova, A., Tolar, M., & Hort, J. (2010). Human analogue of the Morris water maze for testing subjects at risk of Alzheimer's disease. *Neurodegenerative Diseases*, *7*(3), 148–152. doi:10.1159/000289226 PMID:20197695

Laczó, J., Andel, R., Vyhnalek, M., Vlcek, K., Nedelska, Z., Matoska, V., Gazova, I., Mokrisova, I., Sheardova, K., & Hort, J. (2014). APOE and spatial navigation in amnestic MCI: Results from a computer-based test. *Neuropsychology*, *28*(5), 676–684. doi:10.1037/neu0000072 PMID:24749727

Laczó, J., Vlcek, K., Vyhnalek, M., Vajnerova, O., Ort, M., Holmerova, I., Tolar, M., Andel, R., Bojar, M., & Hort, J. (2009). Spatial navigation testing discriminates two types of amnestic mild cognitive impairment. *Behavioural Brain Research*, *202*(2), 252–259. doi:10.1016/j.bbr.2009.03.041 PMID:19463709

Laver, K. E., Lange, B., George, S., Deutsch, J. E., Saposnik, G., & Crotty, M. (2017). Virtual reality for stroke rehabilitation. *Cochrane Database of Systematic Reviews*, *11*(11), 1–183. doi:10.1002/14651858.CD008349.pub4 PMID:29156493

Lawton, C. (1994). Gender differences in way-finding strategies: Relationship to spatial ability and spatial anxiety. *Sex Roles*, *30*(11), 765–779. doi:10.1007/BF01544230

Lawton, M. P., Van Haitsma, K., & Klapper, J. (1999). Observed Emotion Rating Scale. *Journal of Mental Health and Aging*, *5*(1), 69–81.

Lecouvey, G., Morand, A., Gonneaud, J., Pascale, P., Orriols, E., Pélerin, A., & … . (2019). An Impairment of Prospective Memory in Mild Alzheimer's Disease: A Ride in a Virtual Town. *Frontiers in Psychology*, *10*(24), 1–12. doi:10.3389/fpsyg.2019.00241 PMID:30809174

Lipinska, B., & Backman, L. (1997). Encoding-retrieval interactions in mild Alzheimer's disease: The role of access to categorical information. *Brain and Cognition*, *34*(2), 274–286. doi:10.1006/brcg.1997.0916 PMID:9220090

Lithfous, S., Dufour, A., & Després, O. (2013). Spatial navigation in normal aging and the prodromal stage of Alzheimer's disease: Insights from imaging and behavioral studies. *Ageing Research Reviews*, *12*(1), 201–213. doi:10.1016/j.arr.2012.04.007 PMID:22771718

Loewenstein, D. A., Barker, W. W., Chang, J. Y., Apicella, A., Yoshii, F., Kothari, P., Levin, B., & Duara, R. (1989). Predominant left hemisphere metabolic dysfunction in dementia. *Archives of Neurology*, *46*(2), 146–152. doi:10.1001/archneur.1989.00520380046012 PMID:2783845

Manera, V., Chapoulie, E., Bourgeois, J., Guerchouche, R., David, R., Ondre, J., & … . (2016). A Feasibility Study with Image-Based Rendered Virtual Reality in Patients with Mild Cognitive Impairment and Dementia. *PLoS One*, *11*(3), 1–14. doi:10.1371/journal.pone.0151487 PMID:26990298

Mazuryk, T., & Gervautz, M. (1992). *Virtual Reality. History, Applications, Technology and Future*. Institute of Computer Graphics. Technical University of Vienna. Technical Report TR-186-2-96-06.

McNaughton, B. L., Battaglia, F. P., Jensen, O., Moser, E. I., & Moser, M. B. (2006). Path integration and the neural basis of the "cognitive map.". *Nature Reviews. Neuroscience*, *7*(8), 663–678. doi:10.1038/nrn1932 PMID:16858394

Metzler-Baddeley, C., & Snowden, J. S. (2005). Brief report: Errorless versus errorful learning as a memory rehabilitation approach in Alzheimer's Disease. *Journal of Clinical and Experimental Neuropsychology*, *27*(8), 1070–1079. doi:10.1080/13803390490919164 PMID:16207625

Millán-Calenti, J. C., Tubío, J., Pita-Fernández, S., Rochette, S., Lorenzo, T., & Maseda, A. (2012). Cognitive impairment as predictor of functional dependence in an elderly sample. *Archives of Gerontology and Geriatrics*, *54*(1), 197–201. doi:10.1016/j.archger.2011.02.010 PMID:21397345

Monacelli, A. M., Cushman, L. A., Kavcic, V., & Duffy, C. J. (2003). Spatial disorientation in Alzheimer's disease: The remembrance of things passed. *Neurology*, *61*(11), 1491–1497. doi:10.1212/WNL.61.11.1491 PMID:14663030

Morganti, F., Stefanini, S., & Riva, G. (2015). From allo- to egocentric spatial ability in early Alzheimer's disease: A study with virtual reality spatial tasks. *Cognitive Neuroscience*, *4*(4), 171–180. doi:10.1080/17588928.2013.854762 PMID:24251605

Moyle, W., Jones, C., Dwan, T., & Petrovich, T. (2016). Effectiveness of a Virtual Reality Forest on People With Dementia: A Mixed Methods Pilot Study. *The Gerontologist*, *58*(3), 478–487. doi:10.1093/geront/gnw270 PMID:28329867

Optale, G., Urgesi, C., Busato, V., Marin, S., Piron, L., Priftis, K., Gamberini, L., Capodieci, S., & Bordin, A. (2010). Controlling memory impairment in elderly adults using virtual reality memory training: A randomized controlled pilot study. *Neurorehabilitation and Neural Repair*, *24*(4), 348–357. doi:10.1177/1545968309353328 PMID:19934445

Park, E., Yun, B. J., & Jung, T. (2019). Effects of a Mixed Reality-based Cognitive Training System Compared to a Conventional Computer-assisted Cognitive Training System on Mild Cognitive Impairment: A Pilot Study. *Cognitive and Behavioral Neurology*, *32*(3), 172–178. doi:10.1097/WNN.0000000000000197 PMID:31517700

Passini, R., Rainville, C., & Marchand, N. (1998). Wayfinding and dementia: Some research findings and a new look at design. *Journal of Architectural and Planning Research*, *15*(2), 133–151. doi:10.1080/01688639508402431 PMID:8847388

Perri, R., Serra, L., Carlesimo, G. A., & Caltagirone, C. (2007). Amnestic Mild Cognitive Impairment: Difference of Memory Profile in Subjects Who Converted or Did Not Convert to Alzheimer's Disease. *Neuropsychology*, *21*(5), 549–558. doi:10.1037/0894-4105.21.5.549 PMID:17784803

Perry, R. J., Watson, P., & Hodges, J. R. (2000). The nature and staging of attention dysfunction in early (minimal and mild) Alzheimer's disease: Relationship to episodic and semantic memory impairment. *Neuropsychologia*, *38*(3), 252–271. doi:10.1016/S0028-3932(99)00079-2 PMID:10678692

Plancher, G., Barra, J., Orriols, E., & Piolino, P. (2012a). The influence of action on episodic memory: A virtual reality study. *Quarterly Journal of Experimental Psychology*, *66*(5), 895–909. doi:10.1080/17470218.2012.722657 PMID:23025821

Plancher, G., Tirard, A., Gyselinck, V., Nicolas, S., & Piolino, P. (2012). Using virtual reality to characterize episodic memory profiles in amnestic mild cognitive impairment and Alzheimer's disease: Influence of active and passive encoding. *Neuropsychologia*, *50*(5), 592–602. doi:10.1016/j.neuropsychologia.2011.12.013 PMID:22261400

Rainville, C., Passini, R., & Marchand, N. (2001). A multiple case study of wayfinding in dementia of the alzheimertype: Decision making. *Neuropsychology, Development, and Cognition. Section B, Aging, Neuropsychology and Cognition*, *8*(1), 54–71. doi:10.1076/anec.8.1.54.846

Ray, K. D., & Mittelman, M. S. (2017). Music therapy: A nonpharmacological approach to the care of agitation and depressive symptoms for nursing home residents with dementia. *Dementia (London)*, *9*(6), 689–710. doi:10.1177/1471301215613779 PMID:26519453

Rebok, G. W., Ball, K., Guey, L. T., Jones, R. N., Kim, H. Y., King, J. W., Marsiske, M., Morris, J. N., Tennstedt, S. L., Unverzagt, F. W., & Willis, S. L. (2014). Ten year effects of the advanced cognitive training for independent and vital elderly cognitive training trial on cognition and everyday functioning in older adults. *Journal of the American Geriatrics Society*, *62*(1), 16–24. doi:10.1111/jgs.12607 PMID:24417410

Richardson, A. E., Montello, D. R., & Hegarty, M. (1999). Spatial knowledge acquisition from maps and from navigation in real and virtual environments. *Memory & Cognition, Springer*, *27*(4), 741–750. doi:10.3758/BF03211566 PMID:10479831

Riva, G. (1998). Virtual Reality as Assessment Tool in Psychology. *Virtual Reality in Neuro-Psychology*, *44*(9), 71–79. PMID:10175344

Rizzo, A. A., Schultheis, M. T., Kerns, K., & Mateer, C. (2004). Analysis of assets for virtual reality applications in neuropsychology. *Neuropsychological Rehabilitation*, *14*(1), 207–239. doi:10.1080/09602010343000183

Robert, P. H., Konig, A., Amieva, H., Andrieu, S., Bremond, F., Bullock, R., & ... . (2014). Recommendations for the use of serious games in people with alzheimer's disease, related disorders and frailty. *Frontiers in Aging Neuroscience*, *6*(54), 1–13. doi:10.3389/fnagi.2014.00054 PMID:24715864

Sauzeon, H., N'Kaoua, B., Pala, P. A., Taillade, M., Auriacombe, S., & Guitton, P. (2016). Everyday-like memory for objects in ageing and Alzheimer's disease assessed in a visually complex environment: The role of executive functioning and episodic memory. *Journal of Neuropsychology*, *10*(1), 33–58. doi:10.1111/jnp.12055 PMID:25307794

Sauzeon, H., Pala, P. A., Larrue, F., & Wallet, G. (2012). The use of virtual reality for episodic memory assessment: Effects of active navigation. *Experimental Psychology*, *59*(2), 99–108. doi:10.1027/1618-3169/a000131 PMID:22044787

Slobounov, S. M., Ray, W., Johnson, B., Slobounov, E., & Newell, K. M. (2015). Modulation of cortical activity in 2D versus 3D virtual reality environments: An EEG study. *International Journal of Psychophysiology*, *95*(3), 254–260. doi:10.1016/j.ijpsycho.2014.11.003 PMID:25448267

Słyk, S., Zarzycki, M. Z., Kocwa-Karnaś, A., & Domitrz, I. (2019). Virtual reality in the diagnostics and therapy of neurological diseases. *Expert Review of Medical Devices*, *16*(12), 1055–1040. doi:10.1080/17434440.2019.1693892 PMID:31739698

Smith, G., Housen, P., Yaffe, K., Ruff, R., Kennison, R. F., Mahncke, H. W., & Zelinski, E. M. (2009). A cognitive training program based on principles of brain plasticity: Results from the improvement in memory with plasticity-based adaptive cognitive training (IMPACT) study. *Journal of the American Geriatrics Society*, *57*(4), 594–603. doi:10.1111/j.1532-5415.2008.02167.x PMID:19220558

Spiers, H. J., & Maguire, E. A. (2007). A navigational guidance system in the human brain. *Hippocampus*, *17*(8), 618–626. doi:10.1002/hipo.20298 PMID:17492693

Stefanovski, L., Triebkorn, P., Spiegler, A., Diaz-Cortes, M. A., Solodkin, A., Jirsa, V., McIntosh, A. R., & Ritter, P. (2019). Linking Molecular Pathways and Large-Scale Computational Modeling to Assess Candidate Disease Mechanisms and Pharmacodynamics in Alzheimer's Disease for the Alzheimer's Disease. *Frontiers in Computational Neuroscience*, *13*(64), 1–27. doi:10.3389/fncom.2019.00054 PMID:31456676

Tarnanas, I., Tsolaki, M., Nef, T., Muria, R. M., & Mosimann, U. P. (2014). Can a novel computerized cognitive screening test provide additional information for early detection of Alzheimer's disease? *Alzheimer's & Dementia*, *10*(6), 1–9. doi:10.1016/j.jalz.2014.01.002 PMID:24656838

Tost, D., Grau, S., & Ferre, M. (2009). PREVIRNEC: A cognitive telerehabilitation system based on virtual environments. *Virtual Rehabilitation International Conference*, 87-93.

Valdez, P., & Mehrabian, A. (1994). Effects of color on emotions. *Journal of Experimental Psychology. General*, *123*(4), 394–409.

Van der Linden, M., Juillerat, A. C., & Delbeuck, X. (2006). La prise en charge des troubles de la mémoire dans la maladie d'Alzheimer [The management of memory impairments in Alzheimer's disease]. In C. Belin, A. M. Ergis, & O. Moreaud (Eds.), *Actualités sur les démences: Aspects cliniques et neuropsychologiques* (pp. 167–197). Solal.

Van Halteren-van Tilborg, I. A., Scherder, E. J., & Hulstijn, W. (2007). Motor-skill learning in Alzheimer's disease: A review with an eye to the clinical practice. *Neuropsychology Review*, *17*(3), 203–212. doi:10.100711065-007-9030-1 PMID:17680369

Vlc˘ek, K., & Laczò, J. (2014). Neural correlates of spatial navigation changes in mild cognitive impairment and Alzheimer's disease. *Frontiers in Behavioral Neuroscience, 8*(89), 1-6.

Weniger, G., Ruhleder, M., Lange, C., Wolf, S., & Irle, E. (2011). Egocentric and allocentric memory as assessed by virtual reality in individuals with amnestic mild cognitive impairment. *Neuropsychologia*, *49*(3), 518–527. doi:10.1016/j.neuropsychologia.2010.12.031 PMID:21185847

White, P. J. F., & Moussavi, Z. (2016). Neurocognitive Treatment for a Patient with Alzheimer's Disease Using a Virtual Reality Navigational Environment. *Journal of Experimental Neuroscience*, *8*(10), 129–135. doi:10.4137/JEN.S40827 PMID:27840579

Widmann, C. N., Beinhoffa, U., & Riepea, M. W. (2012). Everyday memory deficits in very mild Alzheimer's disease. *Neurobiology of Aging*, *33*(2), 297–303. doi:10.1016/j.neurobiolaging.2010.03.012 PMID:20392540

Wolinsky, F. D., Mahncke, H., Vander Weg, M. W., Martin, R., Unverzagt, F. W., Ball, K. K., Jones, R. N., & Tennstedt, S. L. (2010). Speed of processing training protects self-rated health in older adults: Enduring effects observed in the multi-site ACTIVE randomized controlled trial. *International Psychogeriatrics*, *22*(3), 470–478. doi:10.1017/S1041610209991281 PMID:20003628

Zucchella, C., Capone, A., Codella, V., Vecchione, C., Buccino, G., & Sandrini, G. (2014). Assessing and restoring cognitive functions early after stroke. *Functional Neurology*, *29*(4), 255–262. doi:10.11138/FNeur/2014.29.4.255 PMID:25764255

ADDITIONAL READING

Hill, N. T. M., Mowszowski, L., Psych, D., Naismith, S. L., Psych, D., Chadwick, V. L., & … . (2017). Computerized Cognitive Training in Older Adults With Mild Cognitive Impairment or Dementia: A Systematic Review and Meta-Analysis. *The American Journal of Psychiatry*, *174*(4), 1–13. doi:10.1176/appi.ajp.2016.16030360 PMID:27838936

Rohrbach, N., Gulde, P., Armstrong, A. R., Hartig, L., Abdelrazeq, A., Schröder, S., Neuse, J., Grimmer, T., Diehl-Schmid, J., & Hermsdörfer, J. (2019). An augmented reality approach for ADL support in Alzheimer's disease: A crossover trial. *Journal of Neuroengineering and Rehabilitation*, *16*(66), 1–12. doi:10.118612984-019-0530-z PMID:31159816

Uwajeh, P. C., Iyendo, T. O., & Polay, M. (2019). Therapeutic gardens as a design approach for optimizing the healing environment of patients with Alzheimer's disease and other dementias: A narrative review. *Explore (New York, N.Y.)*, *15*(5), 352–362. doi:10.1016/j.explore.2019.05.002 PMID:31230998

KEY TERMS AND DEFINITIONS

Allocentric Spatial Knowledge: Encoding information about the location of one object or its parts with respect to other objects.

Alzheimer's Disease: Is a neurodegenerative disease that could slowly compromise memory, language, mood, and executive functions.

Augmented Reality: Is an interactive experience where the objects that reside in the real world are enhanced by computer-generated multi-sensory information (e.g., visual, auditory, haptic, somatosensory, and olfactory).

Egocentric Spatial Knowledge: Encoding the objects in the space respect to the body axes of the self (left-right; front-back).

MCI (Mild Cognitive Impairment): Frequent state of cognitive impairment in over 65s which could, but not always, lead to dementia.

Technology-Based Programs: Employment of advanced technologies such as computer and internet in the process of learning or cognitive rehabilitation.

Virtual Reality: An experience that can be similar to or completely different from the real world.

Section 4

Acquired Brain Injury and Stroke

Chapter 12
Cognitive Performance in Immersive Environments After Acquired Brain Injury

Ineke van der Ham
Leiden University, The Netherlands

ABSTRACT

The use of immersive environments such as virtual and augmented reality is quickly developing. For cognitive assessment and training in a neuropsychological setting, this offers a perspective for innovation and improvement of existing methods. Most of the current clinical uses of immersive environments focus on factors such as anxiety, or motor activities for physical therapy. Cognitive applications, concerning, for example, memory, attention, visuospatial processing, are relatively scarce. In this chapter, considerations of using immersive environments for cognitive purposes are presented. In addition to immersion, the individual experience of immersive environments, as expressed by sense of presence, will be discussed. By examining advantages and disadvantages of using immersive environments to measure and train cognitive performance, recommendations for clinical use of these methods are provided.

INTRODUCTION

Immersive technologies like virtual reality (VR) and augmented reality (AR) are growing exponentially and have seemingly endless potential for assessment, learning, and entertainment (Allcoat & von Mühlenen, 2018; Lee et al. 2010; Molina-Carmona et al., 2018, Navarro & Sundstedt, 2020). Applications come in many forms, and are beginning to take on substantial roles in education, training, and healthcare programmes, worldwide. The recent need for social distancing has further stimulated a surge in virtual solutions, for instance for museum visits (Kunjir & Patil, 2020), to stimulate international student collaboration in education (de Back et al., 2020), and to provide healthcare digitally (Papara et al., 2020) Where initial applications mainly concerned entertainment, more recent developments include implementation within education and healthcare settings. For instance, Bogomolova and colleagues (2020) describe an application where medical students can use AR by wearing a HoloLens head mounted display.

DOI: 10.4018/978-1-7998-7430-0.ch012

Through this device, the users can view three dimensional human anatomy and moreover, they are able to interact with the AR projection through hand movement, by e.g. resizing or rotating the image or to tap on certain option buttons. Also specific patient groups can benefit from IEs. A number of studies show that exposure therapy can be highly effective when the object of a specific phobia, e.g. being in an airplane, can be realistically recreated, without actually being exposed to it (Parsons & Rizzo, 2008).

Despite the inherent appeal of these examples, some caution also seems appropriate. Immersive environments are still distinctly different from real environments and therefore present their users with cognitive challenges. Especially neuropsychological patients may present particular challenges in using IEs. Often, immersive learning is used to convey visuospatially complex information, ranging from geometric-shape learning in augmented reality for children (Gecu-Parmaksiz & Delialioglu, 2020) to augmented reality medical education for adult students (Bogomolova et al., 2020). Immersive environments (IEs) also allow for full control over the characteristics of the environment, which can be useful for example, for training navigation ability in virtual environments for stroke patients (van der Kuil et al., 2018) in a secure environment. However, a clear understanding of what drives learning effectiveness in these immersive applications is still lacking.

Reports on IE learning effectiveness are limited and diverse. Immersive learning can even lead to adverse effects in some situations, e.g. when users lack the required spatial skills to accurately process the immersive environment (Price & Lee, 2010), are hindered by stereotypical beliefs about using immersive technologies (Chang et al., 2019), or an entirely different spatial function is trained because of the three dimensional depiction (Kozhevnikov & Dhond, 2012). Moreover, application in vulnerable populations such as patients with acquired brain injury may pose substantial problems, such as cybersickness and cognitive demands that are too high (Weech et al., 2019). It is imperative to understand what is required to obtain a beneficial effect of learning in IEs and how this differs across individuals.

To this end, the current chapter will focus on the use of immersive environments in diagnostics and rehabilitation of patients with acquired brain injury. The number of IE tools that are being developed for this particular population is steadily increasing. After an initial focus mainly on using IEs to train motor skills as part of physical therapy, cognitive applications serving diagnostics as well as rehabilitation are on the rise. Due to the specific profile of such patients, in terms of potential cognitive limitations and often higher age, some caution in the use of novel technology is advisable. Therefore in this chapter, the working mechanisms of immersive environments are explored, within the context of neuropsychological diagnostics and rehabilitation. An in depth discussion of current literature will result in a set of recommendations for the use of IEs in neuropsychological practice, taking into account particular advantages and disadvantages. Furthermore, future directions for research and clinical applications are discussed.

BACKGROUND

The use of immersive technology dates back to the 1960s, when the first multisensory virtual experience was created (Mazuryk & Gervautz, 1996). This was soon followed by the first implementation of AR, with an optical, see-through head-mounted display (Arth et al., 2015). Due to technological challenges that needed to be tackled, it was not until the 1990s that the IE industry started to surge, and became highly popular, but expensive. With further technological innovation and large-scale commercial production in the past decade (e.g. Oculus Rift, HTC Vive, Microsoft Hololens), the use of IEs is now highly accessible and affordable.

From Real to Virtual Environments

Figure 1 depicts the range of IEs, from the fully real environment to the fully virtual environment. In virtual reality (VR), reality is presented completely virtually (Slater & Sanchez-Vives, 2016), where a digital world is created, separate from the existing world. In VR, the most common tool is a head set or projection dome in which the user is fully immersed in a digital environment. Such environments can trigger profound responses, even in the physical domain. One example is the use of a virtual snow world, which is designed to be used in burn victims when their dressings are changed, or wounds are cleaned. In this snow world, the users can participate in a digital snow ball fight. Not only does this distract their attention from the painful medical procedure; it also has been shown to lower pain perception substantially, and distract from common reexperience of trauma (Hoffman, 2004; Wender et al., 2009).

Mixed reality (MR) is an umbrella term that covers the range of applications in which real and virtual worlds are combined to a certain extent (Milgram & Kishino, 1994). Augmented reality (AR) provides a projection of information while the real world is still visible to the user (Azuma, 1997). It should be noted that the definitions MR and AR show some overlap and discrepancies in the literature. AR is typically defined with more detail, as a system that includes real time interaction and enhances real world perception with added virtual elements in a single view (Kaplan et al., 2020). Many applications within healthcare are currently explored within the domain of AR, for instance a simple applications that helps nurses to locate veins when inserting a needle, through near infrared imaging and laser projection onto the skin (AccuVein Inc, Palatine IL) (e.g. Kaddoum et al., 2012).

Figure 1. Visualisation of the different forms of immersive environments, based on the reality-virtuality continuum by Milgram & Kishino (1994)

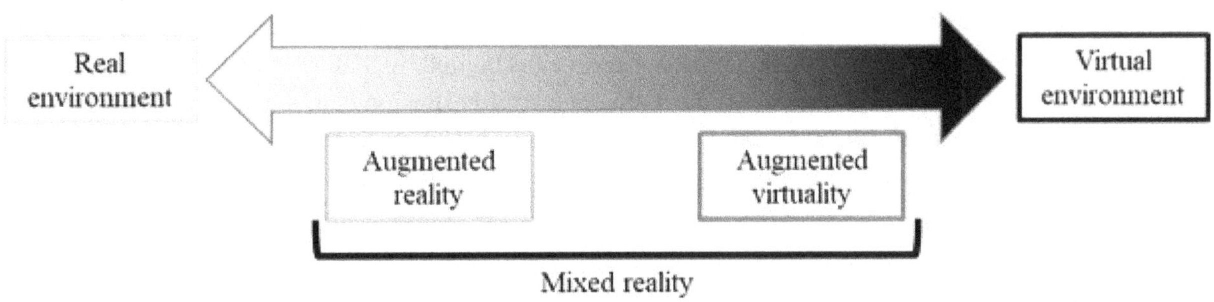

Although only a limited number of applications to the field of neuropsychology have been reported, IEs show great potential for both diagnostics and treatment options. IEs have unique properties that are highly useful in the assessment and training of cognitive performance; information can be presented in a highly controlled manner, information that may be difficult to access due to physical or geographical limitations can be made available, and performance data can be collected at a high level of detail. The main reason why the cognitive applications of IEs, whether it be diagnostics or treatment, is that the cognitive mechanisms of IEs are not yet fully understood. Immersion, and the resulting sense of presence (SoP) may be essential elements to these cognitive mechanisms. IEs are labelled as such because of the property of immersion, which is the objective, technical property of the presentation of digital environments. Depending on the display choice, levels of immersion can vary: it is relatively low when viewing a virtual environment on a regular computer screen and much higher when using projection domes or interactive AR goggles.

Sense of Presence

Where immersion depends on the technical equipment and design of an environment, SoP refers to the subjective experience of the IEs, and reflects the extent to which the observer feels present in the environment. SoP can be described as the *illusion* of being present (Slater, 2018). When immersed in an IE, you are still aware you are witnessing an artificial, digital environment and can typically still perceive the real world to some extent (e.g. auditory and proprioceptive input). However, this illusion of presence captures the essence of IEs, as the illusion is able to mislead our perceptual system and elicit responses, but does not impact our cognitive system in the same way (Slater, 2009). As such, SoP forms a central element to the learning performance in IEs. What constitutes the level of SoP is a matter of debate. While some assume SoP results from immersion, or even use the terms interchangeably, the literature indicates that SoP is the combined result of technical and individual factors. Technical properties like stereoscopy, a high field of view of the display, high control and intuitiveness of interaction with the IE, and multisensory congruency determine immersion and have been shown to increase SoP (Weech et al., 2019; Servotte et al., 2020). Individual factors, such as the elicitation of cognitive, emotional, and behavioural responses can further increase SoP (Parong & Mayer, 2020; Riches et al., 2019). Furthermore, there are reports showing that SoP lowers when diminished agency and physical discomfort such as cybersickness are experienced (Riches et al., 2019). This distinction between technical and individual factors can also be recognised in assessment tools. SoP is often measured through questionnaires, such as the frequently used Igroup Presence Questionnaire (Schubert et al., 2001). Most questions focus on the personal experience of the IE (e.g. I felt present in the virtual space), whereas some questions rely more on technological features (e.g. the virtual world seemed more realistic than the real world). This also appears compatible with the illusion of being present as coined by Slater; at a perceptual level, immersion can lead to place illusion, while cognitively, plausibility illusion can be induced, depending on individual differences in, for instance experience (Slater, 2018). Thus, SoP is central to the IE experience and is the result of technical features that contribute to level of immersion as well as the individual experience (see figure 2).

Figure 2. Sense of presence reflects the experience of immersive environments, based on the level of immersion of the technology used, and how the technology is experienced by the individual user

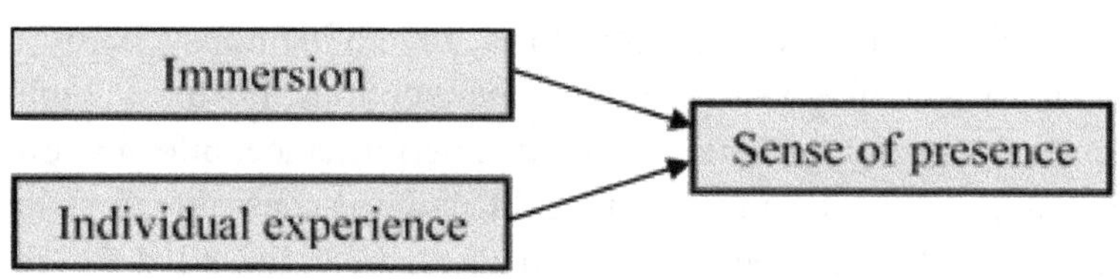

A common assumption is that in order to achieve the best cognitive learning outcomes, immersion should be high (Lee et al., 2010; Allcoat & von Mühlenen, 2018; Molina-Carmona et al., 2018), because this would be accompanied by a high SoP (Bystrom et al., 1999; Parong & Mayer, 2020). Although there are numerous reports in support of this positive relationship between SoP and learning performance (e.g. Lee et al., 2010; Molina-Carmona et al., 2018), several recent publications point in a different direction. The use of display types with higher levels of immersion did not lead to better spatial learning performance and a desktop format may even be slightly favourable (Zhao et al., 2020). An inverse relationship, where SoP was higher in immersive VR, but participants learnt less in this condition. This effect was accompanied by indications of a higher cognitive load (Makransky et al., 2019). Khenak et al. (2020) argue for a relationship between the 'highest degree of physical existence' and best learning performance, favoring learning in the real world, rather than learning with digital materials. Given these recent reports, the relationship between SoP and learning performance cannot simply be regarded as a linear positive relationship. Instead, literature suggests that SoP holds an optimum curve relationship to learning performance in IEs, where with lower levels of SoP, the relation with performance is linear, but with higher levels of SoP, a decline in performance can be present .

Embodiment

In addition to SoP, embodiment can also be considered a key ingredient in how IEs are experienced. Embodiment refers to the extent to which an individual experiences a body as their own. Within the context of using IEs, this refers to the extent to which a virtual body is experienced as the user's own body. Such experiences can also occur without using digital technology. The 'Rubber Hand Illusion', first described by Botvinick & Cohen (1998) clearly illustrates how an external object can be integrated into how the brain represents the body. When a rubber hand is placed in an anatomically correct position in front of someone, with their actual hand placed out of sight next to the rubber hand, and the actual and rubber hand are stroked with a brush simultaneously, the illusion of 'ownership' over the rubber hand typically occurs (e.g. Constantini & Haggard, 2007). Participants subjectively report ownership and also show a spatial drift when they attempt to touch their fingers (e.g. Davies et al., 2013).

With regard to embodiment in IEs, Kilteni, Groten & Slater (2012) have made an important contribution by providing a framework consisting of three elements. Sense of embodiment is defined as sense of self location, sense of agency, and sense of body ownership. In short, feeling present in an IE relies on feeling located inside a physical body, have global motor control over the body, and experiencing self-attribution of a body. This framework is not only highly informative for observing level of embodiment within IES, but also for the potential enhancement of embodiment. Providing an eye level perspective to enhance an egocentric perspective aligned with the virtual body, increasing the similarities in the temporal patterns of movement, and increasing sensory alignment would then all promote a higher sense of embodiment.

Similarly to the line of reasoning used for SoP, enhancing sense of embodiment would similarly enhance performance in IEs. Therefore, when using IEs in the context of cognitive performance, both SoP and sense of embodiment could play important parts and should therefore be considered in task design.

Clinical Use

When exploring the literature concerning IEs within the healthcare setting a wide range of applications can be found, both for healthcare providers and their patients. IEs are increasingly used in medical training, to enhance medical knowledge as well as specific skill training. IEs are particularly useful in this context, as it can provide clear three-dimensional images of complex visuospatial information. Moreover, uncommon situations can be mimicked and skills can be rehearsed without the need for cadavers or other materials that may have limited availability.

Applications with a focus on the patient can play a supportive role in healthcare in various ways. They can play an important part in pain reduction for instance. IEs can provide distraction, through which they can reduce the pain levels experienced during certain procedures (Garrett et al., 2014; Hoffman et al. 2001, Hoffman et al., 2008), and can give the subjective experience of time passing by faster (van der Ham et al., 2019). More specifically, IEs have shown to be highly useful to treat anxiety and trauma related disorders. Due to the realistic visuospatial qualities, a psychophysiological fear response can be evoked and allows for exposure based therapies, for e.g. specific phobias, and posttraumatic stress disorder. All these applications rely strongly on the emotional processing of information presented in the IE.

Within neuropsychology, other approaches are also starting to emerge. Due to the high level of control over the visuospatial information presented, specific movements can be easily rehearsed, in a more motivating, game-like setting, to support interventions aimed at physical therapy (e.g. Alahmari et al., 2013). Furthermore, when daily life activities need to be practiced, IEs allow for a highly controlled setting where all relevant parameters can be manipulated to allow for safe and useful execution of these daily life tasks (Faria et al., 2016).

At this point in the incorporation of IE technology with neuropsychology, many studies are aimed at examining its feasibility, where for instance the accuracy of visuospatial processing or preference for type of VR display in neuropsychological patients is assessed (Parsey & Schmitter-Edgecombe, 2013; Spreij et al, 2020. Now that feasibility is increasingly established, an important next step in the development of IE solutions for neuropsychological diagnostic and treatment procedures is to work towards effective use of IEs. To this end, a thorough understanding of how cognitive performance is affected by doing tasks in IEs is crucial.

Cognitive Performance

The application of IEs to study cognitive functioning is relatively new. As one of the first systematic approaches to neuropsychological assessment Parsons & Rizzo (2008) and Parsons et al. (2008) report that performance in VR is consistent to performance in paper and pencil equivalents, in a sample of young, healthy individuals. They specifically aimed their work at measures of learning and memory and provide evidence that VR can be used for reliable and effective measurements in an ecologically valid environment. IEs provide some clear advantages in the cognitive diagnostic process, over traditional paper and pencil procedures. Behaviour can be observed in a context that reflects everyday life much better than can be achieved on paper. There are reports that this context provides more enjoyment, but could also cause undesired distraction from the task at hand (Elkind et al., 2001). However, potential alternative explanations for the distraction observed are also possible, such as unmatched difficulty level and being unfamiliar with the technology. The distractions found in IEs could also be of use, as a measure of distractibility, that are difficulty to objectively assess in real life (Parsey & Schmitter-Edgecombe, 2013).

Importantly, the different visuospatial context of cognitive measurements as used in IEs allows for potential differences in the precise cognitive construct that is measured. Spatial performance is of particular relevance here, as the digital environments used in IE may very closely resemble real space, but is still clearly distinguishable from it. Navigation performance, for instance, is selectively affected by the absence of full physical involvement while exploring an environment. Route knowledge remains intact, but survey knowledge like drawing a map of the environment is hindered when individuals do not physically engage with a virtual environment (e.g. van der Ham et al., 2015). Furthermore, the use of virtual environments has been shown to lead to distortions in spatial and temporal perception in certain circumstances (e.g., Finnegan et al., 2016; Knapp & Loomis, 2004; Stefanucci et al., 2015; van der Ham et al., 2019). Moreover, the accuracy by which spatial information is perceived can easily be manipulated in VR (e.g., Linkenauger et al., 2015; Cuperus & van der Ham, 2016; Cuperus et al., 2018), which should be considered in interpreting performance in such IEs.

Apart from potentially distorting perception of the visuospatial environments used, the cognitive load involved in IEs, should be noted. Generally, especially AR studies on learning show that providing clear, concrete visuospatial depictions of information can reduce the cognitive load when processing potentially complex information (e.g. Küçük et al., 2016). In contrast the literature also provides evidence that certain properties of IE tools may increase cognitive load, such as a limited field of view (Baumeister et al., 2017), introducing immersive rather than conventional VR viewing (Frederiksen et al., 2020).

Taken together, clear strengths of using IEs to measure cognitive performance include the ease of use, the availability of an ecologically valid setting, compared to traditional paper and pencil alternatives, and the availability of safe and highly controllable settings to work with. In contrast, weaknesses lie with the need for standardized normative data, as traditional measures cannot simply be translated to an immersive alternative (e.g. Parsey & Schmitter-Edgecombe, 2013), a thorough examination of the precise cognitive constructs involved in cognitive tasks, and potential cybersickness particularly in older users (Flynn et al., 2003; Mullen et al., 2010).

Acquired Brain Injury

In this chapter, the focus lies with patients with acquired brain injury (ABI). This particular neuropsychological population is highly relevant in the context of both diagnostic tools and rehabilitation programs. ABI can occur in a wide range of individuals, of varying age and health conditions, as a result of trauma or cardiovascular events for instance. Shortly after the injury occurs, neuropsychological diagnostic tests can be applied to assess the extent and progress of cognitive impairment suffered from the injury. After initial and urgent medical treatment and neuroregenerational processes in the first weeks to months after the injury occurs, there is room for neuropsychological rehabilitation (e.g. Nudo, 2013). Depending on the physical and psychological condition of the patient, a range of restorative or compensatory approaches can be used with the main aim to improve everyday functioning (e.g. Wilson, 2009). Although the use of IE is relatively novel, clinical professionals in this domain show a clear interest and motivation to use IE tool should they be available (van der Ham et al., 2020b). The field shows a clear need to grow beyond the existing feasibility and pilot studies to develop IE tools with sufficient empirical support to their effectiveness and validity. Both diagnostic and rehabilitation tools are of relevance here, as IEs can provide unique contributions to both the assessment of cognitive performance, and potential improvement of cognitive performance through training. To support the development of such tools, a clear understanding of the cognitive processes involved in using IEs is essential. In the next part of this chapter, input is provided to better understand cognitive performance in IEs, by taking into account how IEs are experienced and how this may differ between individuals.

COGNITIVE PERFORMANCE IN VIRTUAL IMMERSIVE ENVIRONMENTS

Especially within a clinical context, IEs provide strong advantages as described earlier. When patients have certain physical limitations, a situation can be created in which they can overcome e.g. motor impairments or fatigue can be reduced. Also, when it is difficult to travel to specific locations, the full control of IE designs allows the creation of any relevant environment while staying in the same place. In line with recent developments, assessment and training of cognitive skills within situations that mimic everyday life can have a clear advantage over traditional paper and pencil testing. For instance, it may be that a patient describe specific problems that occur when going grocery shopping. Reenacting this situation in an IE may help to specifically identify the cause of these problems and specifically train them.

Yet, at this point we know little about what actually happens when cognitive tasks are performed in IEs. There are indications that the immersive nature itself enhances performance (e.g. Ventura et al., 2019), but there are empirical reports showing that performance is similar to more traditional matters, and that differences in e.g. enjoyment and motivation are the main result of using IEs (e.g. Cuperus et al., 2018). If we can better understand how IE affects cognitive performance and through which mechanisms, we are better equipped to design effective diagnostic and rehabilitation tools for ABI patients.

Experience of Immersion

The crucial feature of IEs in relation to cognitive performance is of course immersion. Although immersion is the objective, defining characteristic of IEs, it can result in varying levels of SoP in the environment, or how the IE is subjectively experienced. As argued earlier, SoP shows a clear connection to cognitive performance in IEs, where up to a certain level a higher SoP is linked to better performance. Notably, there are reports indicating that SoP may have an optimum level after which cognitive performance decreases if SoP is too high. Importantly, SoP is the product of immersion and individual experience. Immersion is the result of stable, technical circumstances, whereas the impact of individual experience is highly variable. Therefore, even when the same materials are used, the optimum of the relationship between SoP and learning performance can substantially differ between users.

In this chapter, the individual experience of IEs is further examined as a key element in understanding how IEs may affect cognitive performance. A crucial aspect that has been largely overlooked so far is the subjective and thus individually variable nature of how IEs are experienced. It could well be a crucial factor in understanding contradicting findings in literature concerning IEs and learning performance. As a result, because IEs are now typically applied in the same way for all users, major differences in learning outcome will likely emerge between different users. This one-size-fits-all approach poses a substantial threat to the inclusivity of this booming form of technology. Especially when developing IEs in ABI patients, it is highly important to consider specific needs of this population and individual differences in general that may be relevant within this population. Based on current insights from cognitive neuroscience, computer science, cognitive, and neuropsychology, the characteristics of individual differences in relation to SoP will be discussed here. In particular, spatial ability, gender, and age are presented as central characteristics impacting learning outcome in IEs, through their impact on SoP (see Figure 3).

Figure 3. Proposed relationships between, immersion, sense of presence and cognitive learning outcome, as influenced by the individual experience, involving spatial abilities, gender and age

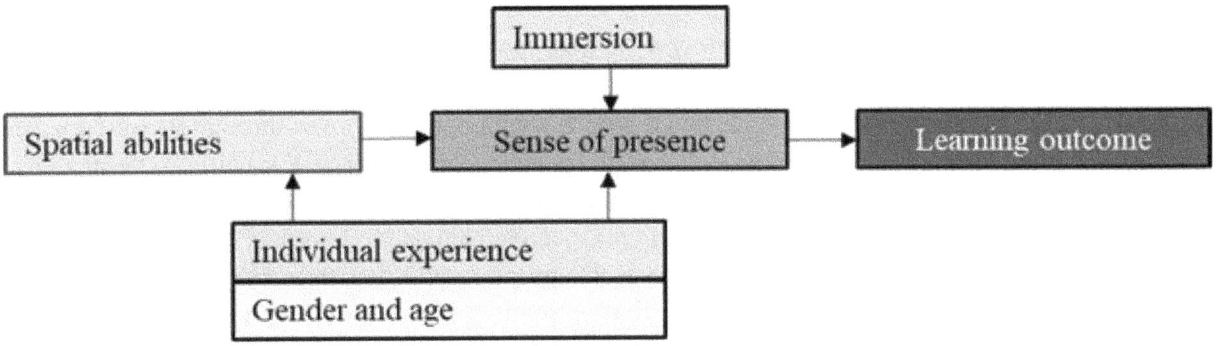

Individual Experience

Spatial Ability

The immersion into the three-dimensional environment of IEs makes visuospatial information its central element. Some researchers argue that visuospatial information is processed at an enhanced level in IEs (Paes et al., 2017), and the interaction with IEs has been shown to have a positive impact on spatial skills (Molina-Carmona et al., 2018). Applications of IEs are particularly fruitful, when the visuospatial information is otherwise less accessible e.g. studying human anatomy without the need for cadavers (Bogomolova et al., 2020), organic structures that are too small to observe without technical support (Allcoat & von Mühlenen, 2018), and spatial navigation in highly controlled and manipulable environments (van der Kuil et al., 2018). Moreover, there are convincing indications that immersive space may be cognitively processed differently from real space, which directly affects the learning quality, e.g. virtual distances are perceived as being compressed under certain circumstances, e.g. IEs may require different image encoding and transformation strategies (Kozhevnikov & Dhond, 2012) also dependent on the specific tasks performed, and some users approach objects in IEs as two-dimensional, rather than three-dimensional objects (Price & Lee, 2010). Therefore, visuospatial functioning can be considered an important factor towards learning quality in IEs and the goal to optimize learning quality.

Spatial ability covers a range of cognitive skills, necessary to process and interact with spatial information, whether real or virtual. Spatial abilities show very high variation across individuals, which has generated many studies assessing the impact of gender, development, aging, and strategy preferences on spatial performance (see for instance Lubinski, 2010; Reilly & Neumann, 2013; van der Ham et al., 2020a; van der Ham & Claessen, 2020). A functional dissociation exists between small-scale and large-scale spatial abilities, which should therefore be considered separately (Hegarty et al., 2006).

Small or 'figural' scale space requires the inspection, imagination or mental transformation of objects, this is relevant, for example, when studying anatomy in AR (Bogomolova et al., 2020). The ability to perform mental rotation is of particular interest to IEs, especially when interacting with virtual objects. In many AR solutions, spatial manipulation of objects is required to study them, e.g. rotating an anatomical structure to fully understand its shape and composition. Mental rotation ability has been extensively studied since the 1970s and displays substantial individual variation between healthy participants, mainly favouring males (Moé, 2009). In recent work, indications were found that especially participants with lower mental rotation abilities perform better in IEs when immersion is high, in comparison to IEs with lower immersion.

Many studies that include measurements of spatial abilities focus on small-scale abilities, however, large-scale spatial functioning may also be of interest, especially when locomotion is involved (Kozhevnikov & Garcia, 2011). When the body is surrounded by a given space and moves through it, we consider this large-scale space. When moving through VR, for instance, to memorize a specific route in a city, large-scale spatial abilities like perspective taking are required. Perspective-taking ability concerns the ability to take on an observer-based or egocentric perspective, and an environment based or allocentric perspective, and to switch between these two types according to task demands. For this spatial ability, large individual differences in skill level as well as strategic preferences exist. A recent initial study highlights the benefits for AR learning of using allocentric views of an environment in initial stages of environment exploration. Moreover, active switching between egocentric and allocentric perspectives promotes the creation of a flexible mental map of the environment, which aids orientation and navigation in the environment (Gardony et al., 2021). In addition to mental maps, perspective taking ability is also highly relevant in IE designs where visual maps are used to help guide users through the digital space, in the form of i.e. simultaneously presented minimaps (Kotlarek, Lin & Ma, 2018).

In short, empirical data is accumulating in support of the relevance of small and large scale spatial abilities to learning outcomes when using IEs.

Age

Very little is known about how aging in adults affects SoP. Immersive environments rely heavily on the ability to take on different spatial perspectives. Spatial perspective-taking changes substantially during our lifespan. In particular, allocentric perspective-taking already shows significant decline in the fifth decade of life, closely linked to hippocampal volume decline (Driscoll et al., 2003). For older adults, the ability to fully grasp three-dimensionality in IEs, and to consider different views of these environments poses a threat to their effectiveness.

In addition to cognitive performance, self-efficacy in older individuals, especially for spatial functions has been found to be lower, compared to young adults (West et al., 2002). Furthermore, a clear increase in anxiety reports for spatial situations has been found with higher age (van der Ham et al., 2020a) (see Figure 4). So, based on cognitive aging patterns and observed indications of lower self-efficacy and higher spatial anxiety, SoP and learning performance in IEs may well be lower with older age. Given the lack of direct investigation, further exploration with empirical studies is in order.

Gender

Similar to age, there is relatively little documentation about the impact of gender on how IEs are experienced. However, the available literature points towards meaningful differences between males and females. It has been suggested that males show higher levels of spatial presence, realness and sense of being there, which cannot be explained by possible differences in computer experience (Felnhofer et al., 2012). Potentially, gaming experience or self-efficacy play a role here. This gender difference was further substantiated by findings indicating that females are less comfortable, less confident and less capable in IEs, especially when the IE design was technical or visually complex (Ausburn et al.,

Figure 4. Spatial anxiety levels are higher in females and older adults, as measured with our validated Wayfinding Questionnaire (see van der Ham et al., 2020).

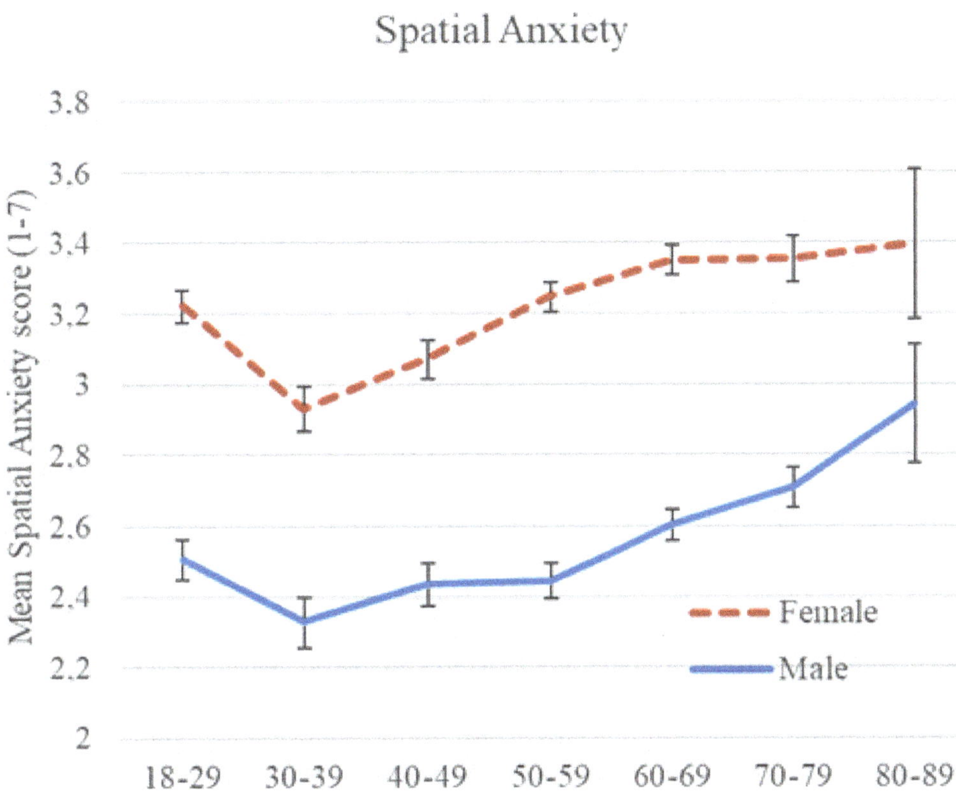

2009). There are also indications that females may suffer more from cybersickness (Shafer, Carbonara & Korpi, 2017), a physiological response which could interfere with SoP. In addition to a direct impact of gender on SoP, gender also has a strong relation to spatial ability levels . Males and females substantially differ in certain spatial skills, especially those related to processing abstract, three-dimensional spatial environments. A strong male advantage in mental rotation is typically found, and clear strategic differences exist in perspective taking. Similar strategic differences also emerge for IEs, where males can acquire better knowledge of an environment due to their IE use, linked to their spatial visualisation ability (Hedge, Weaver & Schnall, 2017). In short, evidence indicates that currently males benefit more from IEs than females.

Crucially, strong stereotypes favouring males exist for spatial abilities, which may also expand to the use of immersive environments. In my lab, we studied gender stereotypes for small-scale spatial abilities and spatial navigation. With a sample of 980 Dutch adult participants (age range 18-94), we found that a male-favouring stereotype for both small-scale and large-scale spatial abilities is very strong, and particularly in young, male adults (see Figure 4). Furthermore, recent findings indicate that IEs itself are linked to a gender-based stereotype favouring males. In a group of 74 young adults (43 females), a significant stereotype was found (mean score= 43.55, on a range of 0 (male advantage) to 100 (female advantage). The gender of the participant did not significantly affect the stereotype score (work in preparation).

Figure 5. Stereotypical belief for small-scale and large scale spatial abilities, for male and female participants across 4 age groups. Overall a significant male advantage is reported, strongest for young, male participants (N=980, work in preparation).

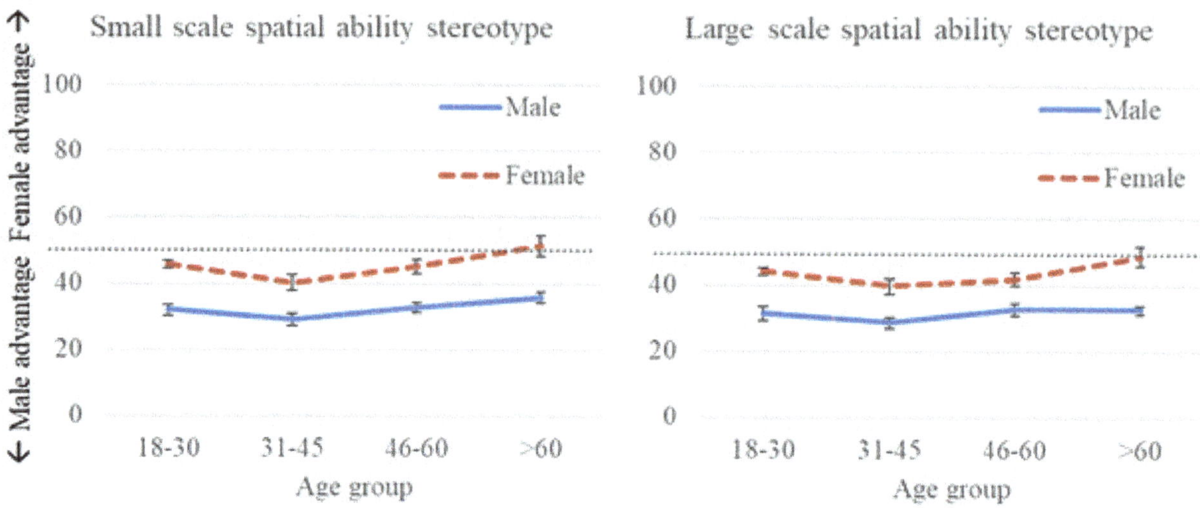

The impact of stereotypical beliefs on cognitive performance can be substantial, with a negative impact through threat (Schmader, 2002), and a positive impact through stereotype boost (Shih, Pittinsky & Ho, 2012). Stereotype threat disrupts performance because processes like a physiological stress response, actively monitoring performance, and efforts to suppress negative thoughts take up executive resources (Schmader, Johns & Forbes, 2008).

Taken together, a male advantage in SoP likely exists, due to higher relevant spatial skill level and self-efficacy. Stereotype beliefs may play a part in spatial skill level and self-efficacy, and thus in turn also affect SoP.

Neuropsychological Context

Goals

The individual experience of IEs has been described above in the context of the general population, but can also be considered specifically for the ABI population. For clinical applications, there are certain characteristics that may make the use of IEs more or less favorable. The initial part of the decision and design process should entail a clear identification of the goals of the diagnostic or rehabilitation tool. It has been shown that not the technology itself, but the emotional consequences of the technology cause certain beneficial effects (e.g. motivation, enjoyment, or distraction). Part of these effects may also be caused by methodological restrictions, where e.g. a VR tool is compared to a very neutral control condition, instead of e.g. similarly arousing 2D video materials. In those cases, it may be advisable to explore other sources of motivation, enjoyment or distraction that may cost less in terms of time and/or money or reduce disadvantages such as cyber sickness. So, it is highly recommended to formulate a clear goal of IE tool use, and to verify whether IE is the most appropriate technology to use to achieve this goal.

Advantages

As described throughout this chapter, the use of IEs offer some clear advantages to more traditional methods of delivering visuospatial information. In particular, for ABI patients, IEs may offer unique opportunities to assess and train cognitive skills that would otherwise be very difficult to create.

Comfort

IEs provide a substantial level of comfort, especially in terms of the availability of visuospatial input. Whatever type of spatial environments or objects that otherwise may not be accessible or available can be created. Without traveling, patients can be exposed to any relevant scenario to practice certain skills. For instance, navigation exercises can be completed in an IE, without physical exercise, allowing for longer training time and ensuring a fully safe experience, as there is no direct interaction with traffic for instance.

Ease of Use

In line with the comfort as experienced by the user, implementing IE tools can be very easy, once the technical development process has been completed. Electronic administration allows for elaborate automated data collection, a clear potential for use online or at home, in case of two-dimensional presentation of IEs. With quickly developing hardware and user interfaces, sufficient ease of use can be ensured. For clinical tools, it is highly recommended to include feasibility as well as usability assessment during the development stage.

Control and Flexibility

An evident advantage of using IEs over real environments or traditional pen and paper exercises is the control the healthcare provider has over de digital material and the flexibility it allows. Often, difficulty levels of exercises or tests can be easily adjusted, or automatically programmed in response to the performance level of the patient. Unpredictable elements in the real environment, such as traffic and weather circumstances can be fully customized in IEs. This provides clear and controlled measurement conditions, while maintaining ecological validity. With a visible trend towards personalization and individualized healthcare, using IEs can provide a very helpful tool. For instance, recognizable objects or streets can be selected, based on a patient's preferences or experience.

Disadvantages

Despite the clear advantages, several disadvantages can also be identified, as mentioned earlier. The advantages and disadvantages should be weighed in the decision whether or not to use IEs for a certain clinical goal.

Cognitive Load

The cognitive load that is imposed by using IEs should be considered. Especially in situations where sensory information is added to the sensory input that would normally be present, this can be an important factor. Even though it may seem that virtual reality may create a separate, fully digital experience, the body itself still experiences its presence in the real world, through e.g. tactile and auditory feedback. A clear assessment of cognitive load, through physiological and behavioral measures prior to using IEs in a clinical context is advisable, preferably in combination with reliable measures of cognitive capabilities of the patient, to ensure these two factors are in balance.

Physical Limitations

Depending on the precise technical tools that are used, there may be physical limitations. For instance, most head mounted displays used for VR or AR presentation have limitations to mobility, as do not allow a user to walk around for a few meters or longer. If involvement of the limbs is of relevance to the tasks used, than additional measurement tools are recommended. One thing to specifically consider in the ABI population is the occurrence of cybersickness. This is heightened in older individuals and moreover brain injury may introduce a higher risk of cybersickness. In such cases, a less immersive set up, by using e.g. a two-dimensional projection on a regular screen may be advisable.

Validity

There are indications that there is substantial overlap between cognitive performance in IEs and in the real world, however, they are not perceived in an identical manner (see e.g. Billger et al., 2004; van der Ham et al., 2019; Cuperus et al., 2018). The potential impact the virtual elements have on cognitive performance concern distortions in spatial perception and potential differences in visual layout compared to the real world. Examples are irrelevant 'noise' that is often not included in virtual designs, such as dynamic features (traffic, people and animals), and additional sensory input, such as sound.

SOLUTIONS AND RECOMMENDATIONS

The use of IEs in healthcare settings has only just started and is developing quickly. For these developments several solutions and recommendations can be made, especially when considering cognitive applications of IEs for ABI patients. First of all, the needs of the intended application should be clearly identified. In the end, IEs are a tool that provide unique opportunities in terms of design, interaction, and data collection, but they are not a goal in itself. Therefore, when considering the options, the problem that needs to be solved should be clearly identified. Should an existing method be replaced or improved? Is there a lack of a specific test and treatment that should be newly developed?

Next, the question whether IEs are the most appropriate method can be addressed. Here, the advantages and disadvantages as described above should be taken into account and the potential added value of using IEs should be actively identified. This added value can concern the availability of stimuli (e.g. a large scale environment cannot be easily accessed in real life), emotional factors (arousal may be heightened when using an IE), or cognitive factors (three-dimensional visuospatial display may further understanding).

Given the state of current literature, more empirical work is needed to better understand how learning performance is affected by IEs. The subjective experience of SoP should be examined in more detail to achieve this goal. In particular, the individual experience of IEs is of importance. As discussed, spatial skills, gender, and age have an impact on the experience of IEs. Up until now, very little attention has been paid to an individualized approach to using IEs. Proceeding towards more personalization will most likely increase the benefits of using IEs.

Recent work provides some useful clues on how to accommodate for individual differences. Avatars, or human characters in the IE, can be designed to overcome impact of stereotypes. This effect is known as the *Proteus effect* – referring to changes in attitudes and behaviour in line with the characteristics of the avatar used (Yee & Bailenson, 2007). It has been demonstrated that stereotypical beliefs can have considerable flexibility and fluidity within individuals (Garcia-Marques, Santos & Mackie, 2006), and using appropriate avatars can thus stimulate changes in stereotypical beliefs. In two recent studies, it has been shown that a stereotype threat effect could be found for both female and male participants, when using an avatar of the stereotypical out-group, in this case female (Peck et al., 2018; Peck, Good & Bourne, 2020). To optimise learning performance in IEs for all users, female performance could be increased by applying avatars to reduce stereotype threat.

Analogously, the impact of spatial anxiety and lower self-efficacy in elderly people could be compensated through a similar pathway, by using younger avatars in the IEs. Such anxiety and self-efficacy effects are also typical for ABI patients. They may benefit from the Proteus effect as well. In related work, the use of elderly avatars in young individuals has been shown to affect physical performance, as it negatively impacts walking speed (Reinhard et al., 2020).

With regard to spatial abilities, cognitive training in preparation of using IE methodology could be effective. Depending on the extent and need of using IEs, this could be a worthwhile application. For instance, mental rotation ability is known for significant training effects, which may benefit those with lower initial spatial abilities. Additionally, the design choices made in IEs can affect the impact of spatial ability of the user. As mentioned in the anatomy learning example above, stereoscopy fully eliminates the difference between users with high and low mental rotation ability. It could therefore well be that stereoscopic applications and augmented reality solutions are more appropriate to use in populations where large variation in spatial may hinder effectiveness of IE tools.

FUTURE RESEARCH DIRECTIONS

In line with the recommendations described above, a number of future research directions can be identified:

1. The role of SoP should be examined, in particular in relation to quality of learning outcome. One key element in this process is to elaborate on ways to measure SoP. This is typically performed with self-report measures such as questionnaires, but more objective, physiological measures could also be applied. It has been shown that skin conductance and heart rate increase with strong SoP (Baumgartner et al., 2006). There are also indications that gait is affected by SoP, due to a bias in spatial perception when SoP is low. In low SoP, gait has been shown to be more subject to the typical distortion in spatial distance estimation in IEs (~90%) (Gonzalez-Franco, Abtahi & Steed, 2019). Thus, the higher the SoP, the more gait patterns resemble those in the real world. A similar case can be made for eye movements as relevant eye-movement parameters have been shown to be related to the extent to which cognitive resources are distributed over the perception of the real world on the one hand, and an internal representation of the world on the other. When the external world becomes more reliable, i.e. when the observer feels more present in the external world,

resources will shift more towards perception of the external world and away from internal, mental representations (Somai, Schut & van der Stigchel, 2020; van der Stigchel, 2020).

2. A stronger focus on the individual is in order. In particular when considering the use of IEs in ABI patients it is worthwhile to identify demographic characteristics and a cognitive profile of the intended user. Age, gender, and spatial ability may impact effectiveness of IEs in specific patients, but also the cognitive load an IE imposes on a user is very important to consider, especially for ABI patients who may suffer from specific cognitive impairments, reducing their ability to effectively .
3. IEs cover a range of different applications, from fully virtual reality to augmented and mixed reality. Moreover, depending on the hardware used, immersion can vary substantially between different set ups. Therefore, findings concerning effective use of IEs should be placed in the perspective of IE characteristics. Given the multidisciplinary nature of this work, as well as variations in definitions used, work towards a clearer and integrated approach to IEs is recommendable.
4. The use of IEs is still relatively new, especially for cognitive applications, whether it concerns assessment or training. For healthcare, developments have been made in fields like anxiety and trauma, and physical therapy solutions. Reliable cognitive tools are still scarce, while healthcare providers indicate they are interested in and motivated to use them (van der Ham et al., 2020b). Therefore, more empirical work specifically focusing on cognitive use of IEs will benefit a possible translation to the clinical neuropsychological setting.

CONCLUSION

Immersive environments are developing quickly in quality and range of applications. Despite numerous reports on their effectiveness in assessing and improving cognitive performance and learning outcome, the underlying cognitive mechanisms are unclear. Especially for ABI patients, a better understanding of such cognitive characteristics would highly benefit diagnostic and training applications. In this chapter, an up to date overview of relevant empirical work is provided, along with a direct link to the field of clinical neuropsychology.

SoP can be considered an important factor towards effectiveness of IE use for cognitive assessment and training. Moreover, individual differences in how IEs are experienced should be considered. Here, age, gender and spatial ability can have substantial impact on individual SoP and as a result also the quality of cognitive measures and training. In particular, for ABI patients, it therefore seems important to consider their cognitive competences and potential threats posed by demographic characteristics.

The use of IEs in this neuropsychological context holds clear advantages in terms of comfort for the patient, ease of use for the healthcare provider and level of control and flexibility. In contract, disadvantages entail a potential threat to performance because of limited cognitive load, physical limitations such as cybersickness, and potential limitations to ecological validity. These advantages and disadvantages are included in the main recommendations. These factors should be considered in the decision process whether or not to use IEs for a specific problem and/or a specific patient. Furthermore, the potential role avatars may play in boosting performance by reducing stereotype threats is worthwhile to explore for the ABI population.

In short, cognitive applications of IEs for ABI patients are highly promising. More empirical exploration is needed for a better understanding of the underlying cognitive mechanisms and how these can be positively impacted to make effective use of IEs for cognitive assessment and training.

REFERENCES

Alahmari, K. A., Sparto, P. J., Marchetti, G. F., Redfern, M. S., Furman, J. M., & Whitney, S. L. (2013). Comparison of virtual reality based therapy with customized vestibular physical therapy for the treatment of vestibular disorders. *IEEE Transactions on Neural Systems and Rehabilitation Engineering*, *22*(2), 389–399. doi:10.1109/TNSRE.2013.2294904 PMID:24608691

Allcoat, D., & von Mühlenen, A. (2018). Learning in virtual reality: Effects on performance, emotion and engagement. *Research in Learning Technology*, *26*(0), 2140. doi:10.25304/rlt.v26.2140

Arth, C., Grasset, R., Gruber, L., Langlotz, T., Mulloni, R., Schmalstieg, D., & Wagner, D. (2015). *The History of Mobile Augmented Reality Developments in Mobile AR over the last almost 50 years.* Academic Press.

Ausburn, L. J., Martens, J., Washington, A., Steele, D., & Washburn, E. (2009). A cross-case analysis of gender issues in desktop virtual reality learning environments. *Journal of STEM Teacher Education*, *46*(3), 6.

Azuma, R. T. (1997). A survey of augmented reality. *Presence (Cambridge, Mass.)*, *6*(4), 355–385. doi:10.1162/pres.1997.6.4.355

Baumeister, J., Ssin, S. Y., ElSayed, N. A., Dorrian, J., Webb, D. P., Walsh, J. A., Simon, T. M., Irlitti, A., Smith, R. T., Kohler, M., & Thomas, B. H. (2017). Cognitive cost of using augmented reality displays. *IEEE Transactions on Visualization and Computer Graphics*, *23*(11), 2378–2388. doi:10.1109/TVCG.2017.2735098 PMID:28809700

Baumgartner, T., Valko, L., Esslen, M., & Jäncke, L. (2006). Neural correlate of spatial presence in an arousing and noninteractive virtual reality: An EEG and psychophysiology study. *Cyberpsychology & Behavior*, *9*(1), 30–45. doi:10.1089/cpb.2006.9.30 PMID:16497116

Billger, M., Heldal, I., Stahre, B., & Renstrom, K. (2004, June). Perception of color and space in virtual reality: a comparison between a real room and virtual reality models. In *Human Vision and Electronic Imaging IX* (Vol. 5292, pp. 90–98). International Society for Optics and Photonics. doi:10.1117/12.526986

Bogomolova, K., van der Ham, I. J., Dankbaar, M. E., van den Broek, W. W., Hovius, S. E., van der Hage, J. A., & Hierck, B. P. (2020). The effect of stereoscopic Augmented Reality visualization on learning anatomy and the modifying effect of visual-spatial abilities: A double-center randomized controlled trial. *Anatomical Sciences Education*, *13*(5), 558–567. doi:10.1002/ase.1941 PMID:31887792

Botvinick, M., & Cohen, J. (1998). Rubber hands 'feel' touch that eyes see. *Nature*, *391*(6669), 756–756. doi:10.1038/35784 PMID:9486643

Bystrom, K. E., Barfield, W., & Hendrix, C. (1999). A conceptual model of the sense of presence in virtual environments. *Presence (Cambridge, Mass.)*, *8*(2), 241–244. doi:10.1162/105474699566107

Chang, F., Luo, M., Walton, G., Aguilar, L., & Bailenson, J. (2019). Stereotype Threat in Virtual Learning Environments: Effects of Avatar Gender and Sexist Behavior on Women's Math Learning Outcomes. *Cyberpsychology, Behavior, and Social Networking*, *22*(10), 634–640. doi:10.1089/cyber.2019.0106 PMID:31580726

Costantini, M., & Haggard, P. (2007). The rubber hand illusion: Sensitivity and reference frame for body ownership. *Consciousness and Cognition*, *16*(2), 229–240. doi:10.1016/j.concog.2007.01.001 PMID:17317221

Cuperus, A. A., Keizer, A., Evers, A. W., van den Houten, M. M., Teijink, J. A., & van der Ham, I. J. (2018). Manipulating spatial distance in virtual reality: Effects on treadmill walking performance in patients with intermittent claudication. *Computers in Human Behavior*, *79*, 211–216. doi:10.1016/j.chb.2017.10.037

Cuperus, A. A., & van der Ham, I. J. (2016). Virtual reality replays of sports performance: Effects on memory, feeling of competence, and performance. *Learning and Motivation*, *56*, 48–52. doi:10.1016/j.lmot.2016.09.005

Davies, A. M. A., White, R. C., & Davies, M. (2013). Spatial limits on the nonvisual self-touch illusion and the visual rubber hand illusion: Subjective experience of the illusion and proprioceptive drift. *Consciousness and Cognition*, *22*(2), 613–636. doi:10.1016/j.concog.2013.03.006 PMID:23644413

de Back, T. T., Tinga, A. M., Nguyen, P., & Louwerse, M. M. (2020). Benefits of immersive collaborative learning in CAVE-based virtual reality. *International Journal of Educational Technology in Higher Education*, *17*(1), 1–18. doi:10.118641239-020-00228-9

Driscoll, I., Hamilton, D. A., Petropoulos, H., Yeo, R. A., Brooks, W. M., Baumgartner, R. N., & Sutherland, R. J. (2003). The aging hippocampus: Cognitive, biochemical and structural findings. *Cerebral Cortex (New York, N.Y.)*, *13*(12), 1344–1351. doi:10.1093/cercor/bhg081 PMID:14615299

Elkind, J. S., Rubin, E., Rosenthal, S., Skoff, B., & Prather, P. (2001). A simulated reality scenario compared with the computerized Wisconsin card sorting test: An analysis of preliminary results. *Cyberpsychology & Behavior*, *4*(4), 489–496. doi:10.1089/109493101750527042 PMID:11708728

Faria, A. L., Andrade, A., Soares, L., & i Badia, S. B. (2016). Benefits of virtual reality based cognitive rehabilitation through simulated activities of daily living: A randomized controlled trial with stroke patients. *Journal of Neuroengineering and Rehabilitation*, *13*(1), 1–12. doi:10.118612984-016-0204-z PMID:27806718

Felnhofer, A., Kothgassner, O. D., Beutl, L., Hlavacs, H., & Kryspin-Exner, I. (2012). Is virtual reality made for men only? Exploring gender differences in the sense of presence. *Proceedings of the International Society on presence research*, 103-112.

Finnegan, D. J., O'Neill, E., & Proulx, M. J. (2016, May). Compensating for distance compression in audiovisual virtual environments using incongruence. In *Proceedings of the 2016 CHI Conference on Human Factors in Computing Systems* (pp. 200-212). 10.1145/2858036.2858065

Flynn, D., Van Schaik, P., Blackman, T., Femcott, C., Hobbs, B., & Calderon, C. (2003). Developing a virtual reality–based methodology for people with dementia: A feasibility study. *Cyberpsychology & Behavior*, *6*(6), 591–611. doi:10.1089/109493103322725379 PMID:14756925

Frederiksen, J. G., Sørensen, S. M. D., Konge, L., Svendsen, M. B. S., Nobel-Jørgensen, M., Bjerrum, F., & Andersen, S. A. W. (2020). Cognitive load and performance in immersive virtual reality versus conventional virtual reality simulation training of laparoscopic surgery: A randomized trial. *Surgical Endoscopy, 34*(3), 1244–1252. doi:10.100700464-019-06887-8 PMID:31172325

Garcia-Marques, L., Santos, A. S. C., & Mackie, D. M. (2006). Stereotypes: Static abstractions or dynamic knowledge structures? *Journal of Personality and Social Psychology, 91*(5), 814–831. doi:10.1037/0022-3514.91.5.814 PMID:17059303

Gardony, A. L., Martis, S. B., Taylor, H. A., & Brunyé, T. T. (2021). Interaction strategies for effective augmented reality geo-visualization: Insights from spatial cognition. *Human-Computer Interaction, 36*(2), 107–149. doi:10.1080/07370024.2018.1531001

Garrett, B., Taverner, T., Masinde, W., Gromala, D., Shaw, C., & Negraeff, M. (2014). A rapid evidence assessment of immersive virtual reality as an adjunct therapy in acute pain management in clinical practice. *The Clinical Journal of Pain, 30*(12), 1089–1098. doi:10.1097/AJP.0000000000000064 PMID:24535053

Gecu-Parmaksiz, Z., & Delialioğlu, Ö. (2020). The effect of augmented reality activities on improving preschool children's spatial skills. *Interactive Learning Environments, 28*(7), 876–889. doi:10.1080/10494820.2018.1546747

Gonzalez-Franco, M., Abtahi, P., & Steed, A. (2019). Individual differences in embodied distance estimation in virtual reality. In *2019 IEEE Conference on Virtual Reality and 3D User Interfaces (VR)* (pp. 941-943). IEEE. 10.1109/VR.2019.8798348

Hedge, C., Weaver, R., & Schnall, S. (2017). Spatial learning and wayfinding in an immersive environment: The digital fulldome. *Cyberpsychology, Behavior, and Social Networking, 20*(5), 327–333. doi:10.1089/cyber.2016.0399 PMID:28459599

Hegarty, M., Montello, D. R., Richardson, A. E., Ishikawa, T., & Lovelace, K. (2006). Spatial abilities at different scales: Individual differences in aptitude-test performance and spatial-layout learning. *Intelligence, 34*(2), 151–176. doi:10.1016/j.intell.2005.09.005

Hoffman, H. G. (2004). Virtual-reality therapy. *Scientific American, 291*(20), 58–65. doi:10.1038cientificamerican0804-58 PMID:15298120

Hoffman, H. G., Patterson, D. R., Carrougher, G. J., & Sharar, S. R. (2001). Effectiveness of virtual reality–based pain control with multiple treatments. *The Clinical Journal of Pain, 17*(3), 229–235. doi:10.1097/00002508-200109000-00007 PMID:11587113

Hoffman, H. G., Patterson, D. R., Seibel, E., Soltani, M., Jewett-Leahy, L., & Sharar, S. R. (2008). Virtual reality pain control during burn wound debridement in the hydrotank. *The Clinical Journal of Pain, 24*(4), 299–304. doi:10.1097/AJP.0b013e318164d2cc PMID:18427228

Kaddoum, R. N., Anghelescu, D. L., Parish, M. E., Wright, B. B., Trujillo, L., Wu, J., Wu, Y., & Burgoyne, L. L. (2012). A randomized controlled trial comparing the AccuVein AV300 device to standard insertion technique for intravenous cannulation of anesthetized children. *Paediatric Anaesthesia, 22*(9), 884–889. doi:10.1111/j.1460-9592.2012.03896.x PMID:22694242

Kaplan, A. D., Cruit, J., Endsley, M., Beers, S. M., Sawyer, B. D., & Hancock, P. A. (2020). The effects of virtual reality, augmented reality, and mixed reality as training enhancement methods: A meta-analysis. *Human Factors*, *63*(4), 706–726. doi:10.1177/0018720820904229 PMID:32091937

Khenak, N., Vézien, J., Théry, D., & Bourdot, P. (2020). Spatial Presence in Real and Remote Immersive Environments and the Effect of Multisensory Stimulation. *PRESENCE: Virtual and Augmented Reality*, *27*(3), 287–308. doi:10.1162/pres_a_00332

Kilteni, K., Groten, R., & Slater, M. (2012). The sense of embodiment in virtual reality. *Presence (Cambridge, Mass.)*, *21*(4), 373–387. doi:10.1162/PRES_a_00124

Knapp, J. M., & Loomis, J. M. (2004). Limited field of view of head-mounted displays is not the cause of distance underestimation in virtual environments. *Presence (Cambridge, Mass.)*, *13*(5), 572–577. doi:10.1162/1054746042545238

Kotlarek, J., Lin, I. C., & Ma, K. L. (2018). Improving spatial orientation in immersive environments. In *Proceedings of the Symposium on Spatial User Interaction* (pp. 79-88). 10.1145/3267782.3267792

Kozhevnikov, M., & Dhond, R. P. (2012). Understanding immersivity: Image generation and transformation processes in 3D immersive environments. *Frontiers in Psychology*, *3*, 284. doi:10.3389/fpsyg.2012.00284 PMID:22908003

Kozhevnikov, M., & Garcia, A. (2011). Visual-spatial learning and training in collaborative design in virtual environments. *Collaborative design in virtual environments*, 17-26.

Küçük, S., Kapakin, S., & Göktaş, Y. (2016). Learning anatomy via mobile augmented reality: Effects on achievement and cognitive load. *Anatomical Sciences Education*, *9*(5), 411–421. doi:10.1002/ase.1603 PMID:26950521

Kunjir, A. R., & Patil, K. R. (2020). Effectiveness of Practicing Social Distancing in Museums and Art Galleries for Visitors Using Mobile Augmented Reality (MAR): SMART—Social Distancing Using Mobile Augmented Reality Technology. *International Journal of Art, Culture and Design Technologies*, *9*(1), 1–14. doi:10.4018/IJACDT.2020010101

Lee, E. A. L., Wong, K. W., & Fung, C. C. (2010). How does desktop virtual reality enhance learning outcomes? A structural equation modeling approach. *Computers & Education*, *55*(4), 1424–1442. doi:10.1016/j.compedu.2010.06.006

Linkenauger, S. A., Bülthoff, H. H., & Mohler, B. J. (2015). Virtual arm' s reach influences perceived distances but only after experience reaching. *Neuropsychologia*, *70*, 393–401. doi:10.1016/j.neuropsychologia.2014.10.034 PMID:25446965

Lubinski, D. (2010). Spatial ability and STEM: A sleeping giant for talent identification and development. *Personality and Individual Differences*, *49*(4), 344–351. doi:10.1016/j.paid.2010.03.022

Makransky, G., Terkildsen, T. S., & Mayer, R. E. (2019). Adding immersive virtual reality to a science lab simulation causes more presence but less learning. *Learning and Instruction*, *60*, 225–236. doi:10.1016/j.learninstruc.2017.12.007

Mazuryk, T., & Gervautz, M. (1996). *Virtual reality-history, applications, technology and future*. Academic Press.

Milgram, P., & Kishino, F. (1994). A taxonomy of mixed reality visual displays. *IEICE Transactions on Information and Systems*, *77*(12), 1321–1329.

Moè, A. (2009). Are males always better than females in mental rotation? Exploring a gender belief explanation. *Learning and Individual Differences*, *19*(1), 21–27. doi:10.1016/j.lindif.2008.02.002

Molina-Carmona, R., Pertegal-Felices, M. L., Jimeno-Morenilla, A., & Mora-Mora, H. (2018). Virtual reality learning activities for multimedia students to enhance spatial ability. *Sustainability*, *10*(4), 1074. doi:10.3390u10041074

Mullen, N. W., Weaver, B., Riendeau, J. A., Morrison, L. E., & Bédard, M. (2010). Driving performance and susceptibility to simulator sickness: Are they related? *The American Journal of Occupational Therapy*, *64*(2), 288–295. doi:10.5014/ajot.64.2.288 PMID:20437916

Navarro, D., & Sundstedt, V. (2020). Biofeedback Methods in Entertainment Games and Virtual Reality: A Review of Physiological Interaction Techniques. *ACM Computing Surveys*.

Nudo, R. J. (2013). Recovery after brain injury: Mechanisms and principles. *Frontiers in Human Neuroscience*, *7*, 887. doi:10.3389/fnhum.2013.00887 PMID:24399951

Paes, D., Arantes, E., & Irizarry, J. (2017). Immersive environment for improving the understanding of architectural 3D models: Comparing user spatial perception between immersive and traditional virtual reality systems. *Automation in Construction*, *84*, 292–303. doi:10.1016/j.autcon.2017.09.016

Papara, R., Galatus, R., & Buzura, L. (2020, July). Virtual Reality as Cost Effective Tool for Distance Healthcare. In *2020 22nd International Conference on Transparent Optical Networks (ICTON)* (pp. 1-6). IEEE. 10.1109/ICTON51198.2020.9203420

Parong, J., & Mayer, R. E. (2020). Cognitive and affective processes for learning science in immersive virtual reality. *Journal of Computer Assisted Learning*. Advance online publication. doi:10.1111/jcal.12482

Parsey, C. M., & Schmitter-Edgecombe, M. (2013). Applications of technology in neuropsychological assessment. *The Clinical Neuropsychologist*, *27*(8), 1328–1361. doi:10.1080/13854046.2013.834971 PMID:24041037

Parsons, T. D., & Rizzo, A. A. (2008). Affective outcomes of virtual reality exposure therapy for anxiety and specific phobias: A meta-analysis. *Journal of Behavior Therapy and Experimental Psychiatry*, *39*(3), 250–261. doi:10.1016/j.jbtep.2007.07.007 PMID:17720136

Parsons, T. D., Silva, T. M., Pair, J., & Rizzo, A. A. (2008). Virtual environment for assessment of neurocognitive functioning: Virtual reality cognitive performance assessment test. *Studies in Health Technology and Informatics*, *132*, 351. PMID:18391320

Peck, T. C., Doan, M., Bourne, K. A., & Good, J. J. (2018). The effect of gender body-swap illusions on working memory and stereotype threat. *IEEE Transactions on Visualization and Computer Graphics*, *24*(4), 1604–1612. doi:10.1109/TVCG.2018.2793598 PMID:29543177

Peck, T. C., Good, J. J., & Bourne, K. A. (2020). Inducing and mitigating stereotype threat through gendered virtual body-swap illusions. In *Proceedings of the 2020 CHI Conference on Human Factors in Computing Systems* (pp. 1-13). ACM.

Price, A., & Lee, H. S. (2010). The effect of two-dimensional and stereoscopic presentation on middle school students' performance of spatial cognition tasks. *Journal of Science Education and Technology*, *19*(1), 90–103. doi:10.100710956-009-9182-2

Reilly, D., & Neumann, D. L. (2013). Gender-role differences in spatial ability: A meta-analytic review. *Sex Roles*, *68*(9-10), 521–535. doi:10.100711199-013-0269-0

Reinhard, R., Shah, K. G., Faust-Christmann, C. A., & Lachmann, T. (2020). Acting your avatar's age: Effects of virtual reality avatar embodiment on real life walking speed. *Media Psychology*, *23*(2), 293–315. doi:10.1080/15213269.2019.1598435

Riches, S., Elghany, S., Garety, P., Rus-Calafell, M., & Valmaggia, L. (2019). Factors affecting sense of presence in a virtual reality social environment: A qualitative study. *Cyberpsychology, Behavior, and Social Networking*, *22*(4), 288–292. doi:10.1089/cyber.2018.0128 PMID:30802148

Schmader, T. (2002). Gender identification moderates stereotype threat effects on women's math performance. *Journal of Experimental Social Psychology*, *38*(2), 194–201. doi:10.1006/jesp.2001.1500

Schmader, T., Johns, M., & Forbes, C. (2008). An integrated process model of stereotype threat effects on performance. *Psychological Review*, *115*(2), 336–356. doi:10.1037/0033-295X.115.2.336 PMID:18426293

Schubert, T., Friedmann, F., & Regenbrecht, H. (2001). The experience of presence: Factor analytic insights. *Presence (Cambridge, Mass.)*, *10*(3), 266–281. doi:10.1162/105474601300343603

Servotte, J. C., Goosse, M., Campbell, S. H., Dardenne, N., Pilote, B., Simoneau, I. L., Guillaume, M., Bragard, I., & Ghuysen, A. (2020). Virtual reality experience: Immersion, sense of presence, and cybersickness. *Clinical Simulation in Nursing*, *38*, 35–43. doi:10.1016/j.ecns.2019.09.006

Shafer, D. M., Carbonara, C. P., & Korpi, M. F. (2017). Modern virtual reality technology: Cybersickness, sense of presence, and gender. *Media Psychology Review*, *11*(2), 1.

Shih, M. J., Pittinsky, T. L., & Ho, G. C. (2012). *Stereotype boost: Positive outcomes from the activation of positive stereotypes*. Academic Press.

Slater, M. (2009). Place illusion and plausibility can lead to realistic behaviour in immersive virtual environments. *Philosophical Transactions of the Royal Society of London. Series B, Biological Sciences*, *364*(1535), 3549–3557. doi:10.1098/rstb.2009.0138 PMID:19884149

Slater, M. (2018). Immersion and the illusion of presence in virtual reality. *British Journal of Psychology*, *109*(3), 431–433. doi:10.1111/bjop.12305 PMID:29781508

Slater, M., & Sanchez-Vives, M. V. (2016). Enhancing our lives with immersive virtual reality. *Frontiers in Robotics and AI*, *3*, 74. doi:10.3389/frobt.2016.00074

Somai, R. S., Schut, M. J., & Van der Stigchel, S. (2020). Evidence for the world as an external memory: A trade-off between internal and external visual memory storage. *Cortex*, *122*, 108-114.

Spreij, L. A., Visser-Meily, J. M., Sibbel, J., Gosselt, I. K., & Nijboer, T. C. (2020). Feasibility and user-experience of virtual reality in neuropsychological assessment following stroke. *Neuropsychological Rehabilitation*, 1–21. doi:10.1080/09602011.2020.1831935 PMID:33138703

Stefanucci, J. K., Creem-Regehr, S. H., Thompson, W. B., Lessard, D. A., & Geuss, M. N. (2015). Evaluating the accuracy of size perception on screen-based displays: Displayed objects appear smaller than real objects. *Journal of Experimental Psychology. Applied*, *21*(3), 215–223. doi:10.1037/xap0000051 PMID:26121374

Van der Ham, I. J., Faber, A. M., Venselaar, M., van Kreveld, M. J., & Löffler, M. (2015). Ecological validity of virtual environments to assess human navigation ability. *Frontiers in Psychology*, *6*, 637. doi:10.3389/fpsyg.2015.00637 PMID:26074831

Van der Ham, I. J., Klaassen, F., van Schie, K., & Cuperus, A. (2019). Elapsed time estimates in virtual reality and the physical world: The role of arousal and emotional valence. *Computers in Human Behavior*, *94*, 77–81. doi:10.1016/j.chb.2019.01.005

van der Ham, I. J., van der Vaart, R., Miedema, A., Visser-Meily, J., & van der Kuil, M. N. (2020b). Healthcare Professionals' Acceptance of Digital Cognitive Rehabilitation. *Frontiers in Psychology*, *11*, 3323. doi:10.3389/fpsyg.2020.617886 PMID:33324309

Van der Ham, I. J. M., & Claessen, M. H. G. (2020). How age relates to spatial navigation performance: Functional and methodological considerations. *Ageing Research Reviews*, *58*, 101020. doi:10.1016/j.arr.2020.101020 PMID:31954190

Van der Ham, I. J. M., van der Kuil, M. N. A., Evers, A. W. M., & Claessen, M. H. G. (2020a). Large-scale assessment of human navigation ability across the lifespan. *Scientific Reports*, *10*(1), 3299. doi:10.103841598-020-60302-0 PMID:32094394

Van der Kuil, M. N., Visser-Meily, J., Evers, A. W., & Van der Ham, I. J. (2018). A usability study of a serious game in cognitive rehabilitation: A compensatory navigation training in acquired brain injury patients. *Frontiers in Psychology*, *9*, 846. doi:10.3389/fpsyg.2018.00846 PMID:29922196

van der Stigchel, S. (2020). An embodied account of visual working memory. *Visual Cognition*, *28*(5-8), 5–8, 414–419. doi:10.1080/13506285.2020.1742827

Ventura, S., Brivio, E., Riva, G., & Baños, R. M. (2019). Immersive versus non-immersive experience: Exploring the feasibility of memory assessment through 360 technology. *Frontiers in Psychology*, *10*, 2509. doi:10.3389/fpsyg.2019.02509 PMID:31798492

Weech, S., Kenny, S., & Barnett-Cowan, M. (2019). Presence and cybersickness in virtual reality are negatively related: A review. *Frontiers in Psychology*, *10*, 158. doi:10.3389/fpsyg.2019.00158 PMID:30778320

Wender, R., Hoffman, H. G., Hunner, H. H., Seibel, E. J., Patterson, D. R., & Sharar, S. R. (2009). Interactivity influences the magnitude of virtual reality analgesia. *Journal of Cyber Therapy and Rehabilitation*, *2*(1), 27–33. PMID:20390047

West, R. L., Welch, D. C., & Knabb, P. D. (2002). Gender and aging: Spatial self-efficacy and location recall. *Basic and Applied Social Psychology*, *24*(1), 71–80. doi:10.1207/S15324834BASP2401_7

Wilson, B. (2009). Evidence for the effectiveness of neuropsychological rehabilitation. *Neuropsychological rehabilitation: Theory, models, therapy and outcome*, 22-36.

Yee, N., & Bailenson, J. (2007). The Proteus effect: The effect of transformed self-representation on behavior. *Human Communication Research, 33*(3), 271–290. doi:10.1111/j.1468-2958.2007.00299.x

Zhao, J., Sensibaugh, T., Bodenheimer, B., McNamara, T. P., Nazareth, A., Newcombe, N., Minear, M., & Klippel, A. (2020). Desktop versus immersive virtual environments: Effects on spatial learning. *Spatial Cognition and Computation, 20*(4), 328–363. doi:10.1080/13875868.2020.1817925

ADDITIONAL READING

Bogomolova, K., van der Ham, I. J., Dankbaar, M. E., van den Broek, W. W., Hovius, S. E., van der Hage, J. A., & Hierck, B. P. (2020). The effect of stereoscopic Augmented Reality visualization on learning anatomy and the modifying effect of visual-spatial abilities: A double-center randomized controlled trial. *Anatomical Sciences Education, 13*(5), 558–567. doi:10.1002/ase.1941 PMID:31887792

Bystrom, K. E., Barfield, W., & Hendrix, C. (1999). A conceptual model of the sense of presence in virtual environments. *Presence (Cambridge, Mass.), 8*(2), 241–244. doi:10.1162/105474699566107

Kaplan, A. D., Cruit, J., Endsley, M., Beers, S. M., Sawyer, B. D., & Hancock, P. A. (2020). The effects of virtual reality, augmented reality, and mixed reality as training enhancement methods: A meta-analysis. *Human Factors, 63*(4), 706–726. doi:10.1177/0018720820904229 PMID:32091937

Milgram, P., & Kishino, F. (1994). A taxonomy of mixed reality visual displays. *IEICE Transactions on Information and Systems, 77*(12), 1321–1329.

Parsey, C. M., & Schmitter-Edgecombe, M. (2013). Applications of technology in neuropsychological assessment. *The Clinical Neuropsychologist, 27*(8), 1328–1361. doi:10.1080/13854046.2013.834971 PMID:24041037

Parsons, T. D., & Rizzo, A. A. (2008). Affective outcomes of virtual reality exposure therapy for anxiety and specific phobias: A meta-analysis. *Journal of Behavior Therapy and Experimental Psychiatry, 39*(3), 250–261. doi:10.1016/j.jbtep.2007.07.007 PMID:17720136

Peck, T. C., Good, J. J., & Bourne, K. A. (2020). Inducing and mitigating stereotype threat through gendered virtual body-swap illusions. In *Proceedings of the 2020 CHI Conference on Human Factors in Computing Systems* (pp. 1-13). 10.1145/3313831.3376419

Slater, M. (2009). Place illusion and plausibility can lead to realistic behaviour in immersive virtual environments. *Philosophical Transactions of the Royal Society of London. Series B, Biological Sciences, 364*(1535), 3549–3557. doi:10.1098/rstb.2009.0138 PMID:19884149

Slater, M. (2018). Immersion and the illusion of presence in virtual reality. *British Journal of Psychology, 109*(3), 431–433. doi:10.1111/bjop.12305 PMID:29781508

Yee, N., & Bailenson, J. (2007). The Proteus effect: The effect of transformed self-representation on behavior. *Human Communication Research*, *33*(3), 271–290. doi:10.1111/j.1468-2958.2007.00299.x

KEY TERMS AND DEFINITIONS

Augmented Reality: Category of immersive environments. In augmented reality the real world is experienced with the addition of interaction computer-generated, multisensory input.

Cognitive Load: The amount of cognitive resources are required to perform a certain task.

Immersive Environments: Environments that are at least in part computer-generated and elicit a feeling of immersion in its users, such as virtual reality, and augmented reality.

Mixed Reality: A general category of immersive environments in which virtual and real reality are both present.

Proteus Effect: The phenomenon in which the behaviour of an individual is affected by the characteristics of an avatar they use in an immersive environment.

Sense of Presence: The individual experience in immersive environments, which reflects the degree to which an individual feels present in the environment.

Virtual Reality: Category of immersive environments in which a complete environment is fully computer-generated.

Chapter 13
The Use of Assistive Technology as a Tool for Family Support and Recovery Post Acquired Brain Injury

Khalida Akbar
Durban University of Technology, South Africa

ABSTRACT

The recovery period post acquired brain injury (ABI) results in individuals becoming vastly dependent on family support and caregivers. Theoretical data and findings suggest that there is a lack of awareness and family support structures surrounding those affected by ABI. The empirical data indicated the need for further research and development aimed at improving conditions for recovery for individuals who are recovering from acquired brain injury. This chapter is aimed at creating awareness of assistive technology that can be used in conjunction with existing family support structures for people who are affected by ABI. The findings of this study have the potential to significantly contribute to practices and policies in society through research by providing a local country-contextual theoretical understanding of what needs to be done for persons with ABI and how AT can be used as a recovery tool within family support structures during the recovery process.

INTRODUCTION

The concept of Acquired Brain injury is a developing form of disability globally. Acquired Brain injury (ABI) can be understood as is a lifelong, chronic health condition, with varying severity of cognitive, physical, and behavioural sequelae (Sakzewski, Lewis, McKinlay, Ziviani, & Boyd, 2016). Acquired brain injury (ABI) refers to brain damage after

birth that may be caused by infection, substance abuse, brain tumours, poisoning, encephalopathy, ischemia, and stroke, or by closed or penetrating head injury (Oliver, Montero, Fernández-Caballero, González, & Molina, 2015). There is currently little evidence to guide occupational therapists in the

DOI: 10.4018/978-1-7998-7430-0.ch013

choice of interventions to address the multi-modal deficits experienced by children with ABI (Sakzewski, Lewis, McKinlay, Ziviani, & Boyd, 2016) .This chapter is aimed at creating awareness of assistive technology that it currently being used and that can be used in conjunction with existing family support structures for people s who are affected by Acquired Brain Injury (ABI). The World Health Organisation has launched a programme to promote Global Cooperation on Assistive Technology (Boot, Owuor, Dinsmore, & MacLachlan, 2018). Lack of education, awareness of the condition and family support structures negatively impacts on recovery and healing. The inclusion and implementation of Assistive Technology (AT) would therefore be highly effective and accessible for these individuals. These AT's will not eliminate family support, but rather aid the recovery process and minimise the level of support that a family would need to provide to the affected person in the household. This is seen as beneficial to both the family the individual recovering post ABI. AT's can be implemented with the use of a range of strategies including use of video-recorded stimuli, communication partner involvement, text message reminders and drawing on metacognitive skills within the group setting were useful for helping people with ABI to set and achieve their goals towards recovery (Behn, Marshall, Togher, & Cruice, 2019). People with severe acquired brain injury often require lifetime support, sometimes received from paid workers if living in shared supported accommodation. Skilled prescription and ongoing support services are necessary to maximise recovery.

This chapter will serve to assist researches in the field, professionals in the field, individuals and family members in gaining insight into the impact of assistive technology and a means of support and recovery post ABI. The existing empirical findings and literature on assistive technology will be analysed and based on finds and discussions the clinical model will be developed. The proposal of the clinical model assists scholars in future research in developing progressive research that incorporates assistive technology, representative of a multi-faceted globalised world was assistive technology will be more vastly accepted and utilised as a means of family support and recovery globally.

BACKGROUND IN UNDERSTANDING ACQUIRED BRAIN INJURY (ABI)

The level of disability in countries and regions is influenced also by physical, human-built, attitudinal and socio-political barriers, including a critical lack of access to assistive products. High-quality and comprehensive disability data are essential to address these trends and challenges.(World Health, 2019). A review of the epidemiology of traumatic brain injury in children and adolescents in North America, Europe, Australia, and New Zealand found a median annual incidence rate of 691 per 100 000 population treated in emergency departments(Sakzewski et al., 2016). Distinctively, prevalence of presbyopia, moderate, and severe vision loss is highest in Armenia and Ukraine compared to Spain and Denmark, with the most substantial difference in prevalence observed for presbyopia and moderate vision loss(Larsson-Lund, Kottorp, & Malinowsky, 2017).

People with severe acquired brain injury often require lifetime support, sometimes received from paid workers if living in shared supported accommodation. People with severe acquired brain injury often require lifetime support, sometimes received from paid workers if living in shared supported accommodation ("Central Nervous System Diseases and Conditions - Brain Injuries; Researchers at Monash University Have Reported New Data on Brain Injuries (Electronic assistive technology used by people with acquired brain injury in shared supported accommodation: Implications for occupational therapy),"

2017). As a consequence of that impairments, the person may present troubles to perform daily-life activities, such as personal care, hygiene, feeding, etc (Gómez et al., 2013).

Electronic assistive technology may offer a less intrusive method of support that can enable autonomous participation and deliver cost savings. However, research on rates, barriers, and facilitators of electronic assistive technology uptake is lacking (Jamwal, Callaway, Ackerl, Farnworth, & Winkler, 2017). Cognitive and psychosocial deficits are frequently more pervasive than motor disabilities, however, persistent deficits in motor function can negatively impact participation in daily life activities(Sakzewski, Lewis, McKinlay, Ziviani, & Boyd, 2016). Overall, there is an increased need for AT to support hearing, vision, and mobility needs in ageing populations. Patients who suffer acquired brain injury may present memory and executive functions deficits. In concrete, some patients could have problems to engage in how to perform activities of daily living, such as doing the laundry or ironing a shirt. This difficulty has motivated us to think about a possible system that may help them in their daily routines (Gómez et al., 2013). Assistive technology can therefore be adapted into their daily routines which in essence will provided the much need support that they require. Tis will not eliminate the family support that these affected individuals will need, but will however minimize the level and amount of effort required from family support.

METHOD OF ANALYSIS

This chapter is based on an appraisal of multidisciplinary scholarship that was conducted and data was collected from internet databases and secondary sources to formulate a theoretical analysis surrounding this research area. This chapter is therefore based on exiting literature and internationally published work by scholars in the field to formulate a framework surrounding adaptive technologies, that can be implemented in family support structures to assist those in need and generally towards transforming the current recovery and family support structures into on that is technologically advanced and affordable to individuals with lower incomes.

ASSISTIVE TECHNOLOGY AS A MEANS OF FAMILY SUPPORT

Assistive technology can be any device that aids functional independence of a person with disabilities, give them greater freedom, and improve their quality of life. It can be classified into various categories based on their primary function: enabling devices, adaptive devices, and rehabilitative devices (Lancioni et al., 2016). Assistive technology for cognition (ATC) can be an effective means of compensating for cognitive impairments following acquired brain injury. Systematic instruction is an evidence-based approach to training a variety of skills and strategies, including the use of ATC (Powell et al., 2015). Nowadays, the assistance for care-dependent people is gaining importance as a research field since it could improve the quality of their lives and those of their relatives (Gómez et al., 2013) Assistive technology devices have also been used to deliver automatic consequences to reduce challenging behaviors (Lancioni et al., 2016). External devices are routinely employed in neurorehabilitation to compensate for a wide range of motor-sensory, cognitive and behavioural impairments (Charters, Gillett, & Simpson, 2015).For example, to remind a person about the stimuli accessible within the context, the computer system may present him or her brief samples (previews) of those stimuli (e.g., songs and video-clips), one every 30 s (Lancioni et al., 2011).

TYPES OF ASSISTIVE TECHNOLOGIES THAT CAN BE USED AS FAMILY SUPPORT

Assistive technologies and ubiquitous computing can be related since both try to help people in their lives (Gómez et al., 2013). Systematic instruction is a comprehensive instructional methodology from the fields of special education and neuropsychological rehabilitation used to teach a broad range of personally relevant facts, concepts, skills, and strategies across disabled and non-disabled populations (Powell et al., 2015). This one of the Assistive technologies being utilized for ABI in some parts of the world.

Another is the Brain-computer interface (BCI) technology which provides Novel neuroengineering solutions to rehabilitation problems caused by amputation or neurologic injury. As a result, neural interfacing techniques are being incur prorated in rehabilitation strategies across patient populations. A review by Bockbrader introduces the concept of BCI, describes how BCls are being used to compensate for lost function or to facilitate rehabilitative therapies, and discusses BCI applications in motor and sensory restoration(Bockbrader et al., 2018).

Snowflake MultiTeach (MT) and Diamond Touch Table (DTT), its an assistive technology that is used in conjunction withs MediqVR virtual reality (VR) platform. At baseline, patients demonstrated social incompetence compared to healthy controls. Post-training evaluations showed that rehabilitation on Snowflake MT improved childrens executive and cooperation skills(Kolk et al., 2019).

Virtual Reality (VR) platforms create a captivating synthetic environment for the user, simu-lating real-world scenarios(Kolk et al., 2019). The explanatory precision of return to work in people with ABI increased minimally by adding the observed ability to use ET and the variables related to ET use when age, perceived ability in ET use and ADL had been taken in account (Larsson-Lund, Kottorp, & Malinowsky, 2017). As one type of external aid, electronic portable assistive devices (EPADs) can be held and transported across environments, and their value as a compensatory tool lies in the capacity to use them in the home, occupational, community and social settings (Charters et al., 2015).

VirtualRehab is a physical rehabilitation system, which uses videogame technology and allows telemonitoring the patients' progress (Oliver et al., 2015). Virtual rehab can be conducted on many different platforms . The most popular platforms currently being used for VirtualRehab is Skype, Zoom, Microsoft Teams .

One innovation currently influencing physical medicine and rehabilitation is brain-computer interface (BCI) technology. BCI systems used for motor control record neural activity associated with thoughts, perceptions, and motor intent; decode brain signals into commands for output devices; and perform the user's intended action through an output device. BCI systems used for sensory augmentation transduce environmental stimuli into neural signals interpretable by the central nervous system. Both types of systems have potential for reducing disability by facilitating a user's interaction with the environment. investigational BCI systems are being used in the rehabilitation setting both as neuroprostheses to replace lost function and as potential plasticity enhancing therapy tools aimed at accelerating neurorecovery (Bockbrader et al., 2018). Alternatively, electronic external memory aids, such as personal data assistants (PDAs), are less conspicuous and have alarms which alert young people to check their reminder systems (Plackett et al., 2016).

Prospective memory impairment, that is memory concerning planning for the future, is one of the most common and debilitating sequelae of acquired brain injury for children and adolescents . Memory impairment can interfere with learning and access to education, everyday adaptive functioning and social participation . Thus, interventions targeted at improving prospective memory are often employed in cognitive rehabilitation, via remedial or compensatory strategies . The most common compensatory strategies used to support memory difficulties are paper and pencil external memory aids (Plackett, Thomas, & Thomas, 2016). A problem is that significant others already bear a huge burden of supporting persons with memory impairment in their everyday life(Olsson, Persson, Bartfai, & Boman, 2017).

METHODS OF BRAIN INJURY REHABILITATION CURRENTLY USED FOR RECOVERY BY PROFESSIONALS IN THE FIELD AND FAMILY SUPPORT STRUCTURES

The general theoretical approach to treatment comprises of various pen and paper exercises, manual apparatus, and computer-based programmes which focus on keeping the mind active and alert, as well as fostering the improvement and compensation of aspects such as short-term and working memory, and utilizing and nurturing inherent talents.

These paper-based exercises are conducted via the aid of The Brainwave Rehabilitation Program which are used extensively to address individualised deficits, which have proven to improved recovery on a functional level. Recovery and rehabilitation focus on different areas of the brain such as attention, memory, motor function and executive functioning and is dependent on the specific needs and injuries of the individual. Part of the job of these specialists consists of, helping patients to acquire a greater level of autonomy in their daily-life activities and adapting and modifying the home environment (Gómez et al., 2013).The main aim to enforce independent living, it is therefore important to incorporate many activities and tasks via the aid of technology as well, such as the use of the internet. Assistive technology devices to support communication in these individuals would improve their quality of life significantly. Therapists create trainings customized to the needs of the patient (Oliver et al., 2015).This means that recovery and treatment can be tailor made to suite each individual in terms of what would be most beneficial to the . This would imply that there is no restriction and evidence stating that pen based treatment is the only form of effective support and treatment that is need post ABI. Setting individualized person-centred goals to address these problems is considered an important aspect of the rehabilitation process, though currently little is known about the process for setting, measuring and achieving goals, particularly within a group context (Behn et al., 2019).

A study fund that "Youth identified the benefits of one-to-one support at home and training of the family compared with typical group training at school(Raghavendra, Newman, Grace, & Wood, 2013). The proliferation of commercially available, mainstream mobile devices and low-cost or free applications(apps) has provided an unprecedented opportunity for individuals with cognitive disabilities associated with ABI. There is a growing interest in smart app technology. This is reflected by the number of websites pertaining to different disciplines and apps relevant to their caseloads (both paediatrics and adults) and goals (therapy, Alternative and Augmentative Communication, mobility, cognition and so forth)(Charters, Gillett, & Simpson, 2015).Assistive technology is also blended into the recovery and treatment of ABI . This is achieved through the utilisation smartphones and technological devices that are able to run applications such as Lumosity, PEAK and Elevate . External devices are routinely employed in neurorehabilitation to compensate for a wide range of motor-sensory, cognitive and behavioural impairments(Charters et al., 2015).

THE IMPORTANCE OF UTILISING ASSISTIVE TECHNOLOGY IN FAMILY SUPPORT AND RECOVERY OF ABI

Assistive technology can be any device that aids functional independence of a person with disabilities, give them greater freedom, and improve their quality of life (Lancioni et al., 2016). Nowadays, the assistance for care-dependent people is gaining importance as a research field since it could improve the quality of their lives and those of their relatives (Gómez et al., 2013). According to news reporting from Frankston, Australia, by NewsRx journalists, research stated, "People with severe acquired brain injury often require lifetime support, sometimes received from paid workers if living in shared supported accommodation ("Central Nervous System Diseases and Conditions - Brain Injuries; Researchers at Monash University Have Reported New Data on Brain Injuries (Electronic assistive technology used by people with acquired brain injury in shared supported accommodation: Implications for occupational therapy)," 2017). Differences in health status are being caused by economic, social or environmental factors beyond the control of individuals. People with disabilites are still generally regarded as a devalued and stigmatised group, where cultural perception can play an important role(Boot et al., 2018). Youth identified the benefits of one-to-one support at home and training of the family compared with typical group training at school (Raghavendra, Newman, Grace, & Wood, 2013). Participants reported that when devices supported multiple functions, such as tablets and smartphones, they were more likely to be used(Alrabiaah et al., 2020).

Children with ABI have deficits in social communication and cooperation skills. After paired neurorehabilitation, we found noticeable increase in patients' ToM skills, communication skills, and cooperation behaviours. Improving social skills is crucial for children for feeling competent in everyday interactions and a better quality of life. Children are easily motivated and their social capital increases by using next-generation devices (MMT/VR) in a playful atmosphere (Kolk et al., 2019).

A study conducted by Lund found that The results showed that the observed ability to use ET, intrapersonal capacities and environmental characteristics related to ET use were significantly associated with return to work in the studied people with ABI, both in the univariate analyses(Larsson-Lund, Kottorp, & Malinowsky, 2017).

A study by Olison The results indicate that sensor technology has potential to increase opportunities for persons with memory impairment to perform and participate in activities and to unburden their partners (Olsson et al., 2017)

CHALLENGES WITH THE IMPLEMENTATION OF ASSISTIVE TECHNOLOGY IN ABI FAMILY SUPPORT

Communication problems are common and pervasive following an ABI and can have a significant impact on a person's life. Setting individualized person-centred goals to address these problems is considered an important aspect of the rehabilitation process, though currently little is known about the process for setting, measuring and achieving goals, particularly within a group context(Behn et al., 2019). The aspect of setting individualised goals is effective in cognitive rehabilitation treatments, but creates challenges when a general assistive technology is used, as the technology was developed holistically for disabilities. It is therefore vital that proper training, induction and monitoring of the use of assistive technologies are carried out in a clear and concise manner . This must be done at a level of communication and exchange that is most suitable to the specific client. This can be integrated into the goals of recovery and daily functioning and routine of the affected person.

Limitations for use in clinical practice, such as financial burden, access to devices and clinician knowledge, currently form barriers for widespread use. Most lower income families do not have private medical insurances and hence to not have access to health care requirements for treatment just as cognitive rehabilitation post ABI . Assistive technology is also seen as an added expense, with many assistive technologies having absorbent costs. These limitations are being addressed through education at a clinical level, advocacy to state services and lobbying for policy changes. A global approach is required to address and allow information sharing to promote achievable service gains(Charters et al., 2015).

The ability to use assistive technology is also concerning as there is a lack of training provided on how these technologies can be used an integrated into daily living. Although smartphones are useful to provide timed-cued reminders, it might be difficult for persons with memory impairment to learn how to use and maintain the device (Olsson et al., 2017). Training therefore should be provide by health care professionals in the field to both the family and client so that once the affected individual is left to function "independently" they are able to use these technologies. Families should also be trained so that they are able to understand the impact ad benefit of using these technologies as well are able to guide there affected family members on how to use the technologies when the need arises

The sensor technology not only supported activities but also influenced the patients by changing behavior, providing a sense of security, independence and increased self-confidence. For the partners, the sensor technology eased daily life, but also gave increased responsibility for maintenance. Technical problems led to frustration and stress for the patients (Olsson et al., 2017). Installing sensor technology with individually pre-recorded voice reminders as memory support in the home had a broad impact on patients' and their families' lives. These effects were both positive and negative. The sensor technology not only supported activities but also influenced the patients by changing behavior, providing a sense of security, independence and increased self-confidence. For the partners, the sensor technology eased daily life, but also gave increased responsibility for maintenance. Technical problems led to frustration and stress for the patients(Olsson, Persson, Bartfai, & Boman, 2017). Based on the abve mentioned theoretical data and reach it is suggested that continuous support and induction to technology is carried out . This will be incorporated into the proposed clinical model with the chapter,

SIGNIFICANCE / CONTRIBUTION TO THE SOCIETY AND KNOWLEDGE

This research will respond to the numerous calls for research in the area of awareness and family support structures following ABI. The current empirical and theoretical findings suggest that minimal research has been conducted in the area of awareness and family support structures of persons post ABI. Therefore this study will contribute to the expansion of knowledge on this issue. There is very little literature on awareness and family support structures of persons following ABI and the use of adaptive technologies in this regard.

The findings of this study have the potential to significantly contribute to practices and policies in society through research by providing a local country-contextual theoretical understanding of what needs to be done for persons with ABI and how AT can be used as a recovery tool within family support structures during the recovery process.

This study further has the potential to contribute to the governance, management, entrepreneurship, psychology and society by exploring an educational perspective on how families currently deal with persons following ABI in South Africa and how they can creatively assist, support and educate families and even communities with the use of adaptive technologies . This study has the potential to make a meaningful contribution in this regard by developing and stimulating a greater interest and improve the interpretation of results of the livelihood and integration in society of persons following ABI in South Africa

RECOMMENDATIONS

The above evidence, analysis and discussions on exiting empirical data and theoretical research indicated that there is a definite lack in awareness, training and funding issues surrounding the adaptability, accessibility and implementation of Assistive Technology in the recovery and family support of people with ABI. The aspect of training can be addressed by professionals in the field who form part of the rehabilitation and recovery treatment of people with ABI. These professionals can provide training to family on how the methods of technology can be used and implemented as well as teach these steps of utilization to their clients. Based Training related to Assistive Technology assessment and acquisition should be included within national health education programmes(Boot et al., 2018). Heath and education programs can be conducted on a introductory based to family so that they become aware of the options of assistive technology and how assistive technology can befit their support to their affected family.

The issue of the lack of awareness of what assistive technology is and the impact that it can have on support to family can be addressed via the use of self-advocacy groups. Self-advocacy groups promote and enhance the participants' personal development and empowerment, giving a greater sense of self determination and autonomy(Boot et al., 2018). These support groups can be formed by affected families and individuals post ABI so that they can meet and provide an awareness and discussions on assistive technologies, the benefits and as well as the support that they have experienced form implementing assistive technology into their daily living. Future research should also focus on triggering of prompting technologies (O'Neill, Best, O'Neill, Ramos, & Gillespie, 2018).

The above mentioned areas can be developed in more depth in future research by scholars in the field who seek to understand the current experiences of families affected by ABI in seeking support, ascertain views held by people affected by ABI regarding the importance of family support, determine the extent to which people affected by ABI are accommodated in society and the way in which support structures could be built using adaptive technology, investigate the level of family support that people affected by ABI experience as part of a society, establish the extent to which people affected by ABI are aware of adaptive technology that can assist them with awareness and support following ABI. The Proposed Clinical Model Family Support Post Acquired Brain Injury (ABI) will therefore assist professionals, scholars and researchers and families in understanding the need and benefit of assistive technology n the family support of ABI. This Clinical Model will also minimise the gap in awareness, training and funding issues surrounding the adaptability, accessibility and implementation of Assistive Technology.

THE PROPOSED CLINICAL MODEL FAMILY SUPPORT POST ACQUIRED BRAIN INJURY (ABI)

Table 1. A Clinical Model

Innovative approaches for the use of Assistive Technologies in Family Support post Acquired Brain Injury			
Clinical model for Family Support post Acquired Brain Injury (ABI)			
Key indicator	**Existing protocol**	**Proposed modification**	**Clinical steps**
Assistive Technology in family support post ABI	Universal acceptance, use and minimal application of Assistive Technology	Integration of Assistive Technology and family support from a diverse range of society, culture and geographical locations	1. Establish local, national and continental and inter-continental relationships/networks between scholars who promote the need for Assistive Technology in family support 2. Create national and continental task teams to advance awareness on Assistive Technology and family support
Playing with boundaries	The use of Assistive Technology for family support s by professional's who adopt a technology based approach that is seen fit for the purposes of development and recovery post ABI	The incorporation of scholarship and processionals in the field of ABI from a diverse range of society, culture and geographical locations	Creating diverse and common practices that can be adopted throughout local, national and continental and inter-continental organizations that will allow diversification and development for future scholars in this area
Transparency of the ideological system	The use of exiting roadmaps of success on Assistive Technology that were used by families and professionals in the field	To create a network and board of scholars with a common understanding of the necessity of transparency and its impact on the successful implementation of Assistive Technology	Develop professional bodies to establish a working group with associates who will function as a means of developing clear and concise information on Assistive Technology so as to ensures that scholars can access. relate to these methods of support wen developing research
Disband the guile system	Dominant Universal acceptance, use and application of Assistive Technology	Development of board and accepting mindsets of scholars towards the future development of Assistive Technology that make room for integration and acceptance in family support	Establish forms where scholars can interact, discuss and develop notions of Assistive Technology so as to disband current guile systems in place
Self-organisation	Personal and opinionated views of scholars in the field of Assistive Technology who expand on research based limited availability of support	Th creation of networks, databases and information sharing of scholars of different continents and cultures	The development of data bases and networks that scholars can readily have access to. Accessibility to guides and protocols by scholars in the field who have provided clarity and transparency of Assistive Technology
Amplified marginalised voices	Assistive Technology that are not being integrated into new and developed research by scholars due to marginalisation and lack of awareness	The development of research teams and networks across national and international boundaries to create an awareness of marginalised voices surrounding the impact of assistive technologies as a means of family support post ABI	Create awareness of the need for inclusivity of practices that are marginalised by integration and adoptability methods established by scholars of local, national and continental and inter-continental bodies
Progressive	Assistive Technology is reconnoitered, and characteristics of related technologies cogitated	Establishing local, national and continental and inter-continental relationships/networks between scholars	Corresponding research and development of scholars in research to work together/ as teams to enhance the impact of assistive technologies on family support post ABI on a global scale who develop guides on the use of Assistive Technology for family support

CONCLUSION

This chapter converges on understanding the concept of assistive technology and family support in the course of theoretical debates in research and recovery and the impact of assistive technology on family support. The discoveries as a result of the theoretical analysis indicate that the notion of assistive technology is reconnoitered, and characteristics of related technologies and methods of recovery cogitated. Assistive technology is thereafter utilised as an analytical stratagem to scrutinize contemporary methods to demonstrate ways in which it has turned out to be undermined and deficient due to its lack of awareness and implementation. The proposal of the clinical model assists scholars in future research in developing progressive research that incorporates improved assistive technology, representative of a multi-faceted globalised world were assistive technology will be more vastly accepted and utilised as a means of family support and recovery globally.

REFERENCES

Behn, N., Marshall, J., Togher, L., & Cruice, M. (2019). Setting and achieving individualized social communication goals for people with acquired brain injury (ABI) within a group treatment. *International Journal of Language & Communication Disorders*, *54*(5), 828–840. doi:10.1111/1460-6984.12488 PMID:31250537

Bockbrader, M. A., Francisco, G., Lee, R., Olson, J., Solinsky, R., & Boninger, M. L. (2018). Brain Computer Interfaces in Rehabilitation Medicine. *PM&R, 10*(9S2), S233-S243. doi:10.1016/j.pmrj.2018.05.028

Boot, F. H., Owuor, J., Dinsmore, J., & MacLachlan, M. (2018). Access to assistive technology for people with intellectual disabilities: A systematic review to identify barriers and facilitators. *Journal of Intellectual Disability Research*, *62*(10), 900–921. doi:10.1111/jir.12532 PMID:29992653

Charters, E., Gillett, L., & Simpson, G. K. (2015). Efficacy of electronic portable assistive devices for people with acquired brain injury: A systematic review. *Neuropsychological Rehabilitation*, *25*(1), 82–121. doi:10.1080/09602011.2014.942672 PMID:25121394

Gómez, J., Montoro, G., Haya, P. A., Alamán, X., Alves, S., & Martínez, M. (2013). Adaptive manuals as assistive technology to support and train people with acquired brain injury in their daily life activities. *Personal and Ubiquitous Computing*, *17*(6), 1117–1126. doi:10.100700779-012-0560-z

Kolk, A., Saard, M., Pertens, L., Kallakas, T., Sepp, K., & Kornet, K. (2019). Structured Model of Neurorehab: A Pilot Study of Modern Multitouch Technology and Virtual Reality Platforms for Training Sociocognitive Deficit in Children with Acquired Brain Injury. *Applied Neuropsychology. Child*, *8*(4), 326–332. doi:10.1080/21622965.2018.1486193 PMID:30295544

Lancioni, G. E., Singh, N. N., O'Reilly, M. F., Sigafoos, J., Alberti, G., & Campodonico, F. (2016). Case Studies of Technology-aided Interventions to Promote Hand Reaching and Standing or Basic Ambulation in Persons with Multiple Disabilities. *Perceptual and Motor Skills*, *122*(1), 200–219. doi:10.1177/0031512516630017 PMID:27420316

Larsson-Lund, M., Kottorp, A., & Malinowsky, C. (2017). Return to work in people with acquired brain injury: Association with observed ability to use everyday technology. *Scandinavian Journal of Occupational Therapy*, *24*(4), 281–289. doi:10.1080/11038128.2016.1194466 PMID:27321247

O'Neill, B., Best, C., O'Neill, L., Ramos, S. D. S., & Gillespie, A. (2018). Efficacy of a Micro-Prompting Technology in Reducing Support Needed by People With Severe Acquired Brain Injury in Activities of Daily Living: A Randomized Control Trial. *The Journal of Head Trauma Rehabilitation*, *33*(5), E33–E41. doi:10.1097/HTR.0000000000000358 PMID:29194177

Oliver, M., Montero, F., Fernández-Caballero, A., González, P., & Molina, J. P. (2015). RGB-D assistive technologies for acquired brain injury: Description and assessment of user experience. *Expert Systems: International Journal of Knowledge Engineering and Neural Networks*, *32*(3), 370–380. doi:10.1111/exsy.12096

Olsson, A., Persson, A.-C., Bartfai, A., & Boman, I.-L. (2017). Sensor technology more than a support. *Scandinavian Journal of Occupational Therapy*, *25*(2), 1–9. doi:10.1080/11038128.2017.1293155 PMID:28276963

Plackett, R., Thomas, S., & Thomas, S. (2016). Professionals' views on the use of smartphone technology to support children and adolescents with memory impairment due to acquired brain injury. *Disability and Rehabilitation. Assistive Technology*, *12*(3), 1–8. doi:10.3109/17483107.2015.1127436 PMID:26730647

Powell, L. E., Glang, A., Pinkelman, S., Albin, R., Harwick, R., Ettel, D., & Wild, M. R. (2015). Systematic instruction of assistive technology for cognition (ATC) in an employment setting following acquired brain injury: A single case, experimental study. *NeuroRehabilitation*, *37*(3), 437–447. doi:10.3233/NRE-151272 PMID:26518534

Raghavendra, P., Newman, L., Grace, E., & Wood, D. (2013). 'I could never do that before': Effectiveness of a tailored Internet support intervention to increase the social participation of youth with disabilities. *Child: Care, Health and Development*, *39*(4), 552–561. doi:10.1111/cch.12048 PMID:23763256

Sakzewski, L., Lewis, M. J., McKinlay, L., Ziviani, J., & Boyd, R. N. (2016). Impact of multi-modal web-based rehabilitation on occupational performance and upper limb outcomes: Pilot randomized trial in children with acquired brain injuries. *Developmental Medicine and Child Neurology*, *58*(12), 1257–1264. doi:10.1111/dmcn.13157 PMID:27230022

Chapter 14
Low Cost, User-Controlled Peroneal Stimulator for Foot Drop in Patients With Stroke:
An Experiment in Indian Rehabilitation Set-Up

Kriti Mishra
https://orcid.org/0000-0002-0047-5933
Independent Researcher, India

Raji Thomas
Christian Medical College, India

ABSTRACT

Foot drop is a common disabling condition following stroke. It has been conventionally managed using an ankle foot orthosis (AFO). An alternate rehabilitation option is the functional electrical stimulation (FES) systems that has undergone numerous improvisations over past few decades to make it more efficient and user friendly. This chapter aims to evaluate a prototype low-cost FES device in an Indian rehabilitation set-up to match the patients' cultural and socio-economic needs. It illustrates a pilot study designed to test the orthotic and clinical efficacy of the device in terms of dynamic ankle angle change during ambulation and comparing the walking speed and endurance with the AFO. A significant change with nearly two-thirds of normal ankle angle change during swing phase of the gait cycle was observed with nearly equivalent orthotic effects in terms of walking endurance and speed. In terms of receptivity, the device received a mixed response from the patients regarding its effectiveness as an orthosis.

INTRODUCTION

Stroke/ Cerebrovascular accident (CVA) is one of the leading causes for acquired neurological disabilities

DOI: 10.4018/978-1-7998-7430-0.ch014

worldwide. In recent decades, a rise in the prevalence of stroke in developing countries like India has been observed (World Health Organization [WHO], 2017). Stroke often results in multiple neurological sequele, impacting not only the patient, but also his/her family resulting in significant financial crisis, thus affecting the quality of life and thereby, adding to the socio-economic burden of the country (WHO, 2017). Hence, rehabilitation of these patients with a context-specific approach is very important.

The spectrum of sequele following stroke range from cognitive and behavioural impairments as well as swallowing and speech deficits to visual dysfunction, motor and sensory impairments (Langhorne et al, 2011). Of these, the motor impairment is the most notable as it affects daily activities and mobility of the patients. Among the motor impairments, weakness of ankle dorsiflexors resulting in foot drop is one of the commonest, leading to difficulty in ground clearance of the foot and consequently, a spectrum of gait impairments (Langhorne et al, 2011). Gait training is hence an important goal of stroke rehabilitation (Jauch et al., 2013; Langhorne et al, 2011). The ankle is supported with an ankle foot orthosis (AFO), which enables the ankle joint to be in neutral position and provides stability to the ankle while the other muscle groups in the affected limb are trained so that the patient can ambulate efficiently (Shahabi et al, 2020). A walking aid like cane or quadripod may be required to assist the ambulation and for safety purposes (Allet et al., 2009).

In past few decades, an alternate option that has been frequently researched and improvised is the Functional Electrical Stimulation (FES) system (Gil-Castillo et al., 2020). In FES system, the electric current is applied to stimulate the nerve or muscle to bring about muscle contraction used for a functional activity. These systems have to be worn by the patient to utilize the muscle contraction and hence, are called neuroprosthesis (Mendes et al, 2020; Takeda et al., 2017). Peroneal Stimulator is the one of the widely explored FES systems for management of foot drop following stroke. This has both orthotic effect by correcting gait abnormalities and also, therapeutic effect by strengthening of muscles and enhancing the voluntary control, promoting recovery in these patients (Kottink et al, 2007, 2008).

Literature reveals that numerous studies have been conducted to compare the efficacy of these systems with traditional AFO in different stages of rehabilitation post-stroke and in different subgroups of patients (Mendes et al, 2020; Prenton et al., 2016). Moreover, research has been conducted to bring about various innovations and improvements in the architectural designs of these systems including trials for non-invasive and invasive devices (Gil-Castillo et al., 2020). Initial trials have been using surface electrodes activated by foot switches. More recently, implantable devices and automatic sensors based on accelerometers and gyroscopes have been tried (Gil-Castillo et al., 2020). Thus, constant attempts have been made to make these devices more user-friendly and with better orthotic efficacy.

However, these available systems are not very cost-effective for a developing country like India, where the cheaper option of AFO is used. Hence, an attempt was made to fabricate a low cost peroneal stimulator in the rehabilitation department of a tertiary care institute in India using an indigenous design. It was also smaller in size and technically simpler than most of the current available devices. After fabrication of the assistive device, a pilot study was conducted to test its efficacy. This chapter elaborates the study conducted with the prototype device. Firstly, it aims to explore the orthotic and clinical efficacy of the device in patients with stroke, comparing it with the standard intervention of AFO in Indian settings. Within Indian context, many patients prefer walking barefoot thereby, avoiding usage of AFOs or footwear within the house. As the device's sensor was mounted on walking aid, it allowed walking bare-foot which is not possible if foot switch based sensor is used. Secondly, as the device was in its pilot phase, its receptivity by the patients was also looked into. Lastly, these findings are discussed in the light of research done so far, providing recommendations for possible future work.

BACKGROUND

Stroke or cerebrovascular accident (CVA) has been defined by World Health Organization as the process of "rapid development of clinical signs and symptoms arising from either a focal or global neurological disturbance of the brain, which lasts for more than 24 hours or longer, may lead to death and has no other apparent cause apart from the vascular origin" (Truelsen et al., 2006). Recently, a newer and broader definition was proposed by the American Stroke Association in 2013 which included both clinical criteria and tissue changes, i.e., the silent pathology (Sacco et al., 2013).

Impact of stroke is based on the affected brain vascular anatomy resulting in specific neurological deficits (Balami et al., 2013). Long term sequelae post-stroke, which can be quite disabling, include mobility problems, sensory problems, urinary and faecal continence problems, neuropathic pain or central post-stroke pain, shoulder pain, fatigue, sexual dysfunction, visual problems, cognitive issues, emotional and mood problems, communication issues like dysphasia, dysarthria etc. (Langhorne et al, 2011; RCP, 2016). All these ultimately impact an individual's activities of daily living (ADL), affecting their financial status and family life, thereby deteriorating the quality of life. (NICE, 2013; RCP, 2016).

Motor impairment restricting mobility is the most easily recognizable impairment post-stroke. These involve changes in motor strength/power, loss of motor control and incoordination, increased tone (spasticity or hypertonia) or contractures. This can result in mobility/gait abnormalities, ataxia, balance issues, movement problems for arm/upper limbs etc. (NICE, 2021; RCP, 2016).

In stroke, there is residual weakness of the limbs with distal muscles being weaker than the proximal. The weakness of the ankle dorsiflexors (muscle groups anterior to the ankle joint) leads to a condition called foot drop (Burridge et al., 2001 as cited in Hwang, 2020, p.1). In normal gait cycle, ankle dorsiflexors keep foot in neutral position at initial contact with the ground during stance phase. They also keep the foot in neutral position and help in clearing the ground for limb advancement during the swing phase (Brockett and Chapman, 2016). In contrast, ankle plantarflexors (muscles posterior to the ankle joint) contract to generate sufficient push-off for the limb advancement during the later stages of stance phase of gait cycle (Brockett and Chapman, 2016). Hence, the ankle plantarflexor spasticity or contracture or overactivity, commonly found in stroke, also contributes to the occurrence of foot drop (Graham, 2010 as cited in Prenton et al., 2016, p.1). This is a common impairment in conditions such as stroke, head injury etc., where upper motor neuronal pathway are affected, collectively called pathologies of central neurological origin (CNO) (Graham, 2010 as cited in Prenton et al., 2016, p.1). In these conditions, the peripheral nerves to the ankle muscles (deep peroneal nerve supplying the dorsiflexors and the tibial nerve for plantarflexors) are intact while the cortical connections are disrupted. In contrast, in lower motor neuron lesions such as peripheral nerve injuries, there is direct damage to these peripheral nerves and cortical connections (corticospinal tracts) are intact (National Health Service [NHS] conditions, 2019).

A number of other typical abnormal movement patterns accompany the foot drop in stroke, namely, reduced knee flexion during swing and stance phases (spastic paretic stiff-legged gait), knee hyperextension (dynamic recurvatum) during stance, and excessive ankle plantar flexion (equinus) during swing and/or stance (Perry and Burnfield, 2010 as cited in Hwang, 2020, p.2). Hence, many stroke survivors develop gait maneuvers to compensate for these impairments (Perry and Burnfield, 2010 as cited in Hwang, 2020, p.2). For instance, hip circumduction, hip hiking, and contralateral vaulting with excessive elevation of the pelvis is often commonly employed to avoid the toe drag and foot drop in these patients. Thus, the foot drop combined with the above gait abnormalities lead to reduction in ambulation speed resulting in slower walk, associated increased energy cost while ambulation, less efficient and potentially unsafe walk due to the associated increased risk of falls and poor quality of life (Graham, 2010 as cited in Prenton et al., 2016, p. 1)

The guidelines by NICE (2013) recommends at least 45 minutes of relevant rehabilitation therapy initially for a period of minimum 5 days per week for people who have the ability to participate, and where functional goals can be achieved. If more therapy is required for later stages, it has to be modified according to the person's needs at that time. Gait training is suggested for patients who can walk, either with or without assistance, in order to improve the endurance and speed of walking (NICE, 2021; RCP, 2016).

Usage of Ankle–foot orthoses (AFO) is recommended for those post-stroke patients who have difficulty in swing-phase foot clearance and/or stance-phase control issues such that it affects their walking (NICE, 2021). It is fabricated from metal/leather, thermoplastics, carbon, graphite, or a hybrid design assembly incorporating some or all the mentioned materials (NICE, 2013; RCP, 2016). It can be of various types, solid ankle, articulated type, leaf spring type, to name a few. AFO provides foot clearance in the swing phase of the gait cycle thereby prevent tripping and falling. It also improves the stance-phase control by preventing knee and ankle collapse or by preventing knee hyper-extension (Shahabi et al, 2020). Effectiveness of AFO is determined in terms of speed, ease of walking and comfort (Shahabi et al, 2020; Tyson and Kent, 2013). Assessment for donning and doffing of AFO, fitting and gait training with AFO must be performed under guidance of rehab professionals as a part of stroke rehabilitation programme (NICE, 2021; RCP, 2016)

Another alternative to AFO that has been repeatedly researched and improvised upon is the FES system or the Drop foot system (NICE, 2021; RCP, 2016). Electrical stimulation can be used for therapeutic or functional purposes in rehabilitation. Therapeutic stimulation induces physiological changes that are persistent even after stimulation is over, thereby, improving voluntary contraction and decreasing or preventing further impairment as a consequence of immobilization or disuse atrophy (Takeda et al., 2017). However, the systems giving electric stimulation to bring about the functional activity have to be donned by the user because their effect lasts till the time the FES application system is switched on. They, therefore, act as replacement for the lost function and are called neuroprosthesis (Melo, 2015 and Popović, 2014 as cited in Mendes et al, 2020, p. 2). Numerous neuroprosthesis have been tried to facilitate functional activity in paralysed lower limbs affected by UMN lesions (like traumatic brain injury, stroke), as the peripheral nervous system is still intact in these patients. One of the most experimented is drop foot stimulator. Drop foot stimulator or peroneal stimulator involves application of electric current to stimulate intact peroneal nerve to generate muscle contraction and enhance gait by improving foot clearance during swing phase and stability during initial stance phase (Takeda et al., 2017).

FES systems have broadly a common architecture comprising of an integrated sensor network or electrodes, a stimulator, and a controller having a control algorithm (Gil-Castillo et al., 2020). The stimulator produces current waveforms for multiple cathodes and this current is delivered to the excitable tissue via the electrodes. The controller regulates the stimulation according to the user. Technical advances have been achieved in each of these components in recent decades. Portable, lightweight stimulation devices with wireless control units, operated through tablet, smartphone or screen are fabricated nowadays (Gil-Castillo et al., 2020). Besides, the stimulation units now consist of a multichannel system providing impulses to multiple muscles groups simultaneously, which are used for management of muscle fatigue or pathologies apart from ankle dorsiflexor weakness (Gil-Castillo et al., 2020). The stimulation parameters determining the waves of current pulses and therefore strength of a muscle contraction include the pulse frequency, amplitude, and duration. The ideal stimulation frequency is the lowest frequency producing a fused contraction. Studies recommend square pulse, symmetrically compensated biphasic-pulses, and trapezoidal-shape wave as the most efficient (Gil-Castillo et al., 2020). Electrodes used include an active electrode or cathode placed near the nerve or muscle motor point to be stimulated and the return electrode or anode over less excitable tissue (tendon or fascia). Additional electrodes are required in multichannel FES systems to bring about simultaneous activation of multiple muscles in a coordinated manner (Gil-Castillo et al., 2020). Based on arrangement of the electrodes, the neuroprosthesis can be categorized as surface type, percutaneous type, or implanted type (Gil-Castillo et al., 2020; Takeda et al., 2017). Limitations related to the surface systems include issues with effort of setup, skin irritation and pain, which in-turn affects the compliance and satisfaction (Taylor, 2010 as cited in Prenton et al., 2016, p. 1). In contrast, the implanted systems addressing these limitations are more costly and not very cost-effective for most of the patients (Prenton et al., 2016). Recently, electrode arrays with self-calibration system allowing proper selection of virtual electrodes have been experimented to attain optimal dorsiflexion. Examples of such a device include ShefStim, DeltaStim etc. that can become an effective non-invasive alternative for future (Gil-Castillo et al., 2020). The controller enables correct detection of gait phase, which is a crucial aspect in FES systems. Different methods can used as a controller ranging from simple switch modulated by the patient such as foot-switches, hand-switches to artificial sensors and recently, natural sensors that record patient's bio-potentials (e.g., EMG or EEG) (Gil-Castillo et al., 2020).

Numerous studies have reported functional and clinical efficacy of FES systems for foot drop. These systems have demonstrated clinically meaningful improvement in walking speed, reduction of effort during walking and spasticity (Street, 2015; Taylor, 2013 as cited in Gil-Castillo et al., 2020). Dunning, 2015; Kottink, 2004 and Prenton 2016 have suggested patients with stroke benefitting from the orthotic effect of PS with task improvements noted while using these systems (as cited in Mendes et al, 2020, p. 8). Cowan 2012; Moss 2011 and Sheffler 2009 found enhanced performance of functional activities in the home and community settings in people with stroke using these devices (as cited in Mendes et al, 2020, p.8). Studies comparing the system with the conventional AFO have proven to have positive equivalent effect on walking (Prenton et al., 2016). However, the evidence that the drop foot system is more beneficial than AFO is lacking (Mendes et al, 2020). The specific, active repetitive movements brought by the FES system induce long-lasting improvements (even when the stimulation is off), by facilitating the neuroplasticity mechanisms, enabling the motor relearning by activating the motor-related areas of the cortex and their residual corticospinal pathways as evidenced in functional MRI (fMRI) studies (Ambrosini 2011; Dunning 2015; Everaert 2010 and Prenton 2016 as cited in Mendes et al, 2020). In most of the trials, the peroneal stimulator has been tried in the chronic phase of the stroke. Only few studies have investigated its use in the acute and sub-acute phases (Dunning et al., 2009; Sabut et al., 2011). Currently, FES systems are being tried outside the clinical settings, on a daily use basis (Mendes et al, 2020).

NICE guidelines, 2013 have recommended the use of FES system. There is adequate evidence on its safety and efficacy in terms of improving gait in drop foot arising from central neurological origin such that its usage can be supported (NICE, 2021). The commercially available devices like ODFS Pace and Pace XL stimulators cost around 670 GBP and 995 GBP, respectively and the overall treatment cost per person is £3,320 and £4,325 over 5 years respectively (NICE, 2016).

Therefore, exploring low cost-effective options for developing countries like India is essential so that both rural and urban population in these regions can avail them uniformly. Moreover, the incidence of stroke has doubled in low- and middle-income countries over past four decades (WHO, 2017). Furthermore, stroke in young is more prevalent for these countries, where on an average, it occurs 15 years earlier as compared to the high-income countries. Thus, the condition mainly affect individuals at the peak of their productive life leading to more disability in them and also, impacting the country's socio-economic development significantly (WHO, 2017). In such a scenario, it is essential to not only improve the acute treatment set-ups, but also strengthen the available rehabilitation services in the country, so that patients irrespective of their socio-economic status can access them (WHO, 2017). Simultaneously, finding context-specific rehabilitation options relevant within the socio-cultural set-up also enhances the chances of continuing these rehabilitative interventions.

Keeping this in mind, the present study is designed for trial of indigenously designed prototype of drop foot (FES) system in an Indian rehabilitation settings. It involved devising a stimulator with hand-switch, making it technically simpler and more adaptable device for use, the sensor being a user-controlled switch. The stimulator was adapted to the Indian settings, mainly in terms of its low cost, small size and no requirement for a foot switch, thereby allowing bare-foot walking that is more prevalent in rural region. The study aimed to test the efficacy of device as an orthosis, followed by its comparison with the conventional treatment of AFO in terms of walking and the response of patients towards the device. Its usage was tested during the rehabilitation of patients in the sub-acute and chronic phases of stroke, which largely is the stroke population admitted in the given rehabilitation set-up.

METHODOLOGY

Settings and Location of the Study

The study was conducted at the Department of Physical Medicine and Rehabilitation at Christian Medical College, located in Vellore town of the southern state Tamil Nadu in India.

Study Design

A pilot study was opted for in order to test the feasibility of the device. A control group was also chosen for comparative analysis with the conventional treatment and randomization was done to reduce the bias. Thus, a pilot phase parallel group study design was opted for.

Participants

Persons with hemiplegia secondary to cerebrovascular accident were chosen.

Inclusion Criteria

1. Age 18 - 70 years (including stroke in young patients)
2. Adequate cognition and communication abilities (> 18/30 on MMSE) to operate the device
3. History of independent mobility function prior to stroke, including walking with assistive device
4. Duration post-stroke: 2 weeks to 1 year
5. Inability to dorsiflex the ankle leading to lack of foot clearance during swing phase of gait
6. Ankle dorsiflexion passive range of motion coming to at least neutral in affected lower limb.
7. Ability to walk 5 meters using AFO and quadripod inside parallel bar, before recruiting

Exclusion Criteria

1. Implants such as cardiac pacemaker or vagal nerve stimulator generating electrical signals or implants in lower limb having metal parts
2. Lower motor neuron disease or injury resulting in inadequate response to stimulation
3. Significant swelling in affected leg extending up to knee
4. Disease limiting wearing of orthosis such as venous stasis or history of lower extremity ulcer, chronic skin condition or peripheral neuropathy
5. Pregnancy
6. Pain in affected leg of more than 5 on a 10-point visual analog scale
7. Pre-existing orthopedic condition or history of pain that could limit ambulatory progress (eg: total hip or knee replacement, limited ROM, arthritis) or Contracture of ankle

Sample Size

20 (10 each in experimental and control group).

Intervention

Indigenously designed Peroneal Nerve Stimulator (PS) having three components, namely, a pair of surface electrodes (square-shaped and re-usable), an electrical stimulator with in-built microprocessor based controller and a hand switch mounted on the quadripod (Figure 1). The stimulator was an in-house development of Bioengineering Department at the institution. It was operated using a small mobile phone battery and had following specifications: frequency= 20 Hertz, pulse amplitude=70 milli-amperes, pulse width= 250 microseconds. The stimulator was controlled by a push-button switch, and was normally off.

The cathode electrode was placed over common peroneal nerve (identified 2 cm below the head of fibula where the nerve winds around the fibular neck) and the anode electrode was placed over the anterior compartment muscles. The position of the electrodes over the nerve and muscle group was adjusted so that maximum ankle dorsiflexion was noticed. The usual inter-electrode distance was around 4 cm. The electrodes were connected through wires to the portable stimulator, which in-turn was kept in the trouser pocket of the participant, if they wanted to. The stimulator was further connected through wires to the hand-switch placed on the quadripod held by the participant on the unaffected side for support and safety while ambulating.

On pressing the switch by the patient during the pre-swing phase of gait of the affected limb, the electric stimuli was generated and transmitted via the electrodes to the common peroneal nerve. This activated the ankle and toes dorsiflexors causing ankle lift resulting in ground clearance during the swing phase for the affected limb. As the limb progressed towards initial contact of the stance phase, the participant would release the switch and stimulation would stop. Since the switch release was done at the initial contact, the stimulation continued till initial loading response and helped in smooth foot contact, thereby preventing the foot slap. Hence, the switch function was co-ordinated manually with different gait-phases and required the patients to voluntarily control their movement.

Of the three weeks training with PS, initial 4 days were given to the patients as 'familiarisation time' to get used to the stimulator and understanding the mechanism of operating and co-ordination of the switch. Thereafter, the patient practised gait training with the PS and quadripod for one hour during

Figure 1. User-controlled Peroneal Nerve Drop Foot System (PS)

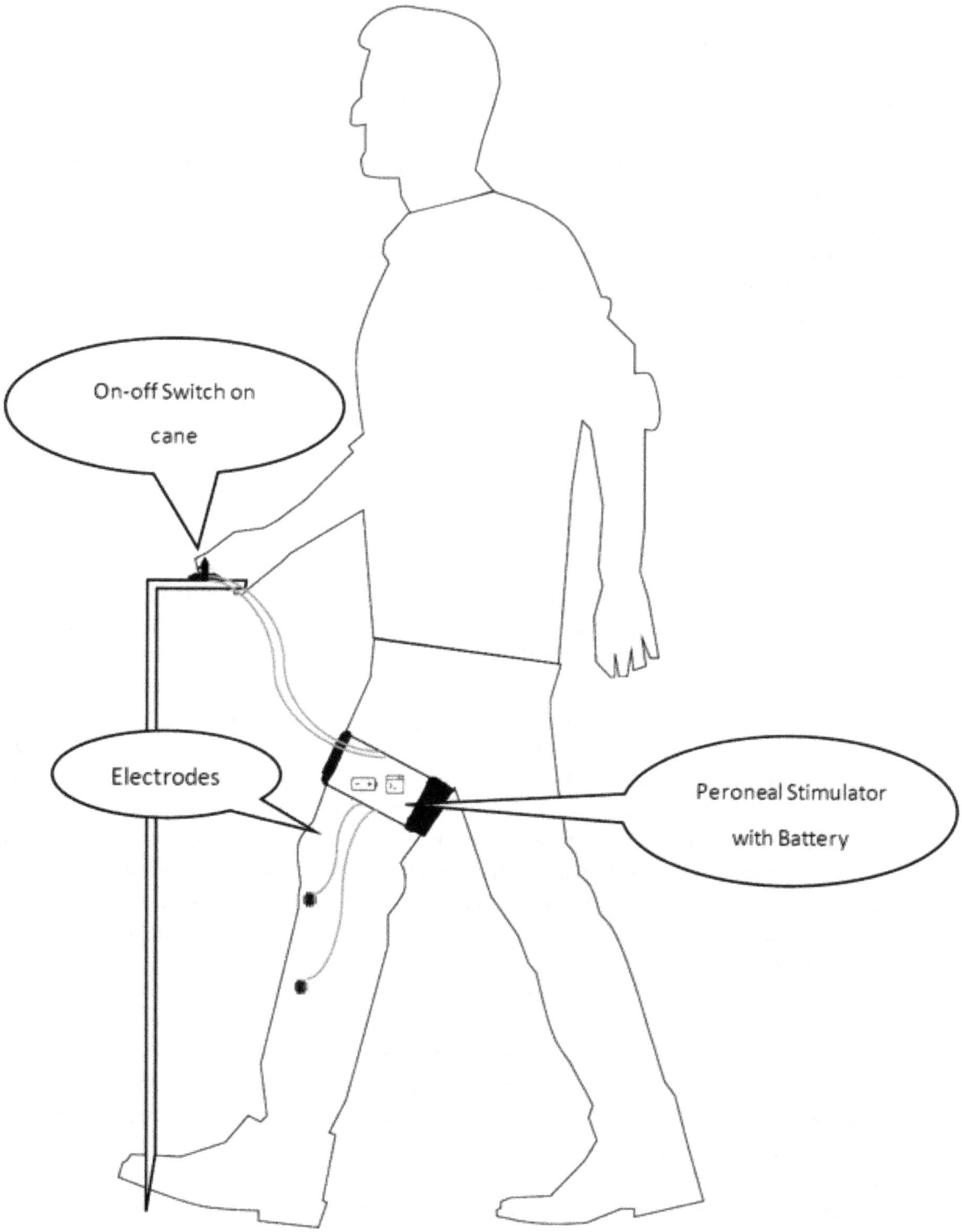

the therapy time, under supervision. For the remaining therapy hours in the day, training was continued with conventional AFO and walking aid, as suitable for the patient's functional requirement. This was done because the patients couldn't be sent home with device in the pilot phase and had to be discharged from the hospital ultimately with an AFO. Hence, it was necessary for them to be used to ambulating with AFO as well.

Control

In this group, patients received gait training using AFO and walking aid all throughout the therapy hours, based on their requirement.

Implementation

Approval was obtained from the Institutional Review Board and Ethics committee. Based on the inclusion/exclusion criteria, participants were recruited by the principal investigator after obtaining an informed written consent. All the participants received rehabilitative therapy (physiotherapy and occupational therapy), so that they are able to ambulate for 5 meters within parallel bars. Being a pilot study, and both stimulator and AFO being applied externally, blinding and masking was difficult. However, the outcome assessor was a neutral person and was not directly involved with the study. A pre-intervention analysis of the outcome measures was done by this neutral assessor. To minimise bias, block randomisation (block size= 5) was done by the statistician and the random allocation sequence was computer generated and concealed in opaque envelopes. Thereafter, the statistician (not involved in the study) disclosed to the principal investigator the group to which the particular patient was assigned to. The participants were accordingly assigned to the respective therapists for the intervention and control group for 3 weeks. At the end of 3 weeks, post-intervention analysis was performed for both groups and a feedback form was used for the intervention group to assess the patients' satisfaction with the device.

Outcome Measures

As aforementioned, the FES systems provide stimulation to ankle dorsiflexors, preventing the ankle drop such that an individual can achieve sufficient ground clearance during the swing phase of gait cycle to avoid any tripping/falls, foot drag or equinus deformity (Melo et al., 2015 as cited in Gil-Castillo et al, 2020, p. 3). Hence, it was decided to evaluate the device orthotic efficacy by measuring the amount of ankle dorsiflexion achieved to provide ground clearance while stimulation is on. Further, its orthotic effectiveness as a substitute for AFO was judged based on its usefulness in gait/ambulation. This was tested through measuring the speed and endurance while walking wearing the device.

Dynamic Range of Motion of Ankle (During Ambulation)

The ankle angle change for the PS group is calculated during the period from switching on of the stimulator up to its switch off time. It was calculated from video analysis of the gait cycle of each participant. The change in ankle angle is timed according to different phases of gait cycle and the difference between maximum plantarflexion during the pre-swing phase and maximum dorsiflexion during the mid-swing phase was taken as the ankle angle change.

The ankle angle in control group using AFO was taken as neutral (0 degrees).

Walking Endurance

The 6 minute walk test (6MWT) was used to measure gait endurance. It assesses the distance walked in time period of 6 minutes over an even surface, at a speed preferred by the participants (Bethoux et al., 2014).

Walking Speed

It was assessed in two ways:

Based on 10 meters walk test (10 Meter WT): In this test, the individual walks a distance of 10 meters with or without assistive device at a self-selected "comfortable speed" and at "as-fast-as-possible" speed. The time taken for initial and last 2 meters is not used for measurement to accommodate for the acceleration and deceleration while walking. The starting time is when foot crosses 2 meters mark and stop time is when the foot crosses 8 meters and this intermediate time duration for the intermediate 6 meters is considered. A total of 3 trials is done and an average of the three time durations is taken. The speed is obtained in meters per second (m/s) by dividing the 6 meters with the calculated average time (Kottink et al., 2007).

Based on 6 min WT: Walking speed was calculated by dividing the distance walked in 6 minutes by 360 seconds (6min = 360s). This was done to note if any changes in speed occurred while walking a larger distance as compared to the 10 meters (Kottink et al., 2007).

Statistical Analysis and Methods

Data collection and outcome assessment was done by a neutral assessor (gait lab co-ordinator) both for pre and post-intervention analysis. The Shapiro-Wilk test was used to calculate the normal distribution of data. The continuous variables within the group were assessed using Wilcoxon Signed-Rank Test to check for the pre and post-intervention effect. For inter-group comparison, Mann-Whitney U Test was used. Spearman's rank correlation coefficient (Spearman's rho) was used for correlation of outcome measures with cognitive function level (MMSE score) and duration after acute stroke event during the subgroup analyses.

RESULTS

Recruitment, Screening and Randomization

In the pilot phase, twenty patients were needed. More than two hundred patients affected with stroke were screened over a period of one year for their eligibility to participate in the study based on the inclusion criteria. Of these, 45 patients were found to match the inclusion criteria. Among them, 13 patients were excluded based on the exclusion criteria and 9 patients refused to consent for the study. Three other patients were found to have significant behavioural issues, which hindered their participation in the rehabilitation programme. The remaining twenty patients were enrolled into the study and randomized into

Table 1. Demographic details of 10 participants each in AFO and PS group

Characteristics		Peroneal stimulator	AFO
Age (mean +/SD)		45.8 +/- 13.73	56.3 +/- 8.95
Gender (Male/Female)		10 / 0	9 / 1
CVA Type	Haemorrhage (H)	2	2
	Ischemic (I)	8	8
Affected side	Right	5	5
	Left	5	5
MMSE score post-stroke	18 - 23	5	5
	24 - 30	5	5
Treatment group (T) in acute phase	T1 (rt-PA)	1	2
	T2 (conservative)	6	2
	T3 (surgical decompression)	2	6
	T4 (rt-PA & decompression)	1	0
Duration since stroke	< 3 months	6	4
	3 – 6 months	1	3
	> 6 months	3	3

intervention group (PS) and control group (AFO), with 10 participants in each group. The participants received treatment for 3 weeks at the rehabilitation institute and were analysed for outcomes measures both pre and post-training. During the study, there were no drop-outs.

Demographic and Clinical Characteristics

The baseline parameters regarding the type of stroke, affected side of motor dysfunction and cognitive level, determined through Mini-Mental State Examination (MMSE) was uniform between the two groups. The details of these parameters are mentioned in table 1. There were differences noted among the participants between the group mainly in terms of the type of treatment received for the acute event and the duration following the acute event. On one hand, 6 patient in the intervention group had acute episode within 3 months, 1 had stroke between 3 to 6 months and 3 had onset of stroke more than six months ago. On the other hand, the control group had a more uniform distribution of patients with 4 patients within 3 months, 3 within 3- 6 months and 3 had the stroke more than six months ago. Among the intervention group, 60% were managed conservatively (non-surgically and no thrombolysis) while 60% of the control group patients were treated with decompressive surgeries.

Outcome Measures

Dynamic Ankle Range of Movement

For 10 patients in PS group, a mean ankle angle change of 11.31 ± 3.56 degrees (between pre-swing to mid-swing phase) was observed while these patients walked using the PS device. This was nearly two-third of the normal ankle angle change of 18 ± 2 degrees (that had been previously determined in the department's gait lab for the normal subjects). Details of the ankle angle change for each patient in PS is enlisted in table 2.

Table 2. Ankle angle change before (Maximum Drop) and during stimulation (Maximum Lift) for 10 patients in PS group

Sl. No	Maximum Drop in Ankle angle from neutral	Maximum Lift in Ankle angle from neutral	Difference
1	-30.08	-15.95	14.13
2	-23.2	-12.03	11.17
3	-26.08	-14.27	11.81
4	-7.88	2.74	10.62
5	-16.49	-2.29	14.2
6	-20.61	-16.41	4.2
7	-19.66	-12	7.66
8	-18.19	-7.62	10.52
9	-26.33	-9.3	17.03
10	-25.02	-13.24	11.78
Mean			11.312
SD			3.56663801

A graphic illustration of the ankle angle change between different phases of gait cycle, (depicted in figure 2) was done for one of the patients in the PS group, which matched nearly the trajectory of the ankle angle change as seen during the gait cycle for a normal individual (shown in figure 3).

Figure 2. Trajectory for ankle change in patient using PS

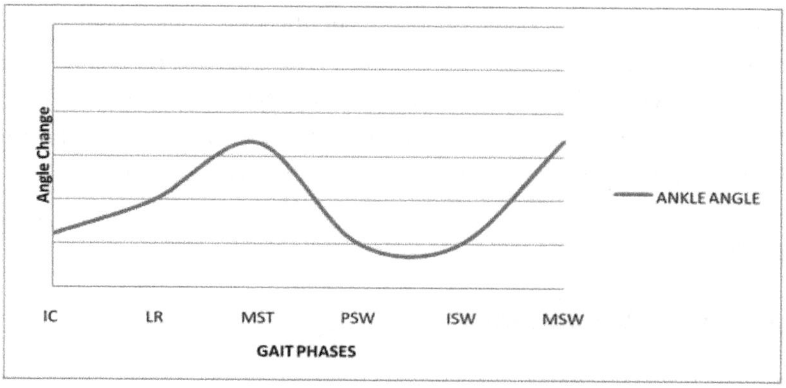

Figure 3. Normal Ankle angle change during gait cycle in normal individuals

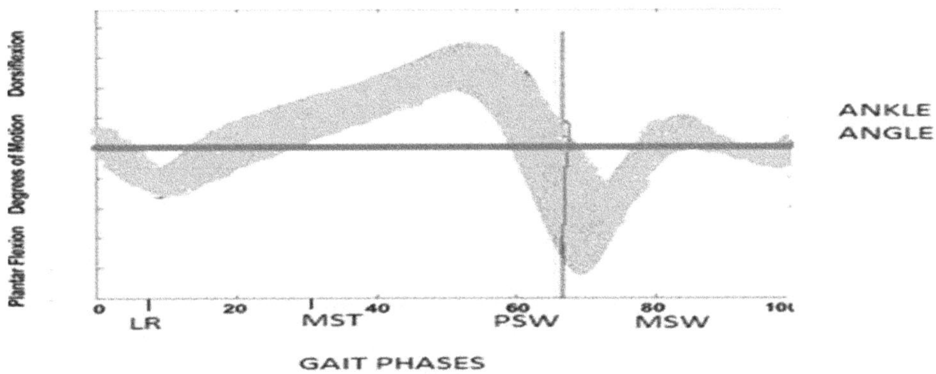

Walking Endurance (6 Minute Walk Test)

At the end of 3 weeks, there was improvement in the mean walking endurance for both the PS and AFO groups (Mean= 18.32, S.D. = 42.76 and Mean: 19.41, S.D. = 29.14, respectively). Further, no statistically significant change in endurance was observed between the PS and the AFO groups (Z-Score: 0.26458, p-value: 0.79486, not significant at $p < .05$, U-value: 46, $p < .05$ is 23). Besides, pre-post intra-group analysis showed statistically insignificant result for PS group (Z score: -1.1722, p-value: 0.242, not significant at $p < .05$) and for the AFO group (Z-score: -1.6818, p-value: 0.09296, not significant at $p < .05$). Details are shown in table 3.

Walking Speed

Based on 6 min Walk Test

At the end of 3 weeks, there was improvement in the mean walking speed for both the PS and AFO groups (Mean= 0.05, S.D. = 0.119 and Mean: 0.05, S.D. = 0.076, respectively. Further, no statistically significant change in speed was observed between the PS and the AFO groups (Z-Score: 0.6425, p-value: 0.522, not significant at $p < .05$, U-value: 41, $p < .05$ is 23). Besides, pre-post intra-group analysis showed no statistically significant difference for both PS group (Z score: -1.172, p-value: 0.242, not significant at $p < .05$) and the AFO group (Z-score: -1.631, p-value: 0.103, not significant at $p < .05$). Details are shown in table 4.

Based on 10 meters Walk Test

An improvement in the mean walking speed was noted for both PS and AFO groups at the end of 3 weeks (Mean= 0.054, S.D. = 0.12 and Mean: 0.074, S.D. = 0.098, respectively). Further, the speed between the groups was not found to be statistically significant (z-score: 0.64254, p-value: 0.522, not significant at $p < .05$, U-value: 41, the critical value of U at $p < .05$ is 23). The within-group analysis for pre-post effect showed no statistically significant change for PS group (Z score: -1.0703, p-value: 0.284, significant at $p < .05$), but statistically significant change for the AFO group (Z score: -1.9876, p-value: 0.0466, significant at $p < .05$). Details for the walking speed are illustrated in table 5.

Table 3. 6 min test for 10 participants in AFO and PS Group. Pre = Pre-study, Post = Post-study, Post-Pre = Difference between Post and Pre Value.

Sl. No		AFO (m)			Stimulator (m)		
		Pre	Post	Post-Pre	Pre	Post	Post-Pre
1		52	95	43	20.5	47.35	26.85
2		150.8	142	-8.8	72	85.2	13.2
3		26	59	33	70.75	66	-4.75
4		61	138	77	54.8	50	-4.8
5		27	55	28	45	46	1
6		23	32	9	66	192	126
7		70	53	-17	74	121.3	47.3
8		36.4	43	6.6	66	59	-7
9		61	95	34	62.6	38	-24.6
10		36.7	26	-10.7	64	74	10
Mean		54.39	73.8	19.41	59.56	77.885	18.32
SD		37.72	41.71	29.14	16.19	46.89	42.75
Within group	Z-Score	-1.6818			-1.1722		
	p-value	0.09296			0.242		
Inter group	Z-Score	0.2645					
	p-value	0.79486					

Additional Analysis of the Data

The dynamic ankle angle change and the walking speed based on 10 meter WT had a statistically significant inverse strong association (r_s = -0.72121, p (2-tailed) = 0.01857). In other words, an increase in ankle change was associated with decrease in speed change. However, the dynamic ankle angle change showed only a moderate inverse correlation with the walking endurance and the walking speed based on 6MWT, which was not statistically significant (r_s = -0.46667, p (2-tailed) = 0.17394). As expected, a statistically significant association was observed for the walking speed obtained from 6 MWT and walking speed based on 10 meter WT for both the intervention and control group (r_s = 0.87879, p (2-tailed) = 0.00081 and r_s = 0.90303, p (2-tailed) = 0.00034, respectively).

Further, subgroup analysis was done to correlate the above outcome measures with the duration since stroke and cognitive level (MMSE score), details of which are mentioned in the table 6 and 7 respectively.

User Feedback

The user feedback about satisfaction with device was administered on the 10 patients in the PS group to know their difficulties and preferences. First, 5 patients preferred PS over AFO, 3 patients liked AFO more and 2 patients were indecisive regarding which of the two is better. Second, of the 10 patients, 6 did not feel any difficulty in using the device; 3 patients felt the coordination of the switch with the ambulation as a difficult feature and the remaining 1 patient found it difficult to re-learn a new walking

Table 4. Walking speed (m/s) based on 6 min Walk test for 10 participants in AFO and PS group. Pre = Pre-study, Post = Post-study, Post-Pre = Difference between Post and Pre Value.

<table>
<tr><th colspan="2" rowspan="2">Sl. No</th><th colspan="3">AFO (m/s)</th><th colspan="3">Stimulator (m/s)</th><th></th></tr>
<tr><th>Pre</th><th>Post</th><th>Post-pre</th><th>Pre</th><th>Post</th><th>Post-pre</th><th></th></tr>
<tr><td colspan="2">1</td><td>0.144</td><td>0.264</td><td>0.12</td><td>0.057</td><td>0.132</td><td>0.075</td><td></td></tr>
<tr><td colspan="2">2</td><td>0.418</td><td>0.394</td><td>-0.024</td><td>0.2</td><td>0.236</td><td>0.036</td><td></td></tr>
<tr><td colspan="2">3</td><td>0.072</td><td>0.164</td><td>0.092</td><td>0.196</td><td>0.183</td><td>-0.013</td><td></td></tr>
<tr><td colspan="2">4</td><td>0.169</td><td>0.383</td><td>0.214</td><td>0.152</td><td>0.139</td><td>-0.013</td><td></td></tr>
<tr><td colspan="2">5</td><td>0.075</td><td>0.153</td><td>0.078</td><td>0.125</td><td>0.128</td><td>0.003</td><td></td></tr>
<tr><td colspan="2">6</td><td>0.064</td><td>0.088</td><td>0.024</td><td>0.183</td><td>0.533</td><td>0.35</td><td></td></tr>
<tr><td colspan="2">7</td><td>0.194</td><td>0.147</td><td>-0.047</td><td>0.205</td><td>0.337</td><td>0.132</td><td></td></tr>
<tr><td colspan="2">8</td><td>0.101</td><td>0.119</td><td>0.018</td><td>0.183</td><td>0.164</td><td>-0.019</td><td></td></tr>
<tr><td colspan="2">9</td><td>0.169</td><td>0.264</td><td>0.095</td><td>0.174</td><td>0.105</td><td>-0.069</td><td></td></tr>
<tr><td colspan="2">10</td><td>0.102</td><td>0.072</td><td>0.03</td><td>0.177</td><td>0.205</td><td>0.028</td><td></td></tr>
<tr><td colspan="2">Mean</td><td>0.15</td><td>0.2</td><td>0.05</td><td>0.17</td><td>0.22</td><td>0.05</td><td></td></tr>
<tr><td colspan="2">SD</td><td>0.105</td><td>0.12</td><td>0.07627</td><td>0.045</td><td>0.1302</td><td>0.11883</td><td></td></tr>
<tr><td rowspan="2">Within group</td><td>Z-Score</td><td colspan="3">-1.631</td><td colspan="4">-1.172</td></tr>
<tr><td>p-value</td><td colspan="3">0.103</td><td colspan="4">0.242</td></tr>
<tr><td rowspan="2">Inter group</td><td>Z-Score</td><td colspan="7">0.6425</td></tr>
<tr><td>p-value</td><td colspan="7">p-value: 0.522 not significant at p < .05</td></tr>
</table>

pattern after having been trained with the AFO. These last 4 patients also felt that the accommodation time of 4 days was too short to adjust to the device. Last, no adverse effects or harms were seen or reported throughout the study in usage of the device.

DISCUSSION

This study aimed to study the orthotic effect of a user-controlled hand-switch based peroneal nerve stimulator and compare it with the conventional management of using AFO in patients with foot drop following stroke. The results brought forth many notable findings and deduction, which are mentioned in the subsequent section.

To begin with, the immediate orthotic effect was demonstrated through the dynamic ankle angle change in the PS group, which was a significant finding of the study. In designed device, the gait phase of pre-swing to mid-swing corresponds to the phase in which stimulation of PS device is on. The database for the normal subjects in the department's gait lab have shown a mean ankle angle of 13 $\pm$ 2 degree in the pre-swing phase and the mean ankle angle of 5 $\pm$ 2 degree in the mid-swing phase, thus making the total ankle angle change from the pre-swing to mid-swing to be 18 $\pm$ 2 degrees. In the current study, the PS group was able to achieve ankle angle change of 11 $\pm$ 3 degrees during this phase of gait cycle, which

Table 5. Walking speed (m/s) based on 10 meter walk test for 10 participants in AFO and PS Group. Pre = Pre-study, Post = Post-study, Post-Pre = Difference between Post and Pre Value.

Sl. No		AFO (m/s)			Stimulator (m/s)			
		Pre	Post	Post-pre	Pre	Post	Post-pre	
1		0.187	0.375	0.188	0.086	0.14	0.054	
2		0.5	0.46	-0.04	0.176	0.24	0.064	
3		0.079	0.177	0.098	0.207	0.2	-0.007	
4		0.19	0.46	0.268	0.167	0.154	-0.0128	
5		0.079	0.182	0.103	0.128	0.113	-0.0145	
6		0.072	0.095	0.023	0.25	0.6	0.35	
7		0.188	0.154	-0.034	0.214	0.353	0.139	
8		0.058	0.11	0.052	0.15	0.154	0.004	
9		0.167	0.25	0.083	0.182	0.107	-0.075	
10		0.11	0.107	-0.003	0.154	0.188	0.034	
Mean		0.163	0.237	0.074	0.171	0.225	0.054	
SD		0.13	0.144	0.098	0.046	0.15	0.12	
Within group	Z-Score	-1.9876			-1.0703			
	p-value	0.046 (significant)			0.284			
Inter group	Z-Score	0.6425						
	p-value	0.522 not significant at $p < .05$						

was nearly two-third of the normal range. This finding is essential for proving the feasibility of the PS as an orthotic device. Most of the previous studies have measured the ankle active and passive ROM using a goniometer and kinematic and kinetic analysis for the dynamic ankle dorsiflexion in the swing phase and plantar flexion in the stance phase. The case series by Sheffler et al. (2013) did not find any device effect on the peak dorsiflexion in swing with statistically insignificant values for the transcutaneous PS, AFO and no device group. In contrast, Kottink et al. (2012) noted a significant change in the minimum

Table 6. Correlation of duration of stroke event to outcome measures

Outcome measures	AFO		PS	
	Correlation co-efficient	Significance (2-tailed)	Correlation co-efficient	Significance (2-tailed)
6-min pre	0.138	0.703	-0.313	0.378
6-min post	0.248	0.49	-0.645	0.044
10 m pre	0.023	0.951	0.014	0.97
10 m post	-0.01	0.979	-0.52	0.123
Ankle angle change	--	--	0.652	0.041

Table 7. Correlation of cognitive level (MMSE score) to outcome measures

Outcome measures	AFO		PS	
	Correlation co-efficient	Significance (2-tailed)	Correlation co-efficient	Significance (2-tailed)
6-min pre	0.064	0.86	-0.441	0.202
6-min post	-0.254	0.479	-0.567	0.087
10 m pre	0.159	0.661	-0.492	0.148
10 m post	-0.131	0.717	-0.686	0.029
Ankle angle change	--	--	0.711	0.021

ankle dorsiflexion angle achieved in the swing phase and thereby, a significantly reduced ankle plantar flexion during swing in the PS group; concluding implantable PS an effective option in providing ankle dorsiflexion during the swing phase of gait cycle. This is similar to the findings in the present study.

In addition, there was no statistically significant difference between the two (PS and AFO) groups in terms of improvement in walking speed and endurance, at the end of 3 weeks of intervention with the respective devices on. Similar findings have been reported by previous studies, although they studied the changes after longer usage of the device and AFO. The studies by Everaert et al. (2013), P. Kluding et al. (2013) and Sheffler et al. (2013) found no significant difference 'between the two groups' at the end of 6 weeks, 30 weeks and 30 weeks respectively. Bethoux et al. (2014, 2015) reported no statistically significant between-group difference for walking speed and 6MWT after 6 months and 12 months of the PS device and AFO usage. A meta-analysis by Prenton et al. (2016) included studies using device in the ward environment and found equivalent orthotic effects of both FES device and AFO on walking speed and endurance for foot drop on stroke participants. A recent review by Mendes et al. (2020) observed both strategies having similar effects on walking speed until six months of device use and low-certainty evidence of no additional benefit on walking speed by using either of the devices between 6 and 12 months of device use. Moreover, there is a low-certainty evidence of motor neuroprosthesis, i.e., PS to be no more beneficial than another assistive device on exercise capacity (Mendes et al., 2020).

A number of factors could be attributed to the 'no difference' seen for 'between the groups' analysis in the present study. Firstly, the device was a pilot design and was still in experimental stages. Hence, patients in PS group received only 1 hour of training with PS and the remaining 3-4 hours of gait training was with AFO. This was mainly due to the fact that patient was planned to be discharged with AFO for community purpose. Secondly, the control group also received electrical stimulation for muscle strengthening, as per the requirement, during the routine physiotherapy sessions, probably averaging the therapeutic effect of stimulation for both the groups. Thirdly, a small sample size of 10 patients in each arm could also possibly contribute to the lack of difference 'between the two groups'. Lastly, these parameters were tested at 3 weeks of interval. Most of the studies have used a time frame of at least 4-6 weeks to evaluate the post-intervention effect (Prenton et al., 2016). Despite that, even in these studies, no significant inter-group differences were noted (Prenton et al., 2016).

Additionally, an improvement in the mean values of walking endurance, as measured by the 6MWT, was noted "within group" for both PS and AFO. A mean change of 30.75% and 35.68% was noted for PS and AFO respectively, although the improvement was not found to be statistically significant for within-group difference. Though the substantial meaningful change has been established by Perera et al. as 50 m, literature also supports other estimates of true clinical change, as compared to statistical or random change (as cited in Bethoux et. al, 2015, p. 919). A 13% change in 6MWT was suggested by Flansbjer et al. as the smallest real difference indicating true clinical change (as cited in Bethoux et. al, 2015, p. 919). Therefore, the present study showed a change in endurance exceeding 13% from the baseline for both the groups, thereby, achieving at least more than the smallest real difference at the end of 3 weeks.

Besides, the current study also evaluated the walking speed for pre-post effect. The walking speed was calculated through two ways, i.e., speed for short distance based on 10 metre walk test and speed for a longer distance from 6MWT, based on a previous study by Kottink et al. (2007). The speed calculated through shorter distance of 10 MWT showed a statistically significant within-group change for AFO with a mean change of 45.39% from baseline while PS group showed a mean change of 31.58% from baseline to 3 weeks, which was not statistically significant. The findings of the present study for the AFO group are similar to Bethoux et al. (2014) who observed the percentage changes in gait speed of 40.0% for the AFO group, but also a change of 41.4% for the PS group at the end of 6 months. Also, the previous research on pre-post intervention analysis of FES device suggests a long-term usage and training with the PS device to demonstrate significant cumulative changes in gait speed. A few examples in support of this are as follows. Stein et al. reported percent increases in speed with FES ranging from 32% at 6 months to 37.8% at 11 months in patients with cardio-vascular accident and multiple sclerosis, respectively (as cited in Beathoux et al, 2014, p. 693). Laufer et al. found 29% improvement in gait speed after 2 months of FES wear to 52% at 12 months. Similarly, Stein et al. noted percentage increase of 15% in gait speed at 3 months, 32% at 6 months, and 47% at 12 months for individuals with chronic hemiplegia post-stroke (as cited in Beathoux et al, 2015, p. 918). Therefore, it is possible that non-significant within-group improvement for the PS group was due to the shorter follow-up evaluation period of 3 weeks in the present study. In contrast, the AFO group was able to demonstrate a significant change in speed on 10 meter WT, since these participants had been using AFO even before the study and continued to do even as control group, thereby, having a longer cumulative effect of training with the AFO, resulting in significant speed change.

An interesting observation in the current study was that the statistically significant change in walking speed as measured on 10-meter WT for the AFO group was no longer significant for speed calculated from longer duration walking as obtained from the 6MWT. Besides, the percentage change of speed was reduced from 45.39% (0.074m/s) to 33.3% (0.05m/s) on walking longer distance or duration. In contrast, the PS group in the present study exhibited a more uniform pattern of speed change on both 10 meter WT and the longer 6minute distance with a similar percentage change of 31.58% (0.054 m/s) and 29.4% (0.05m/s), respectively. Even though both the AFO group and the PS group showed a declining trend in the speed on walking longer duration, the decline in PS group was only 2.1% compared to the 12.1% in the AFO group. There could be a few possible reasons for such an observation. First, it is possible that the AFO group may have experienced a fatigue effect on walking longer duration, as reflected in the declining trend of the speed change for larger distance that was not present for the PS group. Literature shows that PS application has therapeutic effect on the stimulated muscles, which enhances the cortical excitability and facilitates neuromuscular activity (Israel et al, 2011; Kottink et al, 2008). Analyzing this at the current stage was however beyond the scope of this study. Secondly, it is probable that both AFO and PS have a similar orthotic effect on walking longer duration, as was noted by the comparable within-group improvement of 0.05 m/s speed by both the groups from the baseline on walking longer duration, thereby, resulting in a percentage change of 29.4% and 33.3% for PS and AFO, respectively. Lastly, it is likely that the patient might feel higher pressure to perform well during the shorter 10-meter

WT, while the longer duration of the 6MWT reflected a more natural cadence and velocity of a patient (Kottink et al., 2007). This could be supported by the finding in the present study, where a stronger inverse correlation of the ankle change in PS group with the speed of 10 meter WT was noted compared to only a moderate inverse correlation with the walking speed of 6MWT. Hence, it is possible that in shorter distance, the patients were more focused on coordinating the device to obtain the precise ankle angle which averaged out later and became more natural on walking larger distance. However, this would warrant further analysis and research with other gait parameters.

Additional analysis of the data suggested a trend towards significant inverse correlation of the 6 minute walk test with the duration of the stroke in post-phase as compared to the pre-phase within the PS group. This implied that the PS group patients who were within 3 months of stroke (sub-acute phase) had better improvement in walking endurance than those who used the PS in the chronic phase (more than 6 months). However, there was an unequal distribution of the patients in the PS group, i.e., 6 patients, 1 patient and 3 patients for the three time durations taken namely, within 3 months, 3-6 months and more than 6 months, respectively. The allocation of patients was done randomly and could have possibly influenced the result. The control group which had a more uniform distribution in terms of duration with 4, 3, 3 patients in the three time periods respectively, only showed a weak non-significant positive association with the duration of stroke. This suggests that irrespective of the duration from the acute event, patients have similar effect on endurance with the AFO. A previous study by Sabut et al. (2011), which compared the various gait parameters between the sub-acute and chronic period post stroke, had found no statistically significant difference between the two groups in terms of changes observed, suggesting that duration of stroke doesn't affect the gains achieved through the device. Besides, a significant positive association between the ankle angle change and duration in stroke was observed in the current study, suggesting that those in chronic phase were having higher change in foot lift.

Another finding on analysis of sub-groups based on the cognitive level (as determined by MMSE) showed a significant inverse association between the MMSE score and walking speed post-intervention in the PS group. Also, the cognitive ability had a positive significant correlation with ankle angle change. In other words, patients with higher cognitive abilities were inducing more ankle angle change, which was affecting their speed. This could be because the participants with higher MMSE may be putting more conscious effort while walking with the device; higher ankle lift thereby reducing the speed. Further analysis with larger sample size including detailed gait analysis would be needed to substantiate this possibility. Nevertheless, the authors feel that the participants need to be trained more with the device so that they can induce sufficient ankle lift for clearance with minimal impact on their speed.

An essential aspect of the study was to evaluate patient's perception about the device, which brought forward several noteworthy points. Despite being a new and experimental device, it was preferred over AFO by 50% of the patients in the study group and 60% did not feel any difficulty in operating the device. The earlier study by Everaert et al. (2013) found that majority of participants preferred the FES system for reasons such as confidence, comfort, convenience, easy donning and doffing, and safety.

It must be highlighted here that in the current study, the feedback given by the remaining participants enabled the investigators to understand the areas in which the device required improvement to make it more patient-friendly. For instance, one of the patients mentioned that the device made walking a conscious effort since every step had to be synchronised with stimulation. As aforementioned, this point was considered prior to the designing of the device and it was believed that the co-ordination will be a learnt motor task like any other learnt motor behaviour in our day to day activities and this was expected to improve with greater duration of training and use of the device. Another patient stated difficulty in re-learning a new walking pattern with PS after having been trained with the AFO. Though there were no adverse effects of the surface stimulation seen or any untoward events throughout the study, one patient experienced pain in ankle with stimulation (VAS= 4-5) throughout walking for initial 1 week, which later subsided spontaneously.

Limitations

In the end, it is necessary to state the limitations in the study. First, a few technical drawbacks of the device was noted. The stimulator used a simple On/Off of 20Hz stimulation, and had a graded current level. Thus, the transition of current generation was not continuous and so, the movement change produced on changing the current level was abrupt. This was observed as the jerking movement of the foot, during the stimulated foot lift. Moreover, since the device was wired, frequent detachment and breakage of wires was noted requiring re-attachment (an average of 2 times per patient during the 3 week usage). The device also did not have an indicator to show the discharging and recharging status of the battery. Hence, the insufficient generation of ankle lift and gradual decrease in dorsiflexion was taken as an indication for discharging of the battery. Second, being a pilot study, a small sample size of 20 participants with 10 in each arm was enrolled, and use of the AFO had to be continued in the intervention group. There was absence of blinding, because it was necessary to monitor the patients using the device. Third, a non uniform distribution of patients in PS group in terms of duration of the stroke due to random allocation was found. Fourth, a shorter duration of follow-up of 3 weeks was chosen, as compared to previous studies (Prenton et al., 2016). It has been observed in the institute's rehab set-up that the patients with stroke usually required on an average 3-4 weeks to complete gait training with AFO with or without the walking aid, once they have started ambulating 5 meters within the parallel bar. Hence, the follow-up period was kept, in accordance with this protocol of finishing training within the 3 week time frame. Fifth, device is selectively suitable for hemiplegic patients with MMSE level of more than 18 and cannot be used by patients with severe cognitive deficits. This is because a certain level of cognitive ability is required for operating the device and learning the co-ordination and synchronization of the stimulation with the gait cycle. Lastly, no validated questionnaire was used for the patient feed-back.

FUTURE RESEARCH DIRECTIONS

Trials in future can be done after improvisation of the device. This could include exploring a radio-frequency wireless hand-switch for the device, so that the frequent fixing of wires is not there and the device is less cumbersome. Another option could be investigating PS having an automatic stimulation control through accelerometers and gyroscopes determining the swing phase of gait and comparing it to the current the user-based hand-switch PS. Further trials need to evaluate the orthotic effect of PS after longer duration of therapy, thereby, allowing the intervention group patients to use the device for same number of hours as the control group using the AFO. Moreover, trial involving longer follow-up period (minimum 12 weeks), increased sample size and blinding could be done. Studies exploring therapeutic effects of the device and examining feasibility of PS for community use and functional independence in daily activities and other vocational tasks while using the device could be aimed for.

CONCLUSION

To summarise, the study attempted to explore the efficacy of a prototype, low-cost, user-controlled hand-switch peroneal stimulator suitable to the socio-cultural needs of Indian patients, especially the rural population, who preferred walking barefoot and avoided using AFOs or footwear within the house. The device demonstrated training based orthotic effect in terms of dynamic ankle angle change achieved during the ambulation by the patients with foot drop following stroke. The observed change was nearly two-third of normal angle change during the swing phase of the gait and had an advantage of a more physiological form of ground clearance than the traditional management with AFO, where the ankle is in neutral position with no range of movement. Besides, the study also reported nearly equivalent orthotic effects in terms of walking endurance and speed for these patients, when compared with the AFO, although the changes noted were not statistically significant. It is notable here that these assessments were made after rehabilitation training of one hour daily with PS for 3 weeks. Despite being a pilot device and its technical hitches, even with the limited training of a short duration and time, the stimulator group did not show worse results than the AFO in terms of its walking ability. Moreover, the results obtained in the present study were compared to previous studies, which used devices with different sensors (either foot-switches or automatic sensors) or different electrodes (either transcutaneous or implantable). Therefore, the results of the current preliminary design of PS was not expected to yield the same results as for the previous devices, which have undergone recurrent technical improvements. Furthermore, additional analysis showed better orthotic effect for the device for patients in the sub-acute phase of rehabilitation as compared to those in the chronic phase and a more useful option for patients with good cognitive abilities than those with cognitive deficits. Lastly, the device received a mixed response from the patients regarding its effectiveness as an orthosis, with 50% patients preferring the device over the AFO and 60% claiming no difficulty in its usage. This mixed acceptability of the device among the patients was anticipated considering the present study to be a pilot one. In view of the above features, the manually controlled hand-switch PS can be offered as an alternative to an AFO for foot drop correction in selected group of stroke patients having good cognitive abilities within Indian rehabilitation settings. The device definitely requires further modifications in terms of the technical designing to obtain smoother movements and also training of longer duration to prove or disprove its efficacy. Investigating its efficacy on a larger scale for advanced gait skills and community use is also warranted after the technical improvements.

ACKNOWLEDGMENT

Authors would like to acknowledge rehabilitation team of Department of Physical Medicine and Rehabilitation and Bio-engineering Department at Christian Medical College (CMC), Vellore, India for assisting in data collection and implementation of intervention. Please Note: The work presented here was conducted when the first author was affiliated with CMC, Vellore, India

REFERENCES

Allet, L., Leemann, B., Guyen, E., Murphy, L., Monnin, D., Herrmann, F. R., & Schnider, A. (2009). Effect of different walking aids on walking capacity of patients with poststroke hemiparesis. *Archives of Physical Medicine and Rehabilitation*, *90*(8), 1408–1413. doi:10.1016/j.apmr.2009.02.010 PMID:19651276

Balami, J. S., Chen, R. L., & Buchan, A. M. (2013). Stroke syndromes and clinical management. *QJM: An International Journal of Medicine*, *106*(7), 607–615. doi:10.1093/qjmed/hct057 PMID:23483140

Bethoux, F., Rogers, H. L., Nolan, K. J., Abrams, G. M., Annaswamy, T., Brandstater, M., Browne, B., Burnfield, J. M., Feng, W., Freed, M. J., Geis, C., Greenberg, J., Gudesblatt, M., Ikramuddin, F., Jayaraman, A., Kautz, S. A., Lutsep, H. L., Madhavan, S., Meilahn, J., ... Kufta, C. (2015). Long-term follow-up to a randomized controlled trial comparing peroneal nerve functional electrical stimulation to an ankle foot orthosis for patients with chronic stroke. *Neurorehabilitation and Neural Repair*, *29*(10), 911–922. doi:10.1177/1545968315570325 PMID:25653225

Bethoux, F., Rogers, H. L., Nolan, K. J., Abrams, G. M., Annaswamy, T. M., Brandstater, M., Browne, B., Burnfield, J. M., Feng, W., Freed, M. J., Geis, C., Greenberg, J., Gudesblatt, M., Ikramuddin, F., Jayaraman, A., Kautz, S. A., Lutsep, H. L., Madhavan, S., Meilahn, J., ... Kufta, C. (2014). The effects of peroneal nerve functional electrical stimulation versus ankle-foot orthosis in patients with chronic stroke: A randomized controlled trial. *Neurorehabilitation and Neural Repair*, *28*(7), 688–697. doi:10.1177/1545968314521007 PMID:24526708

Brockett, C. L., & Chapman, G. J. (2016). Biomechanics of the ankle. *Orthopaedics and Trauma*, *30*(3), 232–238. doi:10.1016/j.mporth.2016.04.015 PMID:27594929

Dunning, K., Black, K., Harrison, A., McBride, K., & Israel, S. (2009). Neuroprosthesis peroneal functional electrical stimulation in the acute inpatient rehabilitation setting: A case series. *Physical Therapy*, *89*(5), 499–506. doi:10.2522/ptj.20080241 PMID:19270044

Everaert, D. G., Stein, R. B., Abrams, G. M., Dromerick, A. W., Francisco, G. E., Hafner, B. J., Huskey, T. N., Munin, M. C., Nolan, K. J., & Kufta, C. V. (2013). Effect of a foot-drop stimulator and ankle–foot orthosis on walking performance after stroke: A multicenter randomized controlled trial. *Neurorehabilitation and Neural Repair*, *27*(7), 579–591. doi:10.1177/1545968313481278 PMID:23558080

Gil-Castillo, J., Alnajjar, F., Koutsou, A., Torricelli, D., & Moreno, J. C. (2020). Advances in neuroprosthetic management of foot drop: A review. *Journal of Neuroengineering and Rehabilitation*, *17*(1), 1–19. doi:10.118612984-020-00668-4 PMID:32213196

Hwang, Y. I. (2020). Effects of an Elastic AFO on the Walking Patterns of Foot-drop Patients with Stroke. *Journal of the Korean Society of Physical Medicine*, *15*(1), 1–9. doi:10.13066/kspm.2020.15.1.1

Israel, S., Kotowski, S., Talbott, N., Fisher, K., & Dunning, K. (2011). The therapeutic effect of outpatient use of a peroneal nerve functional electrical stimulation neuroprosthesis in people with stroke: A case series. *Topics in Stroke Rehabilitation*, *18*(6), 738–745. doi:10.1310/tsr1806-738 PMID:22436311

Jauch, E. C., Saver, J. L., Adams, H. P. Jr, Bruno, A., Connors, J. J., Demaerschalk, B. M., Khatri, P., McMullan, P. W. Jr, Qureshi, A. I., Rosenfield, K., Scott, P. A., Summers, D. R., Wang, D. Z., Wintermark, M., & Yonas, H. (2013). Guidelines for the early management of patients with acute ischemic stroke: A guideline for healthcare professionals from the American Heart Association/American Stroke Association. *Stroke*, *44*(3), 870–947. doi:10.1161/STR.0b013e318284056a PMID:23370205

Kluding, P. M., Dunning, K., O'Dell, M. W., Wu, S. S., Ginosian, J., Feld, J., & McBride, K. (2013). Foot drop stimulation versus ankle foot orthosis after stroke: 30-week outcomes. *Stroke*, *44*(6), 1660–1669. doi:10.1161/STROKEAHA.111.000334 PMID:23640829

Kottink, A. I., Hermens, H. J., Nene, A. V., Tenniglo, M. J., Groothuis-Oudshoorn, C. G., & IJzerman, M. J. (2008). Therapeutic effect of an implantable peroneal nerve stimulator in subjects with chronic stroke and footdrop: A randomized controlled trial. *Physical Therapy*, *88*(4), 437–448. doi:10.2522/ptj.20070035 PMID:18218825

Kottink, A. I., Hermens, H. J., Nene, A. V., Tenniglo, M. J., van der Aa, H. E., Buschman, H. P., & IJzerman, M. J. (2007). A randomized controlled trial of an implantable 2-channel peroneal nerve stimulator on walking speed and activity in poststroke hemiplegia. *Archives of Physical Medicine and Rehabilitation*, *88*(8), 971–978. doi:10.1016/j.apmr.2007.05.002 PMID:17678657

Kottink, A. I., Tenniglo, M. J., de Vries, W. H., Hermens, H. J., & Buurke, J. H. (2012). Effects of an implantable two-channel peroneal nerve stimulator versus conventional walking device on spatiotemporal parameters and kinematics of hemiparetic gait. *Journal of Rehabilitation Medicine*, *44*(1), 51–57. doi:10.2340/16501977-0909 PMID:22124679

Langhorne, P., Bernhardt, J., & Kwakkel, G. (2011). Stroke rehabilitation. *Lancet*, *377*(9778), 1693–1702. doi:10.1016/S0140-6736(11)60325-5 PMID:21571152

Mendes, L. A., Lima, I. N., Souza, T., do Nascimento, G. C., Resqueti, V. R., & Fregonezi, G. A. (2020). Motor neuroprosthesis for promoting recovery of function after stroke. *Cochrane Database of Systematic Reviews*, *2020*(1), 1. doi:10.1002/14651858.CD012991.pub2

National Health Service Conditions. (2019). *Foot drop*. NHS. https://www.nhs.uk/conditions/foot-drop/

National Institute for Health and Care Excellence (NICE). (2013). *Overview | Stroke rehabilitation in adults | Guidance | NICE*. https://www.nice.org.uk/guidance/cg162

NICE. (2016). *Overview | ODFS Pace and Pace XL functional electrical stimulation devices for treating drop foot | Advice | NICE*. https://www.nice.org.uk/advice/MIB56

NICE. (2021). *Stroke - NICE Pathways*. National Institute for Health and Care Excellence. https://pathways.nice.org.uk/pathways/stroke

Prenton, S., Hollands, K. L., & Kenney, L. P. (2016). Functional electrical stimulation versus ankle foot orthoses for foot-drop: A meta-analysis of orthotic effects. *Journal of Rehabilitation Medicine*, *48*(8), 646–656. doi:10.2340/16501977-2136 PMID:27563700

Royal College of Physicians. (2016). *National clinical guideline for stroke*. https://www.strokeaudit.org/SupportFiles/Documents/Guidelines/2016-National-Clinical-Guideline-for-Stroke-5t-(1).aspx

Sabut, S. K., Sikdar, C., Kumar, R., & Mahadevappa, M. (2011). Clinical use of functional electrical stimulation for correction of foot drop: A comparison between subacute and chronic stroke patients. *Journal of Mechanics in Medicine and Biology*, *11*(05), 1165–1177. doi:10.1142/S0219519411004253

Sacco, R. L., Kasner, S. E., Broderick, J. P., Caplan, L. R., Connors, J. J., Culebras, A., Elkind, M. S. V., George, M. G., Hamdan, A. D., Higashida, R. T., Hoh, B. L., Janis, L. S., Kase, C. S., Kleindorfer, D. O., Lee, J.-M., Moseley, M. E., Peterson, E. D., Turan, T. N., Valderrama, A. L., & Vinters, H. V. (2013). An updated definition of stroke for the 21st century: A statement for healthcare professionals from the American Heart Association/American Stroke Association. *Stroke*, *44*(7), 2064–2089. doi:10.1161/STR.0b013e318296aeca PMID:23652265

Shahabi, S., Shabaninejad, H., Kamali, M., Jalali, M., & Ahmadi Teymourlouy, A. (2020). The effects of ankle-foot orthoses on walking speed in patients with stroke: A systematic review and meta-analysis of randomized controlled trials. *Clinical Rehabilitation*, *34*(2), 145–159. doi:10.1177/0269215519887784 PMID:31822115

Sheffler, L. R., Bailey, S. N., Wilson, R. D., & Chae, J. (2013). Spatiotemporal, kinematic, and kinetic effects of a peroneal nerve stimulator versus an ankle foot orthosis in hemiparetic gait. *Neurorehabilitation and Neural Repair*, *27*(5), 403–410. doi:10.1177/1545968312465897 PMID:23192416

Takeda, K., Tanino, G., & Miyasaka, H. (2017). Review of devices used in neuromuscular electrical stimulation for stroke rehabilitation. *Medical Devices (Auckland, N.Z.)*, *10*, 207–213. doi:10.2147/MDER.S123464 PMID:28883745

Truelsen, T., Begg, S., & Mathers, C. (2006). *The global burden of cerebrovascular disease. WHO Discussion Paper*. World Health Organization. https://www.researchgate.net/profile/Stephen-Begg/publication/228551377_The_Global_Burden_of_Cerebrovascular_Disease/links/0c96051e39e2749573000000/The-Global-Burden-of-Cerebrovascular-Disease.pdf

Tyson, S. F., & Kent, R. M. (2013). Effects of an ankle-foot orthosis on balance and walking after stroke: A systematic review and pooled meta-analysis. *Archives of Physical Medicine and Rehabilitation*, *94*(7), 1377–1385. doi:10.1016/j.apmr.2012.12.025 PMID:23416220

World Health Organization. (2017). *Stroke: A global response is needed*. https://www.who.int/bulletin/volumes/94/9/16-181636/en/

ADDITIONAL READING

Donkor, E. S. (2018). Stroke in the21stCentury: A Snapshot of the Burden, Epidemiology, and Quality of Life. *Stroke Research and Treatment*, *2018*, 1–10. doi:10.1155/2018/3238165 PMID:30598741

Kharb, A., Saini, V., Jain, Y. K., & Dhiman, S. (2011). A review of gait cycle and its parameters. *IJCEM International Journal of Computational Engineering & Management*, *13*, 78–83.

McCrory, P., Bell, S., & Bradshaw, C. (2002). Nerve entrapments of the lower leg, ankle and foot in sport. *Sports Medicine (Auckland, N.Z.)*, *32*(6), 371–391. doi:10.2165/00007256-200232060-00003 PMID:11980501

KEY TERMS AND DEFINITIONS

Ankle Foot Orthosis (AFO): Is a device that is applied externally over ankle and foot to control their position and movement range, thereby, compensating for muscle weakness or fixed joint deformity and facilitating standing and walking.

Functional Electrical Stimulation (FES) Systems: Refers to application of electric current to stimulate nerve or muscle to generate muscle contraction and incorporation of multiple coordinated muscle contractions to bring about functional activity.

Gait Cycle: It is the basic repetitive unit of locomotion with each gait cycle starting from the time when a limb strikes the ground continuing till the whole cycle re-occurs on the same side. Each cycle is divided into stance phase where foot is in contact with ground and swing phase when the foot is in the air for limb advancement.

Peroneal Stimulator: It is a type of FES system used to stimulate the peroneal nerve supplying the ankle and toe dorsiflexors, leading to their contraction and resulting in dorsiflexion while walking.

Rehabilitation: Is the process of reducing the impact of disability in individuals with health conditions using interventions optimizing their functional capacity in a given environmental context.

Stroke: Is defined as a condition having an objective evidence of permanent brain, spinal cord, or retinal cell death caused by vascular aetiology. This evidence can be based on pathological or imaging changes in the presence or absence of clinical symptoms.

Chapter 15
Motor Recovery in Stroke Rehabilitation Supported by Robot-Assisted Therapy

Alex Martino Cinnera
IRCCS Santa Lucia Foundation, Italy

Giovanni Morone
IRCCS Santa Lucia Foundation, Italy

ABSTRACT

This chapter discussed the potential usefulness of robot-assisted therapy for motor recovery after a stroke. An overview of the available literature was performed providing up-to-date information about the use of robot-assistive technology in rehabilitation practice. The chapter discussed the rationale for the use and the different machines in terms of basic engineering principles and the related rehabilitation possibilities. Finally, clinical and rehabilitative implications of the findings were critically discussed.

INTRODUCTION

Stroke is the second leading cause of death and the third leading cause of disability in the world (Johnson, Onuma, Owolabi, & Sachdev, 2016). The global burden of stroke continues to grow, with the stroke prevalence in 2013 reaching almost double than the 1990 prevalence rate (Stinear, 2017). According to the World Health Organization (WHO), cerebrovascular disease is the *'incoming epidemic of the 21st century'* (Sarikaya, Ferro, & Arnold, 2015). Moreover, epidemiological evidence suggests that the incidence of ischaemic stroke has increased in the last years in young adults. These patients have a long-life expectancy after stroke and the costs of long-term care pose huge challenges to health-care systems (Ekker, Boot et al., 2018). The WHO defined stroke as *'rapidly developed clinical signs of focal (or global) disturbance of cerebral function, lasting more than 24 hours or leading to death, with no apparent cause other than of vascular origin'*. Although still widely used, the WHO definition relies heavily on clinical symptoms and is now considered outdated by the American Heart Association and American

DOI: 10.4018/978-1-7998-7430-0.ch015

Stroke Association (AHA) due to significant advances in the 'nature, timing, clinical recognition of stroke and its mimics, and imaging findings that require an updated definition' (Coupland, Thapar, Qureshi, Jenkins, & Davies, 2017). In the last edition - Eleventh Revision - of *WHO International Classification of Diseases* (WHO ICD-11), the definition of stroke, based on tissue definition, has been integrated in addition to clinical symptoms (Feigin, Norrving, Sudlow, & Sacco, 2018). This information clarifies that a cerebrovascular accident to be classified like a stroke if there is a death of brain cells -due to lack of oxygen when the blood flow to the brain is lost by blockage or rupture of an artery to the brain- that involves in permanent clinical symptoms (Johnson, Onuma, Owolabi, & Sachdev, 2016). As defined, the tissue damage can be translated into clinical symptoms that include motor impairment on the right or left side of the body, sensory loss, speech/language problems, behavioural diseases, memory loss and vision problems. Due to the wide range of signs and symptoms, stroke is a highly invalidating disease. For this, impairment due to stroke affects all the domains investigated in The International Classification of Functioning, Disability and Health (ICF). Specifically, a stroke can determine an alteration in more than hundred categories of ICF core set, in regard to the body functions and structures, activities and participation, and in the environmental factors (Geyh, Cieza et al., 2004). The most common and widely recognised impairment caused by stroke is motor impairment, which can result either in a loss or limitation of muscle control or movement or in a limitation of functional mobility (Langhorne, Coupar, & Pollock, 2009). Motor impairment after stroke typically affects the control of movement of the arm, and leg of one side of the body (hemiparesis). Approximately 65% of the hospitalised stroke survivors experience initial motor impairment (Hendricks, van Limbeek, Geurts, & Zwarts, 2002), and the majority of these do not recover to their functional baseline (Claflin, Krishnan, & Khot, 2015). The ability to live independently after stroke critically depends on the recovery of motor function (Stinear, Byblow, & Ward, 2014). It follows that motor recovery is crucial for regaining independence and improving the patients' quality of life (Lieshout, van de Port, Dijkhuizen, & Visser-Meily, 2020; Martino Cinnera, Bonnì et al., 2020). Therefore, much of the focus of stroke rehabilitation, and in particular the work of medical doctors, physiotherapists and occupational therapists, is on the recovery of impaired movement and the associated functions (Langhorne, Coupar, & Pollock, 2009). In view of the high number of patients with permanent motor impairment, it is necessary to research novel neurorehabilitation treatments to minimize long-term disability (Claflin, Krishnan, & Khot, 2015). To maximize motor recovery, alongside conventional therapy, new methods, based on new technologies available, have been developed in the last few decades. Among the new treatments, the potential of using robotic devices to assist patients in motor recovery was explored.

The aim of this chapter is to support the reader with a selective review of the newest evidence-based studies available on the usefulness of robot-assisted therapy for upper and lower limb impairment after a stroke. Specifically, an overview will be provided on the characteristics and therapeutic indications of the various robotic devices and on the new potential in combining robotic therapy with new technologies. This information could be useful to clinicians to expand the possibilities of treating motor disorders due to a stroke.

1 BACKGROUND

The recovery of motor functions after a stroke is mainly due to the modification of the activity and of the structure of the neurons, which takes the name of neuronal plasticity or neuroplasticity. These phenomena, although physiological and necessary for learning and development during life, are massive present following damage to the brain tissue. They can be divided into structural neuroplasticity when a neuron changes its connections, and functional plasticity when the neuron changes its properties. This process has a limited time window which begins immediately after the stroke, peaks approximately in the first 4 weeks, and then tapers off over 6 months (Li, 2017). During this recovery window, new neuronal interconnections occur parallelly with acquiring new functions, and compensating for impairment (Takeuchi & Izumi, 2013). Although stepovers were made in the last decades, mechanisms underlying neuroplasticity dependent recovery are not fully understood, it was learned that plasticity in the adult brain after stroke is enabled by a surprising amount of diffuse and redundant connectivity in the central nervous system (Murphy & Corbett, 2009). In fact, after a stroke, the destruction of neural networks stimulates significant functional and structural plasticity changes that is the base of reorganization of the connection, and this rewiring is highly sensitive to the experience following the damage (Nudo & Friel, 1999, Alia, Spalletti et al., 2017). Although part of the plasticity is intrinsic, the ability of neurons to change in structure and function is strictly subject to activity (activity-dependent plasticity). Simplistically, the neurons that are activated simultaneously to perform a repeated action are likely to bind both structurally and functionally. In motor impairment, specifically, the motor cortex and its descending pathways, can undergo substantial structural and functional reorganization that develop between the perilesional areas, as well as in the ipsilesional and contralesional cortex (Li et al., 2017; Casula, Pellicciari et al., 2021). It follows that the movement is the result of the synchronous activity of a complex network of neurons. Therefore, it is important that motor recovery therapies facilitate a correct neuroplasticity to compensate for functional loss. This information is fundamental because it clarifies that a repeated activity is able to generate permanent changes that can guarantee the execution of that function in the future. This concept is the basis of neurorehabilitation, a correctly repeated motor gesture is learned and determines the creation of specific brain circuits. In this way, neurorehabilitation exploits the concept of activation of experience-dependent neuronal plasticity to augment functional recovery after stroke (Maier et al., 2019). To maximize neuroplasticity processes in stroke rehabilitation programs should include meaningful, repetitive, intensive, and task-specific movement training in an enriched environment to promote neural plasticity and consequently motor recovery (Takeuchi & Izumi, 2013). This assumption is always valid in clinical practice, but it is critical if the patient has moderate or severe impairment that will cause reduced use of the limb in daily living activities and affect the ability to perform numerous exercise repetitions during conventional neuromotor therapy. In this line, the studies regarding the forced use principles in subjects affected by stroke, highlighted that the use of the impaired limb can influence adaptive organizational mechanisms in the intact cerebral cortex and, therefore, promote functional recovery thereby avoiding learning non-use phenomenon (Taub, Uswatte, Mark, & Morris, 2006). Advances in technology are aiding the development of therapies that can augment innate repair mechanisms (Dimyan & Cohen 2011). Among the new therapeutic strategies used to increase activity-dependent neural plasticity, robot-assisted therapy represents an emerging approach that performs highly repetitive, intensive, task oriented and quantifiable neurorehabilitation. In the last decades, it has been increasingly used in a wide range of neurological central nervous system conditions for upper and lower limb paresis. Especially in stroke rehabilitation, the robotic training offers several potential advantages, including good repeatability, precisely controllable assistance or resistance during movements, and objective and quantifiable measures of subject performance (Takeuchi & Izumi, 2013). Although the use of this therapeutic approach is relatively recent, the guidelines of the American Heart and Stroke Association reported that the use of robotic therapy appears to provide some benefit for upper extremity motor abilities and participation. Therefore, it seems to be a promising therapy to use in conjunction with conventional gait training for lower extremity. Moreover, encourage development interventions for individuals with severe stroke (Winstein, Stein et al., 2016). In accord, several national guidelines indicated the potential use of robot-assisted training to increase repetition in more severe subjects (Morone, Palomba et al., 2021). Support for the great advantage of any type of robotic device is mostly related to the warranty of highly repetitive and task-oriented training. These indications are also supported by the Cochrane reviews. In these, a potential benefit has been shown for the use of robot-assisted training for upper and lower limb rehabilitation after a stroke. Specifically, these reviews indicated that people who receive electromechanical and robot-assisted arm training after stroke might improve their activities of daily living, arm function, and arm muscle strength (Mehrholz, Pohl, Platz, Kugler, & Elsner, 2018), while those people who receive electromechanical-assisted gait training in combination with physiotherapy after stroke are more likely to achieve independent walking (Mehrholz, Thomas, Kugler, Pohl, & Elsner, 2020). However, many robotic devices and protocols have been used up to now. This heterogeneity can be justified by the different characteristics of the devices, by the severity of the lesion and demographics characteristics. The wide range of devices and the diversity with which the protocols are applied, even if it is representative of a good therapeutic flexibility, makes it difficult to study the effects and draw totally clear conclusions. It is therefore useful to provide a classification of the most common types of devices and what are the most appropriate clinical indications in relation to the degree of impairment.

2 ROBOT-ASSISTED DEVICES

A robot has been defined as a programmable, multifunctional manipulator which is designed to move material, parts, or specialized devices through variable programmed motions for the performance of a variety of tasks (Xie, 2003). In medical practice, the definition of robotic devices is not totally clear and can be confused with the *'Robotic Surgical Procedures'*. The U.S. National Library of Medicine provided two definitions of robotic devices: 1) *'The application of electronic, computerized control systems to mechanical devices designed to perform human functions. Formerly restricted to industry, but nowadays applied to artificial organs controlled by bionic (bioelectronic) devices, like automated insulin pumps and other prostheses.'; 2) 'Device designed to wear externally to support muscular skeletal system in various movements such as range of motion, weight-bearing, gait, and locomotion.'* Regarding use in neurorehabilitation, Reinkensmeyer (2018) provided a more precise definition of robot: *'Rehabilitation robot, any automatically operated machine that is designed to improve movement in persons with impaired physical functioning'*. In fact, the use of robotic devices for the treatment of motor disorders have the ability to, partially or totally, support the execution of the movement of the impaired limb and to assure its function during a task or during an activity of daily living (i.e., reaching or walking).

In the clinical scenario, robot-assisted devices for upper and lower limb rehabilitation can be divided into end-effector devices and exoskeleton devices:

- The end-effector devices assist the limb during movements from the most distal segment of the extremity. In these devices alignment is not required between patient joints and robot joints. Footplates or handles are used to generate limb movements.

- The exoskeleton devices perform movements through a one-to-one correspondence between patient joints and robot joints. Each single joint is guided along a pre-programed trajectory. The exoskeletons can be classified according to the number of joints controlled and the degree of freedom. Additionally, they can be divided into unilateral and bilateral robots as well as into wearable and grounded robots (Morone, Cocchi, Paolucci, & Iosa, 2020; Molteni, Gasperini, Cannaviello, & Guanziroli, 2018).

Regardless of whether they are end-effector or exoskeleton, these devices can be divided into a four-subgroup classification with respect to the level of weight supported into passive mode, active assisted mode, active mode, and resisted mode (Figure 1) (Zhang, Yue, & Wang, 2017):

- **Passive mode:** The robot supports completely the weight of the limb during a prefixed trajectory. This modality does not require control from the patient or any human-computer interface.
- **Active mode:** The robot will change its trajectory or assistance level according to the patient's movements.
- **Active assist mode:** A partially assisted mode. The patient independently moves the limb, and the robot is activated only when the power overcomes a certain threshold value.
- **Active resist mode:** When the patient initiates the movements, and the robot offers resistance in order to make the exercise more demanding.

Figure 1. Flow diagram of categories and level of assistance of robot devices in rehabilitation

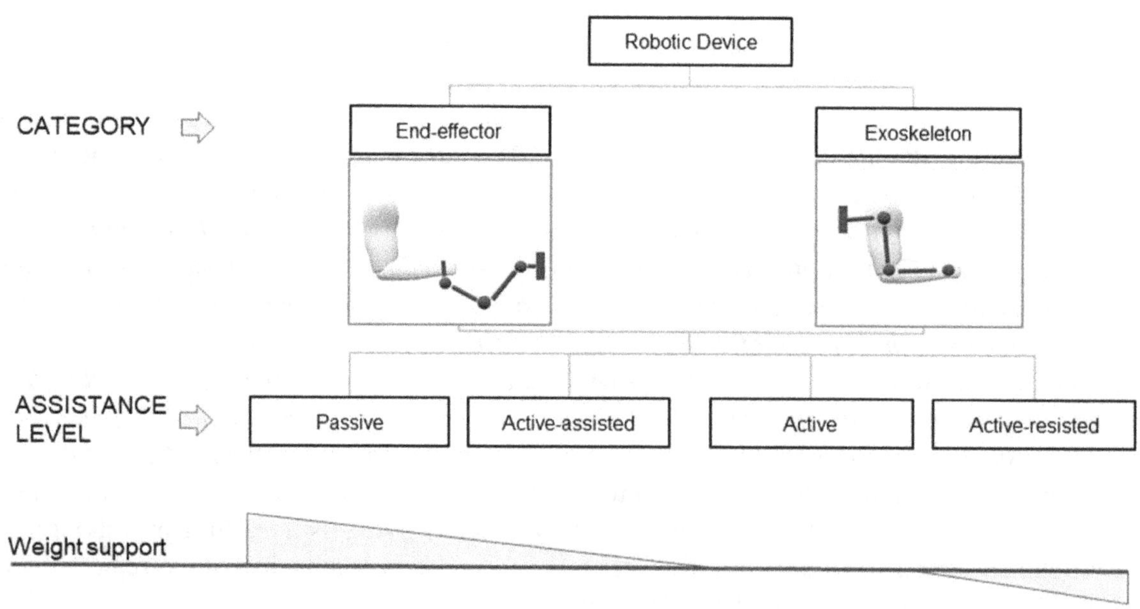

The robot devices can be divided into end-effectors and exoskeletons. Moreover, for the lower limb (specifically for the gait training), it can be perform a further subgroup subdivision (Zhang, Yue, & Wang, 2017):

End-effector:
- Foot plate-based end-effector devices
- Platform-based end-effector devices

Exoskeleton:
- Treadmill-based exoskeletons (grounded)
- Leg orthosis exoskeletons (wearable)

All types of devices can generate the movement in two different modes, independently of human control or in accord to signals obtained from the initiative intention. The control strategy between robot and patients is divided into three modalities:

- **Position control:** in this modality the robot device drives the limb in a pre-fixed trajectory. Any interaction between is needed to trigger the movement by the patient. Moreover, any variables are suitable (i.e. weight support, joints angle etc.)
- **Force signal control:** in this modality the signal to trigger the movement in the robot device is provided by the force of the limb. For this specific robot control, a minimal ability in motor control is required.
- **Biological signal control:** The biological signals generated in the cerebral cortex or in the muscle, can be respectively recorded by electroencephalography (EEG) or electromyography (EMG). Using a transduction system, the signal can be transferred almost in real time to the machine, for triggering the movement.

2.1 Robot Devices for Upper Limb Rehabilitation

Upper limb motor function is often severely affected in stroke patients, and this can limit the patient's activity of daily living, quality of life and re-integration in professional activity (Hatem, Saussez et al., 2016). Recovery of arm and hand functions is one of the primary goals in stroke rehabilitation treatment programs (Franck, Smeets, & Seelen, 2017). Hegemonic function of the upper limb is centred on reaching and grasping as these movements are necessary to hold objects, to perform personal care tasks and for exploring the space. To perform a functional reaching and grasping, the subject needs to be able to move the shoulder and the elbow in three-dimensional space and to carry out at least a whole hand grip. Generally, the target of robot-assisted therapy, and conventional physical therapy is the restoration of these ability skills of the upper limb.

2.1.1 Target of Intervention

Robot devices have been used to increase functional motor recovery of the arm and hand. End-effector devices can increase the movements of the shoulder, elbow and wrist. Like end-effector robots, the exoskeleton device can increase the recovery of motor function of principal joints of the upper limb, some devices can also assist the control of the hand. In consideration of the high specialization of the hand, robots have recently been built that perform neuromotor training only for the hand to be accompanied by robots that perform training for the proximal upper limb (shoulder-elbow) (Calabrò, Accorinti et al., 2019; Sale, Mazzoleni et al., 2014).

2.1.2 Findings and Clinical Indication

Research conducted to date seems to show functional motor recovery of the upper limb in the early stage of stroke (Kim, Lim et al., 2017) and in the chronic patients (Bertani, Melegari et al., 2017). The use of robot-assisted therapy seems to be superior with respect to conventional rehabilitation in improving upper extremity motor impairment in people with severe upper limb hemiplegia and limited potential for spontaneous recovery (Wu, Cheng, Zhang, Yang, & Cai, 2021). Furthermore, the robot-assisted device for the upper limb allows patients to increase the number of repetitions and hence the intensity of practice poststroke, still ensuring the therapy's safety (Veerbeek, Langbroek-Amersfoort, van Wegen, Meskers, & Kwakkel, 2017; Kwakkel, Kollen, & Krebs, 2008). Despite these important findings on functional motor recovery, no other significant conclusion can be found on activity of daily living and muscle tone reduction after use of robot-assisted therapy for the upper limb. Probably the high heterogeneity between studies can be the cause of no significant effects registered (Kwakkel, Kollen, & Krebs, 2008).

Robot-assisted rehabilitation allows more intensive and task-oriented training in particular in more severe subjects in which conventional physiotherapy is not delivered with a high enough intensity because of labor limitations (less active move possibility with repetitive strain injuries and fatigue by therapists). Electromechanical and robotic devices could be used as an adjunct to conventional therapies and in a framework of an individualized written rehabilitation plan. A recently updated Cochrane review including 45 studies with 1619 subjects, indicated that people who receive robot-assisted and electromechanical arm training after stroke might improve their activities of daily living, arm function, and arm muscle strength without an increase of the risk of participant dropout (Mehrholz, Pohl, Platz, Kugler, & Elsner, 2018). Therefore, there is the need to generate evidence to support the selection of specific types of robotic device for specific subgroups of patients according to their severity, sensory deficits, cognitive impairment and considering the goal of the robot-assisted training (i.e., arm or hand recovery). Robot-assisted therapy is particularly suitable and effective for specific subgroups of patients: 1) patients who are less than 3-mo poststroke (subacute stage); 2) patients with moderate and severe lesions might benefit more from robot-assisted training in addition to conventional therapy then conventional therapy alone at a dose metched therapy (Duret, Hutin, Lehenaff, & Gracies, 2015); 3) patients with mild lesions should not be the best candidates for robot-assisted therapy (Morone, Cocchi, Paolucci, & Iosa, 2020). Robot-assisted therapy could mitigate some issues that are related to inconsistent outcomes following conventional physiotherapy such as the variability between therapists; the possibility to measure the amount of subject's performances with high reliability and accuracy; and the possibility to give user-adapted feedback to increase attention and motivation during training (Duret, Hutin, Lehenaff, & Gracies, 2015; Iosa, Morone, Cherubini, & Paolucci, 2016).

2.2 Robot Devices for Lower Limb Rehabilitation

The major functions of the lower limbs are to support the weight of the body and the locomotion. Of the people living with stroke, more than 80% have gait impairment that recovers to some extent in the first 2 months after stroke. However, community ambulation often remains compromised in most survivors. Gait ability has major implications for health as it is an essential predictor for functional independence and long-term survival after stroke (Cirstea, 2020; Li, Francisco, & Zhou, 2018).

2.2.1 Target of Intervention

Gait training is the main focused target during lower limb rehabilitation, the robot devices have been used to increase gait performance. A recent meta-analysis supports the use of robot-assisted gait devices with results like the conventional rehabilitation (Tedla, Dixit, Gular, & Abohashrh, 2019). Moreover, those who receive robot-assisted gait training in combination with conventional rehabilitation after stroke are more likely to achieve independent walking (Mehrholz, Thomas, Kugler, Pohl, & Elsner, 2020).

2.2.2 Findings and Clinical Indication

A recently updated Cochrane Review evaluated the effects of electromechanical and robot-assisted gait training devices for improving walking after stroke (Mehrholz, Thomas, Kugler, Pohl, & Elsner, 2020). In this review, authors included 62 trials involving 2440 participants. Patients who receive electromechanical-assisted gait training in combination with physiotherapy after stroke were more likely to achieve independent walking than people who receive gait training without these devices. Robot-assisted training resulted to be useful for improving walking velocity but not for walking capacity. The role of the different types of devices is not clear (Mehrholz, Thomas, Kugler, Pohl, & Elsner, 2020).

Authors highlighted that people in the subacute phase and people who are non-ambulatory may benefit from this type of training. This outcome was in line with previous hypotheses in which a more severe patient can carry out an adequate training intensity through a greater assistance of the machine in the various articular fulcrums (Mehrholz, Thomas, Kugler, Pohl, & Elsner, 2020).

2.3 Robot-Assisted Therapy Combined with New Technologies

The positive effects of combining two different types of innovative technologies have long been explored. The rationale is that the combination of two technologies could enhance their single effect due to their different mechanisms of action. The combination can boost the effect on functional recovery of the target skill of rehabilitation (Mazzoleni, Duret, Grosmaire, & Battini, 2017).

2.3.1 Immersive and Non-Immersive Virtual Reality

Adding a non-immersive virtual reality system to a simple treadmill during locomotor training might enhance outcome providing a greater subject motivation which results in increased exercise intensity (Mirelman, Rochester et al., 2016). Many robots integrate immersive or non-immersive virtual reality (VR) systems providing online feedback and involving complex cortical mechanisms during planning, execution, and control of the movement. The attention and the executive function during neurorehabilitation are some of the most important cognitive abilities implied in robotic rehabilitation with non-immersive VR feedback that increase top-down components during therapy (Morone, Spitoni et al., 2019). Previous studies reported general improvements in the motor function of patients using the novel interfacing techniques with exoskeletons (i.e., virtual reality, augmented reality, gamification) (Mubin, Alnajjar, Jishtu, Alsinglawi, & Al Mahmud, 2019).

2.3.2 Non-invasive Brain Stimulation

Robot-assisted therapy is often combined with non-invasive brain stimulation by administering the stimulation before robot-assisted training or simultaneously. The use of transcranial direct current stimulation (tDCS) and the transcranial magnetic stimulation (TMS) can be coupled with robot-assisted therapy to increase neural plasticity. Results from recent trials showed that although the approach is feasible, at the moment, there is not enough data about the benefits of non-invasive brain stimulation (NIBS) as an add-on intervention to robot-assisted therapy on upper-limb motor function activity (Reis, Bernardo, Oshiro, Krebs, & Conforto, 2021) or to robot-assisted gait training in patients with subacute stroke (Leon, Cortes et al., 2017). However, in chronic stroke a slight significant motor improvement has been reported in severe upper limb impairment (Di Lazzaro, Capone et al., 2016). By promoting the modulation of excitatory input of the corticospinal tracts on spinal circuits, it may be a promising strategy in improving arm and hand functions.

2.3.3 Botulinum Injection

Botulinum toxin -Type A- (BoNT-A) injections have shown beneficial effects on spasticity and resulted to be a well-tolerated treatment for patients with upper limb spasticity post stroke (Don, Wu, Hu, & Wang 2017). Recent meta-analysis supported the beneficial effects of BoNT-A treatment on improving hypertonicity within 3months post-stroke and added the importance of concomitant neurorehabilitation therapy (Rosales, Efendy et al., 2016). The combined use of robot-assisted therapy and BoNT-A injection has been tested in a limited number of trials. However, there is a hypothesis that a reduction of spacity promoted by the injection, with motor functional therapy performed by robot-assisted device, can increase functional movement recovery. In the upper limb, the combination of robot-assisted therapy with BoNT-A injection has showed a synergistic positive effect in chronic stroke patients (Lee, Jeon, Kim, & Han, 2017; Gandolfi, Valè et al., 2019; Martino Cinnera, Pucello et al., 2019)

2.3.4 Functional Electrical Stimulation

Electric fields excite electrically active tissue by several mechanisms (Roth, 1994). In clinical and research practice, electrical stimulation has been used to perform functional electrical stimulation (FES) (Merrill, Bikson, & Jefferys, 2005). A recent review showed an improvement in motor and gait abilities and in quality of life in stroke patients. Moreover, FES is more effective, if it is associated with other physiotherapy techniques (Romera-De Francisco & Jiménez-Del Barrio, 2016). The combination of robot-assisted therapy with FES, although still not sufficiently explored, showed potential benefits for upper and lower limbs. Specifically, in patients with the same level of arm impairment and corticospinal tract integrity, the use of robot-assisted therapy coupled with FES seemed to induce a higher level of arm recovery (Straudi, Baroni et al., 2020). In the lower limb, the use of FES combined with different walking retraining strategies has shown to result in improvements in hemiplegic gait (Belda-Lois, Mena-del Horno et al., 2011).

3 FUTURE RESEARCH DIRECTIONS

3.1 Closed-Loop Brain Robot Interface

Patients with stroke, especially those with severe motor deficits, cannot execute task-oriented rehabilitation exercises with their affected upper extremity (Grimm & Gharabaghi, 2016). In these cases, a new rehabilitation approach combining robot-assisted therapy and Brain-Computer Interface (BCI) may provide an additional tool for motor recovery, increasing cortical plasticity by means of Hebbian-like learning use (Gomez-Rodriguez, Grosse-Wentrup et al., 2011). Even if it has been limitedly explored, the use of robot-assisted devices, in particular of exoskeletons, allows the formation of closed-loop stimulation circuits (artificial support of the sensorimotor feedback loop). Thanks to the use of the brain-robot-interface (BRI), a subgroup of brain computer interface, it is possible to create protocols that exploit neurophysiological signals (i.e. the EEG or the EMG) (Brauchle, Vukelić, Bauer, & Gharabaghi, 2015) to generate movement and simultaneously stimulate the nervous system. Parallelly, an add-on direct and tailored stimulation can be directed to the central and peripheral nervous system (i.e., NIBS) or direct to the muscles (i.e., FES).

3.2 Neuroprosthesis

In addition to the rehabilitation aspect, motor neuroprostheses could be created by using closed-loops and the use of BRI coupled with wearable exoskeletons. These prostheses can support the movement of the limb in subjects with severe motor disabilities. The biological signal can afford the control of the exoskeleton. In subjects suffering from stroke, in whom the interruption of signal transmission along the cortico-spinal tract occurred, the use of these neuroprosthesis allows to create a neuromotor bypass to control some simple movements. Generally, this system is based on EEG-signal control thanks to which specific frequencies, produced by neuronal pyramids of the cerebral cortex, are translated into activation signals for the wearable exoskeleton. Although these technologies seem complex and difficult to use independently in a domestic environment, to date some experiments seem to demonstrate their practical feasibility and effectiveness (Al-Quraishi, Elamvazuthi, Daud, Parasuraman, & Borboni, 2018).

4 DISCUSSION

The use of robot-assisted therapy has proved effective improvement on functional motor recovery of upper and lower limbs, in patients with both subacute and chronic phase of stroke. The use of robots for the upper limb has as its main objective the recovery of the functions of reaching and grasping, while that of the lower limb has as its objective the recovery of walking. Both of these functions seem to be important to achieve a good level of independence and a good quality of life. The use of robotic devices, also by virtue of the large number of movement repetitions (intensive rehabilitation), proved to be safe for both the patient and the therapist (Duret, Grosmaire, & Krebs, 2019; Mehrholz, Pohl, Platz, Kugler, & Elsner, 2018; Kim, Lim et al., 2017).

Regarding the type of robot, the exoskeleton devices allow a finer control of the joint kinematics allowing even more severely affected subjects to an intensive training as described in robot-assisted walking training (Morone, Paolucci et al 2017). In contrast generally end-effector devices leave the proximal joint of the upper and the lower limb less constricted and exposing them to uncontrolled forces.This feature makes end-effector based robots more usable in mild and moderate patients, while the exoskeletons suitable to in both mild /moderate and severe patients thanks to a more important control of the limbs proximally. (Morone, Cocchi, Paolucci, & Iosa, 2020).

With respect to the level of severity, the subjects with moderate and severe lesions of the lower limbs might benefit more from robot-assisted training in addition to conventional therapy. A large body of literature including Cochrane reviews, support the idea that robot-assisted therapy is more useful for moderate to severe patients, allowing more repetitions in a task specific context and with enriched feedback (Mehrholz, Thomas, Kugler, Pohl, & Elsner, 2020; Duret, Grosmaire, & Krebs, 2019). People with severe impairments often cannot move the limb against the force of gravity and therefore are unable to perform functional movement exercises. In this case the subjects seem to benefit from the use of robot-assisted therapy that makes it possible to perform complete functional movements able to stimulate activity-dependent neuronal plasticity.

The literature available to date offers indications on the effectiveness of the use of robotic devices in neurorehabilitation to improve arm recovery. Specifically, robot-assisted therapy seems to produce an increase in voluntary functional motor recovery and an increase of motor control as well as an improvement of the subject's participation in activities of daily living. Regarding spasticity, the literature shows that there is no improvement with robotic training but that there is not even a worsening after training (Mehrholz, Pohl, Platz, Kugler, & Elsner, 2018). Thus, there is still not enough data to support the improvement in spasticity and quality of life. In addition, there are no findings to support the hypothesis that one type of robotic device is any better or worse than any other device, providing no clear evidence to support the selection of specific types of robotic device to promote hand-arm recovery.

The use of robotic devices coupled with virtual reality (immersive or non-immersive), with neuromodulation techniques, functional electrical stimulation and botulinum toxin injection seem to be valid tools to reduce spasticity in chronic stroke and thus increase voluntary movements in selected cases of stroke subjects (Erbil, Tugbaet al., 2018; Gandolfi, Valè et al., 2019).

Although it is not easy in combined approaches to discern which of the two treatments the improvement is attributable to, further studies may clarify whether this combination can generate a greater recovery than the sum of the effect of the individual treatments.

In the future, the use of wearable exoskeletons could not only favor motor recovery, but also substitute movements where they were not fully recovered. These motor neuroprostheses can be directly controlled by means of biological signals coming from the cortex or muscles not affected by the lesion. At the same time, through the use of non-invasive brain stimulation techniques, closed-loop circuits have been developed that allow us to create customized protocols for each patient. In these complex systems, brain stimulation is generated simultaneously with the movement of the paretic limb by means of the robotic device, whenever the affected brain area has cortical activity close to the physiological one. This mechanism should favor the establishment of normal cortical activation frequencies and favor the phenomena of neuroplasticity at the basis of motor functional recovery (Mondini, Kobler, Sburlea, & Müller-Putz, 2020; Huang, Zhang, Yu, He, & Li, 2019).

Despite this positive finding, the effectiveness of these robots in rehabilitation after stroke is not totally clear (Rodgers, Shaw et al., 2017; Cirstea, 2019), despite the efficacy of the robotic training in upper and lower extremities neurorehabilitation after stroke, has been proven in several trials and by the Cochrane revision. Furthermore, the debate is still open and actually, in current clinical practice, we might perform robot-assisted therapy as add-on to conventional therapy (Morone, Masiero, Werner, & Paolucci, 2014).

Nevertheless, this promising new rehabilitation technique should be a topic for continued research and gains more space in neurorehabilitation year by year. The promise of the robot to improve motor recovery continues to excite patients and caregivers as well as clinicians and researchers (Bernhardt & Mehrholz, 2019) and further investigations are needed to better explore its potential.

5 CONCLUSION

Electromechanical and robot-assisted arm training could increase the intensity of arm and lower limb therapy therapy. Regarding arm training, subjects who receive electromechanical or robot-assisted training in add-on to conventional physiotherapy are more likely to have improvement of the arm function, and of the muscle strength and in their activities of daily living, of the paretic arm." with "...to have improvement of the motor function, muscle strength and in their activities of daily living.

Regarding lower limb training, subjects who receive electronic and robotic devices in add-on to conventional physiotherapy might have more chance to re-walk independently again after a stroke. In particular, people in the first three months after a stroke, as well as people who are unable to walk, might benefit more.

Dose, frequency, time from stroke, type of devices and cost-effective issues should be addressed in future research.

ACKNOWLEDGMENT

The authors thank Enza Leone for English language revision.

REFERENCES

Al-Quraishi, M. S., Elamvazuthi, I., Daud, S. A., Parasuraman, S., & Borboni, A. (2018). EEG-Based Control for Upper and Lower Limb Exoskeletons and Prostheses: A Systematic Review. *Sensors (Basel)*, *18*(10), 3342.

Alia, C., Spalletti, C., Lai, S., Panarese, A., Lamola, G., Bertolucci, F., Vallone, F., Di Garbo, A., Chisari, C., Micera, S., & Caleo, M. (2017). Neuroplastic Changes Following Brain Ischemia and their Contribution to Stroke Recovery: Novel Approaches in Neurorehabilitation. *Frontiers in Cellular Neuroscience*, *11*, 76.

Belda-Lois, J. M., Mena-del Horno, S., Bermejo-Bosch, I., Moreno, J. C., Pons, J. L., Farina, D., Iosa, M., Molinari, M., Tamburella, F., Ramos, A., Caria, A., Solis-Escalante, T., Brunner, C., & Rea, M. (2011). Rehabilitation of gait after stroke: A review towards a top-down approach. *Journal of Neuroengineering and Rehabilitation*, *8*, 66.

Bernhardt, J., & Mehrholz, J. (2019, July 6). Robot-assisted training after stroke: RATULS advances science. *Lancet*, *394*(10192), 6–8.

Bertani, R., Melegari, C., De Cola, M. C., Bramanti, A., Bramanti, P., & Calabrò, R. S. (2017). Effects of robot-assisted upper limb rehabilitation in stroke patients: a systematic review with meta-analysis. *Neurological Sciences, 38*(9), 1561–1569.

Brauchle, D., Vukelić, M., Bauer, R., & Gharabaghi, A. (2015). Brain state-dependent robotic reaching movement with a multi-joint arm exoskeleton: Combining brain-machine interfacing and robotic rehabilitation. *Frontiers in Human Neuroscience*, *9*, 564.

Calabrò, R. S., Accorinti, M., Porcari, B., Carioti, L., Ciatto, L., Billeri, L., Andronaco, V. A., Galletti, F., Filoni, S., & Naro, A. (2019). Does hand robotic rehabilitation improve motor function by rebalancing interhemispheric connectivity after chronic stroke? Encouraging data from a randomised-clinical-trial. *Clinical Neurophysiology*, *130*(5), 767–780.

Casula, E. P., Pellicciari, M. C., Bonnì, S., Spanò, B., Ponzo, V., Salsano, I., Giulietti, G., Martino Cinnera, A., Maiella, M., Borghi, I., Rocchi, L., Bozzali, M., Sallustio, F., Caltagirone, C., & Koch, G. (2021). Evidence for interhemispheric imbalance in stroke patients as revealed by combining transcranial magnetic stimulation and electroencephalography. *Human Brain Mapping*. Advance online publication. doi:10.1002/hbm.25297

Cirstea, C. M. (2019). Are Wearable Robots Effective for Gait Recovery After Stroke? *Stroke*, *50*(12), 3337–3338.

Cirstea, C. M. (2020). Gait Rehabilitation After Stroke: Should We Re-Evaluate Our Practice? *Stroke*, *51*(10), 2892–2894.

Claflin, E. S., Krishnan, C., & Khot, S. P. (2015). Emerging treatments for motor rehabilitation after stroke. *The Neurohospitalist*, *5*(2), 77–88.

Coupland, A. P., Thapar, A., Qureshi, M. I., Jenkins, H., & Davies, A. H. (2017). The definition of stroke. *Journal of the Royal Society of Medicine*, *110*(1), 9–12.

Di Lazzaro, V., Capone, F., Di Pino, G., Pellegrino, G., Florio, L., Zollo, L., Simonetti, D., Ranieri, F., Brunelli, N., Corbetto, M., Miccinilli, S., Bravi, M., Milighetti, S., Guglielmelli, E., & Sterzi, S. (2016). Combining Robotic Training and Non-Invasive Brain Stimulation in Severe Upper Limb-Impaired Chronic Stroke Patients. *Frontiers in Neuroscience*, *10*, 88.

Dimyan, M. A., & Cohen, L. G. (2011). Neuroplasticity in the context of motor rehabilitation after stroke. *Nature Reviews. Neurology*, *7*(2), 76–85.

Dong, Y., Wu, T., Hu, X., & Wang, T. (2017). Efficacy and safety of botulinum toxin type A for upper limb spasticity after stroke or traumatic brain injury: A systematic review with meta-analysis and trial sequential analysis. *European Journal of Physical and Rehabilitation Medicine*, *53*(2), 256–267.

Duret, C., Grosmaire, A. G., & Krebs, H. I. (2019). Robot-Assisted Therapy in Upper Extremity Hemiparesis: Overview of an Evidence-Based Approach. *Frontiers in Neurology*, *10*, 412.

Duret, C., Hutin, E., Lehenaff, L., & Gracies, J. M. (2015). Do all sub acute stroke patients benefit from robot-assisted therapy? A retrospective study. *Restorative Neurology and Neuroscience*, *33*(1), 57–65.

Ekker, M. S., Boot, E. M., Singhal, A. B., Tan, K. S., Debette, S., Tuladhar, A. M., & de Leeuw, F. E. (2018). Epidemiology, aetiology, and management of ischaemic stroke in young adults. *Lancet Neurology, 17*(9), 790–801.

Erbil, D., Tugba, G., Murat, T. H., Melike, A., Merve, A., Cagla, K., Mehmetali, Ç. C., Akay, Ö., & Nigar, D. (2018). Effects of robot-assisted gait training in chronic stroke patients treated by botulinum toxin-a: A pivotal study. *Physiotherapy Research International, 23*(3), e1718.

Feigin, V., Norrving, B., Sudlow, C., & Sacco, R. L. (2018). Updated Criteria for Population-Based Stroke and Transient Ischemic Attack Incidence Studies for the 21st Century. *Stroke, 49*(9), 2248–2255.

Franck, J. A., Smeets, R., & Seelen, H. (2017). Changes in arm-hand function and arm-hand skill performance in patients after stroke during and after rehabilitation. *PLoS One, 12*(6), e0179453.

Gandolfi, M., Valè, N., Dimitrova, E. K., Mazzoleni, S., Battini, E., Filippetti, M., Picelli, A., Santamato, A., Gravina, M., Saltuari, L., & Smania, N. (2019). Effectiveness of Robot-Assisted Upper Limb Training on Spasticity, Function and Muscle Activity in Chronic Stroke Patients Treated With Botulinum Toxin: A Randomized Single-Blinded Controlled Trial. *Frontiers in Neurology, 10*, 41.

Gandolfi, M., Valè, N., Dimitrova, E. K., Mazzoleni, S., Battini, E., Filippetti, M., Picelli, A., Santamato, A., Gravina, M., Saltuari, L., & Smania, N. (2019). Effectiveness of Robot-Assisted Upper Limb Training on Spasticity, Function and Muscle Activity in Chronic Stroke Patients Treated With Botulinum Toxin: A Randomized Single-Blinded Controlled Trial. *Frontiers in Neurology, 10*, 41.

Geyh, S., Cieza, A., Schouten, J., Dickson, H., Frommelt, P., Omar, Z., Kostanjsek, N., Ring, H., & Stucki, G. (2004). ICF Core Sets for stroke. *Journal of Rehabilitation Medicine*, (44), 135–141.

Gomez-Rodriguez, M., Grosse-Wentrup, M., Hill, J., Gharabaghi, A., Scholkopf, B., & Peters, J. (2011). Towards brain-robot interfaces in stroke rehabilitation. *IEEE International Conference on Rehabilitation Robotics, 2011*, 5975385.

Grimm, F., & Gharabaghi, A. (2016). Closed-Loop Neuroprosthesis for Reach-to-Grasp Assistance: Combining Adaptive Multi-channel Neuromuscular Stimulation with a Multi-joint Arm Exoskeleton. *Frontiers in Neuroscience, 10*, 284.

Hatem, S. M., Saussez, G., Della Faille, M., Prist, V., Zhang, X., Dispa, D., & Bleyenheuft, Y. (2016). Rehabilitation of Motor Function after Stroke: A Multiple Systematic Review Focused on Techniques to Stimulate Upper Extremity Recovery. *Frontiers in Human Neuroscience, 10*, 442.

Hendricks, H. T., van Limbeek, J., Geurts, A. C., & Zwarts, M. J. (2002). Motor recovery after stroke: A systematic review of the literature. *Archives of Physical Medicine and Rehabilitation, 83*(11), 1629–1637.

Huang, Q., Zhang, Z., Yu, T., He, S., & Li, Y. (2019). An EEG-/EOG-Based Hybrid Brain-Computer Interface: Application on Controlling an Integrated Wheelchair Robotic Arm System. *Frontiers in Neuroscience, 13*, 1243.

Iosa, M., Morone, G., Cherubini, A., & Paolucci, S. (2016). The Three Laws of Neurorobotics: A Review on What Neurorehabilitation Robots Should Do for Patients and Clinicians. *Journal of Medical and Biological Engineering, 36*, 1–11.

Johnson, W., Onuma, O., Owolabi, M., & Sachdev, S. (2016). Stroke: A global response is needed. *Bulletin of the World Health Organization*, *94*(9), 634–634A.

Kim, G., Lim, S., Kim, H., Lee, B., Seo, S., Cho, K., & Lee, W. (2017). Is robot-assisted therapy effective in upper extremity recovery in early stage stroke? -a systematic literature review. *Journal of Physical Therapy Science*, *29*(6), 1108–1112.

Kwakkel, G., Kollen, B. J., & Krebs, H. I. (2008). Effects of robot-assisted therapy on upper limb recovery after stroke: A systematic review. *Neurorehabilitation and Neural Repair*, *22*(2), 111–121.

Langhorne, P., Coupar, F., & Pollock, A. (2009). Motor recovery after stroke: A systematic review. *Lancet Neurology*, *8*(8), 741–754.

Lee, S. Y., Jeon, Y. T., Kim, B. R., & Han, E. Y. (2017). Combined treatment of botulinumtoxin and robot-assisted rehabilitation therapy on poststroke, upper limb spasticity. *Case Reports in Medicine*, *96*(51), e9468.

Leon, D., Cortes, M., Elder, J., Kumru, H., Laxe, S., Edwards, D. J., Tormos, J. M., Bernabeu, M., & Pascual-Leone, A. (2017). tDCS does not enhance the effects of robot-assisted gait training in patients with subacute stroke. *Restorative Neurology and Neuroscience*, *35*(4), 377–384.

Li, S. (2017). Spasticity, Motor Recovery, and Neural Plasticity after Stroke. *Frontiers in Neurology*, *8*, 120.

Lieshout, E., van de Port, I. G., Dijkhuizen, R. M., & Visser-Meily, J. (2020). Does upper limb strength play a prominent role in health-related quality of life in stroke patients discharged from inpatient rehabilitation? *Topics in Stroke Rehabilitation*, *27*(7), 525–533.

Maier, M., Ballester, B. R., & Verschure, P. (2019). Principles of Neurorehabilitation After Stroke Based on Motor Learning and Brain Plasticity Mechanisms. *Frontiers in Systems Neuroscience*, *13*, 74.

Martino Cinnera, A., Bonnì, S., Pellicciari, M. C., Giorgi, F., Caltagirone, C., & Koch, G. (2020). Health-related quality of life (HRQoL) after stroke: Positive relationship between lower extremity and balance recovery. *Topics in Stroke Rehabilitation*, *27*(7), 534–540.

Martino Cinnera, A., Pucello, A., Lupo, A., Gimigliano, F., Mammucari, E., Cicero, D. L., Iosa, M., Paolucci, S., & Morone, G. (2019). Upper limb motor improvement in chronic stroke after combining botulinum toxin A injection and multi-joints robot-assisted therapy: A case report. *Oxford Medical Case Reports*, *2019*(10), omz097.

Mazzoleni, S., Duret, C., Grosmaire, A. G., & Battini, E. (2017). Combining Upper Limb Robotic Rehabilitation with Other Therapeutic Approaches after Stroke: Current Status, Rationale, and Challenges. *BioMed Research International*, *2017*, 8905637.

Mehrholz, J., Platz, T., Kugler, J., & Pohl, M. (2008). Electromechanical and robot-assisted arm training for improving arm function and activities of daily living after stroke. *Cochrane Database of Systematic Reviews*, (4), CD006876.

Mehrholz, J., Pohl, M., Platz, T., Kugler, J., & Elsner, B. (2018). Electromechanical and robot-assisted arm training for improving activities of daily living, arm function, and arm muscle strength after stroke. *Cochrane Database of Systematic Reviews*, *9*(9), CD006876.

Mehrholz, J., Thomas, S., Kugler, J., Pohl, M., & Elsner, B. (2020). Electromechanical-assisted training for walking after stroke. *Cochrane Database of Systematic Reviews*, *10*(10), CD006185.

Merrill, D. R., Bikson, M., & Jefferys, J. G. (2005). Electrical stimulation of excitable tissue: Design of efficacious and safe protocols. *Journal of Neuroscience Methods*, *141*(2), 171–198.

Mirelman, A., Rochester, L., Maidan, I., Del Din, S., Alcock, L., Nieuwhof, F., Rikkert, M. O., Bloem, B. R., Pelosin, E., Avanzino, L., Abbruzzese, G., Dockx, K., Bekkers, E., Giladi, N., Nieuwboer, A., & Hausdorff, J. M. (2016). Addition of a non-immersive virtual reality component to treadmill training to reduce fall risk in older adults (V-TIME): A randomised controlled trial. *Lancet*, *388*(10050), 1170–1182.

Molteni, F., Gasperini, G., Cannaviello, G., & Guanziroli, E. (2018). Exoskeleton and End-Effector Robots for Upper and Lower Limbs Rehabilitation: Narrative Review. *PM & R*, *10*(9, Suppl 2), S174–S188.

Mondini, V., Kobler, R. J., Sburlea, A. I., & Müller-Putz, G. R. (2020). Continuous low-frequency EEG decoding of arm movement for closed-loop, natural control of a robotic arm. *Journal of Neural Engineering*, *17*(4), 046031.

Morone, G., Cocchi, I., Paolucci, S., & Iosa, M. (2020). Robot-assisted therapy for arm recovery for stroke patients: State of the art and clinical implication. *Expert Review of Medical Devices*, *17*(3), 223–233.

Morone, G., Masiero, S., Werner, C., & Paolucci, S. (2014). Advances in neuromotor stroke rehabilitation. *BioMed Research International*, *2014*, 236043.

Morone, G., Palomba, A., Martino Cinnera, A., Agostini, M., Aprile, I., Arienti, C., Paci, M., Casanova, E., Marino, D., & Rosa, L. A. (2021). Systematic review of guidelines to identify recommendations for upper limb robotic rehabilitation after stroke. *European Journal of Physical and Rehabilitation Medicine, 57*(2), 238–245.

Morone, G., Paolucci, S., Cherubini, A., De Angelis, D., Venturiero, V., Coiro, P., & Iosa, M. (2017). Robot-assisted gait training for stroke patients: Current state of the art and perspectives of robotics. *Neuropsychiatric Disease and Treatment*, *13*, 1303–1311.

Morone, G., Spitoni, G. F., De Bartolo, D., Ghanbari Ghooshchy, S., Di Iulio, F., Paolucci, S., Zoccolotti, P., & Iosa, M. (2019). Rehabilitative devices for a top-down approach. *Expert Review of Medical Devices*, *16*(3), 187–195.

Mubin, O., Alnajjar, F., Jishtu, N., Alsinglawi, B., & Al Mahmud, A. (2019). Exoskeletons With Virtual Reality, Augmented Reality, and Gamification for Stroke Patients' Rehabilitation: Systematic Review. *JMIR Rehabilitation and Assistive Technologies, 6*(2), e12010.

Murphy, T. H., & Corbett, D. (2009). Plasticity during stroke recovery: From synapse to behaviour. *Nature Reviews. Neuroscience*, *10*(12), 861–872.

Nudo, R. J., & Friel, K. M. (1999). Cortical plasticity after stroke: Implications for rehabilitation. *Revue Neurologique*, *155*(9), 713–717.

Reinkensmeyer, D. J. (2018). *Rehabilitation robot*. Encyclopedia Britannica.

Reis, S. B., Bernardo, W. M., Oshiro, C. A., Krebs, H. I., & Conforto, A. B. (2021). Effects of Robotic Therapy Associated With Noninvasive Brain Stimulation on Upper-Limb Rehabilitation After Stroke: Systematic Review and Meta-analysis of Randomized Clinical Trials. *Neurorehabilitation and Neural Repair*, *35*(3), 256–266.

Rodgers, H., Shaw, L., Bosomworth, H., Aird, L., Alvarado, N., Andole, S., Cohen, D. L., Dawson, J., Eyre, J., Finch, T., Ford, G. A., Hislop, J., Hogg, S., Howel, D., Hughes, N., Krebs, H. I., Price, C., Rochester, L., Stamp, E., ... Wilkes, S. (2017). Robot-assisted Training for the Upper Limb after Stroke (RATULS): Study protocol for a randomised controlled trial. *Trials*, *18*(1), 340.

Romera-De Francisco, L., & Jimenez-Del Barrio, S. (2016). Efectividad de la electroestimulacion funcional en pacientes con ictus: Revision sistematica [Effectiveness of functional electrical stimulation in stroke patients: a systematic review]. *Revista de Neurología*, *63*(3), 109–118.

Rosales, R. L., Efendy, F., Teleg, E. S., Delos Santos, M. M., Rosales, M. C., Ostrea, M., Tanglao, M. J., & Ng, A. R. (2016). Botulinum toxin as early intervention for spasticity after stroke or non-progressive brain lesion: A meta-analysis. *Journal of the Neurological Sciences*, *371*, 6–14.

Roth, B. J. (1994). Mechanisms for electrical stimulation of excitable tissue. *Critical Reviews in Biomedical Engineering*, *22*(3-4), 253–305.

Sale, P., Mazzoleni, S., Lombardi, V., Galafate, D., Massimiani, M. P., Posteraro, F., Damiani, C., & Franceschini, M. (2014). Recovery of hand function with robot-assisted therapy in acute stroke patients: A randomized-controlled trial. *International Journal of Rehabilitation Research. Internationale Zeitschrift fur Rehabilitationsforschung. Revue Internationale de Recherches de Readaptation*, *37*(3), 236–242.

Sarikaya, H., Ferro, J., & Arnold, M. (2015). Stroke prevention—medical and lifestyle measures. *European Neurology*, *73*(3-4), 150–157.

Stinear, C. M. (2017). Prediction of motor recovery after stroke: Advances in biomarkers. *Lancet Neurology*, *16*(10), 826–836.

Stinear, C. M., Byblow, W. D., & Ward, S. H. (2014). An update on predicting motor recovery after stroke. *Annals of Physical and Rehabilitation Medicine*, *57*(8), 489–498.

Straudi, S., Baroni, A., Mele, S., Craighero, L., Manfredini, F., Lamberti, N., Maietti, E., & Basaglia, N. (2020). Effects of a Robot-Assisted Arm Training Plus Hand Functional Electrical Stimulation on Recovery After Stroke: A Randomized Clinical Trial. *Archives of Physical Medicine and Rehabilitation*, *101*(2), 309–316.

Takeuchi, N., & Izumi, S. (2013). Rehabilitation with poststroke motor recovery: A review with a focus on neural plasticity. *Stroke Research and Treatment*, *2013*, 128641.

Taub, E., Uswatte, G., Mark, V. W., & Morris, D. M. (2006). The learned nonuse phenomenon: Implications for rehabilitation. *Europa Medicophysica*, *42*(3), 241–256.

Tedla, J. S., Dixit, S., Gular, K., & Abohashrh, M. (2019). Robot-assisted Gait Training Effect on Function and Gait Speed in Subacute and Chronic Stroke Population: A Systematic Review and Meta-Analysis of Randomized Controlled Trials. *European Neurology*, *81*(3-4), 103–111.

The World Health Organization. MONICA Project (Monitoring Trends and Determinants in Cardiovascular Disease): A Major International Collaboration. (1988). *Journal of clinical epidemiology*, *41*(2), 105–114.

Veerbeek, J. M., Langbroek-Amersfoort, A. C., van Wegen, E. E., Meskers, C. G., & Kwakkel, G. (2017). Effects of Robot-Assisted Therapy for the Upper Limb After Stroke. *Neurorehabilitation and Neural Repair*, *31*(2), 107–121.

Winstein, C. J., Stein, J., Arena, R., Bates, B., Cherney, L. R., Cramer, S. C., Deruyter, F., Eng, J. J., Fisher, B., Harvey, R. L., Lang, C. E., MacKay-Lyons, M., Ottenbacher, K. J., Pugh, S., Reeves, M. J., Richards, L. G., Stiers, W., & Zorowitz, R. D. (2016). Guidelines for Adult Stroke Rehabilitation and Recovery: A Guideline for Healthcare Professionals From the American Heart Association/American Stroke Association. *Stroke*, *47*(6), e98–e169.

Wu, J., Cheng, H., Zhang, J., Yang, S., & Cai, S. (2021). Robot-Assisted Therapy for Upper Extremity Motor Impairment After Stroke: A Systematic Review and Meta-Analysis. *Physical Therapy, 101*(4), pzab010.

Xie, M. (2003). *Fundamental of Robotics: Linking Perception to Action*. World Scientific.

Zhang, X., Yue, Z., & Wang, J. (2017). Robotics in Lower-Limb Rehabilitation after Stroke. *Behavioural Neurology*, *2017*, 3731802.

Compilation of References

Adams, L., Gouvousis, A., Vanlue, M., & Waldron, C. (2004). Social Story Intervention: Improving Communication Skills in a Child With an Autism Spectrum Disorder. *Focus on Autism and Other Developmental Disabilities*, *19*(2), 87–94. doi:10.1177/10883576040190020301

Adkins, V. K., & Mathews, R. M. (1997). Prompted voiding to reduce incontinence in community-dwelling older adults. *Journal of Applied Behavior Analysis*, *30*(1), 153–156. doi:10.1901/jaba.1997.30-153 PMID:9103990

Aguirre, G. K., & D'Esposito, M. (1999). Topographical disorientation: A synthesis and taxonomy. *Brain*, *122*(9), 1613–1628. doi:10.1093/brain/122.9.1613 PMID:10468502

Ahmed, R. (2012). *The Effects of Assistive Technology Versus Manual Communication Aids on the Vocabulary Development of Children With Autism* (Doctoral dissertation). San Marcos, CA: California State University.

Aida, T., & Feng, G. (2020). The dawn of non-human primate models for neurodevelopmental disorders. *Current Opinion in Genetics & Development*, *65*, 160–168. doi:10.1016/j.gde.2020.05.040 PMID:32693220

Airaksinen, M., Räsänen, O., Ilén, E., Häyrinen, T., Kivi, A., Marchi, V., Gallen, A., Blom, S., Varhe, A., Kaartinen, N., Haataja, L., & Vanhatalo, S. (2020). Automatic posture and movement tracking of infants with wearable movement sensors. *Scientific Reports*, *10*(1), 169. Advance online publication. doi:10.103841598-019-56862-5 PMID:31932616

Akbas, K., & Mummolo, C. (2021). A computational framework towards the tele-rehabilitation of balance control skills. *Frontiers in Robotics and AI*, *8*, 648485. Advance online publication. doi:10.3389/frobt.2021.648485 PMID:34179106

Akin, N. T. A., & Gokturk, M. (2019). *Comparison of theory of mind tests in augmented reality and 2D environments for children with neurodevelopmental disorders.* . doi:10.1007/978-3-319-94334-3_26

Alahmari, K. A., Sparto, P. J., Marchetti, G. F., Redfern, M. S., Furman, J. M., & Whitney, S. L. (2013). Comparison of virtual reality based therapy with customized vestibular physical therapy for the treatment of vestibular disorders. *IEEE Transactions on Neural Systems and Rehabilitation Engineering*, *22*(2), 389–399. doi:10.1109/TNSRE.2013.2294904 PMID:24608691

Al-Batayneh, O. B., Nazer, T. S., Khader, Y. S., & Owais, A. I. (2020). Effectiveness of a tooth-brushing programme using the picture exchange communication system (PECS) on gingival health of children with autism spectrum disorders. *European Archives of Paediatric Dentistry; Official Journal of the European Academy of Paediatric Dentistry*, *21*(2), 277–283. doi:10.100740368-019-00485-x PMID:31628661

Alcantud, F., Alonso, Y., Coret, J., & Jiménez, E. (2016). Assistive Technologies and Autism Spectrum Disorders. In Human-Computer Interaction: Concepts, Methodologies, Tools, and Applications (pp. 895-924). IGI Global. doi:10.4018/978-1-4666-8789-9.ch041

Alcorn, A. M., Ainger, E., Charisi, V., Mantinioti, S., Petrović, S., Schadenberg, B. R., Tavassoli, T., & Pellicano, E. (2019). Educators' Views on Using Humanoid Robots With Autistic Learners in Special Education Settings in England. *Frontiers in Robotics and AI*, *6*, 107. doi:10.3389/frobt.2019.00107 PMID:33501122

Alhuzimi, T. (2020). Efficacy of Video Modelling (VM) in Developing Social Skills in Children with Autism Spectrum Disorder (ASD) at School in Saudi Arabia. *International Journal of Disability Development and Education*, 1–15. doi:10.1080/1034912X.2020.1716962

Alia, C., Spalletti, C., Lai, S., Panarese, A., Lamola, G., Bertolucci, F., Vallone, F., Di Garbo, A., Chisari, C., Micera, S., & Caleo, M. (2017). Neuroplastic Changes Following Brain Ischemia and their Contribution to Stroke Recovery: Novel Approaches in Neurorehabilitation. *Frontiers in Cellular Neuroscience*, *11*, 76.

Ali, S., Mehmood, F., Dancey, D., Ayaz, Y., Khan, M. J., Naseer, N., Amadeu, R. D. E. C., Sadia, H., & Nawaz, R. (2019). An Adaptive Multi-Robot Therapy for Improving Joint Attention and Imitation of ASD Children. *IEEE Access: Practical Innovations, Open Solutions*, *7*, 7. doi:10.1109/ACCESS.2019.2923678

Allain, P., Foloppe, D. A., Besnard, J., Yamaguchi, T., Etcharry-Bouyx, F., Le Gall, D., Nolin, P., & Richard, P. (2014). Detecting Everyday Action Deficits in Alzheimer's Disease Using a Nonimmersive Virtual Reality Kitchen. *Journal of the International Neuropsychological Society*, *20*(5), 468–477. doi:10.1017/S1355617714000344 PMID:24785240

Allcoat, D., & von Mühlenen, A. (2018). Learning in virtual reality: Effects on performance, emotion and engagement. *Research in Learning Technology*, *26*(0), 2140. doi:10.25304/rlt.v26.2140

Allen, M. L., Hartley, C., & Cain, K. (2016). IPads and the Use of 'Apps' by Children with Autism Spectrum Disorder: Do They Promote Learning? *Frontiers in Phycology*, *7*, 1305. doi:10.3389/fpsyg.2016.01305 PMID:27625621

Allet, L., Leemann, B., Guyen, E., Murphy, L., Monnin, D., Herrmann, F. R., & Schnider, A. (2009). Effect of different walking aids on walking capacity of patients with poststroke hemiparesis. *Archives of Physical Medicine and Rehabilitation*, *90*(8), 1408–1413. doi:10.1016/j.apmr.2009.02.010 PMID:19651276

Allison, S. L., Fagan, A. M., Morris, J. C., & Heada, D. (2016). Spatial Navigation in Preclinical Alzheimer's Disease. *Journal of Alzheimer's Disease*, *52*(1), 77–90. doi:10.3233/JAD-150855 PMID:26967209

Almami, E., Patel, F., Koay, N., Juric, R., & Everiss, C. (2012, June). Towards identifying teaching practices using assistive technologies through ontological reasoning: A Case Study of Pupils with Autism. In *Proceedings of the 17th International Conference on Society for Design and Process Science (SDPS)*, (pp. 10-14). Academic Press.

Alotaibi, M., Long, T., Kennedy, E., & Bavishi, S. (2014). The efficacy of GMFM-88 and GMFM-66 to detect changes in gross motor function in children with cerebral palsy (CP): A literature review. *Disability and Rehabilitation*, *36*(8), 617–627. doi:10.3109/09638288.2013.805820 PMID:23802141

Al-Quraishi, M. S., Elamvazuthi, I., Daud, S. A., Parasuraman, S., & Borboni, A. (2018). EEG-Based Control for Upper and Lower Limb Exoskeletons and Prostheses: A Systematic Review. *Sensors (Basel)*, *18*(10), 3342.

Alrusayni, N. (2017). *The Effectiveness of the High-Tech Speech-Generating Device with Proloquo2Go App in Reducing Echolalia Utterances in a Student with Autism*. Academic Press.

Alves, F. J., De Carvalho, E. A., Aguilar, J., De Brito, L. L., & Bastos, G. S. (2020). Applied behavior analysis for the treatment of autism: A systematic review of assistive technologies. *IEEE Access: Practical Innovations, Open Solutions*, *8*, 118664–118672. doi:10.1109/ACCESS.2020.3005296

Alzahrani, N. S. (2014). *Meta analysis of the effectiveness of using assistive technology to enhance social skills with students diganosed with autism (Master of Special Education Diagnostician Program)*. Lamar University.

Ambrose, C. T. (2012). Neuroangiogenesis: A vascular basis for Alzheimer's disease and cognitive decline during aging. *Journal of Alzheimer's Disease*, *32*(3), 773–778. doi:10.3233/JAD-2012-120067 PMID:22850316

Amir, R. E., Van den Veyver, I. B., Wan, M., Tran, C. Q., Francke, U., & Zoghbi, H. Y. (1999). Rett syndrome is caused by mutations in X-linked MECP2, encoding methyl-CpG-binding protein 2. *Nature Genetics*, *23*(2), 185–188. doi:10.1038/13810 PMID:10508514

Amoako, A. N., & Hare, D. J. (2020). Non-medical interventions for individuals with Rett syndrome: A systematic review. *Journal of Applied Research in Intellectual Disabilities*, *33*(5), 808–827. doi:10.1111/jar.12694 PMID:31833197

Andersen, H. V., & Jensen, R. H. (2018). Assistive Learning Technologies for Learners with ADHD and ASD: A Review 2006-2016. *Læring og Medier*, *11*(19). Advance online publication. doi:10.7146/lom.v11i19.109755

Andersen, K., Levenson, L., & Blumberg, F. C. (2014). The Promise and Limitations of Assistive Technology Use among Children with Autism. In N. R. Silton (Ed.), *Innovative Technologies to Benefit Children on the Autism Spectrum* (pp. 1–19). IGI Global. doi:10.4018/978-1-4666-5792-2.ch001

Anderson, A., Wong, K., Jacoby, P., Downs, J., & Leonard, H. (2014). Twenty years of surveillance in Rett syndrome: What does this tell us? *Orphanet Journal of Rare Diseases*, *9*(1), 87. doi:10.1186/1750-1172-9-87 PMID:24942262

Anopas, D., & Wongsawat, Y. (2014). Virtual reality game for memory skills enhancement based on QEEG. *BMEiCON 2014–7th Biomedical Engineering International Conference.*

Anta˜o, J. Y. F. de L., Abreu, L. C., de, Barbosa, R. T. de A., & Crocetta, T. (2020). Use of Augmented Reality with a Motion-Controlled Game Utilizing Alphabet Letters and Numbers to Improve Performance and Reaction Time Skills for People with Autism Spectrum Disorder. *Cyberpsychology, Behavior, and Social Networking*, *23*(1), 16–22. doi:10.1089/cyber.2019.0103 PMID:31976770

Anttila, M. R., Kivistö, H., Piirainen, A., Kokko, K., Malinen, A., Pekkonen, M., & Sjögren, T. (2019). Cardiac rehabilitees' technology experiences before remote rehabilitation: Qualitative study using a grounded theory approach. *Journal of Medical Internet Research*, *21*(2), e10985. doi:10.2196/10985 PMID:30730298

Arkin, S. (2007). Language-enriched exercise plus socialization slows cognitive decline in Alzheimer's disease. *American Journal of Alzheimer's Disease and Other Dementias*, *22*(1), 62–77. doi:10.1177/1533317506295377 PMID:17534004

Arth, C., Grasset, R., Gruber, L., Langlotz, T., Mulloni, R., Schmalstieg, D., & Wagner, D. (2015). *The History of Mobile Augmented Reality Developments in Mobile AR over the last almost 50 years.* Academic Press.

Arthur-Kelly, M., Foreman, P., Maes, B., Colyvas, K., & Lyons, G. (2018). Observational data on socio-communicative phenomena in classrooms supporting students with profound intellectual and multiple disability (PIMD): Advancing theory development on learning and engagement through data analysis. *Advances in Neurodevelopmental Disorders*, *2*(1), 25–37. doi:10.100741252-017-0045-1

Arthur, M. (2003). Socio-communicative variables and behavior states in students with profound and multiple disabilities: Descriptive data from school settings. *Education and Training in Developmental Disabilities*, *38*, 200–219.

Asano, M., Koh, G. C., Madhukumar, P., Teng, G. Y. H., Liew, P. L. L., Nagalingam, S., Tan, M. L. M., Ng, Y. S., & Tan, B. K. T. (2021). Study protocol: A pilot quasi-experimental trial of tele-rehabilitation and tele-drain care post-mastectomy. *Pilot and Feasibility Studies*, *7*(1), 39. Advance online publication. doi:10.118640814-021-00776-5 PMID:33522962

Asghar, I., Cang, S., & Yu, H. (2018). Usability evaluation of assistive technologies through qualitative research focusing on people with mild dementia. *Computers in Human Behavior*, *79*, 192–201. doi:10.1016/j.chb.2017.08.034

Ashok, J., Bharucha, C., Anand, V., Forlizzi, J., Dew, M. A., & Charles, F. (2009). Reynolds, Scott Stevens, Howard Wactlar, Intelligent Assistive Technology Applications to Dementia Care: Current Capabilities, Limitations, and Future Challenges. *The American Journal of Geriatric Psychiatry*, *17*, 84–88.

Asperger, H. (1944). Die 'Autistischen Psychopathen' im Kindesalter [Autistic Psychopathy of Childhood] [Archives of Psychiatry and Clinical Neuroscience]. *Archiv für Psychiatrie und Nervenkrankheiten*, *117*(1), 76–136. doi:10.1007/BF01837709

Astell, A., Malone, B., Williams, G., Hwang, F., & Ellis, M. (2014). Leveraging everyday technology for people living with dementia: A case study. *Journal of Assistive Technologies*, *8*(4), 164–176. doi:10.1108/JAT-01-2014-0004

Atkin, K., & Lorch, M. P. (2014). An ecological method for the sampling of nonverbal signalling behaviors of young children with profound and multiple learning disabilities (PMLD). *Developmental Neurorehabilitation*, 1–15. PMID:25029100

Ausburn, L. J., Martens, J., Washington, A., Steele, D., & Washburn, E. (2009). A cross-case analysis of gender issues in desktop virtual reality learning environments. *Journal of STEM Teacher Education*, *46*(3), 6.

Autism Speaks Inc. (2021). Retrieved October 13, 2016, from https://www.autismspeaks.org/about-us

Autism Speaks. (2010, April). *What is autism?* Retrieved November 17, 2011, from https://www.educateiowa.gov/sites/files/ed/documents/Parent-Factsheets_April2010_Autism.pdf

Azuma, R. T. (1997). A survey of augmented reality. *Presence (Cambridge, Mass.)*, *6*(4), 355–385. doi:10.1162/pres.1997.6.4.355

Babiloni, C., Del Percio, C., Caroli, A., Salvatore, E., Nicolai, E., Marzano, N., Lizio, R., Cavedo, E., Landau, S., Chen, K., Jagust, W., Reiman, E., Tedeschi, G., Montella, P., De Stefano, M., Gesualdo, L., Frisoni, G. B., & Soricelli, A. (2016). Cortical sources of resting state EEG rhythms are related to brain hypometabolismin subjects with Alzheimer's disease: An EEG-PET study. *Neurobiology Aging Journal*, *48*, 122–134. doi:10.1016/j.neurobiolaging.2016.08.021 PMID:27668356

Bailes, A., Reder, R., & Burch, C. (2009). Development of guidelines for determining frequency of therapy services in a pediatric medical setting. *Pediatric Physical Therapy*, *20*(2), 194–198. doi:10.1097/PEP.0b013e3181728a7b PMID:18480720

Bailey, B., Bryant, L., & Hemsley, B. (2021). Virtual reality and augmented reality for children, adolescents, and adults with communication disability and neurodevelopmental disorders: A systematic review. *Review Journal of Autism and Developmental Disorders*. Advance online publication. doi:10.100740489-020-00230-x

Bai, Z., Blackwell, A. F., & Coulouris, G. (2015). Using Augmented Reality to Elicit Pretend Play for Children with Autism. *IEEE Transactions on Visualization and Computer Graphics*, *21*(5), 598–610.doi:https://doi.org/10.1109/TVCG.2014.2385092

Balami, J. S., Chen, R. L., & Buchan, A. M. (2013). Stroke syndromes and clinical management. *QJM: An International Journal of Medicine*, *106*(7), 607–615. doi:10.1093/qjmed/hct057 PMID:23483140

Bamm, E. L., & Rosenbaum, P. (2008). Family-centered theory: Origins, development, barriers, and supports to implementation in rehabilitation medicine. *Archives of Physical Medicine and Rehabilitation*, *89*(8), 1618–1624. doi:10.1016/j.apmr.2007.12.034 PMID:18586223

Banda, D. R., Dogoe, M. S., & Matuszny, R. M. (2011). Review of Video Prompting Studies with Persons with Developmental Disabilities. *Education and Training in Autism and Developmental Disabilities*, *46*(4), 514–527. http://www.jstor.org/stable/24232363

Bankole, A., Anderson, M., Smith-Jackson, T., Knight, A., Oh, K., Brantley, J., Barth, A., & Lach, J. (2012). Validation of noninvasive body sensor network technology in the detection of agitation in dementia. *American Journal of Alzheimer's Disease and Other Dementias*, *27*(5), 346–354. doi:10.1177/1533317512452036 PMID:22815084

Banta Lavenex, P., & Lavenex, P. (2021). A critical review of spatial abilities in down and williams syndromes: Not all space is created equal. *Frontiers in Psychiatry*, *12*, 669320. Advance online publication. doi:10.3389/fpsyt.2021.669320 PMID:34122185

Barlow, D. H., Andrasik, F., & Hersen, M. (2006). *Single-case experimental designs* (3rd ed.). Allyn & Bacon.

Barnard-Brak, L., Thompson, S., Wei, T., & Richman, D. (2014). Assistive technology as a predictor of general or alternate assessment among elementary-aged students with autism spectrum disorders. *Assistive Technology*, *26*(2), 81–87. doi:10.1080/10400435.2013.833557 PMID:25112052

Baron-Cohen, S. (2009). Autism: The Empathizing-Systemizing (ES) Theory. *Annals of the New York Academy of Sciences*, *1156*(1), 68–80. doi:10.1111/j.1749-6632.2009.04467.x PMID:19338503

Barry, L., Holloway, J., & Mcmahon, J. (2020). A scoping review of the barriers and facilitators to the implementation of interventions in autism education. *Research in Autism Spectrum Disorders*, *78*, 101617. Advance online publication. doi:10.1016/j.rasd.2020.101617

Bassi, M., Cilia, S., Falautano, M., Grobberio, M., Negri, L., Niccolai, C., Pattini, M., Pietrolongo, E., Quartuccio, M. E., Viterbo, R. G., Allegri, B., Amato, M. P., Benin, M., De Luca, G., Gasperini, C., Minacapelli, E., Patti, F., Trojano, M., & Delle Fave, A. (2020). The caring experience in multiple sclerosis: Caregiving tasks, coping strategies and psychological well-being. *Health & Social Care in the Community*, *28*(1), 236–246. doi:10.1111/hsc.12858 PMID:31524966

Baumeister, J., Ssin, S. Y., ElSayed, N. A., Dorrian, J., Webb, D. P., Walsh, J. A., Simon, T. M., Irlitti, A., Smith, R. T., Kohler, M., & Thomas, B. H. (2017). Cognitive cost of using augmented reality displays. *IEEE Transactions on Visualization and Computer Graphics*, *23*(11), 2378–2388. doi:10.1109/TVCG.2017.2735098 PMID:28809700

Baumgartner, T., Valko, L., Esslen, M., & Jäncke, L. (2006). Neural correlate of spatial presence in an arousing and noninteractive virtual reality: An EEG and psychophysiology study. *Cyberpsychology & Behavior*, *9*(1), 30–45. doi:10.1089/cpb.2006.9.30 PMID:16497116

Beals, K. (2017). Remediation and Assistive Technologies for Communication Deficits in Autism Spectrum Disorders. In *Supporting the Education of Children with Autism Spectrum Disorders* (pp. 160–183). IGI Global. doi:10.4018/978-1-5225-0816-8.ch009

Begum, M., Serna, R. W., & Yanco, H. A. (2016). Are Robots Ready to Deliver Autism Interventions? *International Journal of Social Robotics*, *8*, 157–181.doi:https://doi.org/10.1007/s12369-016-0346-y

Behera, C. K., Condell, J., Dora, S., Gibson, D. S., & Leavey, G. (2021). State-of-the-art sensors for remote care of people with dementia during a pandemic: A systematic review. *Sensors (Basel)*, *21*(14), 4688. Advance online publication. doi:10.339021144688 PMID:34300428

Behn, N., Marshall, J., Togher, L., & Cruice, M. (2019). Setting and achieving individualized social communication goals for people with acquired brain injury (ABI) within a group treatment. *International Journal of Language & Communication Disorders*, *54*(5), 828–840. doi:10.1111/1460-6984.12488 PMID:31250537

Belda-Lois, J. M., Mena-del Horno, S., Bermejo-Bosch, I., Moreno, J. C., Pons, J. L., Farina, D., Iosa, M., Molinari, M., Tamburella, F., Ramos, A., Caria, A., Solis-Escalante, T., Brunner, C., & Rea, M. (2011). Rehabilitation of gait after stroke: A review towards a top-down approach. *Journal of Neuroengineering and Rehabilitation*, *8*, 66.

Belić, M., Bobić, V., Badža, M., Šolaja, N., Đurić-Jovičić, M., & Kostić, V. S. (2019). Artificial intelligence for assisting diagnostics and assessment of Parkinson's disease—A review. *Clinical Neurology and Neurosurgery, 184*, 105442. Advance online publication. doi:10.1016/j.clineuro.2019.105442 PMID:31351213

Bellamy, G., Croot, L., Bush, A., Berry, H., & Smith, A. (2010). A study to define: Profound and multiple learning disabilities (PMLD). *Journal of Intellectual Disabilities, 14*(3), 221–235. doi:10.1177/1744629510386290 PMID:21062858

Belleville, S., Gilbert, B., Fontaine, F., Gagnon, L., Menard, E., & Gauthier, S. (2006). Improvement of episodic memory in persons with mild cognitive impairment and healthy older adults: Evidence from a cognitive intervention program. *Dementia and Geriatric Cognitive Disorders, 22*(5-6), 486–499. doi:10.1159/000096316 PMID:17050952

Bell, K. M., Onyeukwu, C., McClincy, M. P., Allen, M., Bechard, L., Mukherjee, A., Hartman, R. A., Smith, C., Lynch, A. D., & Irrgang, J. J. (2019). Verification of a portable motion tracking system for remote management of physical rehabilitation of the knee. *Sensors (Switzerland), 19*(5), 1021. doi:10.339019051021 PMID:30823373

Belva, B. C., Matson, J. L., Sipes, M., & Bamburg, J. W. (2012). An examination of specific communication deficits in adults with profound intellectual disabilities. *Research in Developmental Disabilities, 33*(2), 525–529. doi:10.1016/j.ridd.2011.10.019 PMID:22119701

Ben-Avie, M., Newton, D., & Reichow, B. (2014). Using Handheld Applications to Improve the Transitions of Students with Autism Spectrum Disorders. In N. R. Silton (Ed.), *Innovative Technologies to Benefit Children on the Autism Spectrum* (pp. 105–124). IGI Global. doi:10.4018/978-1-4666-5792-2.ch007

Benedetto, M., Bailes, A., Pandya, S., Edwards, P., & Booker-Feister, C. (2017). *Section on Pediatrics Fact Sheet: Intensity of Service in an Outpatient Setting for Children with Chronic Conditions*. American Physical Therapy Association.

Bennys, K., Rondouin, G., Benattar, E., Gabelle, A., & Touchon, J. (2011). Can event-related potential predict the progression of mild cognitive impairment? *Journal of Clinical Neurophysiology, 28*(6), 625–632. doi:10.1097/WNP.0b013e31823cc2d3 PMID:22146349

Benson, A. (2020). *Math Problem Solving Discussions : Increasing Communication for Students with Autism*. Academic Press.

Berenguer, C., Baixauli, I., Gomez, S., Andrés, M. d., & De Stasio, S. (2020). Exploring the Impact of Augmented Reality in Children and Adolescents with Autism Spectrum Disorder: A Systematic Review. *International Journal of Environmental Research and Public Health, 17*(17), 6143.doi: https://doi.org/10.3390/ijerph17176143

Berenguer, C., Baixauli, I., Gómez, S., Andrés, M. E. P., & De Stasio, S. (2020). Exploring the impact of augmented reality in children and adolescents with autism spectrum disorder: A systematic review. *International Journal of Environmental Research and Public Health, 17*(17), 1–15. doi:10.3390/ijerph17176143 PMID:32847074

Bergh, C., & Wennerholm, U. (2020). Long-term health of children conceived after assisted reproductive technology. *Upsala Journal of Medical Sciences, 125*(2), 152–157. doi:10.1080/03009734.2020.1729904 PMID:32101068

Bernhardt, J., & Mehrholz, J. (2019, July 6). Robot-assisted training after stroke: RATULS advances science. *Lancet, 394*(10192), 6–8.

Bernini, S., Stasolla, F., Panzarasa, S., Quaglini, S., Sinforiani, E., Sandrini, G., Vecchi, T., Tassorelli, C., & Bottiroli, S. (2021). Cognitive telerehabilitation for older adults with neurodegenerative diseases in the COVID-19 era: A perspective study. *Frontiers in Neurology, 11*, 623933. Advance online publication. doi:10.3389/fneur.2020.623933 PMID:33519704

Bertani, R., Melegari, C., De Cola, M. C., Bramanti, A., Bramanti, P., & Calabrò, R. S. (2017). Effects of robot-assisted upper limb rehabilitation in stroke patients: a systematic review with meta-analysis. *Neurological Sciences, 38*(9), 1561–1569.

Bethoux, F., Rogers, H. L., Nolan, K. J., Abrams, G. M., Annaswamy, T. M., Brandstater, M., Browne, B., Burnfield, J. M., Feng, W., Freed, M. J., Geis, C., Greenberg, J., Gudesblatt, M., Ikramuddin, F., Jayaraman, A., Kautz, S. A., Lutsep, H. L., Madhavan, S., Meilahn, J., ... Kufta, C. (2014). The effects of peroneal nerve functional electrical stimulation versus ankle-foot orthosis in patients with chronic stroke: A randomized controlled trial. *Neurorehabilitation and Neural Repair, 28*(7), 688–697. doi:10.1177/1545968314521007 PMID:24526708

Bethoux, F., Rogers, H. L., Nolan, K. J., Abrams, G. M., Annaswamy, T., Brandstater, M., Browne, B., Burnfield, J. M., Feng, W., Freed, M. J., Geis, C., Greenberg, J., Gudesblatt, M., Ikramuddin, F., Jayaraman, A., Kautz, S. A., Lutsep, H. L., Madhavan, S., Meilahn, J., ... Kufta, C. (2015). Long-term follow-up to a randomized controlled trial comparing peroneal nerve functional electrical stimulation to an ankle foot orthosis for patients with chronic stroke. *Neurorehabilitation and Neural Repair, 29*(10), 911–922. doi:10.1177/1545968315570325 PMID:25653225

Biddiss, E., Chan-Viquez, D., Cheung, S. T., & King, G. (2021). Engaging children with cerebral palsy in interactive computer play-based motor therapies: Theoretical perspectives. *Disability and Rehabilitation, 43*(1), 133–147. doi:10.1080/09638288.2019.1613681 PMID:31104517

Billeci, L., Tonacci, A., Narzisi, A., Manigrasso, Z., Varanini, M., Fulceri, F., Lattarulo, C., Calderoni, S., & Muratori, F. (2018). Heart rate variability during a joint attention task in toddlers with autism spectrum disorders. *Frontiers in Physiology, 9*(May), 467. Advance online publication. doi:10.3389/fphys.2018.00467 PMID:29765335

Billger, M., Heldal, I., Stahre, B., & Renstrom, K. (2004, June). Perception of color and space in virtual reality: a comparison between a real room and virtual reality models. In *Human Vision and Electronic Imaging IX* (Vol. 5292, pp. 90–98). International Society for Optics and Photonics. doi:10.1117/12.526986

Billis, A., Mantziari, D., Zilidou, V., & Bamidis, P. D. (2018). Co-Creation of an Innovative Vocational Training Platform to Improve Autonomy in the Context of Alzheimer's Disease. *The American Journal of Geriatric Psychiatry*, 309–323. PMID:29968665

Bimbrahw, J., Boger, J., & Mihailidis, A. (2012). Investigating the Efficacy of a Computerized Prompting Device to Assist Children with Autism Spectrum Disorder with Activities of Daily Living. *Assistive Technology, 24*(4), 286–298. doi:10.1080/10400435.2012.680661

Binder, E. B. (2021). Genotype-Phenotype Predictions in Autism: Are We There Yet? *The American Journal of Psychiatry, 11-12*(1), 11–12. Advance online publication. doi:10.1176/appi.ajp.2020.20111589 PMID:33384006

Bioulac, S., Taillard, J., Philip, P., & Sagaspe, P. (2020). Excessive daytime sleepiness measurements in children with attention deficit hyperactivity disorder. *Frontiers in Psychiatry, 11*, 3. Advance online publication. doi:10.3389/fpsyt.2020.00003 PMID:32174847

Birenboim, A., & Bloom, P. B. (2021). The study of walking, walkability and wellbeing in immersive virtual environments. *International Journal of Environmental Research and Public Health, 18*(2), 1–18. doi:10.3390/ijerph18020364 PMID:33418896

Birks, J. S., & Harvey, R. J. (2018). Donepezil for dementia due to Alzheimer's disease. *Cochrane Database of Systematic Reviews, 8*, 12–13. doi:10.1002/14651858.CD001190.pub3 PMID:29923184

Bockbrader, M. A., Francisco, G., Lee, R., Olson, J., Solinsky, R., & Boninger, M. L. (2018). Brain Computer Interfaces in Rehabilitation Medicine. *PM&R, 10*(9S2), S233-S243. doi:10.1016/j.pmrj.2018.05.028

Bogomolova, K., van der Ham, I. J., Dankbaar, M. E., van den Broek, W. W., Hovius, S. E., van der Hage, J. A., & Hierck, B. P. (2020). The effect of stereoscopic Augmented Reality visualization on learning anatomy and the modifying effect of visual-spatial abilities: A double-center randomized controlled trial. *Anatomical Sciences Education*, *13*(5), 558–567. doi:10.1002/ase.1941 PMID:31887792

Boot, F. H., Owuor, J., Dinsmore, J., & MacLachlan, M. (2018). Access to assistive technology for people with intellectual disabilities: A systematic review to identify barriers and facilitators. *Journal of Intellectual Disability Research*, *62*(10), 900–921. doi:10.1111/jir.12532 PMID:29992653

Botella, C., Fernández-Álvarez, J., Guillén, V., García-Palacios, A., & Baños, R. (2017). Recent Progress in Virtual Reality Exposure Therapy for Phobias: A Systematic Review. *Current Psychiatry Reports*, *19*, 42.doi:https://doi.org/10.1007/s11920-017-0788-4

Bottino, C. M., Carvalho, I. A., Alvarez, A. M., Avila, R., Zukauskas, P. R., Bustamante, S. E. Z., Andrade, F. C., Hototian, S. R., Saffi, F., & Camargo, C. H. P. (2005, December). Cognitive rehabilitation combined with drug treatment in Alzheimer's disease patients: A pilot study. *Clinical Rehabilitation*, *19*(8), 861–864. doi:10.1191/0269215505cr911oa PMID:16323385

Bottiroli, S., Bernini, S., Cavallini, E., Sinforiani, E., Zucchella, C., Pazzi, S., Cristiani, P., Vecchi, T., Tost, D., Sandrini, G., & Tassorelli, C. (2021). The smart aging platform for assessing early phases of cognitive impairment in patients with neurodegenerative diseases. *Frontiers in Psychology*, *12*, 635410. Advance online publication. doi:10.3389/fpsyg.2021.635410 PMID:33790839

Bottiroli, S., Tassorelli, C., Lamonica, M., Zucchella, C., Cavallini, E., Bernini, S., Sinforiani, E., Pazzi, S., Cristiani, P., Vecchi, T., Tost, D., & Sandrini, G. (2017). Smart aging platform for evaluating cognitive functions in aging: A comparison with the MoCA in a normal population. *Frontiers in Aging Neuroscience*, *21*(9), 1–14. doi:10.3389/fnagi.2017.00379 PMID:29209200

Botvinick, M., & Cohen, J. (1998). Rubber hands 'feel' touch that eyes see. *Nature*, *391*(6669), 756–756. doi:10.1038/35784 PMID:9486643

Boucenna, S., Narzisi, A., Tilmont, E., Muratori, F., Pioggia, G., Cohen, D., & Chetouani, M. (2014). Interactive technologies for autistic children: A review. *Cognitive Computation*, *6*(4), 722–740. doi:10.100712559-014-9276-x

Bouck, E. C. (2010). Chapter 6 Technology and students with disabilities: Does it solve all the problems. In F. E. Obiakor, J. P. Bakken, & nthony F. Rotatori (Eds.), Current Issues and Trends in Special Education: Research, Technology, and Teacher Preparation (Vol. 20, pp. 91–104). Emerald Group Publishing Limited. doi:10.1108/S0270-4013(2010)0000020009

Bourrelier, J., Ryard, J., Dion, M., Merienne, F., Manckoundia, P., & Mourey, F. (2016). Use of a virtual environment to engage motor and postural abilities in elderly subjects with and without mild cognitive impairment (MAAMI Project). *IRBM*, *37*(2), 75–80. doi:10.1016/j.irbm.2016.02.007

Bovend'Eerdt, T. J. H., Botell, R. E., & Wade, D. T. (2009). Writing SMART rehabilitation goals and achieving goal attainment scaling: A practical guide. *Clinical Rehabilitation*, *23*(4), 352–361. doi:10.1177/0269215508101741 PMID:19237435

Bowring, D. L., Totsika, V., Hastings, R. P., Toogood, S., & McMahon, M. (2017). Prevalence of psychotropic medication use and association with challenging behavior in adults with an intellectual disability. A total population Study. *Journal of Intellectual Disability Research*, *61*(6), 604–617. doi:10.1111/jir.12359 PMID:28090687

Boyle, E. A., Connolly, T. M., Hainey, T., & Boyle, J. M. (2012). Engagement in digital entertainment games: A systematic review. *Computers in Human Behavior*, *28*(3), 771–780. doi:10.1016/j.chb.2011.11.020

Brandt, Å., Jensen, M. P., Søberg, M. S., Andersen, S. D., & Sund, T. (2020). Information and communication technology-based assistive technology to compensate for impaired cognition in everyday life: A systematic review. *Disability and Rehabilitation. Assistive Technology*, *15*(7), 810–824. doi:10.1080/17483107.2020.1765032 PMID:32407217

Brauchle, D., Vukelić, M., Bauer, R., & Gharabaghi, A. (2015). Brain state-dependent robotic reaching movement with a multi-joint arm exoskeleton: Combining brain-machine interfacing and robotic rehabilitation. *Frontiers in Human Neuroscience*, *9*, 564.

Brockett, C. L., & Chapman, G. J. (2016). Biomechanics of the ankle. *Orthopaedics and Trauma*, *30*(3), 232–238. doi:10.1016/j.mporth.2016.04.015 PMID:27594929

Brodaty, H., Green, A., & Koschera, A. (2003). Meta-analysis of psychosocial interventions for caregivers of people with dementia. *Journal of the American Geriatrics Society*, *51*(5), 657–664. doi:10.1034/j.1600-0579.2003.00210.x PMID:12752841

Brookmeyer, R., Johnson, E., Ziegler-Graham, K., & Arrighi, H. M. (2007). Forecasting the global burden of Alzheimer's disease. *Alzheimer's & Dementia Journal*, *3*(3), 186–191. doi:10.1016/j.jalz.2007.04.381 PMID:19595937

Brownlee, A., & Bruening, L. M. (2012). Methods of communication at end of life for the person with amyotrophic lateral sclerosis. *Topics in Language Disorders*, *32*(2), 168–185. doi:10.1097/TLD.0b013e31825616ef

Brunner, M., Hemsley, B., Togher, L., & Palmer, S. (2017). Technology and its role in rehabilitation for people with cognitive-communication disability following a traumatic brain injury (TBI). *Brain Injury: [BI]*, *31*(8), 1028–1043. doi:10.1080/02699052.2017.1292429 PMID:28471267

Bryant, B. R., Bryant, D. P., Shih, M., & Seok, S. (2010). Assistive technology and supports provision: A selective review of the literature and proposed areas of application. *Exceptionality*, *18*(4), 203–213. doi:10.1080/09362835.2010.513925

Budden, S. (1995). Management of Rett Syndrome: A Ten Year Experience. *Neuropediatrics*, *26*(02), 75–77. doi:10.1055-2007-979727 PMID:7566457

Buggey, T., & Ogle, L. (2012). Video self-modeling. *Psychology in the Schools*, *49*(1), 52–70. doi:10.1002/pits.20618

Byrns, A., Abdessalem, H. B., Cuesta, M., Bruneau, M. A., Belleville, S., & Frasson, C. (2020). Adaptive Music Therapy for Alzheimer's Disease Using Virtual Reality. In V. Kumar & C. Troussas (Eds.), *Intelligent Tutoring Systems*. Springer International Publishing. doi:10.1007/978-3-030-49663-0_25

Bystrom, K. E., Barfield, W., & Hendrix, C. (1999). A conceptual model of the sense of presence in virtual environments. *Presence (Cambridge, Mass.)*, *8*(2), 241–244. doi:10.1162/105474699566107

Cabinio, M., Rossetto, F., Isernia, S., Saibene, F. L., Di Cesare, M., Borgnis, F., Pazzi, S., Migliazza, T., Alberoni, M., Blasi, V., & Baglio, F. (2020). The Use of a Virtual Reality Platform for the Assessment of the Memory Decline and the Hippocampal Neural Injury in Subjects with Mild Cognitive Impairment: The Validity of Smart Aging Serious Game (SASG). *Journal of Clinical Medicine*, *9*(1355), 1–13. doi:10.3390/jcm9051355 PMID:32384591

Caduff, D., & Timpf, S. (2008). On the assessment of landmark salience for human navigation. *Cognitive Processing*, *9*(4), 249–267. doi:10.100710339-007-0199-2 PMID:17999102

Caffò, A. O., Lopez, A., Spano, G., Saracino, G., Stasolla, F., Ciriello, G., Grattagliano, I., Lancioni, G. E., & Bosco, A. (2016). The role of pre-morbid intelligence and cognitive reserve in predicting cognitive efficiency in a sample of italian elderly. *Aging Clinical and Experimental Research*, *28*(6), 1203–1210. doi:10.100740520-016-0580-z PMID:27149863

Caffò, A. O., Lopez, A., Spano, G., Stasolla, F., Serino, S., Cipresso, P., Riva, G., & Bosco, A. (2020). The differential effect of normal and pathological aging on egocentric and allocentric spatial memory in navigational and reaching space. *Neurological Sciences*, *41*(7), 1741–1749. doi:10.100710072-020-04261-4 PMID:32002741

Cage, E., Di Monaco, J., & Newell, V. (2018). Experiences of autism acceptance and mental health in autistic adults. *Journal of Autism and Developmental Disorders*, *48*(2), 473–484. doi:10.100710803-017-3342-7 PMID:29071566

Calabrò, R. S., Accorinti, M., Porcari, B., Carioti, L., Ciatto, L., Billeri, L., Andronaco, V. A., Galletti, F., Filoni, S., & Naro, A. (2019). Does hand robotic rehabilitation improve motor function by rebalancing interhemispheric connectivity after chronic stroke? Encouraging data from a randomised-clinical-trial. *Clinical Neurophysiology*, *130*(5), 767–780.

Calculator, S. (1988). Promoting the acquisition and generalization of conversational skills by individuals with severe disabilities. *Augmentative and Alternative Communication*, *4*(2), 94–103. doi:10.1080/07434618812331274677

Caligari, M., Godi, M., Giardini, M., & Colombo, R. (2019). Development of a new high sensitivity mechanical switch for augmentative and alternative communication access in people with amyotrophic lateral sclerosis. *Journal of Neuroengineering and Rehabilitation*, *16*(1), 152. Advance online publication. doi:10.118612984-019-0626-5 PMID:31783763

Calouro, C., Kwong, M. W., & Gutierrez, M. (2014). An Analysis of State Telehealth Laws and Regulations for Occupational Therapy and Physical Therapy. *International Journal of Telerehabilitation*, *6*(1), 17–24. doi:10.5195/ijt.2014.6141 PMID:25945218

Camilo, M. C. (2009). *Tecnologie quotidiane per la cura della malattia di Alzheimer: risultati della ricerca, direzioni e sfide*. Elsevier.

Caprì, T., Nucita, A., Iannizzotto, G., Stasolla, F., Romano, A., Semino, M., Giannatiempo, S., Canegallo, V., & Fabio, R. A. (2021). Telerehabilitation for Improving Adaptive Skills of Children and Young Adults with Multiple Disabilities: A Systematic Review. *Review Journal of Autism and Developmental Disorders*, *8*(2), 244–252. doi:10.100740489-020-00214-x

Carey, H., Martin, K., Combs-Miller, S., & Heathcock, J. C. (2016). Reliability and Responsiveness of the Timed Up and Go Test in Children With Cerebral Palsy. *Pediatric Physical Therapy*, *28*(4), 401–408. doi:10.1097/PEP.0000000000000301 PMID:27661230

Carlier, S., Van der Paelt, S., Ongenae, F., De Backere, F., & De Turck, F. (2020). Empowering Children with ASD and Their Parents: Design of a Serious Game for Anxiety and Stress Reduction. *Sensors (Basel)*, *20*(4), 966. https://doi.org/10.3390/s20040966

Caro, P., & Derevensky, J. L. (1991). Family-Focused Intervention Model: Implementation and Research Findings. *Topics in Early Childhood Special Education*, *11*(3), 66–91. doi:10.1177/027112149101100307

Carrasco, E., Epelde, G., Moreno, A., Ortiz, A., Garcia, I., Buiza, C., Urdaneta, E., Etxaniz, A., Gonz'alez, M. F., & Arruti, A. (2008). *Natural Interaction between Virtual Characters and Persons with Alzheimer's Disease*. University of the Basque Country.

Carrillo-Avila, A., Melgar-Rodriguez, S., Díaz-Zuñiga, J., & Martínez-Aguilar, V. (2020). Periodontitis and alzheimer´s disease. *Medicina Oral Patología Oral y Cirugia*.

Cass, H., Reilly, S., Owen, L., Wisbeach, A., Weekes, L., Slonims, V., Wigram, T., & Charman, T. (2003). Findings from a multidisciplinary clinical case series of females with Rett syndrome. *Developmental Medicine and Child Neurology*, *45*(5), 325–337. doi:10.1111/j.1469-8749.2003.tb00404.x PMID:12729147

Cassidy, S. A., Stenger, B., Van Dongen, L., Yanagisawa, K., Anderson, R., Wan, V., Baron-Cohen, S., & Cipolla, R. (2016). Expressive visual text-to-speech as an assistive technology for individuals with autism spectrum conditions. *Computer Vision and Image Understanding*, *148*, 193–200. doi:10.1016/j.cviu.2015.08.011 PMID:27375348

Casula, E. P., Pellicciari, M. C., Bonnì, S., Spanò, B., Ponzo, V., Salsano, I., Giulietti, G., Martino Cinnera, A., Maiella, M., Borghi, I., Rocchi, L., Bozzali, M., Sallustio, F., Caltagirone, C., & Koch, G. (2021). Evidence for interhemispheric imbalance in stroke patients as revealed by combining transcranial magnetic stimulation and electroencephalography. *Human Brain Mapping*. Advance online publication. doi:10.1002/hbm.25297

Catania, A. C. (2012). *Learning* (5th ed.). Sloan.

Center for Devices and Radiologial Health. (2014). *Providing Information about pediatric Uses of Medical Devices: Guidance for Industry and Food and Drug Administration Staff.* Washington, DC: U.S. Department of Health and Human Services Retrieved from https://www.fda.gov/regulatory-information/search-fda-guidance-documents/providing-information-about-pediatric-uses-medical-devices

Cerga-Pashoja, A., Gaete, J., Shishkova, A., & Jordanova, V. (2019). Improving Reading in Adolescents and Adults With High-Functioning Autism Through an Assistive Technology Tool: A Cross-Over Multinational Study. *Frontiers in Phychiatry, 10*, 546. doi:10.3389/fpsyt.2019.00546

Chai, X. J., & Jacobs, L. F. (2009). Sex differences in directional cue use in a virtual landscape. *Behavioral Neuroscience*, *123*(3), 276–283. doi:10.1037/a0014722 PMID:19331451

Chalmers, C., Hurst, W., Mackay, M., & Fergus, P. (2019). Identifying behavioral changes for health monitoring applications using the advanced metering infrastructure. *Behaviour & Information Technology*, *38*(11), 1154–1166. doi:10.1080/0144929X.2019.1574900

Chan, D., Gallaher, L. M., Moodley, K., Minati, L., Burgess, N., & Hartley, T. (2016). The 4 Mountains Test: A Short Test of Spatial Memory with High Sensitivity for the Diagnosis of Pre-dementia Alzheimer's Disease. *Journal of Visualized Experiments*, *116*(116), 54–55. doi:10.3791/54454 PMID:27768046

Chandler, W. G. (2014, June). *Assistive Technology and Communication for Students with Autism Spectrum Disorders (ASD).* Retrieved from https://www.wku.edu/cebs/peu/documents/course-syllabi/sped/sped-619.pdf

Chang, F., Luo, M., Walton, G., Aguilar, L., & Bailenson, J. (2019). Stereotype Threat in Virtual Learning Environments: Effects of Avatar Gender and Sexist Behavior on Women's Math Learning Outcomes. *Cyberpsychology, Behavior, and Social Networking*, *22*(10), 634–640. doi:10.1089/cyber.2019.0106 PMID:31580726

Charlop-Christy, M. H., Carpenter, M., Le, L., LeBlanc, L. A., & Kellet, K. (2002). Using the Picture Exchange Communication System (Pecs) With Children With Autism: Assessment of Pecs Acquisition, Speech, Social-Communicative Behavior, and Problem Behavior. *Journal of Applied Behavior Analysis*, *35*(3), 213–231. doi:10.1901/jaba.2002.35-213 PMID:12365736

Charters, E., Gillett, L., & Simpson, G. K. (2015). Efficacy of electronic portable assistive devices for people with acquired brain injury: A systematic review. *Neuropsychological Rehabilitation*, *25*(1), 82–121. doi:10.1080/09602011.2014.942672 PMID:25121394

Chen, W. (2012). Multitouch Tabletop Technology for People with Autism Spectrum Disorder : A review of the Literature. *Proceedings of the 4th International Conference on Software Development for Enhancing Accessibility and Fighting Info-Exclusion*, *14*(1877), 198–207. 10.1016/j.procs.2012.10.023

Chen, C. L., Chen, C. Y., Liaw, M. Y., Chung, C. Y., Wang, C. J., & Hong, W. H. (2013). Efficacy of home-based virtual cycling training on bone mineral density in ambulatory children with cerebral palsy. *Osteoporosis International, 24*(4), 1399–1406. doi:10.100700198-012-2137-0 PMID:23052930

Cheng, Y., Huang, C.-L., & Yang, C.-S. (2015). Using a 3D immersive virtual environment system to enhance social understanding and social skills for children with autism spectrum disorders. *Focus on Autism and Other Development Disabilities, 30*, 4. doi:10.1177/1088357615583473

Cheng, Y., Chiang, H.-C., Ye, J., & Cheng, L.-h. (2010). Enhancing empathy instruction using a collaborative virtual learning environment for children with autistic spectrum conditions. *Computer Education, 55*(4), 1449–1458.doi:https://doi.org/10.1016/j.compedu.2010.06.008

Cheng, Y., Chiang, H., Ye, J., & Cheng, L. (2010). Enhancing empathy instruction using a collaborative virtual learning environment for children with autistic spectrum conditions. *Computers & Education, 55*(4), 1449–1458. doi:10.1016/j.compedu.2010.06.008

Chen, Y., Fanchiang, H. D., & Howard, A. (2018). Effectiveness of Virtual Reality in Children With Cerebral Palsy: A Systematic Review and Meta-Analysis of Randomized Controlled Trials. *Physical Therapy, 98*(1), 63–77. doi:10.1093/ptj/pzx107 PMID:29088476

Cheong, C. K., Lim, K. H., Jang, J. W., & Jhoo, J. H. (2015). The effect of telemedicine on the duration of treatment in dementia patients. *Journal of Telemedicine and Telecare, 21*(4), 214–218. doi:10.1177/1357633X14566571 PMID:25586813

Cherrier, M. M., Mendez, M., & Perryman, K. (2001). Route learning performance in Alzheimer disease patients. *Neuropsychiatry, Neuropsychology, and Behavioral Neurology, 14*(3), 159–168. PMID:11513099

Chetelat, G., Desgranges, B., & Eustache, F. (2006). Brain profile of hypometabolism in early Alzheimer's disease: Relationships with cognitive deficits and atrophy. *Revista de Neurología, 162*(10), 945–951. PMID:17028562

Chia, G. L. C., Anderson, A., & McLean, L. A. (2018). Use of Technology to Support Self-Management in Individuals with Autism: Systematic Review. *Review Journal of Autism and Developmental Disorders, 5*(2), 142–155.https://doi.org/10.1007/s40489-018-0129-5

Chien, M. E., Jheng, C. M., Lin, N. M., Tang, H. H., Taele, P., Tseng, W. S., & Chen, M. Y. (2015). iCAN: A tablet-based pedagogical system for improving communication skills of children with autism. *International Journal of Human-Computer Studies, 73*, 79–90. doi:10.1016/j.ijhcs.2014.06.001

Children's National (Producer). (2020). *PedBot & PedBotHome*. Retrieved from https://drive.google.com/file/d/1sB3t1FuFO6-UFSjs453ST2Kdsn9XZQ5m/view?usp=sharing

Chiu, H. C., Ada, L., & Lee, S. D. (2018). Balance and mobility training at home using Wii Fit in children with cerebral palsy: A feasibility study. *BMJ Open, 8*(5), e019624. doi:10.1136/bmjopen-2017-019624 PMID:29764871

Christiansen, A. S., & Lange, C. (2008). Intermittent versus continuous physiotherapy in children with cerebral palsy. *Developmental Medicine and Child Neurology, 50*(4), 290–293. doi:10.1111/j.1469-8749.2008.02036.x PMID:18279411

Christopher, D. (2018). Assistive Technologies, Inclusion, and Participation for Students with High Functioning ASD. In *Technology and the Curriculum*. Retrieved from https://techandcurriculum.pressbooks.com/chapter/assistive-tech-and-asd/

Chung, J. C., Lai, C. K., Chung, P. M., & French, H. P. (2002). Snoezelen for dementia. *Cochrane Database of Systematic Reviews, 4*, 15–18. PMID:12519587

Cikajlo, I., & Peterlin Potisk, K. (2019). Advantages of using 3D virtual reality-based training in persons with parkinson's disease: A parallel study. *Journal of Neuroengineering and Rehabilitation*, *16*(1), 119. Advance online publication. doi:10.118612984-019-0601-1 PMID:31623622

Cipriani, G., Bianchetti, A., & Trabucchi, M. (2006). Outcomes of a computer based cognitive rehabilitation program on Alzheimer's disease patients compared with those on patients affected by mild cognitive impairment. *Archives of Gerontology and Geriatrics*, *43*(3), 327–335. doi:10.1016/j.archger.2005.12.003 PMID:16451811

Cirino, C. B., Fernandes, A. C., Silva, J. D., & Serra, H. P. (2020, July). ERA-Augmented Reality Teaching-Assistive Technology Developed for the Literacy Process of Children with ASD. In *International Conference on Human-Computer Interaction* (pp. 405-414). Cham: Springer.

Ciro, A., Park, J., Burkhard, G., Yan, N., & Geula, C. (2012). Biochemical differentiation of cholinesterases from normal and Alzheimer's disease cortex. *Current Alzheimer Research*, *9*(1), 138–143. doi:10.2174/156720512799015127 PMID:21244353

Cirstea, C. M. (2019). Are Wearable Robots Effective for Gait Recovery After Stroke? *Stroke*, *50*(12), 3337–3338.

Cirstea, C. M. (2020). Gait Rehabilitation After Stroke: Should We Re-Evaluate Our Practice? *Stroke*, *51*(10), 2892–2894.

Claflin, E. S., Krishnan, C., & Khot, S. P. (2015). Emerging treatments for motor rehabilitation after stroke. *The Neurohospitalist*, *5*(2), 77–88.

Clark, C. C. T., Bisi, M. C., Duncan, M. J., & Stagni, R. (2021). Technology-based methods for the assessment of fine and gross motor skill in children: A systematic overview of available solutions and future steps for effective in-field use. *Journal of Sports Sciences*, *39*(11), 1236–1276. doi:10.1080/02640414.2020.1864984 PMID:33588689

Clay, B., Howett, D., FitzGerald, J., Fletcher, P., Chan, D., & Price, A. (2020). Use of Immersive Virtual Reality in the Assessment and Treatment of Alzheimer's Disease: A Systematic Review. *Journal of Alzheimer's Disease*, *75*(1), 23–43. doi:10.3233/JAD-191218 PMID:32280091

Cleary, K., Monfaredi, R., Salvador, T., Talari, H. F., Coley, C., Kovelman, S., . . . Evans, S. H. (2019). *Pedbothome: Robotically-Assisted Ankle Rehabilitation System For Children With Cerebral Palsy.* Paper presented at the 2019 IEEE 16th International Conference on Rehabilitation Robotics (ICORR). 10.1109/ICORR.2019.8779468

Coffin, A. B., Myles, B. S., Rogers, J., & Szakacs, W. (2016). Supporting the writing skills of individuals with autism spectrum disorder through assistive technologies. In *Technology and the treatment of children with autism spectrum disorder* (pp. 59–73). Springer. doi:10.1007/978-3-319-20872-5_6

Cogné, M., Auriacombe, S., Vasa, L., Tison, F., Klinger, E., Sauzeon, H., Joseph, P.-A., & N'Kaoua, B. (2018). Are Visual Cues Helpful for Virtual Spatial Navigation and Spatial Memory in Patients With Mild Cognitive Impairment or Alzheimer's Disease? *Neuropsychology*, *4*(32), 385–400. doi:10.1037/neu0000435 PMID:29809030

Cogné, M., Taillade, M., N'Kaoua, B., Tarruella, A., Klinger, E., Larrue, F., Sauze'on, H., Joseph, P. A., & Sorita, E. (2017). The contribution of virtual reality to the diagnosis of spatial navigation disorders and to the study of the role of navigational aids: A systematic literature review. *Annals of Physical and Rehabilitation Medicine*, *60*(3), 164–176. doi:10.1016/j.rehab.2015.12.004 PMID:27017533

Cohen, J. (1988). *Statistical Power Analysis for the Behavioral Sciences*. Erlbaum.

Colombini, G., Duradoni, M., Carpi, F., Vagnoli, L., & Guazzini, A. (2021). LEAP motion technology and psychology: A mini-review on hand movements sensing for neurodevelopmental and neurocognitive disorders. *International Journal of Environmental Research and Public Health, 18*(8), 4006. Advance online publication. doi:10.3390/ijerph18084006 PMID:33920362

Columna, L., Prieto, L., Elias-Revolledo, G., & Haegele, J. A. (2020). The perspectives of parents of youth with disabilities toward physical activity: A systematic review. *Disability and Health Journal, 13*(2), 100851. doi:10.1016/j.dhjo.2019.100851 PMID:31679949

Conn, K., Liu, C., Sarkar, N., Stone, W., & Warren, Z. (2008a). Affect-sensitive assistive intervention technologies for children with autism: An individual-specific approach. In *RO-MAN 2008-The 17th IEEE International Symposium on Robot and Human Interactive Communication* (pp. 442-447). Munich: IEEE.

Conn, K., Liu, C., Sarkar, N., Stone, W., & Warren, Z. (2008b). Towards affect-sensitive assistive intervention technologies for children with autism. In *Affective computing: Focus on emotion expression, synthesis and recognition* (pp. 365–390). IntechOpen. doi:10.5772/6171

Costantini, M., & Haggard, P. (2007). The rubber hand illusion: Sensitivity and reference frame for body ownership. *Consciousness and Cognition, 16*(2), 229–240. doi:10.1016/j.concog.2007.01.001 PMID:17317221

Coupland, A. P., Thapar, A., Qureshi, M. I., Jenkins, H., & Davies, A. H. (2017). The definition of stroke. *Journal of the Royal Society of Medicine, 110*(1), 9–12.

Courtenay, K. (2021). The case for removing intellectual disability and autism from the Mental Health Act. *The British Journal of Psychiatry, 218*(1), 64–65. doi:10.1192/bjp.2020.183 PMID:33541473

Coyle, H., Traynor, V., & Solowij, N. (2015). Computerized and virtual reality cognitive training for individuals at high risk of cognitive decline: Systematic review of the literature. *The American Journal of Geriatric Psychiatry, 4*(23), 335–359. doi:10.1016/j.jagp.2014.04.009 PMID:24998488

Craig, A. B. (2013). *Understanding Augmented Reality: Concepts and Applications.* Morgan Kaufmann Publishers.

Cramer, M., Hirano, S. H., Tentori, M., Yeganyan, M. T., & Hayes, G. R. (2011). Classroom-based assistive technology: collective use of interactive visual schedules by students with autism. In *Proceedings of the SIGCHI Conference on Human Factors in Computing Systems* (pp. 1-10). Vancouver: Association for Computing Machinery (ACM). 10.1145/1978942.1978944

Craske, M. G., Treanor, M., Conway, C. C., Zbozinek, T., & Vervliet, B. (2014). Maximizing exposure therapy: An inhibitory learning approach. *Behaviour Research and Therapy, 58*, 10–23. https://doi.org/10.1016/j.brat.2014.04.006

CSDT. (2021). *Center for Self-Determination Theory.* Self-Determination Theory.

Csikszentmihalyi, M. (1990). *Flow: The Psychology of Optimal Experience.* Harper & Row.

Cuhadar, S. (2008). Use of assistive technologies in the education of the children with autism. *The 8th International Educational Technology Conference.* Retrieved from http://ietc2008.home.anadolu.edu.tr/ietc2008/187.doc

Cullen, J. M., Alber-Morgan, S. R., Simmons-Reed, E. A., & Izzo, M. V. (2017). Effects of self-directed video prompting using iPads on the vocational task completion of young adults with intellectual and developmental disabilities. *Journal of Vocational Rehabilitation, 46*(3), 361–375. doi:10.3233/JVR-170873

Cunha, P., Brandão, J., Vasconcelos, J., Soares, F., & Carvalho, V. (2016). Augmented reality for cognitive and social skills improvement in children with ASD. In 13th International Con- ference on Remote Engineering and Virtual Instrumentation (REV). IEEE. https://doi.org/10.1109/REV.2016.7444495.

Cuperus, A. A., Keizer, A., Evers, A. W., van den Houten, M. M., Teijink, J. A., & van der Ham, I. J. (2018). Manipulating spatial distance in virtual reality: Effects on treadmill walking performance in patients with intermittent claudication. *Computers in Human Behavior*, *79*, 211–216. doi:10.1016/j.chb.2017.10.037

Cuperus, A. A., & van der Ham, I. J. (2016). Virtual reality replays of sports performance: Effects on memory, feeling of competence, and performance. *Learning and Motivation*, *56*, 48–52. doi:10.1016/j.lmot.2016.09.005

Cushman, L. A., & Duffy, C. J. (2007). The sex specificity of navigational strategies in Alzheimer disease. *Alzheimer Disease and Associated Disorders*, *21*(2), 122–129. doi:10.1097/WAD.0b013e318047df2f PMID:17545737

Cushman, L. A., Stein, K., & Duffy, C. J. (2008). Detecting navigational deficits in cognitive aging and Alzheimer disease using virtual reality. *Neuorology*, *71*(12), 888–895. doi:10.1212/01.wnl.0000326262.67613.fe PMID:18794491

D'Arrigo, R., Ziviani, J., Poulsen, A. A., Copley, J., & King, G. (2017). Child and parent engagement in therapy: What is the key? *Australian Occupational Therapy Journal*, *64*(4), 340–343. doi:10.1111/1440-1630.12279 PMID:26831473

D'Cunha, N. M., Nguyen, D., Naumovski, N., McKune, A. J., Kellett, J., Georgousopoulou, E. N., Frost, J., & Isbel, S. (2019). A mini-review of virtual reality-based interventions to promote well-being for people living with dementia and mild cognitive impairment. *Gerontology*, *65*(4), 430–440. doi:10.1159/000500040 PMID:31108489

Darejeh, A., & Singh, D. (2013). A review on user interface design principles to increase software usability for users with less computer literacy. *Journal of Computational Science*, *9*(11), 1443–1450.doi:https://doi.org/10.3844/jcssp.2013.1443.1450

David, D. O., Costescu, C. A., Matu, S., Szentagotai, A., & Dobrean, A. (2019). Effects of a Robot-Enhanced Intervention for Children With ASD on Teaching Turn-Taking Skills. *Journal of Educational Computing Research*, *58*(1), 29–62. doi:10.1177/0735633119830344

Davidson, T. M., Bunnell, B. E., Saunders, B. E., Hanson, R. F., Danielson, C. K., Cook, D., Chu, B. C., Dorsey, S., Adams, Z. W., Andrews, A. R. III, Walker, J. H., Soltis, K. E., Cohen, J. A., Deblinger, E., & Ruggiero, K. J. (2019). Pilot evaluation of a tablet-based application to improve quality of care in child mental health treatment. *Behavior Therapy*, *50*(2), 367–379. doi:10.1016/j.beth.2018.07.005 PMID:30824252

Davies, A., Brini, S., Hirani, S., Gathercole, R., Forsyth, K., Henderson, C., Bradley, R., & Davies, L. (2020). The impact of assistive technology on burden and psychological well-being in informal caregivers of people with dementia (ATTILA Study). *Translational Research & Clinical Interventions,* 1-10.

Davies, A. M. A., White, R. C., & Davies, M. (2013). Spatial limits on the nonvisual self-touch illusion and the visual rubber hand illusion: Subjective experience of the illusion and proprioceptive drift. *Consciousness and Cognition*, *22*(2), 613–636. doi:10.1016/j.concog.2013.03.006 PMID:23644413

Davis, O., & Ohman, J. (2017). Wayfinding in Aging and Alzheimer's Disease within a Virtual Senior Residence: Study Protocol. *Journal of Advanced Nursing*, *72*(7), 1677–1688. doi:10.1111/jan.12945 PMID:26915997

Davis, R., Ohman, J. M., & Weisbeck, C. (2017). Salient cues and wayfinding in Alzheimer's disease within a virtual senior residence. *Environment and Behavior*, *49*(9), 1038–1065. doi:10.1177/0013916516677341 PMID:29230067

de Back, T. T., Tinga, A. M., Nguyen, P., & Louwerse, M. M. (2020). Benefits of immersive collaborative learning in CAVE-based virtual reality. *International Journal of Educational Technology in Higher Education*, *17*(1), 1–18. doi:10.118641239-020-00228-9

De Leo, G., Gonzales, C. H., Battagiri, P., & Leroy, G. (2011). A smart-phone application and a companion website for the improvement of the communication skills of children with autism: Clinical rationale, technical development and preliminary results. *Journal of Medical Systems*, *35*(4), 703–711. doi:10.100710916-009-9407-1 PMID:20703781

De Pace, C., & Stasolla, F. (2014). Promoting environmental control, social interaction, and leisure/academy engagement among people with severe/profound multiple disabilities through assistive technology. In *Assistive technologies and computer access for motor disabilities* (pp. 285–319). IGI Global. doi:10.4018/978-1-4666-4438-0.ch010

de Villiers, J. (2021). The case against removing intellectual disability and autism from the Mental Health Act. *The British Journal of Psychiatry*, *218*(1), 63. doi:10.1192/bjp.2020.181 PMID:33541476

Deci, E. L., & Ryan, R. M. (1985). *Intrinsic motivation and self-determination in human behavior*. Plenum Press. doi:10.1007/978-1-4899-2271-7

Déjos, M., Sauzéon, H., & N'kaoua, B. (2012). Virtual reality for clinical assessment of elderly people: Early screening for dementia. *Revue Neurologique*, *168*(5), 404–414. doi:10.1016/j.neurol.2011.09.005 PMID:22137150

Dellazizzo, L., Potvin, S., Luigi, M., & Dumais, A. (2020). Evidence on virtual reality-based therapies for psychiatric disorders: Meta-review of meta-analyses. *Journal of Medical Internet Research*, *22*(8), e20889. Advance online publication. doi:10.2196/20889 PMID:32812889

Deng, L., & Rattadilok, P. (2020). The need for and barriers to using assistive technologies among individuals with Autism Spectrum Disorders in China. *Assistive Technology*, 1–12. doi:10.1080/10400435.2020.1757787 PMID:32310026

Desideri, L., Di Santantonio, A., Varrucciu, N., Bonsi, I., & Di Sarro, R. (2020). Assistive Technology for Cognition to Support Executive Functions in Autism: A Scoping Review. *Advances in Neurodevelopmental Disorders*, *4*(4), 330–343. doi:10.100741252-020-00163-w

Deutsch, J. E., & Westcott McCoy, S. (2017). Virtual Reality and Serious Games in Neurorehabilitation of Children and Adults: Prevention, Plasticity, and Participation. *Pediatr Phys Ther*, *29*(S3), S23-S36. doi:10.1097/PEP.0000000000000387

Devanand, D. P., Pradhaban, G., Liu, X., Khandji, A., De Santi, S., Segal, S., Rusinek, H., Pelton, G. H., Honig, L. S., Mayeux, R., Stern, Y., Tabert, M. H., & de Leon, M. J. (2007). Hippocampal and entorhinal atrophy in mild cognitive impairment: Prediction of Alzheimer disease. *Neurology*, *68*(11), 828–836. doi:10.1212/01.wnl.0000256697.20968.d7 PMID:17353470

Di Lazzaro, V., Capone, F., Di Pino, G., Pellegrino, G., Florio, L., Zollo, L., Simonetti, D., Ranieri, F., Brunelli, N., Corbetto, M., Miccinilli, S., Bravi, M., Milighetti, S., Guglielmelli, E., & Sterzi, S. (2016). Combining Robotic Training and Non-Invasive Brain Stimulation in Severe Upper Limb-Impaired Chronic Stroke Patients. *Frontiers in Neuroscience*, *10*, 88.

Di Nuovo, A., Conti, D., Trubia, G., Buono, S., & Di Nuovo, S. (2018). Deep Learning Systems for Estimating Visual Attention in Robot-Assisted Therapy of Children with Autism and Intellectual Disability. *Robotics*, *7*(2), 25.doi:https://doi.org/10.3390/robotics7020025

Di Palma, S., Tonacci, A., Narzisi, A., Domenici, C., Pioggia, G., Muratori, F., & Billeci, L.The Michelangelo Study Group. (2017). Monitoring of autonomic response to socio-cognitive tasks during treatment in children with autism spectrum disorders by wearable technologies: A feasibility study. *Computers in Biology and Medicine*, *85*, 143–152. doi:10.1016/j.compbiomed.2016.04.001 PMID:27080078

Di Pietro, J., Kelemen, A., Liang, Y., & Sik-Lanyi, C. (2019). Computer- and Robot-Assisted Therapies to Aid Social and Intellectual Functioning of Children with Autism Spectrum Disorder. *Medicina (Kaunas, Lithuania)*, *55*(8), 440. https://doi.org/10.3390/medicina55080440

Diagnostic and Statistical Manual of Mental Disorders (DSM-V) (5th ed.). (2013). American Psychiatric Association (APA).

Diaz-Orueta, U., Etxaniz, A., Gonzalez, M. F., Buiza, C., Urdaneta, E., & Yanguas, J. (2014). Role of cognitive and functional performance in interactions between older people with cognitive decline and an avatar on TV. *Universal Access in the Information Society*, *13*(1), 89–97. doi:10.100710209-013-0288-1

Dimyan, M. A., & Cohen, L. G. (2011). Neuroplasticity in the context of motor rehabilitation after stroke. *Nature Reviews. Neurology*, *7*(2), 76–85.

Dockx, K., Van Remoortel, H., De Buck, E., Schelstraete, C., Vanderheyden, A., Lievens, T., Kinyagu, J. T., Mamuya, S., & Vandekerckhove, P. (2019). Effect of contextualized versus non-contextualized interventions for improving hand washing, sanitation, and health in rural tanzania: Study design of a cluster randomized controlled trial. *International Journal of Environmental Research and Public Health*, *16*(14), 2529. Advance online publication. doi:10.3390/ijerph16142529 PMID:31311186

Dodd, K. J., Taylor, N. F., & Damiano, D. L. (2002). A systematic review of the effectiveness of strength-training programs for people with cerebral palsy. *Archives of Physical Medicine and Rehabilitation*, *83*(8), 1157–1164. doi:10.1053/apmr.2002.34286 PMID:12161840

Doeller, C. F., King, J. A., & Burgess, N. (2008). Parallel striatal and hippocampal systems for landmarks and boundaries in spatial memory. *Proceedings of the National Academy of Sciences of the United States of America*, *105*(15), 5915–5920. doi:10.1073/pnas.0801489105 PMID:18408152

Doherty, A., Bracken, M., & Gormley, L. (2018). Teaching Children with Autism to Initiate and Respond to Peer Mands Using Picture Exchange Communication System (PECS). *Behavior Analysis in Practice*, *11*(4), 279–288. doi:10.100740617-018-00311-8 PMID:30538902

Dong, M., Zhou, Y., Li, J., Rong, X., Fan, W., Zhou, X., & Kong, Y. (2021). State of the art in parallel ankle rehabilitation robot: A systematic review. *Journal of Neuroengineering and Rehabilitation*, *18*(1), 52. doi:10.118612984-021-00845-z PMID:33743757

Dong, Y., Wu, T., Hu, X., & Wang, T. (2017). Efficacy and safety of botulinum toxin type A for upper limb spasticity after stroke or traumatic brain injury: A systematic review with meta-analysis and trial sequential analysis. *European Journal of Physical and Rehabilitation Medicine*, *53*(2), 256–267.

Doniger, G. M., Schnaider Beeri, A., Bahar-Fuchs, A., Gottlieb, A., Tkachov, A., & … . (2018). Virtual reality-based cognitive-motor training for middle-aged adults at high Alzheimer's disease risk: A randomized controlled trial. *Alzheimer's & Dementia: Translational Research & Clinical Interventions*, *4*(4), 118–129. doi:10.1016/j.trci.2018.02.005 PMID:29955655

Doody, R. S., Stevens, J. C., Beck, C., Dubinsky, R. M., Kaye, J. A., Gwyther, L., Mohs, R. C., Thal, L. J., Whitehouse, P. J., DeKosky, S. T., & Cummings, J. L. (2001). Practice parameter: Management of dementia (an evidence-based review). Report of the Quality Standards Subcommittee of the American Academy of Neurology. *Neurology*, *56*(9), 1154–1166. doi:10.1212/WNL.56.9.1154 PMID:11342679

Dooley, P., Wilczenski, F. L., & Torem, C. (2001). Using an activity schedule to smooth school transitions. *Journal of Positive Behavior Interventions*, *3*(1), 57–61. doi:10.1177/109830070100300108

Douard, E., Zeribi, A., Schramm, C., Tamer, P., Loum, M. A., Nowak, S., ... Moreau, C. (2021). Effect sizes of deletions and duplications on autism risk across the genome. *The American Journal of Psychiatry*, *178*(1), 87–98. doi:10.1176/appi.ajp.2020.19080834 PMID:32911998

Dovigo, L., Caprì, T., Iannizzotto, G., Nucita, A., Semino, M., Giannatiempo, S., Zocca, L., & Fabio, R. A. (2021). Social and Cognitive Interactions Through an Interactive School Service for RTT Patients at the COVID-19 Time. *Frontiers in Psychology*, *12*, 2417. doi:10.3389/fpsyg.2021.676238 PMID:34248774

Downs, J. A., Bebbington, A., Jacoby, P., Msall, M. E., McIlroy, O., Fyfe, S., ... Leonard, H. (2008). Gross motor profile in Rett syndrome as determined by video analysis. *Neuropediatrics*, *39*(04), 205–210. doi:10.1055-0028-1104575 PMID:19165708

Downs, J., Rodger, J., Li, C., Tan, X., Hu, N., Wong, K., de Klerk, N., & Leonard, H. (2018). Environmental enrichment intervention for Rett syndrome: An individually randomised stepped wedge trial. *Orphanet Journal of Rare Diseases*, *13*(1), 3. doi:10.118613023-017-0752-8 PMID:29321033

Downs, J., Torode, I., Wong, K., Ellaway, C., Elliott, E. J., Christodoulou, J., Jacoby, P., Thomson, M. R., Izatt, M. T., Askin, G. N., McPhee, B. I., Bridge, C., Cundy, P., & Leonard, H. (2016). The natural history of scoliosis in females with rett syndrome. *Spine*, *41*(10), 856–863. doi:10.1097/BRS.0000000000001399 PMID:26679887

Drahota, A., Wood, J. J., Sze, K. M., & Van Dyke, M. (2011). Effects of cognitive behavioral therapy on daily living skills in children with high-functioning autism and concurrent anxiety disorders. *Journal of Autism and Developmental Disorders*, *41*(3), 257–265.doi:https://doi.org/10.1007/s10803-010-1037-4

Drasgow, E., Wolery, M., Chezan, L. C., Halle, J., & Hajiaghamohseni, Z. (2017). Systematic instruction of students with significant cognitive disabilities. In *Handbook of special education* (pp. 632–648). Taylor and Francis Inc. doi:10.4324/9781315517698-49

Driscoll, I., Hamilton, D. A., Petropoulos, H., Yeo, R. A., Brooks, W. M., Baumgartner, R. N., & Sutherland, R. J. (2003). The aging hippocampus: Cognitive, biochemical and structural findings. *Cerebral Cortex (New York, N.Y.)*, *13*(12), 1344–1351. doi:10.1093/cercor/bhg081 PMID:14615299

Dubois, B., Feldman, H. H., Jacova, C., Hampel, H., Molinuevo, J. L., Blennow, K., DeKosky, S. T., Gauthier, S., Selkoe, D., Bateman, R., Cappa, S., Crutch, S., Engelborghs, S., Frisoni, G. B., Fox, N. C., Galasko, D., Habert, M.-O., Jicha, G. A., Nordberg, A., ... Cummings, J. L. (2014). Advancing research diagnostic criteria for Alzheimer's disease: The IWG-2 criteria. *Lancet Neurology*, *13*(6), 614–629. doi:10.1016/S1474-4422(14)70090-0 PMID:24849862

Duff, P., & Dolphin, C. (2007). Cost-benefit analysis of assistive technology to support independence for people with dementia – part 2. Results from employing the ENABLE cost-benefit model in practice. *Technology and Disability*, *19*(2-3), 79–90. doi:10.3233/TAD-2007-192-305

Dunning, K., Black, K., Harrison, A., McBride, K., & Israel, S. (2009). Neuroprosthesis peroneal functional electrical stimulation in the acute inpatient rehabilitation setting: A case series. *Physical Therapy*, *89*(5), 499–506. doi:10.2522/ptj.20080241 PMID:19270044

Dunn, J., & Clare, L. (2007). Learning face–name associations in early-stage dementia: Comparing the effects of errorless learning and effortful processing. *Neuropsychological Rehabilitation*, *17*(6), 735–754. doi:10.1080/09602010701218317 PMID:17852759

Dunst, C. J., Trivette, C. M., Davis, M., & Cornwell, J. (1988). Enabling and Empowering Families of Children With Health Impairments. *Children's Health Care*, *17*(2), 71–81. doi:10.120715326888chc1702_2

Durand, V. M. (1999). Functional Communication Training Using Assistive Devices: Recruiting Natural Communities of Reinforcement. *Journal of Applied Behavior Analysis*, *32*(3), 247–267. doi:10.1901/jaba.1999.32-247 PMID:10513023

Duret, C., Grosmaire, A. G., & Krebs, H. I. (2019). Robot-Assisted Therapy in Upper Extremity Hemiparesis: Overview of an Evidence-Based Approach. *Frontiers in Neurology*, *10*, 412.

Duret, C., Hutin, E., Lehenaff, L., & Gracies, J. M. (2015). Do all sub acute stroke patients benefit from robot-assisted therapy? A retrospective study. *Restorative Neurology and Neuroscience*, *33*(1), 57–65.

Edwards, S., Rudaizky, D., Toner, M., & Chen, W. (2021). A qualitative study of factors perceived by parents as promoting personal recovery in children and young people with attention deficit hyperactivity disorder. *Advances in Neurodevelopmental Disorders*, *5*(1), 102–115. doi:10.100741252-020-00187-2

Ekker, M. S., Boot, E. M., Singhal, A. B., Tan, K. S., Debette, S., Tuladhar, A. M., & de Leeuw, F. E. (2018). Epidemiology, aetiology, and management of ischaemic stroke in young adults. *Lancet Neurology*, *17*(9), 790–801.

el Kaliouby, R., & Robinson, P. (2007). *Therapeutic versus prosthetic assistive technologies: The case of autism.* Retrieved from Computer Laboratory, University of Cambridge: https://www.cl.cam.ac.uk/~pr10/publications/at07.pdf

Elefant, C. (2001). Speechless yet communcative: revealing the person behind the disablity of Rett syndrome through clinical research on songs in music therapy. In D. Aldridge, G. Di Franco, E. Ruud, & T. Wigram (Eds.), *Music Therapy in Europe. The 5th European Music Therapy Congress (Napoli, April 2001)* (pp. 113–128). Ismez.

Elkind, J. S., Rubin, E., Rosenthal, S., Skoff, B., & Prather, P. (2001). A simulated reality scenario compared with the computerized Wisconsin card sorting test: An analysis of preliminary results. *Cyberpsychology & Behavior*, *4*(4), 489–496. doi:10.1089/109493101750527042 PMID:11708728

El-Seoud, S. A., Halabi, O., & Geroimenko, V. (2019). Assisting Individuals with Autism and Cognitive Disorders: An Augmented Reality-Based Framework. *International Journal of Online Biomedical Engineering*, *15*(04), 28.doi:http://dx.doi.org/10.3991/ijoe.v15i04.9835

Epstein, L. G. (1995). Rett Syndrome--Clinical and Biological Aspects: Studies on 130 Swedish Females. In Archives of Neurology (Vol. 52, Issue 4). Cambridge University Press. doi:10.1001/archneur.1995.00540280025011

Erbil, D., Tugba, G., Murat, T. H., Melike, A., Merve, A., Cagla, K., Mehmetali, Ç. C., Akay, Ö., & Nigar, D. (2018). Effects of robot-assisted gait training in chronic stroke patients treated by botulinum toxin-a: A pivotal study. *Physiotherapy Research International, 23*(3), e1718.

Escobedo, L., Tentori, M., Quintana, E., Favela, J., & Garcia-Rosas, D. (2014). Using Augmented Reality to Help Children with Autism Stay Focused. *IEEE CS*, 38–46.

Escobedo, L., Nguyen, D. H., Boyd, L., Hirano, S., Rangel, A., Garcia-Rosas, D., Tentori, M., & Hayes, G. (2012). MOSOCO: A Mobile Assistive Tool to Support Children with Autism Practicing Social Skills in Real-Life Situations. *Proceedings of the SIGCHI Conference on Human Factors in Computing Systems*, 2589–2598. 10.1145/2207676.2208649

Esteban, P. B. (2017). How to Build a Supervised Autonomous System for Robot-Enhanced Therapy for Children with Autism Spectrum Disorder. *Paladyn: Journal of Behavioral Robotics*, *8*(1), 18–38.doi:https://doi.org/10.1515/pjbr-2017-0002

Everaert, D. G., Stein, R. B., Abrams, G. M., Dromerick, A. W., Francisco, G. E., Hafner, B. J., Huskey, T. N., Munin, M. C., Nolan, K. J., & Kufta, C. V. (2013). Effect of a foot-drop stimulator and ankle–foot orthosis on walking performance after stroke: A multicenter randomized controlled trial. *Neurorehabilitation and Neural Repair*, *27*(7), 579–591. doi:10.1177/1545968313481278 PMID:23558080

Fabio, R. A., Billeci, L., Crifaci, G., Troise, E., Tortorella, G., & Pioggia, G. (2016). Cognitive training modifies frequency EEG bands and neuropsychological measures in Rett syndrome. *Research in Developmental Disabilities*, *53-54*, 73–85. doi:10.1016/j.ridd.2016.01.009 PMID:26859707

Fabio, R. A., Gangemi, A., Semino, M., Vignoli, A., Canevini, M. P., Priori, A., ... Caprì, T. (2020). Effects of combined transcranial direct current stimulation with cognitive training in girls with Rett syndrome. *Brain Sciences*, *10*(5), 276. Advance online publication. doi:10.3390/brainsci10050276 PMID:32370253

Fabio, R. A., Giannatiempo, S., & Caprì, T. (2019). Attention and identification of the same and the similar visual stimuli in Rett syndrome. *Life Span and Disability*, *22*, 113–127.

Fabricatore, C. (2002). *Learning and Videogames: An Unexploited Synergy*. Springer Science & Business Media.

Fage, C., Consel, C. Y., Balland, E., Etchegoyhen, K., Amestoy, A., Bouvard, M., & Sauzéon, H. (2018). Tablet apps to support first school inclusion of children with autism spectrum disorders (ASD) in mainstream classrooms: A pilot study. *Frontiers in Psychology*, *9*, 2020. doi:10.3389/fpsyg.2018.02020 PMID:30405498

Fan, T. (2012, May). *Enhancing Learning with the Use of Assistive Technology for Children on the Autism Spectrum* (Master of Science in Education). San Rafael, CA: Dominican University of California.

Faria, A. L., Andrade, A., Soares, L., & i Badia, S. B. (2016). Benefits of virtual reality based cognitive rehabilitation through simulated activities of daily living: A randomized controlled trial with stroke patients. *Journal of Neuroengineering and Rehabilitation*, *13*(1), 1–12. doi:10.118612984-016-0204-z PMID:27806718

Farias, S. T., Harrell, E., Neumann, C., & Houtz, A. (2003). The relationship between neuropsychological performance and daily functioning in individuals with Alzheimer's disease: Ecological validity of neuropsychological tests. *Archives of Clinical Neuropsychology*, *18*(6), 655–672. doi:10.1093/arclin/18.6.655 PMID:14591439

Fasilis, T., Patrikelis, P., Siatouni, A., Alexoudi, A., Veretzioti, A., Zachou, L., & Gatzonis, S.-S. (2018). A pilot study and brief overview of rehabilitation via virtual environment in patients suffering from dementia. *Psychiatriki*, *29*(1), 42–51. doi:10.22365/jpsych.2018.291.42 PMID:29754119

Fau, D. (2020). *FDA U.S. Food & Drug & Devices Administration*. Retrieved from https://wku.edu/research/documents/covid-19_nih_an_fda_afternoon_webinar.pdf

Fazana, F., Alsadoon, A., Prasad, P. W., Costadopoulos, N., Elchouemi, A., & Sreedharan, S. (2017, July). Integration of assistive and wearable technology to improve communication, social interaction and health monitoring for children with autism spectrum disorder (ASD). In *Region 10 Symposium (TENSYMP)* (pp. 1-5). Cochin: IEEE. 10.1109/TENCONSpring.2017.8070018

Fehlings, D., Switzer, L., Findlay, B., & Knights, S. (2013). Interactive computer play as "motor therapy" for individuals with cerebral palsy. *Seminars in Pediatric Neurology*, *20*(2), 127–138. doi:10.1016/j.spen.2013.06.003 PMID:23948687

Feigin, V., Norrving, B., Sudlow, C., & Sacco, R. L. (2018). Updated Criteria for Population-Based Stroke and Transient Ischemic Attack Incidence Studies for the 21st Century. *Stroke*, *49*(9), 2248–2255.

Felce, D., & Perry, J. (1995). Quality of life: Its definition and measurement. *Research in Developmental Disabilities*, *16*(1), 51–74. doi:10.1016/0891-4222(94)00028-8 PMID:7701092

Felnhofer, A., Kothgassner, O. D., Beutl, L., Hlavacs, H., & Kryspin-Exner, I. (2012). Is virtual reality made for men only? Exploring gender differences in the sense of presence. *Proceedings of the International Society on presence research*, 103-112.

Finnegan, D. J., O'Neill, E., & Proulx, M. J. (2016, May). Compensating for distance compression in audiovisual virtual environments using incongruence. In *Proceedings of the 2016 CHI Conference on Human Factors in Computing Systems* (pp. 200-212). 10.1145/2858036.2858065

Flewitt, R., Kucirkova, N., & Messer, D. (2014). Touching the virtual, touching the real: iPads and enabling literacy for students experiencing disability. *Australian Journal of Language and Literacy, 37*(2), 107–116.

Flynn, D., van Schaik, P., Blackman, T., Femcott, C., Hobbs, B., & Calderon, C. (2003). Developing a virtual reality-based methodology for people with dementia: A feasibility study. *Cyberpsychology Behavior Journal, 6*(6), 591–611. doi:10.1089/109493103322725379 PMID:14756925

Foloppe, D., Richard, P., Yamaguchi, T., Etcharry-Bouyx, F., & Allain, P. (2018). The potential of virtual reality-based training to enhance the functional autonomy of Alzheimer's disease patients in cooking activities: A single case study. *Neuropsychological Rehabilitation, 28*(5), 709–733. doi:10.1080/09602011.2015.1094394 PMID:26480838

Fombonne, E. (2018). The rising prevalence of autism. *Journal of Child Psychology and Psychiatry, and Allied Disciplines, 59*(7), 717–720. doi:10.1111/jcpp.12941 PMID:29924395

Fonzo, M., Sirico, F., & Corrado, B. (2020). Evidence-based physical therapy for individuals with rett syndrome: A systematic review. In Brain Sciences (Vol. 10, Issue 7, pp. 1–20). MDPI AG. doi:10.3390/brainsci10070410

Francis, P. (2004, October). *Techniques to include users with autism in the design of assistive technologies* (Honor's thesis). University of Melbourne.

Francis, P., Firth, L., & Mellor, D. (2005, September). Reducing the risk of abandonment of assistive technologies for people with autism. In *International Federation for Information Processing (IFIP) Conference on Human-Computer Interaction* (pp. 1104-1107). Berlin: Springer.

Francis, P., Mellor, D., & Firth, L. (2009). Techniques and recommendations for the inclusion of users with autism in the design of assistive technologies. *Assistive Technology, 21*(2), 57–68. doi:10.1080/10400430902945561 PMID:19715250

Franck, J. A., Smeets, R., & Seelen, H. (2017). Changes in arm-hand function and arm-hand skill performance in patients after stroke during and after rehabilitation. *PLoS One, 12*(6), e0179453.

Franki, I., Desloovere, K., De Cat, J., Feys, H., Molenaers, G., Calders, P., ... Van Broeck, C. (2012). The evidence-base for conceptual approaches and additional therapies targeting lower limb function in children with cerebral palsy: A systematic review using the ICF as a framework. *Journal of Rehabilitation Medicine, 44*(5), 396–405. doi:10.2340/16501977-0984 PMID:22549647

Frauenberger, C., Good, J., Alcorn, A., & Pain, H. (2012). Supporting the design contributions of children with autism spectrum conditions. In IIDC '12: Proceedings of the 11th International Conference on Interaction Design and Children. Association for Computing Machinery. https://doi.org/10.1145/2307096.2307112.

Frederiksen, J. G., Sørensen, S. M. D., Konge, L., Svendsen, M. B. S., Nobel-Jørgensen, M., Bjerrum, F., & Andersen, S. A. W. (2020). Cognitive load and performance in immersive virtual reality versus conventional virtual reality simulation training of laparoscopic surgery: A randomized trial. *Surgical Endoscopy, 34*(3), 1244–1252. doi:10.100700464-019-06887-8 PMID:31172325

Freeman, D., Reeve, S., Robinson, A., Ehlers, A., Clark, D., Spanlang, B., & Slater, M. (2017). Virtual reality in the assessment, understanding, and treatment of mental health disorders. *Psychological Medicine, 47*(14), 2393–2400. doi:10.1017/S003329171700040X PMID:28325167

Freyhoff, G., Hess, G., Kerr, L., Menzel, E., Tronbacke, B., & Van Der Veken, K. (1998). *Make it Simple - European Guidelines for the Production of Easy-to-Read Informationfor People with Learning Disability for authors, editors, information providers,translators and other interested persons.* Brussels: ILSMH European Association. Retrieved from https://moodle2.units.it/pluginfile.php/303860/mod_resource/content/1/ILSMH%201998%20or%20Freyhoff%20Make%20it%20simple.pdf

Fried-Oken, M., Mooney, A., & Peters, B. (2015). Supporting communication for patients with neurodegenerative disease. *NeuroRehabilitation*, *37*(1), 69–87. doi:10.3233/NRE-151241 PMID:26409694

Frith, U. (1989). *Autism: Explaining the Enigma*. Blackwell Publishing.

Frith, U. (2003). *Autism: Explaining the enigma* (2nd ed.). Blackwell Publishing. Retrieved from https://psycnet.apa.org/record/2003-00578-000

Fteiha, M. A. (2017). Effectiveness of assistive technology in enhancing language skills for children with autism. *International Journal of Developmental Disabilities*, *63*(1), 36–44. doi:10.1080/20473869.2015.1136129

Gal, E., Lamash, L., Bauminger-Zviely, N., Zancanaro, M., & Weiss, P. L. (2016). Using Multitouch Collaboration Technology to Enhance Social Interaction of Children with High-Functioning Autism. *Physical & Occupational Therapy in Pediatrics*, *36*(1), 46–58. doi:10.3109/01942638.2015.1040572 PMID:26422262

Gallego, M. G., & García, J. G. (2017). Music therapy and Alzheimer's disease: Cognitive, psy-chological, and behavioural effects. *Neurologia (Barcelona, Spain)*, *32*(5), 300–308. PMID:26896913

Gal, N., Andrei, D., Nemeş, D. I., Nədəşan, E., & Stoicu-Tivadar, V. (2015). A Kinect based intelligent e-rehabilitation system in physical therapy. *Studies in Health Technology and Informatics*, *210*, 489–493. doi:10.3233/978-1-61499-512-8-489 PMID:25991195

Gandolfi, M., Valè, N., Dimitrova, E. K., Mazzoleni, S., Battini, E., Filippetti, M., Picelli, A., Santamato, A., Gravina, M., Saltuari, L., & Smania, N. (2019). Effectiveness of Robot-Assisted Upper Limb Training on Spasticity, Function and Muscle Activity in Chronic Stroke Patients Treated With Botulinum Toxin: A Randomized Single-Blinded Controlled Trial. *Frontiers in Neurology*, *10*, 41.

Gannotti, M. E. (2017). Coupling Timing of Interventions With Dose to Optimize Plasticity and Participation in Pediatric Neurologic Populations. *Pediatr Phys Ther, 29* (S3), S37-S47. doi:10.1097/PEP.0000000000000383

Garcı'a-Betances, R. I., Jime'nez-Mixco, V., Arredondo, M. T., & Cabrera-Umpie'rrez, M. F. (2015). Using Virtual Reality for Cognitive Training of the Elderly. *American Journal of Alzheimer's Disease and Other Dementias*, *30*(1), 49–54. doi:10.1177/1533317514545866 PMID:25107931

Garcia-Marques, L., Santos, A. S. C., & Mackie, D. M. (2006). Stereotypes: Static abstractions or dynamic knowledge structures? *Journal of Personality and Social Psychology*, *91*(5), 814–831. doi:10.1037/0022-3514.91.5.814 PMID:17059303

Gardiner, E., Miller, A. R., & Lach, L. M. (2020). Service adequacy and the relation between child behavior problems and negative family impact reported by primary caregivers of children with neurodevelopmental conditions. *Research in Developmental Disabilities*, *104*, 103712. Advance online publication. doi:10.1016/j.ridd.2020.103712 PMID:32554267

Gardony, A. L., Martis, S. B., Taylor, H. A., & Brunyé, T. T. (2021). Interaction strategies for effective augmented reality geo-visualization: Insights from spatial cognition. *Human-Computer Interaction*, *36*(2), 107–149. doi:10.1080/07370024.2018.1531001

Garrett, B., Taverner, T., Masinde, W., Gromala, D., Shaw, C., & Negraeff, M. (2014). A rapid evidence assessment of immersive virtual reality as an adjunct therapy in acute pain management in clinical practice. *The Clinical Journal of Pain*, *30*(12), 1089–1098. doi:10.1097/AJP.0000000000000064 PMID:24535053

Gecu-Parmaksiz, Z., & Delialioğlu, Ö. (2020). The effect of augmented reality activities on improving preschool children's spatial skills. *Interactive Learning Environments*, *28*(7), 876–889. doi:10.1080/10494820.2018.1546747

Gentry, T., Kriner, R., Sima, A., McDonough, J., & Wehman, P. (2015, March 1). Reducing the need for personal supports among workers with autism using an iPod touch as an assistive technology: Delayed randomized control trial. *Journal of Autism and Developmental Disorders*, *45*(3), 669–684. doi:10.100710803-014-2221-8 PMID:25212414

Gentry, T., Wallace, J., Kvarfordt, C., & Lynch, K. B. (2010). Personal digital assistants as cognitive aids for high school students with autism: Results of a community-based trial. *Journal of Vocational Rehabilitation*, *32*(2), 101–107. doi:10.3233/JVR-2010-0499

Georgescu, A. L., Kuzmanovic, B., Roth, D., Bente, G., & Vogeley, K. (2014). The use of virtual characters to assess and train non-verbal communication in high-functioning autism. *Frontiers in Human Neuroscience*, *8*(Oct). Advance online publication. doi:10.3389/fnhum.2014.00807 PMID:25360098

Gerhardt, P. F., & Lainer, I. (2011). Addressing the Needs of Adolescents and Adults with Autism: A Crisis on the Horizon. *Journal of Contemporary Psychotherapy*, *41*, 37–45. doi:10.100710879-010-9160-2

Geschwind, D. H. (2009). Advances in autism. *Annual Review of Medicine*, *60*(1), 367–380. doi:10.1146/annurev.med.60.053107.121225 PMID:19630577

Geyh, S., Cieza, A., Schouten, J., Dickson, H., Frommelt, P., Omar, Z., Kostanjsek, N., Ring, H., & Stucki, G. (2004). ICF Core Sets for stroke. *Journal of Rehabilitation Medicine*, (44), 135–141.

Ghai, S., & Ghai, I. (2019). Virtual Reality Enhances Gait in Cerebral Palsy: A Training Dose-Response Meta-Analysis. *Frontiers in Neurology*, *10*, 236. doi:10.3389/fneur.2019.00236 PMID:30984095

Ghanouni, P., Jarus, T., Zwicker, J. G., Lucyshyn, J., Mow, K., & Ledingham, A. (2019). Social stories for children with autism spectrum disorder: Validating the content of a virtual reality program. *Journal of Autism and Developmental Disorders*, *49*(2), 660–668. doi:10.100710803-018-3737-0 PMID:30203311

Gibson, G., Dickinson, C., & Brittain, K. (2015). The everyday use of assistive technology by people with dementia and their family carers: A qualitative study. *BMC Geriatrics*, *15*, 89.

Giesbers, S., Didden, R., Radstaake, M., Korzilius, H., Gontard, A., & Lang, R. (2012). Incontinence in individuals with Rett syndrome: A comparative study. *Journal of Developmental and Physical Disabilities*, *24*(3), 287–300. doi:10.100710882-012-9271-7 PMID:22639525

Gil-Castillo, J., Alnajjar, F., Koutsou, A., Torricelli, D., & Moreno, J. C. (2020). Advances in neuroprosthetic management of foot drop: A review. *Journal of Neuroengineering and Rehabilitation*, *17*(1), 1–19. doi:10.118612984-020-00668-4 PMID:32213196

Gil-González, I., Pérez-San-Gregorio, M. Á., Conrad, R., & Martín-Rodríguez, A. (2021). Predicting improvement of quality of life and mental health over 18-months in multiple sclerosis patients. *Multiple Sclerosis and Related Disorders*, *53*, 103093. Advance online publication. doi:10.1016/j.msard.2021.103093 PMID:34175814

Gillespie-Lynch, K., Kapp, S. K., Brooks, P. J., Pickens, J., & Schwartzman, B. (2017, March 28). Whose expertise is it? Evidence for autistic adults as critical autism experts. *Frontiers in Psychology*, *8*. Advance online publication. doi:10.3389/fpsyg.2017.00438 PMID:28400742

Gillner, S., & Mallot, H. A. (1998). Navigation and acquisition of spatial knowledge in a virtual maze. *Journal of Cognitive Neuroscience*, *10*(4), 445–463. doi:10.1162/089892998562861 PMID:9712675

Giullian, N., Ricks, D., Atherton, A., Colton, M., Goodrich, M., & Brinton, B. (2010). Detailed Requirements for Robots in Autism Therapy. In *International Conference on Systems, Man and Cybernetics* (pp. 2595-2602). Istanbul: IEEE. doi:10.1109/ICSMC.2010.5641908

Glaesar, B. C., Pierson, M. R., & Fritschmann, N. (2003). Comic Strip Conversations: A positive behavioral support strategy. *Teaching Exceptional Children, 36*(2), 14–19. doi:10.1177/004005990303600202

Glaze, D. G., Percy, A. K., Skinner, S., Motil, K. J., Neul, J. L., Barrish, J. O., Lane, J. B., Geerts, S. P., Annese, F., Graham, J., McNair, L., & Lee, H. S. (2010). Epilepsy and the natural history of Rett syndrome. *Neurology, 74*(11), 909–912. doi:10.1212/WNL.0b013e3181d6b852 PMID:20231667

Gmmash, A. S., Effgen, S. K., Skubik-Peplaski, C., & Lane, J. D. (2021). Parental Adherence to Home Activities in Early Intervention for Young Children With Delayed Motor Development. *Physical Therapy, 101*(4), pzab023. Advance online publication. doi:10.1093/ptj/pzab023 PMID:33481991

Gobeil, G., Pigot, H., Laliberté, C., Dépelteau, A., Laverdière, O., Grégoire, M.A.D., Laprise, N., Beauchamp, I., Couture, M., Adelise, Y., & Bier, N. (n.d.). Facilitating day-to-day life management of older people with Alzheimer's disease: A revelatory single-case study on the acceptability. *AMELIS Interactive Calendar, 18*, 241-257.

Golledge, R. G. (1999). *Wayfinding Behavior: Cognitive Mapping and Other Spatial Processes.* The Johns Hopkins University Press.

Gómez, J., Montoro, G., Haya, P. A., Alamán, X., Alves, S., & Martínez, M. (2013). Adaptive manuals as assistive technology to support and train people with acquired brain injury in their daily life activities. *Personal and Ubiquitous Computing, 17*(6), 1117–1126. doi:10.100700779-012-0560-z

Gomez-Rodriguez, M., Grosse-Wentrup, M., Hill, J., Gharabaghi, A., Scholkopf, B., & Peters, J. (2011). Towards brain-robot interfaces in stroke rehabilitation. *IEEE International Conference on Rehabilitation Robotics, 2011*, 5975385.

Góngora Alonso, S., Hamrioui, S., De La Torre Díez, I., Motta Cruz, E., López-Coronado, M., & Franco, M. (2019). Social robots for people with aging and dementia: A systematic review of literature. *Telemedicine Journal and e-Health, 25*(7), 533–540. doi:10.1089/tmj.2018.0051 PMID:30136901

Gonzalez-Franco, M., Abtahi, P., & Steed, A. (2019). Individual differences in embodied distance estimation in virtual reality. In *2019 IEEE Conference on Virtual Reality and 3D User Interfaces (VR)* (pp. 941-943). IEEE. 10.1109/VR.2019.8798348

Goode, P. S., Burgio, K. L., Richter, H. E., & Markland, A. D. (2010). Incontinence in older women. *Journal of the American Medical Association, 303*(21), 2172–2181. doi:10.1001/jama.2010.749 PMID:20516418

Goosen, L. (2019b). Information Systems and Technologies Opening New Worlds for Learning to Children with Autism Spectrum Disorders. Smart Innovation, Systems and Technologies, 111, 134-143. doi:10.1007/978-3-030-03577-8_16

Goosen, L. (2019a). Research on Technology-Supported Teaching and Learning for Autism. In L. Makewa, B. Ngussa, & J. Kuboja (Eds.), *Technology-Supported Teaching and Research Methods for Educators* (pp. 88–110). IGI Global. doi:10.4018/978-1-5225-5915-3.ch005

Goosen, L. (2020). Technology Opening New Worlds for Those with Autism – an Overview. In M. Clasquin-Johnson, D. Mahlo, & M. Clasquin-Johnson (Eds.), *Autism: Perspectives from Africa* (Vol. 1, pp. 135–168). UNISA Press.

Goo, T. (2007). Medical music therapy based on baby science (baby-science-based music therapy) and assistive technology for children. *Current Pediatric Reviews, 3*(3), 198–206. doi:10.2174/157339607781369573

Grandgeorge, M., & Masataka, N. (2016). Atypical Color Preference in Children with Autism Spectrum Disorder. *Frontiers in Psychology, 7*. doi:10.3389/fpsyg.2016.01976

Greathead, S., Yates, R., Hill, V., Kenny, L., Croydon, A., & Pellicano, E. (2016). Supporting children with severe-to-profound learning difficulties and complex communication needs to make their views known. *Topics in Language Disorders*, *36*(3), 217–244. doi:10.1097/TLD.0000000000000096

Greeno, J. G. (1994). Gibson's affordances. *Psychological Review*, *101*(2), 336–342. doi:10.1037/0033-295X.101.2.336 PMID:8022965

Gregg, L., & Tarrier, N. (2007). Virtual reality in mental health: A review of the literature. *Social Psychiatry and Psychiatric Epidemiology*, *42*(5), 343–354. doi:10.100700127-007-0173-4 PMID:17431528

Grimm, F., & Gharabaghi, A. (2016). Closed-Loop Neuroprosthesis for Reach-to-Grasp Assistance: Combining Adaptive Multi-channel Neuromuscular Stimulation with a Multi-joint Arm Exoskeleton. *Frontiers in Neuroscience*, *10*, 284.

Grindrod, K. A., Li, M., & Gates, A. (2014). Evaluating user perceptions of mobile medication management applications with older adults: A usability study. *JMIR mHealth and uHealth*, *2*(1), 11. doi:10.2196/mhealth.3048 PMID:25099993

Groba, B., Nieto-Riveiro, L., Canosa, N., Concheiro-Moscoso, P., Miranda-Duro, M., & Pereira, J. (2021). Stakeholder Perspectives to Support Graphical User Interface Design for Children with Autism Spectrum Disorder: A Qualitative Study. *International Journal of Environmental Research and Public Health*, *18*(9), 4631. https://doi.org/10.3390/ijerph18094631

Gronseth, G. S., Cox, J., Gloss, D., Merillat, S., Dittman, J., Armstrong, M. J., & Getchius, T. S. D. (2017). *Clinical Practice Guideline Process Manual*. American Academy of Neurology.

Grove, J., Ripke, S., Als, T. D., Mattheisen, M., Walters, R. K., Won, H., ... Awashti, S. (2019). Identification of common genetic risk variants for autism spectrum disorder. *Nature Genetics*, *51*(3), 431–444. doi:10.103841588-019-0344-8 PMID:30804558

Grynszpan, O., Weiss, P. L. T., Perez, F., & Gal, E. (2014). Innovative technology-based interventions for autism spectrum disorders : A meta-analysis. *Autism*, *18*(4), 346–361. doi:10.1177/1362361313476767 PMID:24092843

Gualniera, L., Singh, J., Fiori, F., & Santosh, P. (2021). Emotional behavioural and autonomic dysregulation (EBAD) in Rett syndrome – EDA and HRV monitoring using wearable sensor technology. *Journal of Psychiatric Research*, *138*, 186–193. doi:10.1016/j.jpsychires.2021.03.052 PMID:33862302

Gupta, S., Mishra, C., Katyayan, P., & Joshi, N. (2018). Assistive Technology for Neurological Disorders. SSRN *Electronic Journal, January*. doi:10.2139/ssrn.3166499

Hadders-Algra, M., Boxum, A. G., Hielkema, T., & Hamer, E. G. (2017). Effect of early intervention in infants at very high risk of cerebral palsy: A systematic review. *Developmental Medicine and Child Neurology*, *59*(3), 246–258. doi:10.1111/dmcn.13331 PMID:27925172

Halabi, O., El-Seoud, S. A., Alja'am, J. M., Alpona, H., Al-Hemadi, M., & Al-Hassan, D. (2017). Design of Immersive Virtual Reality System to Improve Communication Skills in Individuals with Autism. *International Jouranl of Emerging Technologies in Learning*, *12*(5), 50. doi:10.3991/ijet.v12i05.6766

Hampshire, P. K., & Allred, K. W. (2018). A Parent-Implemented, Technology-Mediated Approach to Increasing Self-Management Homework Skills in Middle School Students with Autism. *Exceptionality*, *26*(2), 119–136. doi:10.1080/09362835.2016.1216848

Harris, J. F., Janvier, Y. M., Mandell, D., & Cidav, Z. (2021, January). Validation of the developmental check-in tool for low-literacy autism screening. *Pediatrics*, *147*(1), e20193659. Advance online publication. doi:10.1542/peds.2019-3659 PMID:33303635

Hashim, R., & Yussof, H. (2017, October). Preparation for adulthood: Benefits of assistive technologies in social skills training of children with autism. In *International Symposium on Robotics and Intelligent Sensors (IRIS)* (pp. 374-378). Ottawa: IEEE. 10.1109/IRIS.2017.8250151

Hatem, S. M., Saussez, G., Della Faille, M., Prist, V., Zhang, X., Dispa, D., & Bleyenheuft, Y. (2016). Rehabilitation of Motor Function after Stroke: A Multiple Systematic Review Focused on Techniques to Stimulate Upper Extremity Recovery. *Frontiers in Human Neuroscience, 10*, 442.

Hedge, C., Weaver, R., & Schnall, S. (2017). Spatial learning and wayfinding in an immersive environment: The digital fulldome. *Cyberpsychology, Behavior, and Social Networking, 20*(5), 327–333. doi:10.1089/cyber.2016.0399 PMID:28459599

Hegarty, M., Montello, D. R., Richardson, A. E., Ishikawa, T., & Lovelace, K. (2006). Spatial abilities at different scales: Individual differences in aptitude-test performance and spatial-layout learning. *Intelligence, 34*(2), 151–176. doi:10.1016/j.intell.2005.09.005

Hendricks, H. T., van Limbeek, J., Geurts, A. C., & Zwarts, M. J. (2002). Motor recovery after stroke: A systematic review of the literature. *Archives of Physical Medicine and Rehabilitation, 83*(11), 1629–1637.

Hermes, E. D. A., Lyon, A. R., Schueller, S. M., & Glass, J. E. (2019). Measuring the implementation of behavioral intervention technologies: Recharacterization of established outcomes. *Journal of Medical Internet Research, 21*(1), e11752. Advance online publication. doi:10.2196/11752 PMID:30681966

Hervás, R., Francisco, V., Méndez, G., & Bautista, S. (2019, September). A User-Centred Methodology for the Development of Computer-Based Assistive Technologies for Individuals with Autism. In *IFIP Conference on Human-Computer Interaction* (pp. 85-106). Cham: Springer. 10.1007/978-3-030-29381-9_6

Hetzroni, O., Rubin, C., & Konkol, O. (2002). The use of assistive technology for symbol identification by children with Rett syndrome. *Journal of Intellectual & Developmental Disability, 27*(1), 57–71. doi:10.1080/13668250120119626-1

Hickie, I. B., Scott, E. M., Cross, S. P., Iorfino, F., Davenport, T. A., Guastella, A. J., Naismith, S. L., Carpenter, J. S., Rohleder, C., Crouse, J. J., Hermens, D. F., Koethe, D., Markus Leweke, F., Tickell, A. M., Sawrikar, V., & Scott, J. (2019). Right care, first time: A highly personalized and measurement-based care model to manage youth mental health. *The Medical Journal of Australia, 211*(S9), S3–S46. doi:10.5694/mja2.50383 PMID:31679171

Higashida, N. (2013). *Jump: The Inner Voice of a Theirteen-Year-Old Boy with Autism.* New York: Penguin Random House.

Hill, N. T., Mowszowski, L., Naismith, S. L., Chadwick, V. L., Valenzuela, M., & Lampit, A. (2017). Computerized cognitive training in older adults with mild cognitive impairment or dementia: A systematic review and meta-analysis. *The American Journal of Psychiatry, 174*(4), 329–340. doi:10.1176/appi.ajp.2016.16030360 PMID:27838936

Ho, D., Quake, S. R., McCabe, E. R. B., Chng, W. J., Chow, E. K., Ding, X., Gelb, B. D., Ginsburg, G. S., Hassenstab, J., Ho, C.-M., Mobley, W. C., Nolan, G. P., Rosen, S. T., Tan, P., Yen, Y., & Zarrinpar, A. (2020). Enabling Technologies for Personalized and Precision Medicine. *Trends in Biotechnology, 38*(5), 497–518. doi:10.1016/j.tibtech.2019.12.021 PMID:31980301

Hoenig, H. (2004). Assistive technology and mobility aids for the older patient with disability. *The Annals of Long-Term Care: the Official Journal of the American Medical Directors Association, 12*, 12–13.

Hoffman, H. G. (2004). Virtual-reality therapy. *Scientific American, 291*(20), 58–65. doi:10.1038cientificameric an0804-58 PMID:15298120

Hoffman, H. G., Patterson, D. R., Carrougher, G. J., & Sharar, S. R. (2001). Effectiveness of virtual reality–based pain control with multiple treatments. *The Clinical Journal of Pain, 17*(3), 229–235. doi:10.1097/00002508-200109000-00007 PMID:11587113

Hoffman, H. G., Patterson, D. R., Seibel, E., Soltani, M., Jewett-Leahy, L., & Sharar, S. R. (2008). Virtual reality pain control during burn wound debridement in the hydrotank. *The Clinical Journal of Pain, 24*(4), 299–304. doi:10.1097/AJP.0b013e318164d2cc PMID:18427228

Holthe, T., & Wulff-Jacobsen, I. (2016). Matching user needs to technology in dementia care: Experiences with the alma supervisor educational program. *Family Medicine and Primary Care Review, 18*, 492–496. doi:10.5114/fmpcr.2016.63710

Hong, J. A. (2008). A review on high-tech assistive technologies in language education for the students with autism spectrum disorders. *Special Education Research, 7*(1).

Hornof, A., Whitman, H., Sutherland, M., Gerendasy, S., & McGrenere, J. (2017). Designing for the "universe of one": Personalized interactive media systems for people with the severe cognitive impairment associated with Rett syndrome. *Conference on Human Factors in Computing Systems - Proceedings*, 2137-2148. 10.1145/3025453.3025904

Hort, J., Laczo, J., Vyhnalek, M., Bojar, M., Bures, J., & Vlcek, K. (2007). Spatial navigation deficit in amnestic mild cognitive impairment. *Proceedings of the National Academy of Sciences of the United States of America, 104*(10), 4042–4047. doi:10.1073/pnas.0611314104 PMID:17360474

Howett, D., Castegnaro, A., Krzywicka, K., Hagman, J., Marchment, D., Henson, R., Rio, M., King, J. A., Burgess, N., & Chan, D. (2019). Differentiation of mild cognitive impairment using an entorhinal cortex-based test of virtual reality navigation. *Brain, 142*(6), 1751–1766. doi:10.1093/brain/awz116 PMID:31121601

Howorth, S. K., Rooks-ellis, D., Flanagan, S., & Ok, M. W. (2019). Augmented Reality Supporting Reading Skills of Students with Autism Spectrum Disorder. *Intervention in School and Clinic, 55*(2), 71–77. doi:10.1177/1053451219837635

Huang, J. S., Yang, F. C., Chien, W. C., Yeh, T. C., Chung, C. H., Tsai, C. K., Tsai, S.-J., Yang, S.-S., Tzeng, N.-S., Chen, M.-H., & Liang, C. S. (2021, January 4). Risk of Substance Use Disorder and Its Associations with Comorbidities and Psychotropic Agents in Patients with Autism. *JAMA Pediatrics, 175*(2), e205371. Advance online publication. doi:10.1001/jamapediatrics.2020.5371 PMID:33394019

Huang, Q., Zhang, Z., Yu, T., He, S., & Li, Y. (2019). An EEG-/EOG-Based Hybrid Brain-Computer Interface: Application on Controlling an Integrated Wheelchair Robotic Arm System. *Frontiers in Neuroscience, 13*, 1243.

Huffman, J. M., Bross, L. A., Watson, E. K., Wills, H. P., & Mason, R. A. (2019). Preliminary Investigation of a Self-monitoring Application for a Postsecondary Student with Autism. *Advances in Neurodevelopmental Disorders, 3*(4), 423–433. doi:10.100741252-019-00124-y

Hull, L., Petrides, K. V., Allison, C., Smith, P., Baron-Cohen, S., Lai, M. C., & Mandy, W. (2017). "Putting on my best normal": Social camouflaging in adults with autism spectrum conditions. *Journal of Autism and Developmental Disorders, 47*(8), 2519–2534. doi:10.100710803-017-3166-5 PMID:28527095

Hung, K. N. G., & Fong, K. N. K. (2019). Effects of telerehabilitation in occupational therapy practice: A systematic review. *Hong Kong Journal of Occupational Therapy, 32*(1), 3–21. doi:10.1177/1569186119849119 PMID:31217758

Hutchinson, N., & Bodicoat, A. (2015). The effectiveness of intensive interaction, a systematic literature review. *Journal of Applied Research in Intellectual Disabilities, 28*(6), 437–454. doi:10.1111/jar.12138 PMID:25565017

Hutton, J. L., Colver, A. F., & Mackie, P. C. (2000). Effect of severity of disability on survival in north east England cerebral palsy cohort. *Archives of Disease in Childhood, 83*(6), 468–474. doi:10.1136/adc.83.6.468 PMID:11087278

Hwang, Y. I. (2020). Effects of an Elastic AFO on the Walking Patterns of Foot-drop Patients with Stroke. *Journal of the Korean Society of Physical Medicine*, *15*(1), 1–9. doi:10.13066/kspm.2020.15.1.1

Iannizzotto, G., Nucita, A., Fabio, R. A., Caprì, T., & Bello, L. L. (2020). Remote eye-tracking for cognitive telerehabilitation and interactive school tasks in times of COVID-19. *Information (Switzerland)*, *11*(6), 296. Advance online publication. doi:10.3390/info11060296

Ibrahim, Z., & Alias, M. (2018). A review on using assistive technology to enhance social skills competence among children with autism spectrum disorder (ASD). *Advanced Science Letters*, *24*(6), 4250–4254. doi:10.1166/asl.2018.11582

IDEA. (n.d.). https://sites.ed.gov/idea/statute-chapter-33/subchapter-i/1401

Imbeault, H., Langlois, F., Bocti, C., Gagnon, L., & Bier, N. (2018). Can people with Alzheimer's disease improve their day-to-day functioning with a tablet computer? *Neuropsychological Rehabilitation*, *28*(5), 779–796. doi:10.1080/09602011.2015.1133431 PMID:28278593

IMPACT. (2021). *Training Featuring Real Case Studies*. Retrieved from https://idea2impact.org/

Institute for Patient- and Family-Centered Care. (2011). *Advancing the practice of patient- and family-centered care in hospitals - how to get started* (Vol. 20814, Issue 301). Author.

Investigators, A. and D. D. M. N. S. Y. 2008 P. (2012). Prevalence of Autism Spectrum Disorders — Autism and Developmental Disabilities Monitoring Network, 14 Sites, United States, 2008. *Morbidity and Mortality Weekly Report: Surveillance Summaries, 61*(3), 1–19. http://www.jstor.org/stable/24806043

Iosa, M., Morone, G., Cherubini, A., & Paolucci, S. (2016). The Three Laws of Neurorobotics: A Review on What Neurorehabilitation Robots Should Do for Patients and Clinicians. *Journal of Medical and Biological Engineering*, *36*, 1–11.

Irvin, D. W., Crutchfield, S. A., Greenwood, C. R., Simpson, R. L., Sangwan, A., & Hansen, J. H. L. (2017). Exploring classroom behavioral imaging: Moving closer to effective and data-based early childhood inclusion planning. *Advances in Neurodevelopmental Disorders*, *1*(2), 95–104. doi:10.100741252-017-0014-8

Israel, S., Kotowski, S., Talbott, N., Fisher, K., & Dunning, K. (2011). The therapeutic effect of outpatient use of a peroneal nerve functional electrical stimulation neuroprosthesis in people with stroke: A case series. *Topics in Stroke Rehabilitation*, *18*(6), 738–745. doi:10.1310/tsr1806-738 PMID:22436311

Jagos, H., David, V., Haller, M., Kotzian, S., Hofmann, M., Schlossarek, S., Eichholzer, K., Winkler, M., Frohner, M., Reichel, M., Mayr, W., & Rafolt, D. (2015). A framework for (tele-) monitoring of the rehabilitation progress in stroke patients. *Applied Clinical Informatics*, *6*(4), 757–768. doi:10.4338/ACI-2015-03-RA-0034 PMID:26767068

Jak, A. J. (2012). The impact of physical and mental activity on cognitive aging. *Current Topics in Behavioral Neurosciences*, *10*, 273–291. doi:10.1007/7854_2011_141 PMID:21818703

Jamal, H. A. (2020, May). Developing the Language Ability of Children with Autism Spectrum Disorder (ASD) Using Assistive Technology and a Picture Exchange Communication System (PECS) through Adapting Elements of the Australian Educational Environment on Inclusive Public Schools. *Journal of Special Education and Rehabilitation*, *10*(36), 1–47. doi:10.12816/0055786

Jauch, E. C., Saver, J. L., Adams, H. P. Jr, Bruno, A., Connors, J. J., Demaerschalk, B. M., Khatri, P., McMullan, P. W. Jr, Qureshi, A. I., Rosenfield, K., Scott, P. A., Summers, D. R., Wang, D. Z., Wintermark, M., & Yonas, H. (2013). Guidelines for the early management of patients with acute ischemic stroke: A guideline for healthcare professionals from the American Heart Association/American Stroke Association. *Stroke*, *44*(3), 870–947. doi:10.1161/STR.0b013e318284056a PMID:23370205

Jheng, S. S., & Pai, M. C. (2009). Cognitive map in patients with mild Alzheimer's disease: A computer-generated arena study. *Behavioural Brain Research, 200*(1), 42–47. doi:10.1016/j.bbr.2008.12.029 PMID:19162077

Johnson, L. (2018). For people with dementia, virtual reality can be life-changing. *Wired.* https://www.wired.co.uk/article/virtual-reality-dementia-technology

Johnson, J. J., Rahn, N. L., & Bricker, D. (2015). *An activity-based approach to early intervention* (4th ed.). Paul H. Brookes Publishing Co.

Johnson, W., Onuma, O., Owolabi, M., & Sachdev, S. (2016). Stroke: A global response is needed. *Bulletin of the World Health Organization, 94*(9), 634–634A.

Jusoh, W., & Majid, R. A. (2017). Using Picture Exchange Communication System To Improve Speech Utterance Among Children With Autism. *Journal of ICSAR, 1*(1), 46–49. doi:10.17977/um005v1i12017p046

Kaddoum, R. N., Anghelescu, D. L., Parish, M. E., Wright, B. B., Trujillo, L., Wu, J., Wu, Y., & Burgoyne, L. L. (2012). A randomized controlled trial comparing the AccuVein AV300 device to standard insertion technique for intravenous cannulation of anesthetized children. *Paediatric Anaesthesia, 22*(9), 884–889. doi:10.1111/j.1460-9592.2012.03896.x PMID:22694242

Kakkar, D. (2019). Diagnostic assessment techniques and non-invasive biomarkers for Autism Spectrum Disorder. *International Journal of E-Health and Medical Communications, 10*(3), 79–95. doi:10.4018/IJEHMC.2019070105

Kakkar, D., & Tanu, T. (2018). Strengthening risk prediction using statistical learning in children with autism spectrum disorder. *Advances in Autism, 4*(3), 141–152. doi:10.1108/AIA-06-2018-0022

Kalová, E., Vlcek, K., Jarolímová, E., & Bures, J. (2005). Allothetic orientation and sequential ordering of places is impaired in early stages of Alzheimer's disease: Corresponding results in real space tests and computer tests. *Behavioural Brain Research, 159*(2), 175–186. doi:10.1016/j.bbr.2004.10.016 PMID:15817181

Kaplan, A. D., Cruit, J., Endsley, M., Beers, S. M., Sawyer, B. D., & Hancock, P. A. (2020). The effects of virtual reality, augmented reality, and mixed reality as training enhancement methods: A meta-analysis. *Human Factors, 63*(4), 706–726. doi:10.1177/0018720820904229 PMID:32091937

Kats, Y., & Stasolla, F. (Eds.). (2021). *Education and Technology Support for Children and Young Adults With ASD and Learning Disabilities*. IGI Global. doi:10.4018/978-1-7998-7053-1

Kavcic, V., & Duffy, C. (2003). Attentional dynamics and visual perception: Mechanisms of spatial disorientation in Alzheimer's disease. *Brain, 126*(5), 1173–1181. doi:10.1093/brain/awg105 PMID:12690056

Kayabinar, B., Alemdaroğlu-Gürbüz, İ., & Yilmaz, Ö. (2021). The effects of virtual reality augmented robot-assisted gait training on dual-task performance and functional measures in chronic stroke: A randomized controlled single-blind trial. *European Journal of Physical and Rehabilitation Medicine, 57*(2), 227–237. doi:10.23736/S1973-9087.21.06441-8 PMID:33541040

Kazdin, A. E. (2001). *Behavior modification in applied settings*. Wadsworth: Thomson Learning.

Kazdin, A. E. (2001). *Behavior modification in applied settings* (6th ed.). Wadsworth.

Ke, F., Moon, J., & Sokolikj, Z. (2020). Virtual Reality–Based Social Skills Training for Children With Autism Spectrum Disorder. *Journal of Special Education Technology*, 1–14. doi:10.1177/0162643420945603

Kellstedt, D. K., Spengler, J. O., Foster, M., Lee, C., & Maddock, J. E. (2021). A scoping review of bikeability assessment methods. *Journal of Community Health, 46*(1), 211–224. doi:10.100710900-020-00846-4 PMID:32419079

Kennedy, K. (2005). *Single case designs for educational research.* Allyn & Bacon.

Kenney, S. (2013). *The Impact of Using Assistive Technology on Writing Productivity of Young Writers with Autism* (Ph.D. thesis). Fairfax, VA: George Mason University. Retrieved January 22, 2021, from https://www.learntechlib.org/p/119919/

Kerr, A. (2007). *Understanding Rett Disorder: A Guide for Professionals.* University of Glasgow.

Khan, M. (2021). Balancing non-discrimination and risk management in mental health legislation for autism. *The British Journal of Psychiatry, 218*(1), 63–64. doi:10.1192/bjp.2020.182 PMID:33541470

Khantreejitranon, A. (2018). Using a social story intervention to decrease inappropriate behavior of preschool children with autism. *Kasetsart Journal of Social Sciences, 39*(1), 90–97. doi:10.1016/j.kjss.2017.12.019

Khanuja, K., Joki, J., Bachmann, G., & Cuccurullo, S. (2018). Gait and balance in the aging population: Fall prevention using innovation and technology. *Maturitas, 110*, 51–56. doi:10.1016/j.maturitas.2018.01.021 PMID:29563035

Khenak, N., Vézien, J., Théry, D., & Bourdot, P. (2020). Spatial Presence in Real and Remote Immersive Environments and the Effect of Multisensory Stimulation. *PRESENCE: Virtual and Augmented Reality, 27*(3), 287–308. doi:10.1162/pres_a_00332

Kilteni, K., Groten, R., & Slater, M. (2012). The sense of embodiment in virtual reality. *Presence (Cambridge, Mass.), 21*(4), 373–387. doi:10.1162/PRES_a_00124

Kim, E. S., Laird, L., Wilson, C., Bieg, T., Mildner, P., Möller, S., Schatz, R., Schwarz, S., Spang, R., Voigt-Antons, J.-N., & Rochon, E. (2021). Implementation and effects of an information technology-based intervention to support speech and language therapy among stroke patients with aphasia: Protocol for a virtual randomized controlled trial. *JMIR Research Protocols, 10*(7), e30621. Advance online publication. doi:10.2196/30621 PMID:34255727

Kim, G., Lim, S., Kim, H., Lee, B., Seo, S., Cho, K., & Lee, W. (2017). Is robot-assisted therapy effective in upper extremity recovery in early stage stroke? -a systematic literature review. *Journal of Physical Therapy Science, 29*(6), 1108–1112.

King, S., Teplicky, R., King, G., & Rosenbaum, P. (2004). Family-Centered Service for Children with Cerebral Palsy and Their Families: A Review of the Literature. In Seminars in Pediatric Neurology (Vol. 11, Issue 1, pp. 78–86). W.B. Saunders. doi:10.1016/j.spen.2004.01.009

Kiresuk, T. J., & Sherman, R. E. (1968). Goal attainment scaling: A general method for evaluating comprehensive community mental health programs. *Community Mental Health Journal, 4*(6), 443–453. doi:10.1007/BF01530764 PMID:24185570

Klimova, B., Valis, M., & Kuca, K. (2018). Exploring assistive technology as a potential beneficial intervention tool for people with Alzheimer's disease – a systematic review. *Neuropsychiatric Disease and Treatment, 14*, 3151–3158. doi:10.2147/NDT.S181849 PMID:30532546

Klingberg, T. (2010). Training and plasticity of working memory. *Trends in Cognitive Sciences, 14*(7), 317–324. doi:10.1016/j.tics.2010.05.002 PMID:20630350

Kluding, P. M., Dunning, K., O'Dell, M. W., Wu, S. S., Ginosian, J., Feld, J., & McBride, K. (2013). Foot drop stimulation versus ankle foot orthosis after stroke: 30-week outcomes. *Stroke, 44*(6), 1660–1669. doi:10.1161/STROKEAHA.111.000334 PMID:23640829

Knapp, J. M., & Loomis, J. M. (2004). Limited field of view of head-mounted displays is not the cause of distance underestimation in virtual environments. *Presence (Cambridge, Mass.), 13*(5), 572–577. doi:10.1162/1054746042545238

Kober, S. E., Wood, G., Hofer, D., Kreuzig, W., Kiefer, M., & Neuper, C. (2013). Virtual reality in neurologic rehabilitation of spatial disorientation. *Journal of Neuroengineering and Rehabilitation*, *10*(1), 1–13. doi:10.1186/1743-0003-10-17 PMID:23394289

Koch, A. (2012). *Assistive technologies for children with autism spectrum disorders*. Division of Science and Mathematics, University of Minnesota.

Koegel, L. K., Koegel, R. L., Frea, W., & Green-Hopkins, I. (2003). Priming as a method of coordinating educational services for students with autism. *Language, Speech, and Hearing Services in Schools*, *34*(3), 228–235. doi:10.1044/0161-1461(2003/019) PMID:27764324

Koldrack, P., Luplow, M., Kirste, T., & Teipel, S. (2013). Cognitive assistance to support social integration in Alzheimer's disease. *Geriatric Mental Health Care*, *1*(2), 39–45. doi:10.1016/j.gmhc.2013.04.005

Kolk, A., Saard, M., Pertens, L., Kallakas, T., Sepp, K., & Kornet, K. (2019). Structured Model of Neurorehab: A Pilot Study of Modern Multitouch Technology and Virtual Reality Platforms for Training Sociocognitive Deficit in Children with Acquired Brain Injury. *Applied Neuropsychology. Child*, *8*(4), 326–332. doi:10.1080/21622965.2018.1486193 PMID:30295544

Kõlves, K., Fitzgerald, C., Nordentoft, M., Wood, S. J., & Erlangsen, A. (2021, January 12). Assessment of Suicidal Behaviors Among Individuals With Autism Spectrum Disorder in Denmark. *JAMA Network Open*, *4*(1), e2033565. Advance online publication. doi:10.1001/jamanetworkopen.2020.33565 PMID:33433599

Koly, K. N., Martin-Herz, S. P., Islam, M. S., Sharmin, N., Blencowe, H., & Naheed, A. (2021). Parent mediated intervention programmes for children and adolescents with neurodevelopmental disorders in South Asia: A systematic review. *PLoS One, 16*(3). . doi:10.1371/journal.pone.0247432

Kotipalli, P., Praveen Kumar, E. R., Mohan Raju, M. A. S., & Murali Krishna, D. (2019). *Supportive communication system for the elderly disabled people*. . doi:10.1007/978-981-13-1921-1_45

Kotlarek, J., Lin, I. C., & Ma, K. L. (2018). Improving spatial orientation in immersive environments. In *Proceedings of the Symposium on Spatial User Interaction* (pp. 79-88). 10.1145/3267782.3267792

Kottink, A. I., Hermens, H. J., Nene, A. V., Tenniglo, M. J., Groothuis-Oudshoorn, C. G., & IJzerman, M. J. (2008). Therapeutic effect of an implantable peroneal nerve stimulator in subjects with chronic stroke and footdrop: A randomized controlled trial. *Physical Therapy*, *88*(4), 437–448. doi:10.2522/ptj.20070035 PMID:18218825

Kottink, A. I., Hermens, H. J., Nene, A. V., Tenniglo, M. J., van der Aa, H. E., Buschman, H. P., & IJzerman, M. J. (2007). A randomized controlled trial of an implantable 2-channel peroneal nerve stimulator on walking speed and activity in poststroke hemiplegia. *Archives of Physical Medicine and Rehabilitation*, *88*(8), 971–978. doi:10.1016/j.apmr.2007.05.002 PMID:17678657

Kottink, A. I., Tenniglo, M. J., de Vries, W. H., Hermens, H. J., & Buurke, J. H. (2012). Effects of an implantable two-channel peroneal nerve stimulator versus conventional walking device on spatiotemporal parameters and kinematics of hemiparetic gait. *Journal of Rehabilitation Medicine*, *44*(1), 51–57. doi:10.2340/16501977-0909 PMID:22124679

Koumakis, L., Chatzaki, C., Kazantzaki, E., Maniadi, E., & Tsiknakis, M. (2019). Dementia care frameworks and assistive technologies for their implementation: A review. *IEEE Reviews in Biomedical Engineering*, *12*, 4–18. doi:10.1109/RBME.2019.2892614 PMID:30640629

Koumpouros, Y. (2021). An "all-in-one" wearable application for assisting children with autism spectrum disorder. *Technology and Disability*, *33*(1), 65–75. doi:10.3233/TAD-200291

Kozhevnikov, M., & Garcia, A. (2011). Visual-spatial learning and training in collaborative design in virtual environments. *Collaborative design in virtual environments*, 17-26.

Kozhevnikov, M., & Dhond, R. P. (2012). Understanding immersivity: Image generation and transformation processes in 3D immersive environments. *Frontiers in Psychology*, *3*, 284. doi:10.3389/fpsyg.2012.00284 PMID:22908003

Kozima, H., Nakagawa, C., & Yasuda, Y. (2007). Children–robot interaction: a pilot study in autism therapy. In C. von Hofsten & K. B. T.-P. In B. R. Rosander (Ed.), *From Action to Cognition* (Vol. 164, pp. 385–400). Elsevier. doi:10.1016/S0079-6123(07)64021-7

Kroesch, A. M., Douglas, K. H., Jozwik, S., Uphold, N. M., & Chung, Y. (2020). Teaching american government content to students with developmental disabilities using technology and constant time delay. *Journal of Developmental and Physical Disabilities*, *32*(6), 925–941. doi:10.100710882-019-09726-9

Küçük, S., Kapakin, S., & Göktaş, Y. (2016). Learning anatomy via mobile augmented reality: Effects on achievement and cognitive load. *Anatomical Sciences Education*, *9*(5), 411–421. doi:10.1002/ase.1603 PMID:26950521

Kulkarni, M. (2017, January 15). *Assistive technologies for autism, cerebral palsy, multiple disabilities, and intellectual disabilities.* An invited report submitted to The National Trust, Ministry of Social Justice and Empowerment, Government of India. Retrieved from https://repository.iimb.ac.in/handle/2074/13855

Kumazaki, H., Muramatsu, T., Yoshikawa, Y., Matsumoto, Y., Miyao, M., Ishiguro, H., ... Kikuchi, M. (2019). How the Realism of Robot Is Needed for Individuals With Autism Spectrum Disorders in an Interview Setting. *Frontiers in Psychiatry*, *10*, 486.doi:https://doi.org/10.3389/fpsyt.2019.00486

Kumazaki, H., Warren, Z., Corbett, B. A., Yoshikawa, Y., Matsumoto, Y., Higashida, H., ... Kikuchi, M. (2017). Android Robot-Mediated Mock Job Interview Sessions for Young Adults with Autism Spectrum Disorder: A Pilot Study. *Frontiers in Psychiatry*, *8*, 169.doi:https://doi.org/10.3389/fpsyt.2017.00169

Kunjir, A. R., & Patil, K. R. (2020). Effectiveness of Practicing Social Distancing in Museums and Art Galleries for Visitors Using Mobile Augmented Reality (MAR): SMART—Social Distancing Using Mobile Augmented Reality Technology. *International Journal of Art, Culture and Design Technologies*, *9*(1), 1–14. doi:10.4018/IJACDT.2020010101

Kwakkel, G., Kollen, B. J., & Krebs, H. I. (2008). Effects of robot-assisted therapy on upper limb recovery after stroke: A systematic review. *Neurorehabilitation and Neural Repair*, *22*(2), 111–121.

Laczó, J., Andel, R., Vyhnálek, M., Vlcek, K., Magerova, H., Varjassyova, A., Tolar, M., & Hort, J. (2010). Human analogue of the Morris water maze for testing subjects at risk of Alzheimer's disease. *Neurodegenerative Diseases*, *7*(3), 148–152. doi:10.1159/000289226 PMID:20197695

Laczó, J., Andel, R., Vyhnalek, M., Vlcek, K., Nedelska, Z., Matoska, V., Gazova, I., Mokrisova, I., Sheardova, K., & Hort, J. (2014). APOE and spatial navigation in amnestic MCI: Results from a computer-based test. *Neuropsychology*, *28*(5), 676–684. doi:10.1037/neu0000072 PMID:24749727

Laczó, J., Vlcek, K., Vyhnalek, M., Vajnerova, O., Ort, M., Holmerova, I., Tolar, M., Andel, R., Bojar, M., & Hort, J. (2009). Spatial navigation testing discriminates two types of amnestic mild cognitive impairment. *Behavioural Brain Research*, *202*(2), 252–259. doi:10.1016/j.bbr.2009.03.041 PMID:19463709

Lancini, G., Singh, N.N., O'Reilly, M.F., Sigafoos, J., Bosco, A., Zonno, N., & Badagliacca, F. (2011). Persons with mild or moderate Alzheimer's disease learn to use urine alarms and prompts to avoid large urinary accidents. *Research in Developmental Disabilities, 32,* 1998-2004.

Lancioni, G., De Caro, M.F., Singh, N.N., O'Reilly, M.F., Sigafoos, J., & Buono, S. (2014). Further evaluation of programs for promoting daily activities and indoor orientation and travel in persons with moderate Alzheimer's disease. *Life Span and Disability, 2,* 245-263..

Lancioni, G., Perrilli, V., Singh, N.N., O'Reilly, M.F., Sigafoos, J., Bosco, A., De Caro, M.F., Cassano, G., Pinto, K., & Minervini, M. (2011). *Persons with mild or moderate Alzheimer's disease use a basic orientation technology to travel to different rooms within a day center*. Academic Press.

Lancioni, G. E., Belardinelli, M. O., Chiapparino, C., Angelillo, M. T., Stasolla, F., Singh, N. N., O'Reilly, M. F., Sigafoos, J., & Oliva, D. (2008). Learning in post-coma persons with profound multiple disabilities: Two case evaluations. *Journal of Developmental and Physical Disabilities, 20*(3), 209–216. doi:10.100710882-008-9105-9

Lancioni, G. E., Bosco, A., De Caro, M. F., Singh, N. N., O'reilly, M. F., Green, V. A., Ferlisi, G., Zullo, V., D'Amico, F., Addante, L. M., Denitto, F., & Zonno, N. (2015). Effects of response-related music stimulation versus general music stimulation on positive participation of patients with Alzheimer's disease. *Developmental Neurorehabilitation, 18*(3), 169–176. doi:10.3109/17518423.2013.802388 PMID:23869934

Lancioni, G. E., O' Reilly, M. F., Singh, N. N., Sigafoos, J., Didden, R., Oliva, D., & Montironi, G. (2007). Persons with multiple disabilities and minimal motor behavior using small forehead movements and new microswitch technology to control environmental stimuli. *Perceptual and Motor Skills, 104*(3), 870–878. doi:10.2466/pms.104.3.870-878 PMID:17688142

Lancioni, G. E., O'Reilly, M. F., Singh, N. N., Groeneweg, J., Bosco, A., Tota, A., Smaldone, A., Stasolla, F., Manfredi, F., Baccani, S., & Pidala, S. (2006). A social validation assessment of microswitch-based programs for persons with multiple disabilities employing teacher trainees and parents as raters. *Journal of Developmental and Physical Disabilities, 18*(4), 383–391. doi:10.100710882-006-9024-6

Lancioni, G. E., O'Reilly, M. F., Singh, N. N., Sigafoos, J., Didden, R., Oliva, D., Campodonico, F., de Pace, C., Chiapparino, C., & Groeneweg, J. (2009). Persons with multiple disabilities accessing stimulation and requesting social contact via microswitch and VOCA devices: New research evaluation and social validation. *Research in Developmental Disabilities, 30*(5), 1084–1094. doi:10.1016/j.ridd.2009.03.004 PMID:19361954

Lancioni, G. E., O'Reilly, M. F., Singh, N. N., Sigafoos, J., Oliva, D., & Severini, L. (2008a). Enabling two persons with multiple disabilities to access environmental stimuli and ask for social contact through microswitches and a VOCA. *Research in Developmental Disabilities, 29*(1), 21–28. doi:10.1016/j.ridd.2006.10.001 PMID:17174529

Lancioni, G. E., O'Reilly, M. F., Singh, N. N., Sigafoos, J., Oliva, D., & Severini, L. (2008b). Three persons with multiple disabilities accessing environmental stimuli and asking for social contact through microswitch and VOCA technology. *Journal of Intellectual Disability Research, 52*(4), 327–336. doi:10.1111/j.1365-2788.2007.01024.x PMID:18339095

Lancioni, G. E., O'Reilly, M. F., Singh, N. N., Sigafoos, J., Tota, A., Antonucci, M., & Oliva, D. (2006). Children with multiple disabilities and minimal motor behavior using chin movements to operate microswitches to obtain environmental stimulation. *Research in Developmental Disabilities, 27*(3), 290–298. doi:10.1016/j.ridd.2005.02.003 PMID:16005183

Lancioni, G. E., O'Reilly, M. F., Singh, N. N., Stasolla, F., Manfredi, F., & Oliva, D. (2004). Adapting a grid into a microswitch to suit simple hand movements of a child with profound multiple disabilities. *Perceptual and Motor Skills, 99*(2), 724–728. doi:10.2466/pms.99.2.724-728 PMID:15560365

Lancioni, G. E., Olivetti, M., Singh, N. N., O'Reilly, M., Sigafoos, J., & Alberti, G. (2019). Recent technology-aided programs to support adaptive responses, functional activities, and leisure and communication in people with significant disabilities. *Frontiers in Neurology, 10*, 643. doi:10.3389/fneur.2019.00643 PMID:31312169

Lancioni, G. E., Perilli, V., Singh, N. N., O'Reilly, M. F., & Cassano, G. (2011). A man with severe Alzheimer's disease stops wandering during a picture coloring activity. *Developmental Neurorehabilitation, 14*(4), 242–246. doi:10.3109/17518423.2011.575439 PMID:21732808

Lancioni, G. E., Simone, I. L., De Caro, M. F., Singh, N. N., O'Reilly, M. F., Sigafoos, J., Ferlisi, G., Zullo, V., Schirone, S., Denitto, F., & Zonno, N. (2015). Assisting persons with advanced amyotrophic lateral sclerosis in their leisure engagement and communication needs with a basic technology-aided program. *NeuroRehabilitation, 36*(3), 355–365. doi:10.3233/NRE-151224 PMID:26409339

Lancioni, G. E., & Singh, N. N. (2014). *Assistive technologies for people with diverse abilities*. Springer. doi:10.1007/978-1-4899-8029-8

Lancioni, G. E., Singh, N. N., O'Reilly, M. F., Green, V. A., Ferlisi, G., Ferrarese, G., Zullo, V., Perilli, V., Cassano, G., Cordiano, N., Pinto, K., & Zonno, N. (2013). Self-regulated music stimulation for persons with Alzheimer's disease: Impact assessment and social validation. *Developmental Neurorehabilitation, 16*(1), 17–26. doi:10.3109/17518423.2012.707693 PMID:23030807

Lancioni, G. E., Singh, N. N., O'Reilly, M. F., Sigafoos, J., Alberti, G., & Campodonico, F. (2016). Case Studies of Technology-aided Interventions to Promote Hand Reaching and Standing or Basic Ambulation in Persons with Multiple Disabilities. *Perceptual and Motor Skills, 122*(1), 200–219. doi:10.1177/0031512516630017 PMID:27420316

Lancioni, G. E., Singh, N. N., O'Reilly, M. F., Sigafoos, J., Chiapparino, C., Stasolla, F., Bosco, A., De Pace, C., & Oliva, D. (2007). Enabling a young man with minimal motor behavior to manage independently his leisure television engagement. *Perceptual and Motor Skills, 105*(1), 47–54. doi:10.2466/pms.105.1.47-54 PMID:17918548

Lancioni, G. E., Singh, N. N., O'Reilly, M. F., Sigafoos, J., Chiapparino, C., Stasolla, F., & Oliva, D. (2007b). Using an optic sensor and a scanning keyboard emulator to facilitate writing by persons with pervasive motor disabilities. *Journal of Developmental and Physical Disabilities, 19*(6), 593–603. doi:10.100710882-007-9073-5

Lancioni, G. E., Singh, N. N., O'Reilly, M. F., Sigafoos, J., D'Amico, F., Pinto, K., & Chiapparino, C. (2017). Supporting simple activity engagement in persons with moderate to severe Alzheimer's disease through a technology-aided program. *American Journal of Alzheimer's Disease and Other Dementias, 32*(3), 137–144. doi:10.1177/1533317517698793 PMID:28423935

Lancioni, G., Nirbhay, N. S., O'Reilly, M. F., Sigafoos, J., D'Amico, F., Ferlisi, G., Denitto, F., De Vanna, F., & Belardinelli, M. O. (2015). Patients with moderate Alzheimer's disease engage in verbal reminiscence with the support of a computer-aided program: A pilot study. *Frontiers in Aging Neuroscience, 7*, 1–9. doi:10.3389/fnagi.2015.00109 PMID:26089797

Lancioni, G., Nirbhay, N. S., O'Reilly, M. F., Sigafoos, J., D'Amico, F., Sasanellli, G., De Vanna, F., & Signorino, M. (2015). Persons with Alzheimer's disease engage in leisure and mild physical activity with the support of technology-aided programs. *Research in Developmental Disabilities, 37*, 55–63. doi:10.1016/j.ridd.2014.11.004 PMID:25460220

Lancioni, G., Nirbhay, N. S., O'Reilly, M. F., Sigafoos, J., Renna, C., Ventrella, M., Pinto, K., & Minervini, M. G. (2014). Supporting daily activities and indoor travel of persons with moderate Alzheimer's disease through standard technology resources. *Research in Developmental Disabilities, 34*(8), 2351–2359. doi:10.1016/j.ridd.2013.04.020 PMID:23711628

Lancioni, G., O'Reilly, M. F., Nirbhay, N., Singh, C., Sigafoos, J., Grumo, G., Pinto, K., Stasolla, F., Signorino, M., & Groeneweg, J. (2013). Assessing the impact and social perception of self-regulated music stimulation with patients with Alzheimer's disease. *Research in Developmental Disabilities, 34*(1), 139–146. doi:10.1016/j.ridd.2012.07.026 PMID:22944256

Lancioni, G., O'Reilly, M. F., Singh, N. N., Sigafoos, J., Rigante, V., De Franciscis, L., Stasolla, F., Perilli, V., & Lang, R. (2013). A Further Evaluation of the Impact of Self-regulated Music Stimulation on Positive Participation of Patients with Alzheimer's Disease. *Journal of Developmental and Physical Disabilities*, *25*(3), 273–283. doi:10.100710882-012-9301-5

Lancioni, G., Perilli, V., O'Reilly, M. F., Nirbhay, N., Singh, C., Sigafoos, J., Bosco, A., Caffò, A., Picucci, L., Cassano, G., & Groeneweg, J. (2013). Technology-based orientation programs to support indoor travel by persons with moderate Alzheimer's disease: Impact assessment and social validation. *Research in Developmental Disabilities*, *34*(1), 286–293. doi:10.1016/j.ridd.2012.08.016 PMID:22982468

Lancioni, G., Perilli, V., Singh, N. N., O'Reilly, M. F., & Sigafoos, J. (2016). Technology-Aided Programs to Support Positive Verbal and Physical Engagement in Persons with Moderate or Severe Alzheimer's Diseas. *Frontiers in Aging Neuroscience*, *8*, 1–8. doi:10.3389/fnagi.2016.00087 PMID:27148050

Lancioni, G., Perilli, V., Singh, N. N., O'Reilly, M. F., Sigafoos, J., Cassano, G., Pinto, K., Minervini, M. G., & Oliva, D. (2012). Technology-aided pictorial cues to support the performance of daily activities by persons with moderate Alzheimer's disease. *Research in Developmental Disabilities*, *33*(1), 265–273. doi:10.1016/j.ridd.2011.09.017 PMID:22093673

Lancioni, G., Perilli, V., Singh, N. N., O'Reilly, M. F., Sigafoos, J., D'Amico, F., Laporta, D., Cattaneo, M. G., Scordamaglia, A., & Pinto, K. (2018). Technology-Based Behavioral Interventions for Daily Activities and Supported Ambulation in People With Alzheimer's Disease. *American Journal of Alzheimer's Disease and Other Dementias*, *33*(5), 318–326. doi:10.1177/1533317518775038 PMID:29742903

Lancioni, G., Perilli, V., Singh, N. N., O'Reilly, M. F., Sigafoos, J., D'Amico, F., Turnone, B., Laporta, D., Scordamaglia, A., & Pinto, K. (2019). Smartphone-Based Interventions to Foster Simple Activity and Personal Satisfaction in People With Advanced Alzheimer's Disease. *American Journal of Alzheimer's Disease and Other Dementias*, *34*(7-8), 478–485. doi:10.1177/1533317519844144 PMID:31014071

Lancioni, G., Sigafoos, J., O'Reilly, M. F., & Singh, N. N. (2013). *Assistive technology: Interventions for individuals with severe/profound and multiple disabilities*. Springer Science & Business Media. doi:10.1007/978-1-4614-4229-5

Lancioni, G., Singh, N., O'Reilly, M. F., Renna, C., Pinto, K., De Vanna, F., Caffò, A., & Stasolla, F. (2014). Persons with moderate Alzheimer's disease use simple technology aids to manage daily activities and leisure occupation. *Research in Developmental Disabilities*, *35*(9), 2117–2128. doi:10.1016/j.ridd.2014.05.002 PMID:24881006

Lancioni, G., Singh, N., O'Reilly, M. F., Sigafoos, J., Ferlisi, G., Zullo, V., Schirone, S., Prisco, R., & Denitto, F. (2014). A computer-aided program for helping patients with moderate Alzheimer's disease engage in verbal reminiscence. *Research in Developmental Disabilities*, *35*(11), 3026–3033. doi:10.1016/j.ridd.2014.07.047 PMID:25124700

Landau, R., Werner, S., Auslander, G. K., Shoval, N., & Heinik, J. (2009). Attitudes of family members and care professionals towards the use of GPS for monitoring patients with dementia: An exploratory study. *British Journal of Social Work*, *39*, 670–692. doi:10.1093/bjsw/bcp037

Langer, A., Gassner, L., Flotz, A., Hasenauer, S., Gruber, J., Wizany, L., Pokan, R., Maetzler, W., & Zach, H. (2021). How COVID-19 will boost remote exercise-based treatment in Parkinson's disease: A narrative review. *NPJ Parkinson's Disease*, *7*(1), 25. Advance online publication. doi:10.103841531-021-00160-3 PMID:33686074

Langhorne, P., Bernhardt, J., & Kwakkel, G. (2011). Stroke rehabilitation. *Lancet*, *377*(9778), 1693–1702. doi:10.1016/S0140-6736(11)60325-5 PMID:21571152

Langhorne, P., Coupar, F., & Pollock, A. (2009). Motor recovery after stroke: A systematic review. *Lancet Neurology*, *8*(8), 741–754.

Lang, R., Ramdoss, S., Raulston, T., Carnet, A., Sigafoos, J., Didden, R., & O'Reilly, M. F. (2014). Assistive technology for people with autism spectrum disorders. In *Assistive Technologies for People with Diverse Abilities* (pp. 157–190). Springer. doi:10.1007/978-1-4899-8029-8_6

Larsson-Lund, M., Kottorp, A., & Malinowsky, C. (2017). Return to work in people with acquired brain injury: Association with observed ability to use everyday technology. *Scandinavian Journal of Occupational Therapy*, *24*(4), 281–289. doi:10.1080/11038128.2016.1194466 PMID:27321247

Lattimore, L. P., Parsons, M. B., & Reid, D. H. (2008). Simulation Training of Community Job Skills for Adults with Autism: A Further Analysis. *Behavior Analysis in Practice*, *1*, 24–29.doi:https://doi.org/10.1007/BF03391717

Laufer, Y., & Weiss, P. L. (2011). Virtual reality in assessment and treatment of children with motor impairments: A systematic review. *Journal, Physical Therapy Education*, *25*(1), 59–71. doi:10.1097/00001416-201110000-00011

Lauriks, S., Reinersmann, A., Van der Roest, H. G., Meiland, F. J., Davies, R. J., Moelaert, F., Mulvenna, M. D., Nugent, C. D., & Dröes, R. M. (2007). Review of ICT-based services for identified unmet needs in people with dementia. *Ageing Research Reviews*, *6*(3), 223–246. doi:10.1016/j.arr.2007.07.002 PMID:17869590

Lau-Zhu, A., Lau, M. P. H., & McLoughlin, G. (2019). Mobile EEG in research on neurodevelopmental disorders: Opportunities and challenges. *Developmental Cognitive Neuroscience*, *36*, 100635. Advance online publication. doi:10.1016/j.dcn.2019.100635 PMID:30877927

Laver, K. E., Lange, B., George, S., Deutsch, J. E., Saposnik, G., & Crotty, M. (2017). Virtual reality for stroke rehabilitation. *Cochrane Database of Systematic Reviews*, *11*(11), 1–183. doi:10.1002/14651858.CD008349.pub4 PMID:29156493

Law, M., Darrah, J., Pollock, N., King, G., Rosenbaum, P., Russell, D., Palisano, R., Harris, S., Armstrong, R., & Watt, J. (1998). Family-centred functional therapy for children with cerebral palsy: An emerging practice model. *Physical & Occupational Therapy in Pediatrics*, *18*(1), 83–102. doi:10.1080/J006v18n01_06

Lawton, C. (1994). Gender differences in way-finding strategies: Relationship to spatial ability and spatial anxiety. *Sex Roles*, *30*(11), 765–779. doi:10.1007/BF01544230

Lawton, M. P., Van Haitsma, K., & Klapper, J. (1999). Observed Emotion Rating Scale. *Journal of Mental Health and Aging*, *5*(1), 69–81.

Lazarou, I., Parastatidis, T., Tsolaki, A., Gkioka, M., Karakostas, A., Douka, S., & Tsolaki, M. (2017). International ballroom dancing against neurodegeneration: A randomized controlled trial in Greek community-dwelling elders with mild cognitive impairment. *American Journal of Alzheimer's Disease and Other Dementias*, *32*(8), 489–499. doi:10.1177/1533317517725813 PMID:28840742

Lecouvey, G., Morand, A., Gonneaud, J., Pascale, P., Orriols, E., Pélerin, A., & ... . (2019). An Impairment of Prospective Memory in Mild Alzheimer's Disease: A Ride in a Virtual Town. *Frontiers in Psychology*, *10*(24), 1–12. doi:10.3389/fpsyg.2019.00241 PMID:30809174

Lee, E. A. L., Wong, K. W., & Fung, C. C. (2010). How does desktop virtual reality enhance learning outcomes? A structural equation modeling approach. *Computers & Education*, *55*(4), 1424–1442. doi:10.1016/j.compedu.2010.06.006

Lee, F. K. I., Lee, T. F. D., & So, W. K. W. (2016). Effects of a tailor-made exercise program on exercise adherence and health outcomes in patients with knee osteoarthritis: A mixed-methods pilot study. *Clinical Interventions in Aging*, *11*, 1391–1402. doi:10.2147/CIA.S111002 PMID:27785001

Lee, I. F. K., Yau, F. N., Yim, S. S. H., & Lee, D. T. F. (2018). Evaluating the impact of a home-based rehabilitation service on older people and their caregivers: A matched-control quasi-experimental study. *Clinical Interventions in Aging, 13*, 1727–1737. doi:10.2147/CIA.S172871 PMID:30254432

Lee, I.-J., Chen, C.-H., Wang, C.-P., & Chung, C.-H. (2018). Augmented Reality Plus Concept Map Technique to Teach Children with ASD to Use Social Cues When Meeting and Greeting. *The Asia-Pacific Education Researcher, 27*(3), 227–243. doi:10.100740299-018-0382-5

Lee, J. H., Kim, J. H., Jhoo, J. H., Lee, K. U., Kim, K. W., Lee, D. Y., & Woo, J. I. (2008). A telemedicine system as a care modality for dementia patients in Korea. *Alzheimer Disease and Associated Disorders, 14*(2), 94–101. doi:10.1097/00002093-200004000-00007 PMID:10850748

Lee, J., Kim, D., Ryoo, H., & Shin, B.-S. (2016). Sustainable wearables: Wearable technology for enhancing the quality of human life. *Sustainability (Switzerland), 8*(5), 466. Advance online publication. doi:10.3390u8050466

Lee, S. Y., Jeon, Y. T., Kim, B. R., & Han, E. Y. (2017). Combined treatment of botulinumtoxin and robot-assisted rehabilitation therapy on poststroke, upper limb spasticity. *Case Reports in Medicine, 96*(51), e9468.

Leonard, H., Fyfe, S., Leonard, S., & Msall, M. (2001). Functional status, medical impairments, and rehabilitation resources in 84 females with Rett syndrome: A snapshot across the world from the parental perspective. *Disability and Rehabilitation, 23*(3–4), 107–117. doi:10.1080/09638280150504180 PMID:11247006

Leon, D., Cortes, M., Elder, J., Kumru, H., Laxe, S., Edwards, D. J., Tormos, J. M., Bernabeu, M., & Pascual-Leone, A. (2017). tDCS does not enhance the effects of robot-assisted gait training in patients with subacute stroke. *Restorative Neurology and Neuroscience, 35*(4), 377–384.

Leuty, V., Boger, J., Young, L., Hoey, J., & Mihailidis, A. (2013). Engaging older adults with dementia in creative occupations using artificially intelligent assistive technology. *Assistive Technology, 25*(2), 72–79. doi:10.1080/10400435.2012.715113 PMID:23923689

Levac, D., Rivard, L., & Missiuna, C. (2012). Defining the active ingredients of interactive computer play interventions for children with neuromotor impairments: A scoping review. *Research in Developmental Disabilities, 33*(1), 214–223. doi:10.1016/j.ridd.2011.09.007 PMID:22093667

Leyzberg, D., Spaulding, S., Toneva, M., & Scassellati, B. (2012). The Physical Presence of a Robot Tutor Increases Cognitive Learning Gains. *Proceedings of the Annual Meeting of the Cognitive Science Society, 34*(34).

Li, R., Lu, B., & McDonald-Maier, K.D. (2015). Cognitive assisted living ambient system: a survey. *The Digital Competence Framework 2.0, 1*, 229-252.

Lieshout, E., van de Port, I. G., Dijkhuizen, R. M., & Visser-Meily, J. (2020). Does upper limb strength play a prominent role in health-related quality of life in stroke patients discharged from inpatient rehabilitation? *Topics in Stroke Rehabilitation, 27*(7), 525–533.

Lillo-Navarro, C., Medina-Mirapeix, F., Escolar-Reina, P., Montilla-Herrador, J., Gomez-Arnaldos, F., & Olivera-Sousa, S. L. (2015). Parents of children with physical disabilities perceive that characteristics of home exercise programs and physiotherapists' teaching styles influence adherence: A qualitative study. *Journal of Physiotherapy, 61*(2), 81–86. doi:10.1016/j.jphys.2015.02.014 PMID:25804826

Lim, J., Greenspoon, D., Hunt, A., & McAdam, L. (2020). Rehabilitation interventions in Rett syndrome: a scoping review. In Developmental Medicine and Child Neurology (Vol. 62, Issue 8, pp. 906–916). Blackwell Publishing Ltd. doi:10.1111/dmcn.14565

Lim, F. S., Wallace, T., Luszcz, M. A., & Reynolds, K. J. (2013). Usability of tablet computers by people with early-stage dementia. *Gerontology*, *59*(2), 174–182. doi:10.1159/000343986 PMID:23257664

Linkenauger, S. A., Bülthoff, H. H., & Mohler, B. J. (2015). Virtual arm′ s reach influences perceived distances but only after experience reaching. *Neuropsychologia*, *70*, 393–401. doi:10.1016/j.neuropsychologia.2014.10.034 PMID:25446965

Lipinska, B., & Backman, L. (1997). Encoding-retrieval interactions in mild Alzheimer's disease: The role of access to categorical information. *Brain and Cognition*, *34*(2), 274–286. doi:10.1006/brcg.1997.0916 PMID:9220090

Li, R., Lindholm, K., Yang, L. B., Yue, X., Citron, M., Yan, R., Beach, T., Sue, L., Sabbagh, M., Cai, H., Wong, P., Price, D., & Shen, Y. (2004). Amyloid beta peptide load is correlated with increased beta-secretase activity in sporadic Alzheimer's disease patients. *Proceedings of the National Academy of Sciences*, 101.

Li, S. (2017). Spasticity, Motor Recovery, and Neural Plasticity after Stroke. *Frontiers in Neurology*, *8*, 120.

Lithfous, S., Dufour, A., & Després, O. (2013). Spatial navigation in normal aging and the prodromal stage of Alzheimer's disease: Insights from imaging and behavioral studies. *Ageing Research Reviews*, *12*(1), 201–213. doi:10.1016/j.arr.2012.04.007 PMID:22771718

Liu, R., Salisbury, J. P., Vahabzadeh, A., & Sahin, N. T. (2017). Feasibility of an autism-focused augmented reality smart-glasses system for social communication and behavioral coaching. *Frontiers in Pediatrics*, *5*, 145. Advance online publication. doi:10.3389/fped.2017.00145 PMID:28695116

Loewenstein, D. A., Barker, W. W., Chang, J. Y., Apicella, A., Yoshii, F., Kothari, P., Levin, B., & Duara, R. (1989). Predominant left hemisphere metabolic dysfunction in dementia. *Archives of Neurology*, *46*(2), 146–152. doi:10.1001/archneur.1989.00520380046012 PMID:2783845

Loomes, R., Hull, L., & Mandy, W. (2017). What Is the Male-to-Female Ratio in Autism Spectrum Disorder? A Systematic Review and Meta-Analysis. *Journal of the American Academy of Child and Adolescent Psychiatry*, *56*(6), 466–474. https://doi.org/10.1016/j.jaac.2017.03.013

Lopes, S., Magalhães, P., Pereira, A., Martins, J., Magalhães, C., Chaleta, E., & Rosário, P. (2018). Games Used With Serious Purposes: A Systematic Review of Interventions in Patients With Cerebral Palsy. *Frontiers in Psychology*, *9*, 1712. doi:10.3389/fpsyg.2018.01712 PMID:30283377

López-Sastre, R. J., Baptista-Ríos, M., Acevedo-Rodríguez, F. J., Pacheco-Da-costa, S., Maldonado-Bascón, S., & Lafuente-Arroyo, S. (2021). A low-cost assistive robot for children with neurodevelopmental disorders to aid in daily living activities. *International Journal of Environmental Research and Public Health*, *18*(8), 3974. Advance online publication. doi:10.3390/ijerph18083974 PMID:33918839

LoPresti, E., Bodine, C., & Lewis, C. (2008). Assistive technology for cognition: Understanding the needs of persons with disabilities. *IEEE Engineering in Medicine and Biology Magazine*, *27*(2), 29–39. doi:10.1109/EMB.2007.907396 PMID:18463019

Lorah, E. R., Tincani, M., Dodge, J., Gilroy, S., Hickey, A., & Hantula, D. (2013). *Evaluating Picture Exchange and the iPad ™ as a Speech Generating Device to Teach Communication to Young Children with Autism.* doi:10.1007/s10882-013-9337-1

Lorah, E. R., Parnell, A., Schaefer Whitby, P., & Hantula, D. (2015). A systematic review of tablet computers and portable media players as speech generating devices for individuals with autism spectrum disorder. *Journal of Autism and Developmental Disorders*, *45*(12), 3792–3804. doi:10.100710803-014-2314-4

Lord, C., Brugha, T. S., Charman, T., Cusack, J., Dumas, G., Frazier, T., ... Taylor, J. L. (2020, January 16). Autism spectrum disorder. *Nature Reviews. Disease Primers*, *6*(5), 1–23. doi:10.103841572-019-0138-4 PMID:31949163

Lord, C., Rapley, T., Marcroft, C., Pearse, J., & Basu, A. (2018). Determinants of parent-delivered therapy interventions in children with cerebral palsy: A qualitative synthesis and checklist. *Child: Care, Health and Development*, *44*(5), 659–669. doi:10.1111/cch.12592 PMID:30033521

Lorish, C. D., Abraham, N., Austin, J., Bradley, L. A., & Alarcon, G. S. (1991). Disease and psychosocial factors related to physical functioning in rheumatoid arthritis. *The Journal of Rheumatology*, *18*(8), 1150–1157. PMID:1834844

Lorusso, M. L., Giorgetti, M., Travellini, S., Greci, L., Zangiacomi, A., Mondellini, M., Sacco, M., & Reni, G. (2018). Giok the Alien: An AR-Based Integrated System for the Empowerment of Problem-Solving, Pragmatic, and Social Skills in Pre-School Children. In Sensors (Vol. 18, Issue 7). doi:10.339018072368

Lotan, M. (2006). Management of Rett Syndrome in the Controlled Multisensory (Snoezelen) Environment. A Review with Three Case Stories. *The Scientific World Journal*, *6*, 791–807. doi:10.1100/tsw.2006.159 PMID:16830051

Lotan, M., Schenker, R., Wine, J., & Downs, J. (2012). The conductive environment enhances gross motor function of girls with Rett syndrome. A pilot study. *Developmental Neurorehabilitation*, *15*(1), 19–25. doi:10.3109/17518423.2011.629374 PMID:22256830

Lubinski, D. (2010). Spatial ability and STEM: A sleeping giant for talent identification and development. *Personality and Individual Differences*, *49*(4), 344–351. doi:10.1016/j.paid.2010.03.022

Lumbreras, M. A. M., de Lourdes, M.-T. M., & Ariel, S.-R. (2018). Aura: Augmented Reality in Mobile Devices for the Learning of Children With ASD – Augmented Reality in the Learning of Children With Autism. In G. R. Ruiz & M. H. Hernández (Eds.), *Augmented Reality for Enhanced Learning Environments* (pp. 142–169). IGI Global. doi:10.4018/978-1-5225-5243-7.ch006

LuxAI. (n.d.). https://luxai.com/blog/robot-for-autism-hardware-design/

Macdonald, R., Clark, M., Garrigan, E., & Vangala, M. (2005). Using video modeling to teach pretend play to children with autism. *Behavioral Interventions*, *20*(4), 225–238. doi:10.1002/bin.197

MacDuff, G. S., Krantz, P. J., & McClannahan, L. E. (1993). Teaching Children With Autism To Use Photographic Activity Schedules: Maintenance and Generalization of Complex Response Chains. *Journal of Applied Behavior Analysis*, *26*(1), 89–97. doi:10.1901/jaba.1993.26-89 PMID:8473261

Macedo, L. G., Elkins, M. R., Maher, C. G., Moseley, A. M., Herbert, R. D., & Sherrington, C. (2010). There was evidence of convergent and construct validity of Physiotherapy Evidence Database quality scale for physiotherapy trials. *Journal of Clinical Epidemiology*, *63*(8), 920–925. doi:10.1016/j.jclinepi.2009.10.005 PMID:20171839

Maenner, M. J., Yeargin-Allsopp, M., Van Naarden Braun, K., Christensen, D. L., & Schieve, L. A. (2016). Development of a Machine Learning Algorithm for the Surveillance of Autism Spectrum Disorder. *PLoS One*, *11*(12), e0168224. doi:10.1371/journal.pone.0168224

Maes, B., Lambrechts, G., Hostyn, I., & Petry, K. (2007). Quality-enhancing interventions for people with profound intellectual and multiple disabilities: A review of the empirical research literature. *Journal of Intellectual & Developmental Disability*, *32*(3), 163–178. doi:10.1080/13668250701549427 PMID:17885894

Ma, H.-H. (2009). The effectiveness of intervention on the behavior of individuals with autism: A meta-analysis using percentage of data points exceeding the median of baseline phase (PEM). *Behavior Modification*, *33*(3), 339–359. doi:10.1177/0145445509333173 PMID:19282505

Maher, C. A., Williams, M. T., & Olds, T. S. (2008). The six-minute walk test for children with cerebral palsy. *International Journal of Rehabilitation Research. Internationale Zeitschrift fur Rehabilitationsforschung. Revue Internationale de Recherches de Readaptation*, *31*(2), 185–188. doi:10.1097/MRR.0b013e32830150f9 PMID:18467936

Maier, M., Ballester, B. R., & Verschure, P. (2019). Principles of Neurorehabilitation After Stroke Based on Motor Learning and Brain Plasticity Mechanisms. *Frontiers in Systems Neuroscience*, *13*, 74.

Mailloux, Z., May-Benson, T. A., Summers, C. A., Miller, L. J., Brett-Green, B., Burke, J. P., Cohn, E. S., Koomar, J. A., Parham, L. D., Roley, S. S., Schaaf, R. C., & Schoen, S. A. (2007). Goal attainment scaling as a measure of meaningful outcomes for children with sensory integration disorders. *The American Journal of Occupational Therapy*, *61*(2), 254–259. doi:10.5014/ajot.61.2.254 PMID:17436848

Makransky, G., Terkildsen, T. S., & Mayer, R. E. (2019). Adding immersive virtual reality to a science lab simulation causes more presence but less learning. *Learning and Instruction*, *60*, 225–236. doi:10.1016/j.learninstruc.2017.12.007

Mancioppi, G., Fiorini, L., Timpano Sportiello, M., & Cavallo, F. (2019). Novel technological solutions for assessment, treatment, and assistance in mild cognitive impairment. *Frontiers in Neuroinformatics*, *13*, 58. Advance online publication. doi:10.3389/fninf.2019.00058 PMID:31456679

Man, D. W., Chung, J. C., & Lee, G. Y. (2012). Evaluation of a virtual reality-based memory training programme for Hong Kong Chinese older adults with questionable dementia: A pilot study. *International Journal of Geriatric Psychiatry*, *27*(5), 513–520. doi:10.1002/gps.2746 PMID:21681818

Manera, V., Chapoulie, E., Bourgeois, J., Guerchouche, R., David, R., Ondre, J., & … . (2016). A Feasibility Study with Image-Based Rendered Virtual Reality in Patients with Mild Cognitive Impairment and Dementia. *PLoS One*, *11*(3), 1–14. doi:10.1371/journal.pone.0151487 PMID:26990298

Manera, V., Petit, P. D., Derreumaux, A., Orvieto, I., Romagnoli, M., Lyttle, G., David, R., & Robert, P. H. (2015). 'Kitchen and cooking,' a serious game for mild cognitive impairment and Alzheimer's disease: A pilot study. *Frontiers in Aging Neuroscience*, *7*, 24. doi:10.3389/fnagi.2015.00024 PMID:25852542

Mani, S., Sharma, S., Omar, B., Paungmali, A., & Joseph, L. (2017). Validity and reliability of Internet-based physiotherapy assessment for musculoskeletal disorders: A systematic review. *Journal of Telemedicine and Telecare*, *23*(3), 379–391. doi:10.1177/1357633X16642369 PMID:27036879

Manoli, D. S., & State, M. W. (2021). Autism Spectrum Disorder Genetics and the Search for Pathological Mechanisms. *The American Journal of Psychiatry*, *178*(1), 30–38. doi:10.1176/appi.ajp.2020.20111608 PMID:33384012

Mansouri-Benssassi, E., Gomez, J. C., Boyd, L. E., Hayes, G. R., & Ye, J. (2018). Wearable assistive technologies for autism: Opportunities and challenges. *IEEE Pervasive Computing*, *17*(2), 11–21. doi:10.1109/MPRV.2018.022511239

Manta, O., Androutsou, T., Anastasiou, A., Koumpouros, Y., Matsopoulos, G., & Koutsouris, D. (2020). Innovative technological advancements to improve cognitive and social skills of students with neurodevelopmental disorders. *Technology and Disability*, *32*(4), 243–253. doi:10.3233/TAD-200288

Mantovani, E., Zucchella, C., Bottiroli, S., Federico, A., Giugno, R., Sandrini, G., Chiamulera, C., & Tamburin, S. (2020). Telemedicine and virtual reality for cognitive rehabilitation: A roadmap for the COVID-19 pandemic. *Frontiers in Neurology*, *11*, 926. Advance online publication. doi:10.3389/fneur.2020.00926 PMID:33041963

Maresova, P., Tomsone, S., Lameski, P., Madureira, J., Mendes, A., Zdravevski, E., Chorbev, I., Trajkovik, V., Ellen, M., & Rodile, K. (2018). Technological Solutions for Older People with Alzheimer's Disease [Review]. *Current Alzheimer Research*, *15*(10), 975–983. doi:10.2174/1567205015666180427124547 PMID:29701154

Margari, L., Craig, F., Margari, F., Legrottaglie, A., Palumbi, R., & De Giambattista, C. (2016). A review of executive function deficits in autism spectrum disorder and attention-deficit/hyperactivity disorder. *Neuropsychiatric Disease and Treatment, 12*, 1191. doi:10.2147/NDT.S104620 PMID:27274255

Martino Cinnera, A., Bonnì, S., Pellicciari, M. C., Giorgi, F., Caltagirone, C., & Koch, G. (2020). Health-related quality of life (HRQoL) after stroke: Positive relationship between lower extremity and balance recovery. *Topics in Stroke Rehabilitation, 27*(7), 534–540.

Martino Cinnera, A., Pucello, A., Lupo, A., Gimigliano, F., Mammucari, E., Cicero, D. L., Iosa, M., Paolucci, S., & Morone, G. (2019). Upper limb motor improvement in chronic stroke after combining botulinum toxin A injection and multi-joints robot-assisted therapy: A case report. *Oxford Medical Case Reports, 2019*(10), omz097.

Marz, K., Eisenberg, G., Diener, P., Amadio, G., Foreman, M. H., & Engsberg, J. R. (2016). The effects of virtual reality on the upper extremity skills of girls with Rett syndrome: A single case study. *Journal of Intellectual Disability - Diagnosis and Treatment, 4,* 152-159.

Maskey, M., Lowry, J., Rodgers, J., McConachie, H., & Parr, J. R. (2014). Reducing specific phobia/fear in young people with autism spectrum disorders (ASDs) through a virtual reality environment intervention. *PLoS One, 9*(7).https://doi.org/10.1371/journal.pone.0100374

Maskey, M., Rodgers, J., Grahame, V., Glod, M., Honey, E., Kinnear, J., ... Parr, J. R. (2019). A Randomised Controlled Feasibility Trial of Immersive Virtual Reality Treatment with Cognitive Behaviour Therapy for Specific Phobias in Young People with Autism Spectrum Disorder. *Journal of Autism and Developmental Disorders, 49*(5), 1912–1927. doi:https://doi.org/10.1007/s10803-018-3861-x

Mason, R. A., Ganz, J. B., Parker, R. I., Burke, M. D., & Camargo, S. P. (2012). Moderating factors of video-modeling with other as model: A meta-analysis of single-case studies. *Research in Developmental Disabilities, 33*(4), 1076–1086. doi:10.1016/j.ridd.2012.01.016 PMID:22502832

Matamala-Gomez, M., Bottiroli, S., Realdon, O., Riva, G., Galvagni, L., Platz, T., Sandrini, G., De Icco, R., & Tassorelli, C. (2021). Telemedicine and virtual reality at time of COVID-19 pandemic: An overview for future perspectives in neurorehabilitation. *Frontiers in Neurology, 12*, 646902. Advance online publication. doi:10.3389/fneur.2021.646902 PMID:33841313

Matamala-Gomez, M., Donegan, T., Bottiroli, S., Sandrini, G., Sanchez-Vives, M. V., & Tassorelli, C. (2019). Immersive virtual reality and virtual embodiment for pain relief. *Frontiers in Human Neuroscience, 13*, 279. Advance online publication. doi:10.3389/fnhum.2019.00279 PMID:31551731

Matthews, K. A., Xu, W., Gaglioti, A. H., Holt, J. B., Croft, J. B., Mack, D., & McGuire, L. C. (2019). Racial and ethnic estimates of Alzheimer's disease and related dementias in the United States (2015-2060) in adults aged ³65 years. *Alzheimer's & Dementia, 15*(1), 17–24. doi:10.1016/j.jalz.2018.06.3063 PMID:30243772

Mayes, S. D., Calhoun, S. L., Aggarwal, R., Baker, C., Mathapati, S., Molitoris, S., & Mayes, R. D. (2013). Unusual fears in children with autism. *Research in Autism Spectrum Disorders, 7*, 151–158.doi:https://doi.org/10.1016/j.rasd.2012.08.002

Mazuryk, T., & Gervautz, M. (1992). *Virtual Reality. History, Applications, Technology and Future.* Institute of Computer Graphics. Technical University of Vienna. Technical Report TR-186-2-96-06.

Mazuryk, T., & Gervautz, M. (1996). *Virtual reality-history, applications, technology and future.* Academic Press.

Mazzoleni, S., Duret, C., Grosmaire, A. G., & Battini, E. (2017). Combining Upper Limb Robotic Rehabilitation with Other Therapeutic Approaches after Stroke: Current Status, Rationale, and Challenges. *BioMed Research International, 2017*, 8905637.

McCarron, H., Zmora, R., & Gaugler, J.E. (n.d.). A Web-Based Mobile App With a Smartwatch to Support Social Engagement in Persons With Memory Loss: Pilot Randomized Controlled Trial. *JIMIR Aging, 2*, 1-15.

McMurray, K. R. (2016). *A comparison of two types of augmentative and alternative communication systems (iPad and PECS) for children with autism spectrum disorder: The benefits of integrating assistive technology into the ASD classroom* (Doctoral dissertation). Fullerton, CA: California State University.

McMurray, K., & Pierson, M. R. (2016). The importance of assistive technology in the classroom for males and females with autism spectrum disorder. *Journal of Gender and Power*, *5*(1), 59–78.

McNaughton, B. L., Battaglia, F. P., Jensen, O., Moser, E. I., & Moser, M. B. (2006). Path integration and the neural basis of the "cognitive map.". *Nature Reviews. Neuroscience*, *7*(8), 663–678. doi:10.1038/nrn1932 PMID:16858394

Mechling, L. C., Gast, D. L., & Seid, N. H. (2010). Evaluation of a personal digital assistant as a self-prompting device for increasing multi-step task completion by students with moderate intellectual disabilities. *Education and Training in Autism and Developmental Disabilities*, 422–439.

Medina-Mirapeix, F., Lillo-Navarro, C., Montilla-Herrador, J., Gacto-Sánchez, M., Franco-Sierra, M., & Escolar-Reina, P. (2017). Predictors of parents' adherence to home exercise programs for children with developmental disabilities, regarding both exercise frequency and duration: A survey design. *European Journal of Physical and Rehabilitation Medicine*, *53*(4), 545–555. doi:10.23736/S1973-9087.17.04464-1 PMID:28466627

Mehrholz, J., Platz, T., Kugler, J., & Pohl, M. (2008). Electromechanical and robot-assisted arm training for improving arm function and activities of daily living after stroke. *Cochrane Database of Systematic Reviews*, (4), CD006876.

Mehrholz, J., Pohl, M., Platz, T., Kugler, J., & Elsner, B. (2018). Electromechanical and robot-assisted arm training for improving activities of daily living, arm function, and arm muscle strength after stroke. *Cochrane Database of Systematic Reviews*, *9*(9), CD006876.

Mehrholz, J., Thomas, S., Kugler, J., Pohl, M., & Elsner, B. (2020). Electromechanical-assisted training for walking after stroke. *Cochrane Database of Systematic Reviews*, *10*(10), CD006185.

Meiland, F. (2007). COGKNOW: Development of an ICT device to support people with dementia. *The Journal on Information Technology in Healthcare*, *5*, 324–334.

Melander, C., Martinsson, J., & Gustafsson, S. (2017). Measuring electrodermal activity to improve the identification of agitation in individuals with dementia. *Dementia and Geriatric Cognitive Disorders*, *7*(3), 430–409. doi:10.1159/000484890 PMID:29430245

Mendes, L. A., Lima, I. N., Souza, T., do Nascimento, G. C., Resqueti, V. R., & Fregonezi, G. A. (2020). Motor neuroprosthesis for promoting recovery of function after stroke. *Cochrane Database of Systematic Reviews*, *2020*(1), 1. doi:10.1002/14651858.CD012991.pub2

Merrill, D. R., Bikson, M., & Jefferys, J. G. (2005). Electrical stimulation of excitable tissue: Design of efficacious and safe protocols. *Journal of Neuroscience Methods*, *141*(2), 171–198.

Mesa-Gresa, P., Gil-Gómez, H., Lozano-Quilis, J., & Gil-Gómez, J.-A. (2018). Effectiveness of virtual reality for children and adolescents with autism spectrum disorder: An evidence-based systematic review. *Sensors (Switzerland)*, *18*(8), 2486. Advance online publication. doi:10.339018082486 PMID:30071588

Metzler-Baddeley, C., & Snowden, J. S. (2005). Brief report: Errorless versus errorful learning as a memory rehabilitation approach in Alzheimer's Disease. *Journal of Clinical and Experimental Neuropsychology*, *27*(8), 1070–1079. doi:10.1080/13803390490919164 PMID:16207625

Milgram, P., & Kishino, F. (1994). A taxonomy of mixed reality visual displays. *IEICE Transactions on Information and Systems*, *77*(12), 1321–1329.

Millán-Calenti, J. C., Tubío, J., Pita-Fernández, S., Rochette, S., Lorenzo, T., & Maseda, A. (2012). Cognitive impairment as predictor of functional dependence in an elderly sample. *Archives of Gerontology and Geriatrics*, *54*(1), 197–201. doi:10.1016/j.archger.2011.02.010 PMID:21397345

Mira, M. (1992). Book Review: Autism and Asperger syndrome. *Focus on Autistic Behavior*, *7*(3), 13–15. doi:10.1177/108835769200700302

Mirelman, A., Rochester, L., Maidan, I., Del Din, S., Alcock, L., Nieuwhof, F., Rikkert, M. O., Bloem, B. R., Pelosin, E., Avanzino, L., Abbruzzese, G., Dockx, K., Bekkers, E., Giladi, N., Nieuwboer, A., & Hausdorff, J. M. (2016). Addition of a non-immersive virtual reality component to treadmill training to reduce fall risk in older adults (V-TIME): A randomised controlled trial. *Lancet*, *388*(10050), 1170–1182.

Mirenda, P. (2001). Autism, augmentative communication, and assistive technology what do we really know? *Focus on Autism and Other Developmental Disabilities*, *16*(3), 141–151. http://foa.sagepub.com/content/16/3/141.short. doi:10.1177/108835760101600302

Miskelly, F. (2005). Tracciamento elettronico di pazienti con demenza e vagabondi utilizzando la tecnologia dei telefoni cellulari. *Age and Ageing*, *34*, 497–499. doi:10.1093/ageing/afi145 PMID:16107453

Mitchell, L. C., Engleman, M., & Linden, M. T. (2012). *The effectiveness of assistive technology (TAP-it® and VizZle®) to enhance progress of young children with autism spectrum disorders*. Retrieved from https://www.teachsmart.org/pdf/the-effectiveness-of-assistive-technology-to-enhance-progress-of-young-children-with-autism-spectrum-disorders.pdf

Moè, A. (2009). Are males always better than females in mental rotation? Exploring a gender belief explanation. *Learning and Individual Differences*, *19*(1), 21–27. doi:10.1016/j.lindif.2008.02.002

Mokashi, S., Yarosh, S., & Abowd, G. D. (2013). Exploration of videochat for children with autism. In IIDC '13: Proceedings of the 12th International Conference on Interaction Design and Children. Association for Computing Machinery. https://doi.org/10.1145/2485760.2485839.

Moktar, M. N., Fikry, A., Musa, R., Hassan, H., Ahmad, S. S., Ismail, Z., ... Hashim, R. (2014, December). Extending cultural model of assistive technology design for autism treatment. In *International Symposium on Robotics and Manufacturing Automation (ROMA)* (pp. 172-175). Kuala Lumpur: IEEE. 10.1109/ROMA.2014.7295882

Mold, M., Umar, D., King, A., & Exley, C. (2018). Aluminium in brain tissue in autism. *Journal of Trace Elements in Medicine and Biology*, *46*, 76–82. doi:10.1016/j.jtemb.2017.11.012 PMID:29413113

Molina-Carmona, R., Pertegal-Felices, M. L., Jimeno-Morenilla, A., & Mora-Mora, H. (2018). Virtual reality learning activities for multimedia students to enhance spatial ability. *Sustainability*, *10*(4), 1074. doi:10.3390u10041074

Molteni, F., Gasperini, G., Cannaviello, G., & Guanziroli, E. (2018). Exoskeleton and End-Effector Robots for Upper and Lower Limbs Rehabilitation: Narrative Review. *PM & R*, *10*(9, Suppl 2), S174–S188.

Monacelli, A. M., Cushman, L. A., Kavcic, V., & Duffy, C. J. (2003). Spatial disorientation in Alzheimer's disease: The remembrance of things passed. *Neurology*, *61*(11), 1491–1497. doi:10.1212/WNL.61.11.1491 PMID:14663030

Mondini, V., Kobler, R. J., Sburlea, A. I., & Müller-Putz, G. R. (2020). Continuous low-frequency EEG decoding of arm movement for closed-loop, natural control of a robotic arm. *Journal of Neural Engineering*, *17*(4), 046031.

Monfaredi, R., Fooladi, H., Tabrizi, P. R., Kovelman, S., Salvador, T., Coley, C., . . . Evans, S. (2018). *PedBot: Robotically assisted ankle robot and video game for children with neuromuscular disorders*. Paper presented at the SPIE Medical Imaging Conference. 10.1117/12.2295031

Moorcroft, A., Scarinci, N., & Meyer, C. (2018). A systematic review of the barriers and facilitators to the provision and use of low-tech and unaided AAC systems for people with complex communication needs and their families. *Disability and Rehabilitation. Assistive Technology*, *0*(0), 1–22. doi:10.1080/17483107.2018.1499135 PMID:30070927

Moore, D., Cheng, Y., McGrath, P., & Powell, N. (2005). Avatars and Autism, Assistive Technologies. In A. Pruski & H. Knops (Eds.), *Virtuality to Reality* (pp. 442–448). IOS Press.

Moreau, N. G., Bodkin, A. W., Bjornson, K., Hobbs, A., Soileau, M., & Lahasky, K. (2016). Effectiveness of rehabilitation interventions to improve gait speed in children with cerebral palsy: Systematic review and meta-analysis. *Physical Therapy*, *96*(12), 1938–1954. doi:10.2522/ptj.20150401 PMID:27313240

Morganti, F., Stefanini, S., & Riva, G. (2015). From allo- to egocentric spatial ability in early Alzheimer's disease: A study with virtual reality spatial tasks. *Cognitive Neuroscience*, *4*(4), 171–180. doi:10.1080/17588928.2013.854762 PMID:24251605

Morone, G., Palomba, A., Martino Cinnera, A., Agostini, M., Aprile, I., Arienti, C., Paci, M., Casanova, E., Marino, D., & Rosa, L. A. (2021). Systematic review of guidelines to identify recommendations for upper limb robotic rehabilitation after stroke. *European Journal of Physical and Rehabilitation Medicine, 57*(2), 238–245.

Morone, G., Cocchi, I., Paolucci, S., & Iosa, M. (2020). Robot-assisted therapy for arm recovery for stroke patients: State of the art and clinical implication. *Expert Review of Medical Devices*, *17*(3), 223–233.

Morone, G., Masiero, S., Werner, C., & Paolucci, S. (2014). Advances in neuromotor stroke rehabilitation. *BioMed Research International*, *2014*, 236043.

Morone, G., Paolucci, S., Cherubini, A., De Angelis, D., Venturiero, V., Coiro, P., & Iosa, M. (2017). Robot-assisted gait training for stroke patients: Current state of the art and perspectives of robotics. *Neuropsychiatric Disease and Treatment*, *13*, 1303–1311.

Morone, G., Spitoni, G. F., De Bartolo, D., Ghanbari Ghooshchy, S., Di Iulio, F., Paolucci, S., Zoccolotti, P., & Iosa, M. (2019). Rehabilitative devices for a top-down approach. *Expert Review of Medical Devices*, *16*(3), 187–195.

Morris, M., Lundell, J., & Dishman, E. (2004). Catalyzing social interaction with ubiquitous computing: a needs assessment of elders coping with cognitive decline. *Human Factors in Computing Systems*, 5-6.

Morrison, K. E., Pinkham, A. E., Kelsven, S., Ludwig, K., Penn, D. L., & Sasson, N. J. (2019). Psychometric Evaluation of Social Cognitive Measures for Adults with Autism. *Autism Research: Official Journal of the International Society for Autism Research, 12*(5), 766–778. doi:10.1002/aur.2084

Morrison, R. S., Sainato, D. M., Benchaaban, D., & Endo, S. (2002). Increasing play skills of children with autism using activity schedules and correspondence training. *Journal of Early Intervention*, *25*(1), 58–72. doi:10.1177/105381510202500106

Moxley-Haegert, L., & Serbin, L. A. (1983). Developmental education for parents of delayed infants: Effects on parental motivation and children's development. *Child Development*, *54*(5), 1324–1331. doi:10.2307/1129685 PMID:6194944

Moyle, W., Jones, C., Dwan, T., & Petrovich, T. (2016). Effectiveness of a Virtual Reality Forest on People With Dementia: A Mixed Methods Pilot Study. *The Gerontologist*, *58*(3), 478–487. doi:10.1093/geront/gnw270 PMID:28329867

Mubin, O., Alnajjar, F., Jishtu, N., Alsinglawi, B., & Al Mahmud, A. (2019). Exoskeletons With Virtual Reality, Augmented Reality, and Gamification for Stroke Patients' Rehabilitation: Systematic Review. *JMIR Rehabilitation and Assistive Technologies, 6*(2), e12010.

Muhle, R., Trentacoste, S. V., & Rapin, I. (2004). The genetics of autism. *Pediatrics, 113*(5), e472–e486. doi:10.1542/peds.113.5.e472 PMID:15121991

Mullen, N. W., Weaver, B., Riendeau, J. A., Morrison, L. E., & Bédard, M. (2010). Driving performance and susceptibility to simulator sickness: Are they related? *The American Journal of Occupational Therapy, 64*(2), 288–295. doi:10.5014/ajot.64.2.288 PMID:20437916

Murphy, T. H., & Corbett, D. (2009). Plasticity during stroke recovery: From synapse to behaviour. *Nature Reviews. Neuroscience, 10*(12), 861–872.

Nakken, H., & Vlaskamp, C. (2007). A Need for a Taxonomy for Profound Intellectual and Multiple Disabilities. *Journal of Policy and Practice in Intellectual Disabilities, 4*(2), 83–87. doi:10.1111/j.1741-1130.2007.00104.x

National Health Service Conditions. (2019). *Foot drop.* NHS. https://www.nhs.uk/conditions/foot-drop/

National Institute for Health and Care Excellence (NICE). (2013). *Overview | Stroke rehabilitation in adults | Guidance | NICE.* https://www.nice.org.uk/guidance/cg162

National Research Council. (2001). *Educating children with autism.* National Academies Press.

Navarro, D., & Sundstedt, V. (2020). Biofeedback Methods in Entertainment Games and Virtual Reality: A Review of Physiological Interaction Techniques. *ACM Computing Surveys.*

Neul, J. L., Kaufmann, W. E., Glaze, D. G., Christodoulou, J., Clarke, A. J., Bahi-Buisson, N., ... Percy, A. K. (2010). Rett syndrome: Revised diagnostic criteria and nomenclature. *Annals of Neurology, 68*(6), 944–950. doi:10.1002/ana.22124 PMID:21154482

Neven, A., Janssens, D., Alders, G., Wets, G., Wijmeersch, B. V., & Feys, P. (2013). Documenting outdoor activity and travel behaviour in persons with neurological conditions using travel diaries and GPS tracking technology: A pilot study in multiple sclerosis. *Disability and Rehabilitation, 35*(20), 1718–1725. doi:10.3109/09638288.2012.751137 PMID:23343357

Neville, R. D., Draper, C. E., Cooper, T. J., Abdullah, M. M., & Lakes, K. D. (2021). Association between engagement in physical activity and adaptive behavior in young children with autism spectrum disorder. *Mental Health and Physical Activity, 20*, 100389. Advance online publication. doi:10.1016/j.mhpa.2021.100389

Newell, A. F., Carmichael, A., Gregor, P., & Alm, N. (2007). *Information technology for the cognitive support.* Lawrence Erlbaum Associates.

NICE. (2016). *Overview | ODFS Pace and Pace XL functional electrical stimulation devices for treating drop foot | Advice | NICE.* https://www.nice.org.uk/advice/MIB56

NICE. (2021). *Stroke - NICE Pathways.* National Institute for Health and Care Excellence. https://pathways.nice.org.uk/pathways/stroke

Nijhof, N., Van Hoof, J., Van Rijn, H., & Van Gemert-Pijnen, J. E. (2013). The behavioral outcomes of a technology-supported leisure activity in people with dementia. *Technology and Disability, 25*(4), 263–273. doi:10.3233/TAD-140398

Nikopoulos, C. K., & Keenan, M. (2004). Effects of Video Modelling on Training and Generalisation of Social Initiation and Reciprocal Play by Children With Autism. *European Journal of Behavior Analysis, 5*(1), 1–13. doi:10.1080/15021149.2004.11434227

Nikopoulos, C. K., & Keenan, M. (2007). Using Video Modeling to Teach Complex Social Sequences to Children with Autism. *Journal of Autism and Developmental Disorders*, *37*(4), 678–693. doi:10.100710803-006-0195-x PMID:16897375

Nikopoulou-Smyrni, P., Halder, S., Mackeogh, T., & Dillenburger, K. (2012). *Registration for a Systematic Review: Electronic Assistive Technology for Improving Social and Behavioral Outcomes for Individuals with Autism Spectrum Disorder (ASD).* Retrieved from Campbell Systematic Reviews: https://www.campbellcollaboration.org/lib/project/248/

Nind, M., & Hewett, D. (1988). Interaction as curriculum. *British Journal of Special Education*, *15*(2), 55–57. doi:10.1111/j.1467-8578.1988.tb00314.x

Nind, M., & Hewett, D. (2012). *Access to communication: Developing the basics of communication with people with severe learning difficulties through intensive interaction.* Routledge. doi:10.4324/9780203462409

Nind, M., & Thomas, G. (2005). Reinstating the value of teachers' tacit knowledge for the benefit of learners: Using 'intensive interaction'. *Journal of Research in Special Educational Needs*, *5*(3), 97–100. doi:10.1111/j.1471-3802.2005.00048.x

Noel, J., Lakshminarasimhan, K. J., Park, H., & Angelaki, D. E. (2020). Increased variability but intact integration during visual navigation in autism spectrum disorder. *Proceedings of the National Academy of Sciences of the United States of America*, *117*(20), 11158-11166. 10.1073/pnas.2000216117

Noriega, D. B., & Savelkoul, H. F. J. (2014). Immune dysregulation in autism spectrum disorder. *European Journal of Pediatrics*, *173*(1), 33–43. doi:10.100700431-013-2183-4 PMID:24297668

Norman, J. M., Collins, B. C., & Schuster, J. W. (2001). Using an instructional package including video technology to teach self-help skills to elementary students with mental disabilities. *Journal of Special Education Technology*, *16*(3), 5–18. doi:10.1177/016264340101600301

Novak, I. (2014). Evidence-based diagnosis, health care, and rehabilitation for children with cerebral palsy. Journal of child neurology. *Journal of Child Neurology*, *29*(8), 1141–1156. doi:10.1177/0883073814535503 PMID:24958005

Novak, I., Morgan, C., Adde, L., Brunstrom-Hernandez, J., Blackman, J., Boyd, R. N., & Badawi, N. (2017). *Early Detection and Diagnosis of Cerebral Palsy and "High-Risk of Cerebral Palsy" International Clinical Practice Guideline.* Academic Press.

Nudo, R. J. (2013). Recovery after brain injury: Mechanisms and principles. *Frontiers in Human Neuroscience*, *7*, 887. doi:10.3389/fnhum.2013.00887 PMID:24399951

Nudo, R. J., & Friel, K. M. (1999). Cortical plasticity after stroke: Implications for rehabilitation. *Revue Neurologique*, *155*(9), 713–717.

O'Brolcháin, F., & Gordijn, B. (2017, January). Risks of Stigmatisation Resulting from Assistive Technologies for People with Autism Spectrum Disorder. *Studies in Health Technology and Informatics*, *242*, 265–268. PMID:28873808

O'Brolcháin, F., & Gordijn, B. (2018). Risks of stigmatisation resulting from assistive technologies for persons with autism spectrum disorder. *Technologies*, *6*(1), 27. Advance online publication. doi:10.3390/technologies6010027

O'Brolcháin, F., & Gordijn, B. (2020). Responsibility-enhancing assistive technologies and people with autism. *Cambridge Quarterly of Healthcare Ethics*, *29*(4), 607–616. doi:10.1017/S0963180120000353 PMID:32892779

O'Connor, K. (2012). Auditory processing in autism spectrum disorder: a review. *Elsevier, 36*, 836-854. doi:10.1016/j.neubiorev.2011.11.008

O'Malley, P., Lewis, M. E., Donehower, C., & Stone, D. (2014). Effectiveness of Using iPads to Increase Academic Task Completion by Students with Autism. *Universal Journal of Educational Research*, *2*(1), 90–97. doi:10.13189/ujer.2014.020111

O'Neill, B., Best, C., O'Neill, L., Ramos, S. D. S., & Gillespie, A. (2018). Efficacy of a Micro-Prompting Technology in Reducing Support Needed by People With Severe Acquired Brain Injury in Activities of Daily Living: A Randomized Control Trial. *The Journal of Head Trauma Rehabilitation*, *33*(5), E33–E41. doi:10.1097/HTR.0000000000000358 PMID:29194177

O'Neill, S. J., Smyth, S., Smeaton, A., & O'Connor, N. E. (2020). Assistive technology: Understanding the needs and experiences of individuals with autism spectrum disorder and/or intellectual disability in Ireland and the UK. *Assistive Technology*, *32*(5), 251–259. doi:10.1080/10400435.2018.1535526 PMID:30668926

O'Neil, M. E., Fragala-Pinkham, M. A., Westcott, S. L., Martin, K., Chiarello, L. A., Valvano, J., & Rose, R. U. (2006). Physical therapy clinical management recommendations for children with cerebral palsy - spastic diplegia: Achieving functional mobility outcomes. *Pediatric Physical Therapy*, *18*(1), 49–72. doi:10.1097/01.pep.0000202099.01653.a9

O'Reilly, M. F., Renzaglia, A., Hutchins, M., Koterba-Buss, L., Clayton, M., Halle, J. W., & Izen, C. (1992). Teaching systematic instruction competencies to special education student teachers: An applied behavioral supervision model. *Research and Practice for Persons with Severe Disabilities*, *17*, 104–111.

Obeid, R., Brooks, P. J., Powers, K. L., Gillespie-lynch, K., & Lum, J. A. G. (2016). Statistical Learning in Specific Language Impairment and Autism Spectrum Disorder : A Meta-Analysis. *Frontiers in Psychology*, *7*, 1–18. doi:10.3389/fpsyg.2016.01245 PMID:27602006

Oksnebjerg, L., Woods, B., & Waldemar, G. (2019). Designing the ReACT app to support self-management of people with dementia: An iterative user-involving process. *Gerontology*, *65*(6), 673–685. doi:10.1159/000500445 PMID:31266031

Oliver, M., Montero, F., Fernández-Caballero, A., González, P., & Molina, J. P. (2015). RGB-D assistive technologies for acquired brain injury: Description and assessment of user experience. *Expert Systems: International Journal of Knowledge Engineering and Neural Networks*, *32*(3), 370–380. doi:10.1111/exsy.12096

Olsson, A., Persson, A.-C., Bartfai, A., & Boman, I.-L. (2017). Sensor technology more than a support. *Scandinavian Journal of Occupational Therapy*, *25*(2), 1–9. doi:10.1080/11038128.2017.1293155 PMID:28276963

Optale, G., Urgesi, C., Busato, V., Marin, S., Piron, L., Priftis, K., Gamberini, L., Capodieci, S., & Bordin, A. (2010). Controlling memory impairment in elderly adults using virtual reality memory training: A randomized controlled pilot study. *Neurorehabilitation and Neural Repair*, *24*(4), 348–357. doi:10.1177/1545968309353328 PMID:19934445

Oskoui, M., Coutinho, F., Dykeman, J., Jetté, N., & Pringsheim, T. (2013). An update on the prevalence of cerebral palsy: A systematic review and meta-analysis. *Developmental Medicine and Child Neurology*, *55*(6), 509–519. doi:10.1111/dmcn.12080 PMID:23346889

Ozanne, J. L., & Saatcioglu, B. (2008). Participatory action research. *The Journal of Consumer Research*, *35*(3), 423–439. doi:10.1086/586911

Ozturk, E., van Iersel, M., van Loon, K., den Rooijen, C., van Dongen, E., & van Wijngaarden, R. D. (2018). Interactive online learning on perioperative management of elderly patients. *Frontiers in Aging Neuroscience*, *5*, 45–48. PMID:29502855

Paes, D., Arantes, E., & Irizarry, J. (2017). Immersive environment for improving the understanding of architectural 3D models: Comparing user spatial perception between immersive and traditional virtual reality systems. *Automation in Construction*, *84*, 292–303. doi:10.1016/j.autcon.2017.09.016

Palmen, A., Didden, R., & Verhoeven, L. (2012). A personal digital assistant for improving independent transitioning in adolescents with high-functioning autism spectrum disorder. *Developmental Neurorehabilitation*, *15*(6), 401–413. doi:10.3109/17518423.2012.701240 PMID:23030628

Papara, R., Galatus, R., & Buzura, L. (2020, July). Virtual Reality as Cost Effective Tool for Distance Healthcare. In *2020 22nd International Conference on Transparent Optical Networks (ICTON)* (pp. 1-6). IEEE. 10.1109/ICTON51198.2020.9203420

Parens, E., & Asch, A. (1999). Special Supplement: The Disability Rights Critique of Prenatal Genetic Testing Reflections and Recommendations. *The Hastings Center Report*, *29*(5), S1–S2. doi:10.2307/3527746 PMID:10587809

Park, E.-Y. (2016). Effect of physical therapy frequency on gross motor function in children with cerebral palsy. *Journal of Physical Therapy Science*, *28*(6), 1888–1891. doi:10.1589/jpts.28.1888 PMID:27390440

Park, E., Yun, B. J., & Jung, T. (2019). Effects of a Mixed Reality-based Cognitive Training System Compared to a Conventional Computer-assisted Cognitive Training System on Mild Cognitive Impairment: A Pilot Study. *Cognitive and Behavioral Neurology*, *32*(3), 172–178. doi:10.1097/WNN.0000000000000197 PMID:31517700

Parong, J., & Mayer, R. E. (2020). Cognitive and affective processes for learning science in immersive virtual reality. *Journal of Computer Assisted Learning*. Advance online publication. doi:10.1111/jcal.12482

Parra, E., Chicchi Giglioli, I. A., Philip, J., Carrasco-Ribelles, L. A., Marín-Morales, J., & Alcañiz Raya, M. (2021). Combining virtual reality and organizational neuroscience for leadership assessment. *Applied Sciences (Switzerland)*, *11*(13), 5956. Advance online publication. doi:10.3390/app11135956

Parsey, C. M., & Schmitter-Edgecombe, M. (2013). Applications of technology in neuropsychological assessment. *The Clinical Neuropsychologist*, *27*(8), 1328–1361. doi:10.1080/13854046.2013.834971 PMID:24041037

Parsons, T. D., & Rizzo, A. A. (2008). Affective outcomes of virtual reality exposure therapy for anxiety and specific phobias: A meta-analysis. *Journal of Behavior Therapy and Experimental Psychiatry*, *39*(3), 250–261. doi:10.1016/j.jbtep.2007.07.007 PMID:17720136

Parsons, T. D., Silva, T. M., Pair, J., & Rizzo, A. A. (2008). Virtual environment for assessment of neurocognitive functioning: Virtual reality cognitive performance assessment test. *Studies in Health Technology and Informatics*, *132*, 351. PMID:18391320

Passini, R., Rainville, C., & Marchand, N. (1998). Wayfinding and dementia: Some research findings and a new look at design. *Journal of Architectural and Planning Research*, *15*(2), 133–151. doi:10.1080/01688639508402431 PMID:8847388

Pastorino, G. M. G., Operto, F. F., Padovano, C., Vivenzio, V., Scuoppo, C., Pastorino, N., Roccella, M., Vetri, L., Carotenuto, M., & Coppola, G. (2021). Social cognition in neurodevelopmental disorders and epilepsy. *Frontiers in Neurology*, *12*, 658823. Advance online publication. doi:10.3389/fneur.2021.658823 PMID:33935956

Patel, S., Park, H., Bonato, P., Chan, L., & Rodgers, M. (2012). A review of wearable sensors and systems with application in rehabilitation. *Journal of Neuroengineering and Rehabilitation*, *9*(1), 1–17. doi:10.1186/1743-0003-9-21 PMID:22520559

Pavlov, N. (2014). User interface for people with autism spectrum disorders. *Journal of Software Engineering and Applications*, *7*(2), 7. doi:10.4236/jsea.2014.72014

Peck, T. C., Doan, M., Bourne, K. A., & Good, J. J. (2018). The effect of gender body-swap illusions on working memory and stereotype threat. *IEEE Transactions on Visualization and Computer Graphics*, *24*(4), 1604–1612. doi:10.1109/TVCG.2018.2793598 PMID:29543177

Peck, T. C., Good, J. J., & Bourne, K. A. (2020). Inducing and mitigating stereotype threat through gendered virtual body-swap illusions. In *Proceedings of the 2020 CHI Conference on Human Factors in Computing Systems* (pp. 1-13). ACM.

Perilli, V., Stasolla, F., Caffò, A. O., Albano, V., & D'Amico, F. (2019). Microswitch-cluster technology for promoting occupation and reducing hand biting of six adolescents with fragile X syndrome: New evidence and social rating. *Journal of Developmental and Physical Disabilities*, *31*(1), 115–133. doi:10.100710882-018-9634-9

Perri, R., Serra, L., Carlesimo, G. A., & Caltagirone, C. (2007). Amnestic Mild Cognitive Impairment: Difference of Memory Profile in Subjects Who Converted or Did Not Convert to Alzheimer's Disease. *Neuropsychology*, *21*(5), 549–558. doi:10.1037/0894-4105.21.5.549 PMID:17784803

Perry, R. J., Watson, P., & Hodges, J. R. (2000). The nature and staging of attention dysfunction in early (minimal and mild) Alzheimer's disease: Relationship to episodic and semantic memory impairment. *Neuropsychologia*, *38*(3), 252–271. doi:10.1016/S0028-3932(99)00079-2 PMID:10678692

Peterson, C. M., Mikal, J. P., McCarron, H. R., Finlay, J. M., Mitchell, L. L., & Gaugler, J. E. (2020). The Feasibility and Utility of a Personal Health Record for Persons With Dementia and Their Family Caregivers for Web-Based Care Coordination: Mixed Methods Study. *JMIRI Aging*, *3*(1), 1–16. doi:10.2196/17769 PMID:32589158

Petry, K., & Maes, B. (2007). Description of the support needs of people with profound multiple disabilities using the 2002 AAMR system: An overview of literature. *Education and Training in Developmental Disabilities*, *42*, 130–143.

Petry, K., Maes, B., & Vlaskamp, C. (2005). Domains of quality of life of people with profound multiple disabilities: The perspective of parents and direct support staff. *Journal of Applied Research in Intellectual Disabilities*, *18*(1), 35–46. doi:10.1111/j.1468-3148.2004.00209.x

Pezzuoli, F., Tafaro, D., Pane, M., Corona, D., & Corradini, M. L. (2020). Development of a New Sign Language Translation System for People with Autism Spectrum Disorder. *Advances in Neurodevelopmental Disorders*, *4*(4), 439–446. doi:10.100741252-020-00175-6

Pimentel, L., & Teixeira, K. (1995). *Virtual reality: Through the new looking glass*. McGraw Hill.

Pino, M., Granata, C., Legouverneur, G., & Rigaud, A. S. (2012). Assessing design features of a graphical user interface for a social assistive robot for older adults with cognitive impairment. *International Symposium of Automation and Robotics in Construction*, *7*, 55-86. 10.22260/ISARC2012/0085

Pizzamiglio, M. R., Vitturini, C., Piccardi, L., & Spitoni, G. (2008). Sensor-Motor Rehabilitation in Rett Syndrome: A Case Report. *Focus on Autism and Other Developmental Disabilities*, *23*(1), 49–62. doi:10.1177/1088357607311446

Plackett, R., Thomas, S., & Thomas, S. (2016). Professionals' views on the use of smartphone technology to support children and adolescents with memory impairment due to acquired brain injury. *Disability and Rehabilitation. Assistive Technology*, *12*(3), 1–8. doi:10.3109/17483107.2015.1127436 PMID:26730647

Plancher, G., Barra, J., Orriols, E., & Piolino, P. (2012a). The influence of action on episodic memory: A virtual reality study. *Quarterly Journal of Experimental Psychology*, *66*(5), 895–909. doi:10.1080/17470218.2012.722657 PMID:23025821

Plancher, G., Tirard, A., Gyselinck, V., Nicolas, S., & Piolino, P. (2012). Using virtual reality to characterize episodic memory profiles in amnestic mild cognitive impairment and Alzheimer's disease: Influence of active and passive encoding. *Neuropsychologia*, *50*(5), 592–602. doi:10.1016/j.neuropsychologia.2011.12.013 PMID:22261400

Pliasa, S., & Fachantidis, N. (2019, October). Mobile Technologies Serious Games for the Development of Social Skills in Children with Autism Spectrum Disorders. In *Interactive Mobile Communication, Technologies and Learning* (pp. 618–628). Springer.

Plow, M., & Finlayson, M. (2013). Potential benefits of nintendo wii fit among people with multiple sclerosis: A longitudinal pilot study. *International Journal of MS Care*, *15*(S1, SUPPL.1), 13–23. doi:10.7224/1537-2073-15.S1.13 PMID:24453702

Pop, C. A., Simut, R. E., Pintea, S., Saldien, J., Rusu, A. S., Vanderfaeillie, J., David, D. O., Lefeber, D., & Vanderborght, B. (2013). Social robots vs. computer display: Does the way social stories are delivered make a difference for their effectiveness on ASD children. *Journal of Educational Computing Research*, *49*(3), 381–401. doi:10.2190/EC.49.3.f

Powell, L. E., Glang, A., Pinkelman, S., Albin, R., Harwick, R., Ettel, D., & Wild, M. R. (2015). Systematic instruction of assistive technology for cognition (ATC) in an employment setting following acquired brain injury: A single case, experimental study. *NeuroRehabilitation*, *37*(3), 437–447. doi:10.3233/NRE-151272 PMID:26518534

Prenton, S., Hollands, K. L., & Kenney, L. P. (2016). Functional electrical stimulation versus ankle foot orthoses for foot-drop: A meta-analysis of orthotic effects. *Journal of Rehabilitation Medicine*, *48*(8), 646–656. doi:10.2340/16501977-2136 PMID:27563700

Price, A., & Lee, H. S. (2010). The effect of two-dimensional and stereoscopic presentation on middle school students' performance of spatial cognition tasks. *Journal of Science Education and Technology*, *19*(1), 90–103. doi:10.100710956-009-9182-2

Puglia, M. H., Krol, K. M., Missana, M., Williams, C. L., Lillard, T. S., Morris, J. P., Connelly, J. J., & Grossmann, T. (2020). Epigenetic tuning of brain signal entropy in emergent human social behavior. *BMC Medicine*, *18*(1), 244. Advance online publication. doi:10.118612916-020-01683-x PMID:32799881

Qi, C. H., Barton, E. E., Collier, M., & Lin, Y. (2017). A Systematic Review of Single-Case Research Studies on Using Video Modeling Interventions to Improve Social Communication Skills for Individuals With Autism Spectrum Disorder. *Focus on Autism and Other Developmental Disabilities*, •••, 1–9. doi:10.1177/1088357617741282

Quick, V. B., Wang, B., & State, M. W. (2021). Leveraging large genomic datasets to illuminate the pathobiology of autism spectrum disorders. *Neuropsychopharmacology*, *46*(1), 55–69. doi:10.103841386-020-0768-y PMID:32668441

Rabins, P. V., Blacker, D., & Rovner, B. W. (2007). (Steering Committee on Practice Guidelines) "American Psychiatric Association practice guideline for the treatment of patients with Alzheimer's disease and other dementias. *The American Journal of Psychiatry*, *164*, 5–56. PMID:18340692

Radwan, A., & Cataltepe, Z. (2016). Using assistive technology to enhance teaching for students with autism spectrum disorders. *International E-Journal of Advances in Education*, *2*(4), 112–121. doi:10.18768/ijaedu.15760

Raghavendra, P., Newman, L., Grace, E., & Wood, D. (2013). ' I could never do that before': Effectiveness of a tailored Internet support intervention to increase the social participation of youth with disabilities. *Child: Care, Health and Development*, *39*(4), 552–561. doi:10.1111/cch.12048 PMID:23763256

Rainville, C., Passini, R., & Marchand, N. (2001). A multiple case study of wayfinding in dementia of the alzheimertype: Decision making. *Neuropsychology, Development, and Cognition. Section B, Aging, Neuropsychology and Cognition*, *8*(1), 54–71. doi:10.1076/anec.8.1.54.846

Ramey, C. T., & Ramey, S. L. (1998). Early Intervention and Early Experience. *The American Psychologist*, *53*(2), 109–120. doi:10.1037/0003-066X.53.2.109 PMID:9491742

Ranasinghe, K. G., Cha, J., Iaccarino, L., Hinkley, L. B., Beagle, A. J., Pham, J., Jagust, W. J., Miller, B. L., Rankin, K. B., Rabinovici, G. D., Vossel, K. A., & Nagarajan, N. N. (2020). Neurophysiological signatures in Alzheimer's disease are distinctly associated with TAU, amyloid-β accumulation, and cognitive decline. *Journal of Translational Medicine*, 12. PMID:32161102

Randström, K. B., Asplund, K., Svedlund, M., & Paulson, M. (2013). Activity and participation in home rehabilitation: Older people's and family members' perspectives. In Journal of Rehabilitation Medicine (Vol. 45, Issue 2, pp. 211–216). doi:10.2340/16501977-1085

Rauch, A., Cieza, A., & Stucki, G. (2008). How to apply the international classification of functioning, disability and health (ICF) for rehabilitation management in clinical practice. *European Journal of Physical and Rehabilitation Medicine, 44*(3), 329–342. PMID:18762742

Ray, K. D., & Mittelman, M. S. (2017). Music therapy: A nonpharmacological approach to the care of agitation and depressive symptoms for nursing home residents with dementia. *Dementia (London), 9*(6), 689–710. doi:10.1177/1471301215613779 PMID:26519453

Reason, P., & Bradbury, H. (2001). *Handbook of action research: Participative inquiry and practice*. Sage.

Rebok, G. W., Ball, K., Guey, L. T., Jones, R. N., Kim, H. Y., King, J. W., Marsiske, M., Morris, J. N., Tennstedt, S. L., Unverzagt, F. W., & Willis, S. L. (2014). Ten year effects of the advanced cognitive training for independent and vital elderly cognitive training trial on cognition and everyday functioning in older adults. *Journal of the American Geriatrics Society, 62*(1), 16–24. doi:10.1111/jgs.12607 PMID:24417410

Reichle, J. (2011). Evaluating assistive technology in the education of persons with severe disabilities. *Journal of Behavioral Education, 20*(1), 77–85. doi:10.100710864-011-9121-1

Reid, D. T. (2002). Benefits of a virtual play rehabilitation environment for children with cerebral palsy on perceptions of self-efficacy: A pilot study. *Pediatric Rehabilitation, 5*(3), 141–148. doi:10.1080/1363849021000039344 PMID:12581476

Reilly, D., & Neumann, D. L. (2013). Gender-role differences in spatial ability: A meta-analytic review. *Sex Roles, 68*(9-10), 521–535. doi:10.100711199-013-0269-0

Reinhard, R., Shah, K. G., Faust-Christmann, C. A., & Lachmann, T. (2020). Acting your avatar's age: Effects of virtual reality avatar embodiment on real life walking speed. *Media Psychology, 23*(2), 293–315. doi:10.1080/15213269.2019.1598435

Reinkensmeyer, D. J. (2018). *Rehabilitation robot*. Encyclopedia Britannica.

Reis, S. B., Bernardo, W. M., Oshiro, C. A., Krebs, H. I., & Conforto, A. B. (2021). Effects of Robotic Therapy Associated With Noninvasive Brain Stimulation on Upper-Limb Rehabilitation After Stroke: Systematic Review and Meta-analysis of Randomized Clinical Trials. *Neurorehabilitation and Neural Repair, 35*(3), 256–266.

Remmele, J., Helm, P. C., Oberhoffer-Fritz, R., Bauer, U. M. M., Pickardt, T., Ewert, P., & Tutarel, O. (2021). A national comparative investigation of twins with congenital heart defects for neurodevelopmental outcomes and quality of life (same same, but different?): Protocol for a prospective observational study. *JMIR Research Protocols, 10*(5), e26404. Advance online publication. doi:10.2196/26404 PMID:33983133

Ren, Z., & Wu, J. (2019). The Effect of Virtual Reality Games on the Gross Motor Skills of Children with Cerebral Palsy: A Meta-Analysis of Randomized Controlled Trials. *International Journal of Environmental Research and Public Health, 16*(20), 3885. Advance online publication. doi:10.3390/ijerph16203885 PMID:31614990

Rett, A. (1966). Uber ein eigenartigers himatrophisches syndrom bei hyperamonaemie im kinsalter. *Wiener Medizinische Wochenschrift, 116*, 723–728. PMID:5300597

Reuten, A., van Dam, M., & Naber, M. (2018). Pupillary Responses to Robotic and Human Emotions: The Uncanny Valley and Media Equation Confirmed. *Frontiers in Psychology, 9*, 774. https://doi.org/10.3389/fpsyg.2018.00774

Rice, L. M., Wall, C. A., Fogel, A., & Shic, F. (2015). Computer-Assisted Face Processing Instruction Improves Emotion Recognition, Mentalizing, and Social Skills in Students with ASD. *Journal of Autism and Developmental Disorders, 45*(7), 2176–2186. Advance online publication. doi:10.100710803-015-2380-2 PMID:25694364

Richardson, A. E., Montello, D. R., & Hegarty, M. (1999). Spatial knowledge acquisition from maps and from navigation in real and virtual environments. *Memory & Cognition, Springer, 27*(4), 741–750. doi:10.3758/BF03211566 PMID:10479831

Riches, S., Elghany, S., Garety, P., Rus-Calafell, M., & Valmaggia, L. (2019). Factors affecting sense of presence in a virtual reality social environment: A qualitative study. *Cyberpsychology, Behavior, and Social Networking, 22*(4), 288–292. doi:10.1089/cyber.2018.0128 PMID:30802148

Ringland, K. E., Wolf, C. T., Boyd, L. E., Baldwin, M. S., & Hayes, G. R. (2016, October). Would you be mine: Appropriating minecraft as an assistive technology for youth with autism. In *Proceedings of the 18th International ACM SIGACCESS Conference on Computers and Accessibility* (pp. 33-41). Reno: ACM. 10.1145/2982142.2982172

Riva, G. (1998). Virtual Reality as Assessment Tool in Psychology. *Virtual Reality in Neuro-Psychology, 44*(9), 71–79. PMID:10175344

Rizzo, A. A., Schultheis, M. T., Kerns, K., & Mateer, C. (2004). Analysis of assets for virtual reality applications in neuropsychology. *Neuropsychological Rehabilitation, 14*(1), 207–239. doi:10.1080/09602010343000183

Robert, P. H., Konig, A., Amieva, H., Andrieu, S., Bremond, F., Bullock, R., & … . (2014). Recommendations for the use of serious games in people with alzheimer's disease, related disorders and frailty. *Frontiers in Aging Neuroscience, 6*(54), 1–13. doi:10.3389/fnagi.2014.00054 PMID:24715864

Robertson, C. E., & Baron-Cohen, S. (2017, September 29). Sensory perception in autism. *Nature Reviews. Neuroscience, 18*(11), 671–684. doi:10.1038/nrn.2017.112 PMID:28951611

Robins, B., Dautenhahn, K., & Dubowski, J. (2006). Does appearance matter in the interaction of children with autism with a humanoid robot? *Interaction Studies: Social Behaviour and Communication in Biological and Artificial Systems, 7*(3), 479–512.doi:https://doi.org/10.1075/is.7.3.16rob

Robinson, H. (2012). *Suitability of healthcare robots for a dementia unit and suggested improvements.* Elsevier.

Roche, L., Sigafoos, J., Lancioni, G. E., O'Reilly, M. F., & Green, V. (2015). Microswitch technology for enabling self-determined responding in children with profound and multiple disabilities: A systematic review. *Augmentative and Alternative Communication, 31*(3), 246–258. doi:10.3109/07434618.2015.1024888 PMID:25791421

Rodgers, H., Shaw, L., Bosomworth, H., Aird, L., Alvarado, N., Andole, S., Cohen, D. L., Dawson, J., Eyre, J., Finch, T., Ford, G. A., Hislop, J., Hogg, S., Howel, D., Hughes, N., Krebs, H. I., Price, C., Rochester, L., Stamp, E., ... Wilkes, S. (2017). Robot-assisted Training for the Upper Limb after Stroke (RATULS): Study protocol for a randomised controlled trial. *Trials, 18*(1), 340.

Rohrbach, N., Gulde, P., Armstrong, A. R., Hartig, L., Abdelrazeq, A., Schröder, S., Neuse, J., Grimmer, T., Diehl-Schmid, J., & Hermsdörfer, J. (2019). An augmented reality approach for ADL support in Alzheimer's disease: A crossover trial. *Journal of Neuroengineering and Rehabilitation, 16*(1), 66. Advance online publication. doi:10.118612984-019-0530-z PMID:31159816

Roldán-Álvarez, D., Gomez, J., Márquez-Fernández, A., Martín, E., & Montoro, G. (2016, July). Mobile devices as assistive technologies for ASD: Experiences in the classroom. In *International Conference of Design, User Experience, and Usability* (pp. 187-197). Cham: Springer.

Romera-De Francisco, L., & Jimenez-Del Barrio, S. (2016). Efectividad de la electroestimulacion funcional en pacientes con ictus: Revision sistematica [Effectiveness of functional electrical stimulation in stroke patients: a systematic review]. *Revista de Neurología*, *63*(3), 109–118.

Romero-Ayuso, D., Alcántara-Vázquez, P., Almenara-García, A., Nuñez-Camarero, I., Triviño-Juárez, J. M., Ariza-Vega, P., Molina, J.-P., & González, P. (2020). Self-regulation in children with neurodevelopmental disorders "SR-MRehab: Un colegio emocionante": A protocol study. *International Journal of Environmental Research and Public Health*, *17*(12), 1–23. doi:10.3390/ijerph17124198 PMID:32545534

Rosales, R. L., Efendy, F., Teleg, E. S., Delos Santos, M. M., Rosales, M. C., Ostrea, M., Tanglao, M. J., & Ng, A. R. (2016). Botulinum toxin as early intervention for spasticity after stroke or non-progressive brain lesion: A meta-analysis. *Journal of the Neurological Sciences*, *371*, 6–14.

Rose, A. S., Djukic, A., Janjowski, J., Feldman, J. F., Fishman, I., & McDermott, M. V. (2012). Rett syndrome: An eye-tracking study of attention and recognition memory. *Developmental Medicine and Child Neurology*, *8*, 301–302. PMID:23488948

Rosello, B., Berenguer, C., Baixauli, I., Colomer, C., & Miranda, A. (2018). ADHD symptoms and learning behaviors in children with ASD without intellectual disability. A mediation analysis of executive functions. *PLoS One*, *13*(11).doi: https://doi.org/10.1371/journal.pone.0207286

Rosenberg, L., & Nygård, L. (2017). Learning and knowing technology as lived experience in people with Alzheimer's disease: A phenomenological study. *Aging & Mental Health*, *21*(12), 1272–1279. doi:10.1080/13607863.2016.1222347 PMID:27592720

Rosenbloom, R., Mason, R. A., Wills, H. P., & Mason, B. A. (2016). Technology delivered self-monitoring application to promote successful inclusion of an elementary student with autism. *Assistive Technology*, *28*(1), 9–16. doi:10.1080/10400435.2015.1059384 PMID:26151808

Rose, S. A., Wass, S., Jankowski, J. J., Feldman, J. F., & Djukic, A. (2017). Sustained attention in the face of distractors: A study of children with Rett syndrome. *Neuropsychology*, *31*(4), 403–410. doi:10.1037/neu0000369 PMID:28383972

Rosset, D. B., Rondan, C., Da Fonseca, D., Santos, A., Assouline, B., & Christine, D. (2008). Typical emotion processing for cartoon but not for real faces in children with autistic spectrum disorders. *Journal of Autism and Developmental Disorders*, *38*(5), 919–925.doi:https://doi.org/10.1007/s10803-007-0465-2

Roth, B. J. (1994). Mechanisms for electrical stimulation of excitable tissue. *Critical Reviews in Biomedical Engineering*, *22*(3-4), 253–305.

Royal College of Physicians. (2016). *National clinical guideline for stroke*. https://www.strokeaudit.org/SupportFiles/Documents/Guidelines/2016-National-Clinical-Guideline-for-Stroke-5t-(1).aspx

Rusakova, I. (2021). *Designing for the autistic community*. Retrieved from UX Collective: https://uxdesign.cc/inclusive-design-guide-7-principles-of-designing-for-the-autistic-community-1e6dcd4bae85

Rushton, P. W., & Miller, W. C. (2002). Goal Attainment Scaling in the rehabilitation of patients with lower-extremity amputations: A pilot study. *Archives of Physical Medicine and Rehabilitation*, *83*(6), 771–775. doi:10.1053/apmr.2002.32636 PMID:12048654

Rutter, M., Le Couteur, A., & Lord, C. (2003). *Autism diagnostic interview-revised*. Western Psychological Services. Retrieved from https://www.academia.edu/download/2163587/8j7zpy2k00w44i8.pdf

Ryan, R. M., & Deci, E. L. (2000). Self-determination theory and the facilitation of intrinsic motivation, social development, and well-being. *The American Psychologist*, *55*(1), 68–78. doi:10.1037/0003-066X.55.1.68 PMID:11392867

Sabut, S. K., Sikdar, C., Kumar, R., & Mahadevappa, M. (2011). Clinical use of functional electrical stimulation for correction of foot drop: A comparison between subacute and chronic stroke patients. *Journal of Mechanics in Medicine and Biology*, *11*(05), 1165–1177. doi:10.1142/S0219519411004253

Sacco, R. L., Kasner, S. E., Broderick, J. P., Caplan, L. R., Connors, J. J., Culebras, A., Elkind, M. S. V., George, M. G., Hamdan, A. D., Higashida, R. T., Hoh, B. L., Janis, L. S., Kase, C. S., Kleindorfer, D. O., Lee, J.-M., Moseley, M. E., Peterson, E. D., Turan, T. N., Valderrama, A. L., & Vinters, H. V. (2013). An updated definition of stroke for the 21st century: A statement for healthcare professionals from the American Heart Association/American Stroke Association. *Stroke*, *44*(7), 2064–2089. doi:10.1161/STR.0b013e318296aeca PMID:23652265

Sakzewski, L., Lewis, M. J., McKinlay, L., Ziviani, J., & Boyd, R. N. (2016). Impact of multi-modal web-based rehabilitation on occupational performance and upper limb outcomes: Pilot randomized trial in children with acquired brain injuries. *Developmental Medicine and Child Neurology*, *58*(12), 1257–1264. doi:10.1111/dmcn.13157 PMID:27230022

Sale, P., Mazzoleni, S., Lombardi, V., Galafate, D., Massimiani, M. P., Posteraro, F., Damiani, C., & Franceschini, M. (2014). Recovery of hand function with robot-assisted therapy in acute stroke patients: A randomized-controlled trial. *International Journal of Rehabilitation Research. Internationale Zeitschrift fur Rehabilitationsforschung. Revue Internationale de Recherches de Readaptation*, *37*(3), 236–242.

Salminen, A.-L., Hiekkala, S., & Stenberg, J.-H. (2016). *Remote rehabilitation. Research of the Social Insurance Institution of Finland*. KELA.

Sampath, H., Agarwal, R., & Indurkhya, B. (2013, September). Assistive technology for children with autism-lessons for interaction design. In *Proceedings of the 11th Asia Pacific Conference on Computer Human Interaction* (pp. 325-333). Bangalore: ACM. 10.1145/2525194.2525300

Sandlund, M., Dock, K., Häger, C. K., & Waterworth, E. L. (2012). Motion interactive video games in home training for children with cerebral palsy: Parents' perceptions. *Disability and Rehabilitation*, *34*(11), 925–933. doi:10.3109/09638288.2011.626489 PMID:22066685

Sandlund, M., McDonough, S., & Häger-Ross, C. (2009). Interactive computer play in rehabilitation of children with sensorimotor disorders: A systematic review. *Developmental Medicine and Child Neurology*, *51*(3), 173–179. doi:10.1111/j.1469-8749.2008.03184.x PMID:19191834

Sandlund, M., Waterworth, E. L., & Hager, C. K. (2011). Using motion interactive games to promote physical activity and enhance motor performance in chldren with cerebral palsy. *Developmental Neurorehabilitation*, *14*(1), 15–21. doi:10.3109/17518423.2010.533329 PMID:21241174

Santos, A. V. F., Licursi, L. A., Amaral, M. F., Cavalcanti, A., & Silveira, Z. C. (2019). User-centered design of a customized assistive device to support feeding. *Procedia CIRP, 84,* 743-748.

Santosh, P., Lievesley, K., Fiori, F., & Singh, J. (2017). Development of the tailored Rett intervention and assessment longitudinal (TRIAL) database and the Rett evaluation of symptoms and treatments (REST) questionnaire. *BMJ Open*, *7*(6), e015342. Advance online publication. doi:10.1136/bmjopen-2016-015342 PMID:28637735

Sarikaya, H., Ferro, J., & Arnold, M. (2015). Stroke prevention—medical and lifestyle measures. *European Neurology*, *73*(3-4), 150–157.

Sauzeon, H., N'Kaoua, B., Pala, P. A., Taillade, M., Auriacombe, S., & Guitton, P. (2016). Everyday-like memory for objects in ageing and Alzheimer's disease assessed in a visually complex environment: The role of executive functioning and episodic memory. *Journal of Neuropsychology, 10*(1), 33–58. doi:10.1111/jnp.12055 PMID:25307794

Sauzeon, H., Pala, P. A., Larrue, F., & Wallet, G. (2012). The use of virtual reality for episodic memory assessment: Effects of active navigation. *Experimental Psychology, 59*(2), 99–108. doi:10.1027/1618-3169/a000131 PMID:22044787

Savvidis, T. P., Konstantinidis, E. I., Dias, S. B., Diniz, J. A., Hadjileontiadis, L. J., & Bamidis, P. D. (2018). *Exergames for Parkinson's disease patients: How participatory design led to technology adaptation.* doi:10.3233/978-1-61499-880-8-78

Scassellati, B., Admoni, H., & Matarić, M. (2012). Robots for Use in Autism Research. *Annual Review of Biomedical Engineering, 14*, 275–294. https://www.annualreviews.org/doi/abs/10.1146/annurev-bioeng-071811-150036

Scassellati, B., Boccanfuso, L., Huang, C. M., Mademtzi, M., Qin, M., Salomons, N., Ventola, P., & Shic, F. (2018). Improving social skills in children with ASD using a long-term, in-home social robot. *Science Robotics, 3*(21), eaat7544. Advance online publication. doi:10.1126cirobotics.aat7544 PMID:33141724

Schaefer, C., & Norah, L. J. (2014). Fostering Ambulation for a Preschool Child with Rett Syndrome: A Case Report. *College of Nursing Faculty Research and Publications, 323*, 1–12.

Schafer, E. C., Wright, S., Anderson, C., Jones, J., Pitts, K., Bryant, D., Watson, M., Box, J., Neve, M., Mathews, L., & Reed, M. P. (2016). Assistive technology evaluations: Remote-microphone technology for children with Autism Spectrum Disorder. *Journal of Communication Disorders, 64*, 1–17. doi:10.1016/j.jcomdis.2016.08.003 PMID:27592101

Schischlevskij, P., Cordts, I., Günther, R., Stolte, B., Zeller, D., Schröter, C., Weyen, U., Regensburger, M., Wolf, J., Schneider, I., Hermann, A., Metelmann, M., Kohl, Z., Linker, R. A., Koch, J. C., Stendel, C., Müschen, L. H., Osmanovic, A., Binz, C., ... Schreiber-Katz, O. (2021). Informal caregiving in amyotrophic lateral sclerosis (als): A high caregiver burden and drastic consequences on caregivers' lives. *Brain Sciences, 11*(6), 748. Advance online publication. doi:10.3390/brainsci11060748 PMID:34200087

Schladen, M. M., & Choong, E. A. (2021). Preferences of adolescents with CP for design of performance feed from a gamified, robotic home ankle therapy system. Manuscript in Process. Department of Biomedical Engineering. The Catholic University of America.

Schladen, M. M., Koumpouros, Y., & Lum, P. (2021). *Factors Mediating Use of Advanced Rehabilitation Technologies in the Home.* Paper presented at the Advances in Human Factors and Ergonomics in Healthcare and Medical Devices, Cham.

Schladen, M. M., Cleary, K., Koumpouros, Y., Monfaredi, R., Salvador, T., Talari, H. F., Slagle, J., Coley, C., Kovelman, S., Belschner, J., & Evans, S. H. (2020). Toward Evaluation of the Subjective Experience of a General Class of User-Controlled, Robot-Mediated Rehabilitation Technologies for Children with Neuromotor Disability. *Informatics (MDPI), 7*(4), 45. Advance online publication. doi:10.3390/informatics7040045

Schladen, M. M., Rounds, A. K., McManus, T., Bennewith, A., Claypool, H., & Groah, S. L. (2021). Intermittent Catheter Reimbursement in the United States: The Experience of Nine Stakeholders Through the Lens of Actor-Network Theory. *Qualitative Report, 26*(2), 443–464. doi:10.46743/2160-3715/2021.4660

Schlosser, R. W., & Wendt, O. (2008, August). Effects of augmentative and alternative communication intervention on speech production in children with autism: A systematic review. *American Journal of Speech-Language Pathology, 17*(3), 212–230. doi:10.1044/1058-0360(2008/021) PMID:18663107

Schmader, T. (2002). Gender identification moderates stereotype threat effects on women's math performance. *Journal of Experimental Social Psychology, 38*(2), 194–201. doi:10.1006/jesp.2001.1500

Schmader, T., Johns, M., & Forbes, C. (2008). An integrated process model of stereotype threat effects on performance. *Psychological Review*, *115*(2), 336–356. doi:10.1037/0033-295X.115.2.336 PMID:18426293

Schubert, T., Friedmann, F., & Regenbrecht, H. (2001). The experience of presence: Factor analytic insights. *Presence (Cambridge, Mass.)*, *10*(3), 266–281. doi:10.1162/105474601300343603

Schweigert, P., & Rowland, C. (1992). Early communication and microtechnology: Instructional sequence and case studies of children with severe multiple disabilities. *Augmentative and Alternative Communication*, *8*(4), 273–286. doi:10.1080/07434619212331276313

Schwickert, L., Becker, C., Lindemann, U., Maréchal, C., Bourke, A., Chiari, L., Helbostad, J. L., Zijlstra, W., Aminian, K., Todd, C., Bandinelli, S., & Klenk, J. (2013). Fall detection with body-worn sensors: A systematic review. *Zeitschrift für Gerontologie und Geriatrie*, *46*(8), 706–719. doi:10.100700391-013-0559-8 PMID:24271251

Scientific Foresight Unit. (2018). *Part IV: Legal and socio-ethical perspectives*. Retrieved from https://www.europarl.europa.eu/RegData/etudes/IDAN/2018/603218/EPRS_IDA(2018)603218(ANN4)_EN.pdf

Seitz, R. J., & Donnan, G. A. (2015). Recovery potential after acute stroke. *Frontiers in Neurology*, *6*. Advance online publication. doi:10.3389/fneur.2015.00238 PMID:26617568

Selander, H., Strand, N., Almberg, M., & Lidestam, B. (2021). Ready for a Learner's permit? clinical neuropsychological off-road tests and driving behaviors in a simulator among adolescents with ADHD and ASD. *Developmental Neurorehabilitation*, *24*(4), 256–265. doi:10.1080/17518423.2020.1869339 PMID:33459571

Servotte, J. C., Goosse, M., Campbell, S. H., Dardenne, N., Pilote, B., Simoneau, I. L., Guillaume, M., Bragard, I., & Ghuysen, A. (2020). Virtual reality experience: Immersion, sense of presence, and cybersickness. *Clinical Simulation in Nursing*, *38*, 35–43. doi:10.1016/j.ecns.2019.09.006

Sgandurra, G., Beani, E., Giampietri, M., Rizzi, R., Cioni, G., Cecchi, F., & … . (2018). Early intervention at home in infants with congenital brain lesion with CareToy revised: A RCT protocol. *BMC Pediatrics*, *18*(1), 295. Advance online publication. doi:10.118612887-018-1264-y PMID:30185165

Shafer, D. M., Carbonara, C. P., & Korpi, M. F. (2017). Modern virtual reality technology: Cybersickness, sense of presence, and gender. *Media Psychology Review*, *11*(2), 1.

Shahabi, S., Shabaninejad, H., Kamali, M., Jalali, M., & Ahmadi Teymourlouy, A. (2020). The effects of ankle-foot orthoses on walking speed in patients with stroke: A systematic review and meta-analysis of randomized controlled trials. *Clinical Rehabilitation*, *34*(2), 145–159. doi:10.1177/0269215519887784 PMID:31822115

Sharan, D., Rajkumar, J. S., & Balakrishnan, R. (2016). Efficacy of an activity monitor as a biofeedback device in cerebral palsy. *Journal of Rehabilitation and Assistive Technologies Engineering*, *3*. doi:10.1177/2055668316676032 PMID:31186915

Shattuck, P. T., Roux, A. M., Hudson, L. E., Lounds Taylor, J., Maenner, M. J., & Trani, J.-F. (2012). Services for adults with an autism spectrum disorder. *Canadian Journal of Psychiatry*, *57*(5), 284–291. doi:10.1177/070674371205700503

Sheffler, L. R., Bailey, S. N., Wilson, R. D., & Chae, J. (2013). Spatiotemporal, kinematic, and kinetic effects of a peroneal nerve stimulator versus an ankle foot orthosis in hemiparetic gait. *Neurorehabilitation and Neural Repair*, *27*(5), 403–410. doi:10.1177/1545968312465897 PMID:23192416

Sherzai, A., & Sherzai, D. (2017). *The Alzheimer's Solution: A Breakthrough Program to Prevent and Reverse the Symptoms of Cognitive Decline at Every Age*. HarperOne.

Shih, M. J., Pittinsky, T. L., & Ho, G. C. (2012). *Stereotype boost: Positive outcomes from the activation of positive stereotypes*. Academic Press.

Shikako-Thomas, K., Shevell, M., Lach, L., Law, M., Schmitz, N., Poulin, C., & Majnemer, A. (2015). Are you doing what you want to do? Leisure preferences of adolescents with cerebral palsy. *Developmental Neurorehabilitation, 18*(4), 234–240. doi:10.3109/17518423.2013.794166 PMID:23869565

Shillingsburg, M. A., Marya, V., Bartlett, B. L., & Thompson, T. M. (2019). Teaching mands for information using speech generating devices: A replication and extension. *Journal of Applied Behavior Analysis, 52*(3), 756–771. doi:10.1002/jaba.579 PMID:31157409

Siebes, R. C., Wijnroks, L., Ketelaar, M., van Schie, P. E. M., Gorter, J. W., & Vermeer, A. (2007). Parent participation in paediatric rehabilitation treatment centres in the Netherlands: A parents' viewpoint. *Child: Care, Health and Development, 33*(2), 196–205. doi:10.1111/j.1365-2214.2006.00636.x PMID:17291324

Siegel, S., & Castellan, N. J. (1988). *Non parametric statistics* (2nd ed.). Mc Graw Hill.

Sigafoos, J., O'Reilly, M. F., Ledbetter-Cho, K., Lim, N., Lancioni, G. E., & Marschik, P. B. (2019). Addressing sequelae of developmental regression associated with developmental disabilities: A systematic review of behavioral and educational intervention studies. *Neuroscience and Biobehavioral Reviews, 96*, 56–71. doi:10.1016/j.neubiorev.2018.11.014 PMID:30481529

Sigafoos, J., Reilly, M. O., Ganz, J. B., Lancioni, G. E., & Schlosser, R. W. (2005). Supporting self-determination in AAC interventions by assessing preference for communication devices. *Technology and Disability, 17*(3), 143–153. doi:10.3233/TAD-2005-17302

Sigafoos, J., Roche, L., & Tait, K. (2021). Challenges in providing AAC intervention to people with profound intellectual and multiple disabilities. In B. T. Ogletree (Ed.), *Augmentative and Alternative Communication: Challenges and Solutions* (pp. 229–252). Plural Publishing.

Sigafoos, J., Woodyatt, G., Keen, D., Tait, K., Tucker, M., Roberts-Pennell, D., & Pittendreigh, N. (2000). Identifying potential communicative acts in children with developmental and physical disabilities. *Communication Disorders Quarterly, 21*(2), 77–86. doi:10.1177/152574010002100202

Silberman, S. (2015). *NeuroTribes: The Legacy of Autism and the Future of Neurodiversity*. Avery Pub Group.

Simacek, J., Dimian, A. F., & McComas, J. J. (2017). Communication intervention for young children with severe neurodevelopmental disabilities via telehealth. *Journal of Autism and Developmental Disorders, 47*(3), 744–767. doi:10.100710803-016-3006-z PMID:28093677

Simacek, J., Pennington, B., Reichle, J., & Parker-McGowan, Q. (2018). Aided AAC for people with severe to profound and multiple disabilities: A systematic review of interventions and treatment intensity. *Advances in Neurodevelopmental Disorders, 2*(1), 100–115. doi:10.100741252-017-0050-4

Simeoli, R., Milano, N., Rega, A., & Marocco, D. (2021). Using technology to identify children with autism through motor abnormalities. *Frontiers in Psychology, 12*, 635696. Advance online publication. doi:10.3389/fpsyg.2021.635696 PMID:34113283

Simões, M., Bernardes, M., Barros, F., & Castelo-Branco, M. (2018). Virtual travel training for autism spectrum disorder: Proof-of-concept interventional study. *JMIR Serious Games, 20*(3), e5. Advance online publication. doi:10.2196/games.8428 PMID:29559425

Siniscalco, D., Cirillo, A., Bradstreet, J. J., & Antonucci, N. (2013). Epigenetic findings in autism: New perspectives for therapy. *International Journal of Environmental Research and Public Health, 10*(9), 4261–4273. doi:10.3390/ijerph10094261 PMID:24030655

Siriaraya, P., & Ang, C. S. (2014). Recreating living experiences from past memories through virtual worlds for people with dementia. *Proceedings of the SIGCHI Conference on Human Factors in Computing Systems.* 10.1145/2556288.2557035

Slater, M. (2009). Place illusion and plausibility can lead to realistic behaviour in immersive virtual environments. *Philosophical Transactions of the Royal Society of London. Series B, Biological Sciences, 364*(1535), 3549–3557. doi:10.1098/rstb.2009.0138 PMID:19884149

Slater, M. (2018). Immersion and the illusion of presence in virtual reality. *British Journal of Psychology, 109*(3), 431–433. doi:10.1111/bjop.12305 PMID:29781508

Slater, M., & Sanchez-Vives, M. V. (2016). Enhancing our lives with immersive virtual reality. *Frontiers in Robotics and AI, 3*, 74. doi:10.3389/frobt.2016.00074

Slobounov, S. M., Ray, W., Johnson, B., Slobounov, E., & Newell, K. M. (2015). Modulation of cortical activity in 2D versus 3D virtual reality environments: An EEG study. *International Journal of Psychophysiology, 95*(3), 254–260. doi:10.1016/j.ijpsycho.2014.11.003 PMID:25448267

Słyk, S., Zarzycki, M. Z., Kocwa-Karnaś, A., & Domitrz, I. (2019). Virtual reality in the diagnostics and therapy of neurological diseases. *Expert Review of Medical Devices, 16*(12), 1055–1040. doi:10.1080/17434440.2019.1693892 PMID:31739698

Smith, G., Housen, P., Yaffe, K., Ruff, R., Kennison, R. F., Mahncke, H. W., & Zelinski, E. M. (2009). A cognitive training program based on principles of brain plasticity: Results from the improvement in memory with plasticity-based adaptive cognitive training (IMPACT) study. *Journal of the American Geriatrics Society, 57*(4), 594–603. doi:10.1111/j.1532-5415.2008.02167.x PMID:19220558

Smith, M. J., Fleming, M. F., Wright, M. A., Losh, M., Boteler Humm, L., Olsen, D., & Bell, M. D. (2015). Brief report: Vocational outcomes for young adults with autism spectrum disorders at six months after virtual reality job interview training. *Journal of Autism and Developmental Disorders, 45*(10), 3364–3369.doi:https://doi.org/10.1007/s10803-015-2470-1

Smith, M. J., Ginger, E. J., Wright, K., Wright, M. A., Lounds Taylor, J., Boteler Humm, L., ... Fleming, M. F. (2014). Virtual reality job interview training in adults with autism spectrum disorder. *Journal of Autism and Developmental Disorders, 44*, 2450–2463.doi:https://doi.org/10.1007/s10803-014-2113-y

Smith, M. J., Smith, J. D., Fleming, M. F., Jordan, N., Brown, H. C., Humm, L., ... Bell, M. D. (2017). Mechanism of Action for Obtaining Job Offers With Virtual Reality Job Interview Training. *Psychiatric Services (Washington, D.C.), 68*(7), 747–750.doi:https://doi.org/10.1176/appi.ps.201600217

Smith, T. J., & Bernardini, S. (2014). ECHOES : An intelligent serious game for fostering social communication in children with autism. *Information Sciences, 264*, 41–60. doi:10.1016/j.ins.2013.10.027

Snell, M. E. (1987). *Systematic instruction of people with severe handicaps.* Prentice Hall.

Somai, R. S., Schut, M. J., & Van der Stigchel, S. (2020). Evidence for the world as an external memory: A trade-off between internal and external visual memory storage. *Cortex, 122*, 108-114.

Span, M., Hettinga, M., Groen-van de Ven, L., Jukema, J., Janssen, R., Vernooij-Dassen, M., Eefsting, J., & Smits, C. (2018). Involving people with dementia in developing an interactive web tool for shared decision-making: Experiences with a participatory design approach. *Disability and Rehabilitation*, *40*(12), 1410–1412. doi:10.1080/09638288.2017.1298162 PMID:28286969

Sparrow, S. S., Balla, D. A., & Cicchetti, D. V. (2005). *Vineland-II Adaptive Behavior Scales* (2nd ed.). Pearson.

Spector, A., Thorgrimsen, L., Woods, B., Royan, L., Davies, S., Butterworth, M., & Orrell, M. (2003). Efficacy of an evidence-based cognitive stimulation therapy programme for people with dementia: Randomised controlled trial. *The British Journal of Psychiatry*, *183*(3), 248–254. doi:10.1192/bjp.183.3.248 PMID:12948999

Spence-Cochran, K., & Pearl, C. (2012). Assistive technology to support people with autism spectrum disorders. In *Educating students with autism spectrum disorders: Research-based principles and practices* (pp. 295–311). Routledge.

Spencer, V., Simpson, C. G., Day, M., Buster, E., Spencer, V. G., & Simpson, C. G. (2008). Using the Power Card Strategy to Teach Social Skills to a Child with Autism. *TEACHING Exceptional Children Plus*, *5*(1), 1–10.

Spiers, H. J., & Maguire, E. A. (2007). A navigational guidance system in the human brain. *Hippocampus*, *17*(8), 618–626. doi:10.1002/hipo.20298 PMID:17492693

Spreij, L. A., Visser-Meily, J. M., Sibbel, J., Gosselt, I. K., & Nijboer, T. C. (2020). Feasibility and user-experience of virtual reality in neuropsychological assessment following stroke. *Neuropsychological Rehabilitation*, 1–21. doi:10.1080/09602011.2020.1831935 PMID:33138703

Sriram, V., Jenkinson, C., & Peters, M. (2019). Informal carers' experience of assistive technology use in dementia care at home: A systematic review. *BMC Geriatrics*, *14*(1), 160. doi:10.118612877-019-1169-0 PMID:31196003

Stamford, J. A., Schmidt, P. N., & Friedl, K. E. (2015). What engineering technology could do for quality of life in Parkinson's disease: A review of current needs and opportunities. *IEEE Journal of Biomedical and Health Informatics*, *19*(6), 1862–1872. doi:10.1109/JBHI.2015.2464354 PMID:26259205

Stanger, C., Mims, P., Wood, L., & Ahlgrim-Delzell, L. (2016). Supporting Literacy Achievement for Students with Intellectual Disability and Autism through Curricular Programs that Incorporate Assistive Technology. *Assistive Technology Outcomes & Benefits*, *10*(1), 51–73.

Stasolla, F., Perilli, V., & Boccasini, A. (2019). Assistive Technology for Supporting Communication, Occupation, and Leisure by Children with Severe to Profound Developmental Disabilities. In Advanced Methodologies and Technologies in Artificial Intelligence, Computer Simulation, and Human-Computer Interaction (pp. 237-249). IGI Global.

Stasolla, F. (2021). Virtual reality and wearable technologies to support adaptive responding of children and adolescents with neurodevelopmental disorders: A critical comment and new perspectives. *Frontiers in Psychology*, *12*, 720626. Advance online publication. doi:10.3389/fpsyg.2021.720626 PMID:34322073

Stasolla, F., Boccasini, A., & Perilli, V. (2017). Assistive Technology-Based Programs to Support Adaptive Behaviors by Children with Autism Spectrum Disorders: A Literature Overview. In Y. Kats (Ed.), *Supporting the Education of Children with Autism Spectrum Disorders* (pp. 140–159). IGI Global. doi:10.4018/978-1-5225-0816-8.ch008

Stasolla, F., Boccasini, A., Perilli, V., Caffò, A. O., Damiani, R., & Albano, V. (2014). A selective overview of microswitch-based programs for promoting adaptive behaviors of children with developmental disabilities. *International Journal of Ambient Computing and Intelligence*, *6*(2), 56–74. doi:10.4018/IJACI.2014070104

Stasolla, F., Boccasini, A., Perilli, V., Damiani, R., & Albano, V. (2015a). Assistive technology for promoting adaptive skills of children with autism spectrum disorders: A literature overview. *International Journal of Psychology and Psychoanalysis*, *1*(2). Advance online publication. doi:10.23937/2572-4037.1510008

Stasolla, F., & Caffò, A. O. (2013). Promoting adaptive behaviors by two girls with Rett syndrome through a microswitch-based program. *Research in Autism Spectrum Disorders*, *7*(10), 1265–1272. doi:10.1016/j.rasd.2013.07.010

Stasolla, F., Caffò, A. O., Damiani, R., Perilli, V., Di Leone, A., & Albano, V. (2015b). Assistive technology-based programs to promote communication and leisure activities by three children emerged from a minimal conscious state. *Cognitive Processing*, *16*(1), 69–78. doi:10.100710339-014-0625-1 PMID:25077461

Stasolla, F., Caffò, A. O., & Perilli, V. (2018). Assistive Technology-Based Programs and Cognitive-Behavioral Interventions for Helping Adaptive Responding of Children and Adolescents with Rett Syndrome: A Selective Overview. In Y. Kats & F. Stasolla (Eds.), *Education and Technology Support for Children and Young Adults with ASD and Learning Disabilities* (pp. 167–188). IGI Global.

Stasolla, F., Caffò, A. O., & Perilli, V. (2020). Fostering inclusion of children and adolescents with autism spectrum disorders in daily settings through technological supports: A selective overview. In Y. Kats & F. Stasolla (Eds.), *Education and technology support for children and young adults with ASD and learning disabilities* (pp. 224–245). IGI Global.

Stasolla, F., Caffò, A. O., Perilli, V., & Albano, V. (2019). Experimental Examination and Social Validation of a Microswitch Intervention to Improve Choice-Making and Activity Engagement for Six Girls with Rett Syndrome. *Developmental Neurorehabilitation*, *22*(8), 527–541. doi:10.1080/17518423.2019.1624655 PMID:31169045

Stasolla, F., Caffò, A. O., Perilli, V., Boccasini, A., Damiani, R., & D'Amico, F. (2019). Assistive technology for promoting adaptive skills of children with cerebral palsy: Ten cases evaluation. *Disability and Rehabilitation. Assistive Technology*, *14*(5), 489–502. doi:10.1080/17483107.2018.1467972 PMID:29732901

Stasolla, F., Caffò, A. O., Perilli, V., Boccasini, A., Stella, A., Damiani, R., & Damato, C. (2017). A microswitch-based program for promoting initial ambulation responses: An evaluation with two girls with multiple disabilities. *Journal of Applied Behavior Analysis*, *50*(2), 345–356. doi:10.1002/jaba.374 PMID:28128442

Stasolla, F., Caffò, A. O., Perrilli, V., Boccasini, A., Damiani, R., & D'Amico, F. (2017). Fostering Locomotion Fluency of Five Adolescents with Rett Syndrome through a Microswitch-Based Program: Contingency Awareness and Social Rating. *Journal of Developmental and Physical Disabilities*, *30*(2), 239–258. doi:10.100710882-017-9582-9

Stasolla, F., & Ciarmoli, D. (2020). Supporting Adaptive Responding and Reducing Challenging Behaviors of Children with Rare Genetic Syndromes and Severe to Profound Developmental Disabilities Through Assistive Technology-Based Programs. *International Journal of Behavioral Research & Psychology*, *8*, 1–3. doi:10.19070/2332-3000-2000010e

Stasolla, F., Damiani, R., Perilli, V., Di Leone, A., Albano, V., Stella, A., & Damato, C. (2014). Technological supports to promote choice opportunities by two boys with fragile X syndrome and severe to profound developmental disabilities. *Research in Developmental Disabilities*, *35*(11), 2993–3000. doi:10.1016/j.ridd.2014.07.045 PMID:25118066

Stasolla, F., & De Pace, C. (2014). Assistive technology to promote leisure and constructive engagement by two boys emerged from a minimal conscious state. *NeuroRehabilitation*, *35*(2), 253–259. doi:10.3233/NRE-141112 PMID:24990021

Stasolla, F., De Pace, C., Damiani, R., Di Leone, A., Albano, V., & Perrilli, V. (2014). Comparing PECS and VOCA to promote communication opportunities and to reduce stereotyped behaviors by three girls with Rett syndrome. *Research in Autism Spectrum Disorders*, *8*(10), 1269–1278. doi:10.1016/j.rasd.2014.06.009

Stasolla, F., Matamala-Gomez, M., Bernini, S., Caffò, A. O., & Bottiroli, S. (2021). Virtual reality as a technological-aided solution to support communication in persons with neurodegenerative diseases and acquired brain injury during COVID-19 pandemic. *Frontiers in Public Health*, *8*, 635426. Advance online publication. doi:10.3389/fpubh.2020.635426 PMID:33665181

Stasolla, F., & Passaro, A. (2020). Enhancing Life Skills of Chidren and Adolescents with Autism Spectrum Disorders and Intellectual Disabilities through Technological Supports: A selective overview. In T. Wadhera & D. Kakkar (Eds.), *Interdisciplinary Approaches to Altering Neurodevelopmental Disorders* (pp. 41–62). IGI Global. doi:10.4018/978-1-7998-3069-6.ch004

Stasolla, F., & Perilli, V. (2015). Assistive technology to promote communication, leisure, occupation skills by children with Rett syndrome and severe to profound developmental disabilities: A literature overview. In D. Kolby (Ed.), *Rett syndrome and other communication disorders: Symptoms, treatments and Prognosis* (pp. 32–48). Nova Publisher.

Stasolla, F., & Perilli, V. (2015). Microswitch-based programs (MBP) to promote communication, occupation, and leisure skills for children with multiple disabilities: a literature overview. In N. R. Silton (Ed.), *Recent advances in assistive technologies to support children with developmental disorders* (pp. 195–216). Nova Science Publishers. doi:10.4018/978-1-4666-8395-2.ch009

Stasolla, F., Perilli, V., & Boccasini, A. (2016). Assistive Technologies for Persons with Multiple Disabilities. In J. Luiselli & A. J. Fisher (Eds.), *Computer-Assisted and Web-Based Innovations in Psychology, Special Education, and Health* (pp. 287–310). Elsevier. doi:10.1016/B978-0-12-802075-3.00011-5

Stasolla, F., Perrilli, V., Di Leone, A., Damiani, R., Albano, V., Stella, A., & Damato, C. (2015). Technological aids to support choice strategies by three girls with Rett syndrome. *Research in Developmental Disabilities*, *36*, 36–44. doi:10.1016/j.ridd.2014.09.017 PMID:25310833

Steenbergen, B., van der Kamp, J., Verneau, M., Jongbloed-Pereboom, M., & Masters, R. S. (2010). Implicit and explicit learning: Applications from basic research to sports for individuals with impaired movement dynamics. *Disability and Rehabilitation*, *32*(18), 1509–1516. doi:10.3109/09638288.2010.497035 PMID:20575752

Stefanovski, L., Triebkorn, P., Spiegler, A., Diaz-Cortes, M. A., Solodkin, A., Jirsa, V., McIntosh, A. R., & Ritter, P. (2019). Linking Molecular Pathways and Large-Scale Computational Modeling to Assess Candidate Disease Mechanisms and Pharmacodynamics in Alzheimer's Disease for the Alzheimer's Disease. *Frontiers in Computational Neuroscience*, *13*(64), 1–27. doi:10.3389/fncom.2019.00054 PMID:31456676

Stefanucci, J. K., Creem-Regehr, S. H., Thompson, W. B., Lessard, D. A., & Geuss, M. N. (2015). Evaluating the accuracy of size perception on screen-based displays: Displayed objects appear smaller than real objects. *Journal of Experimental Psychology. Applied*, *21*(3), 215–223. doi:10.1037/xap0000051 PMID:26121374

Steiner, W. A., Ryser, L., Huber, E., Uebelhart, D., Aeschlimann, A., & Stucki, G. (2002). Use of the ICF model as a clinical problem-solving tool in physical therapy and rehabilitation medicine. *Physical Therapy*, *82*(11), 1098–1107. doi:10.1093/ptj/82.11.1098 PMID:12405874

Stinear, C. M. (2017). Prediction of motor recovery after stroke: Advances in biomarkers. *Lancet Neurology*, *16*(10), 826–836.

Stinear, C. M., Byblow, W. D., & Ward, S. H. (2014). An update on predicting motor recovery after stroke. *Annals of Physical and Rehabilitation Medicine*, *57*(8), 489–498.

Stoccoro, A., & Coppedè, F. (2018). Role of epigenetics in Alzheimer's disease pathogenesis. *Neurodegenerative Disease Management*, *8*(3), 181–193. doi:10.2217/nmt-2018-0004 PMID:29888987

Straudi, S., Baroni, A., Mele, S., Craighero, L., Manfredini, F., Lamberti, N., Maietti, E., & Basaglia, N. (2020). Effects of a Robot-Assisted Arm Training Plus Hand Functional Electrical Stimulation on Recovery After Stroke: A Randomized Clinical Trial. *Archives of Physical Medicine and Rehabilitation, 101*(2), 309–316.

Strickland, D. C., Coles, C. D., & Southern, L. B. (2013). JobTIPS: A transition to employment program for individuals with autism spectrum disorders. *Journal of Autism and Developmental Disorders, 43*(10), 2472–2483.doi:https://doi.org/10.1007/s10803-013-1800-4

Stucki, G., & Sangha, O. (1998). Principles of rehabilitation. *Rheumatology, 1*, 517–530.

Stummer, C., Dibilio, V., Overeem, S., Weerdesteyn, V., Bloem, B. R., & Nonnekes, J. (2015). The walk-bicycle: A new assistive device for Parkinson's patients with freezing of gait? *Parkinsonism & Related Disorders, 21*(7), 755–757. doi:10.1016/j.parkreldis.2015.04.025 PMID:25983112

Sula, A., & Bushti, J. (2014, February). Using Assistive Technologies (AT) as form of technology based intervention to foster and promote Albanian language development in children with autism. *International Journal of Science, Innovation & New Technology, 1*(9), 33–41.

Sula, A., & Spaho, E. (2014). Using assistive technologies in autism care centers to support children develop communication and language skills. A case study: Albania. *Academic Journal of Interdisciplinary Studies, 3*(1), 203–212. doi:10.5901/ajis.2014.v3n1p203

Syriopoulou-Delli, C. K., & Gkiolnta, E. (2020). Review of assistive technology in the training of children with autism spectrum disorders. *International Journal of Developmental Disabilities*, 1–13. doi:10.1080/20473869.2019.1706333

Szpak, A., Michalski, S. C., Saredakis, D., Chen, C. S., & Loetscher, T. (2019). Beyond Feeling Sick: The Visual and Cognitive Aftereffects of Virtual Reality. *IEEE Access: Practical Innovations, Open Solutions, 7*, 130883–130892. doi:10.1109/ACCESS.2019.2940073

Takahashi, H., Nakahachi, T., Komatsu, S., Ogino, K., Iida, Y., & Kamio, Y. (2014). Hyperreactivity to weak acoustic stimuli and prolonged acoustic startle latency in children with autism spectrum disorders. *Molecular Autism, 5*, 23.doi:https://doi.org/10.1186/2040-2392-5-23

Takeda, K., Tanino, G., & Miyasaka, H. (2017). Review of devices used in neuromuscular electrical stimulation for stroke rehabilitation. *Medical Devices (Auckland, N.Z.), 10*, 207–213. doi:10.2147/MDER.S123464 PMID:28883745

Takeuchi, N., & Izumi, S. (2013). Rehabilitation with poststroke motor recovery: A review with a focus on neural plasticity. *Stroke Research and Treatment, 2013*, 128641.

Tanaka, J. W., Wolf, J. M., Klaiman, C., Koenig, K., Cockburn, J., Herlihy, L., Brown, C., Stahl, S., Kaiser, M. D., & Schultz, R. T. (2010). Using computerized games to teach face recognition skills to children with autism spectrum disorder: The Let's Face It! program. *Journal of Child Psychology and Psychiatry, and Allied Disciplines, 51*(8), 944–952. doi:10.1111/j.1469-7610.2010.02258.x PMID:20646129

Tang, W., Wang, A., Ramkumar, S., & Nair, R. K. R. (2020). Signal identification system for developing rehabilitative device using deep learning algorithms. *Artificial Intelligence in Medicine, 102*. doi:10.1016/j.artmed.2019.101755

Tarnanas, I., Tsolaki, M., Nef, T., Muria, R. M., & Mosimann, U. P. (2014). Can a novel computerized cognitive screening test provide additional information for early detection of Alzheimer's disease? *Alzheimer's & Dementia, 10*(6), 1–9. doi:10.1016/j.jalz.2014.01.002 PMID:24656838

Tatla, S. K., Sauve, K., Jarus, T., Virji-Babul, N., & Holsti, L. (2014). The effects of motivating interventions on rehabilitation outcomes in children and youth with acquired brain injuries: A systematic review. *Brain Injury: [BI]*, *28*(8), 1022–1035. doi:10.3109/02699052.2014.890747 PMID:24661000

Tatla, S. K., Sauve, K., Virji-Babul, N., Holsti, L., Butler, C., & Van Der Loos, H. F. (2013). Evidence for outcomes of motivational rehabilitation interventions for children and adolescents with cerebral palsy: An American Academy for Cerebral Palsy and Developmental Medicine systematic review. *Developmental Medicine and Child Neurology*, *55*(7), 593–601. doi:10.1111/dmcn.12147 PMID:23550896

Taub, E., Uswatte, G., Mark, V. W., & Morris, D. M. (2006). The learned nonuse phenomenon: Implications for rehabilitation. *Europa Medicophysica*, *42*(3), 241–256.

Taylor, N. F., Dodd, K. J., McBurney, H., & Graham, H. K. (2004). Factors influencing adherence to a home-based strength-training programme for young people with cerebral palsy. *Physiotherapy*, *90*(2), 57–53. doi:10.1016/j.physio.2003.09.001

Tedla, J. S., Dixit, S., Gular, K., & Abohashrh, M. (2019). Robot-assisted Gait Training Effect on Function and Gait Speed in Subacute and Chronic Stroke Population: A Systematic Review and Meta-Analysis of Randomized Controlled Trials. *European Neurology*, *81*(3-4), 103–111.

Tentori, M., Escobedo, L., & Balderas, G. (2015). A Smart Environment for Children with Autism. *IEEE Pervasive Computing*, *14*(2), 42–50. doi:10.1109/MPRV.2015.22

The World Health Organization. MONICA Project (Monitoring Trends and Determinants in Cardiovascular Disease): A Major International Collaboration. (1988). *Journal of clinical epidemiology*, *41*(2), 105–114.

Tiger, J. H., Hanley, G. P., & Bruzek, J. (2008). Functional communication training: A review and practical guide. *Behavior Analysis in Practice*, *1*(1), 16–23. doi:10.1007/BF03391716 PMID:22477675

Tost, D., Grau, S., & Ferre, M. (2009). PREVIRNEC: A cognitive telerehabilitation system based on virtual environments. *Virtual Rehabilitation International Conference*, 87-93.

Treangen, T. J., & Salzberg, S. L. (2012). Repetitive DNA and next-generation sequencing: Computational challenges and solutions. *Nature Reviews. Genetics*, *13*(1), 36–46. doi:10.1038/nrg3117 PMID:22124482

Truelsen, T., Begg, S., & Mathers, C. (2006). *The global burden of cerebrovascular disease. WHO Discussion Paper*. World Health Organization. https://www.researchgate.net/profile/Stephen-Begg/publication/228551377_The_Global_Burden_of_Cerebrovascular_Disease/links/0c96051e39e2749573000000/The-Global-Burden-of-Cerebrovascular-Disease.pdf

Tse, M. M. Y., Kwan, R. Y. C., & Lau, J. L. (2018). Ageing in individuals with intellectual disability: Issues and concerns in Hong Kong. *Hong Kong Medical Journal*, *24*(1), 68–72. doi:10.12809/hkmj166302 PMID:29326402

Turner-Stokes, L. (2009). Goal attainment scaling (GAS) in rehabilitation: A practical guide. *Clinical Rehabilitation*, *23*(4), 362–370. doi:10.1177/0269215508101742 PMID:19179355

Tyson, S. F., & Kent, R. M. (2013). Effects of an ankle-foot orthosis on balance and walking after stroke: A systematic review and pooled meta-analysis. *Archives of Physical Medicine and Rehabilitation*, *94*(7), 1377–1385. doi:10.1016/j.apmr.2012.12.025 PMID:23416220

U.S. Food & Drug Administration. (2017). *Deciding When to Submit a 510(k) for a Change to an Existing Device: Guidance for Industry and Food and Drug Administration Staff*. Washington, DC: Center for Devices and Radiological Health, Center for Biologics Evaluation and Research Retrieved from https://www.fda.gov/media/99812/download

U.S. Food & Drug Administration. (2020). *Premarket Notification 510(k)*. Retrieved from https://www.fda.gov/medical-devices/premarket-submissions/premarket-notification-510k#s

Ueda, R., Okada, T., Kita, Y., Ozawa, Y., Inoue, H., Shioda, M., Kono, Y., Kono, C., Nakamura, Y., Amemiya, K., Ito, A., Sugiura, N., Matsuoka, Y., Kaiga, C., Kubota, M., & Ozawa, H. (2021). The quality of life of children with neurodevelopmental disorders and their parents during the coronavirus disease 19 emergency in japan. *Scientific Reports*, *11*(1), 3042. Advance online publication. doi:10.103841598-021-82743-x PMID:33589663

Ulrich, D. A., Lloyd, M. C., Tiernan, C. W., Looper, J. E., & Angulo-Barroso, R. M. (2008). Effects of intensity of treadmill training on developmental outcomes and stepping in infants with Down syndrome: A randomized trial. *Physical Therapy*, *88*(1), 114–122. doi:10.2522/ptj.20070139 PMID:17940103

Ustad, T., Sorsdahl, A. B., & Ljunggren, A. E. (2009). Effects of intensive physiotherapy in infants newly diagnosed with cerebral palsy. *Pediatric Physical Therapy*, *21*(2), 140–148. doi:10.1097/PEP.0b013e3181a3429e PMID:19440122

UX Collective. (n.d.). https://uxdesign.cc/inclusive-design-guide-7-principles-of-designing-for-the-autistic-community-1e6dcd4bae85

Valadão, C. T., Goulart, C., Rivera, H., Caldeira, E., Bastos Filho, T. F., Frizera-Neto, A., & Carelli, R. (2016). Analysis of the use of a robot to improve social skills in children with autism spectrum disorder. *Revista Brasileira de Engenharia Biomédica*, *32*(2), 161–175. doi:10.1590/2446-4740.01316

Valdez, P., & Mehrabian, A. (1994). Effects of color on emotions. *Journal of Experimental Psychology. General*, *123*(4), 394–409.

Valentine, A. Z., Brown, B. J., Groom, M. J., Young, E., Hollis, C., & Hall, C. L. (2020). A systematic review evaluating the implementation of technologies to assess, monitor and treat neurodevelopmental disorders: A map of the current evidence. *Clinical Psychology Review*, *80*, 101870. Advance online publication. doi:10.1016/j.cpr.2020.101870 PMID:32712216

Van der Ham, I. J. M., & Claessen, M. H. G. (2020). How age relates to spatial navigation performance: Functional and methodological considerations. *Ageing Research Reviews*, *58*, 101020. doi:10.1016/j.arr.2020.101020 PMID:31954190

Van der Ham, I. J. M., van der Kuil, M. N. A., Evers, A. W. M., & Claessen, M. H. G. (2020a). Large-scale assessment of human navigation ability across the lifespan. *Scientific Reports*, *10*(1), 3299. doi:10.103841598-020-60302-0 PMID:32094394

Van der Ham, I. J., Faber, A. M., Venselaar, M., van Kreveld, M. J., & Löffler, M. (2015). Ecological validity of virtual environments to assess human navigation ability. *Frontiers in Psychology*, *6*, 637. doi:10.3389/fpsyg.2015.00637 PMID:26074831

Van der Ham, I. J., Klaassen, F., van Schie, K., & Cuperus, A. (2019). Elapsed time estimates in virtual reality and the physical world: The role of arousal and emotional valence. *Computers in Human Behavior*, *94*, 77–81. doi:10.1016/j.chb.2019.01.005

van der Ham, I. J., van der Vaart, R., Miedema, A., Visser-Meily, J., & van der Kuil, M. N. (2020b). Healthcare Professionals' Acceptance of Digital Cognitive Rehabilitation. *Frontiers in Psychology*, *11*, 3323. doi:10.3389/fpsyg.2020.617886 PMID:33324309

Van der Kuil, M. N., Visser-Meily, J., Evers, A. W., & Van der Ham, I. J. (2018). A usability study of a serious game in cognitive rehabilitation: A compensatory navigation training in acquired brain injury patients. *Frontiers in Psychology*, *9*, 846. doi:10.3389/fpsyg.2018.00846 PMID:29922196

Van der Linden, M., Juillerat, A. C., & Delbeuck, X. (2006). La prise en charge des troubles de la mémoire dans la maladie d'Alzheimer [The management of memory impairments in Alzheimer's disease]. In C. Belin, A. M. Ergis, & O. Moreaud (Eds.), *Actualités sur les démences: Aspects cliniques et neuropsychologiques* (pp. 167–197). Solal.

van der Meer, L., Achmadi, D., Cooijmans, M., Didden, R., Lancioni, G. E., O'Reilly, M. F., Roche, L., Stevens, M., Carnett, A., Hodis, F., Green, V. A., Sutherland, D., Lang, R., Rispoli, M., Marschik, P. B., & Sigafoos, J. (2014). An iPad-Based Intervention for Teaching Picture and Word Matching to a Student with ASD and Severe Communication Impairment. *Journal of Developmental and Physical Disabilities*, *27*(1), 67–78. doi:10.100710882-014-9401-5

van der Meer, L., Matthews, T., Ogilvie, E., Berry, A., Waddington, H., Balandin, S., ... Sigafoos, J. (2017). Training direct-care staff to provide communication intervention to adults with intellectual disability: A systematic review. *American Journal of Speech-Language Pathology*, *26*, 1279–1295.

van der Stigchel, S. (2020). An embodied account of visual working memory. *Visual Cognition*, *28*(5-8), 5–8, 414–419. doi:10.1080/13506285.2020.1742827

Van Halteren-van Tilborg, I. A., Scherder, E. J., & Hulstijn, W. (2007). Motor-skill learning in Alzheimer's disease: A review with an eye to the clinical practice. *Neuropsychology Review*, *17*(3), 203–212. doi:10.100711065-007-9030-1 PMID:17680369

van Stenseel, F. J., Zegers, V., & Bögels, S. M. (2016). Predictors of Treatment Effectiveness for Youth with ASD and Comorbid Anxiety Disorders: It all Depends on the Family? *Journal of Autism and Developmental Disorders*, *47*, 636–645. doi:10.100710803-016-2956-5

Vanderborght, B., Simut, R., Saldien, J., A. Pop, C., Rusu, A. S., Pintea, S., Lefeber, D., & David, D. O. (2012). Using the social robot probo as a social story telling agent for children with ASD. *Interaction Studies. Social Behaviour and Communication in Biological and Artificial SystemsInteraction Studies / Social Behaviour and Communication in Biological and Artificial SystemsInteraction Studies*, *13*(3), 348–372. doi:10.1075/is.13.3.02van

Veerbeek, J. M., Langbroek-Amersfoort, A. C., van Wegen, E. E., Meskers, C. G., & Kwakkel, G. (2017). Effects of Robot-Assisted Therapy for the Upper Limb After Stroke. *Neurorehabilitation and Neural Repair*, *31*(2), 107–121.

Ventura, S., Brivio, E., Riva, G., & Baños, R. M. (2019). Immersive versus non-immersive experience: Exploring the feasibility of memory assessment through 360 technology. *Frontiers in Psychology*, *10*, 2509. doi:10.3389/fpsyg.2019.02509 PMID:31798492

Venturoli, A. (2016). *Autismo e lavoro. Una breve rassegna bibliografica internazionale.* Rome: ISFOL. Retrieved from https://isfoloa.isfol.it/xmlui/handle/123456789/1268

Vlcˇek, K., & Laczò, J. (2014). Neural correlates of spatial navigation changes in mild cognitive impairment and Alzheimer's disease. *Frontiers in Behavioral Neuroscience, 8*(89), 1-6.

Vrana-Diaz, C. J., Balasubramanian, P., Kayadjanian, N., Bohonowych, J., & Strong, T. V. (2020). Variability and change over time of weight and BMI among adolescents and adults with Prader-Willi syndrome: A 6-month text-based observational study. *Orphanet Journal of Rare Diseases*, *15*(1), 233. Advance online publication. doi:10.118613023-020-01504-7 PMID:32883323

Wadhera, T., & Kakkar, D. (2019). Eye Tracker: An Assistive Tool in Diagnosis of Autism Spectrum Disorder. In Emerging Trends in the Diagnosis and Intervention of Neurodevelopmental Disorders (pp. 125-152). IGI Global.

Wadhera, T., & Kakkar, D. (2020). Big Data-Based System: A Supportive Tool in Autism Spectrum Disorder Analysis. In Interdisciplinary Approaches to Altering Neurodevelopmental Disorders (pp. 303-319). IGI Global. doi:10.4018/978-1-7998-3069-6.ch017

Wadhera, T., & Kakkar, D. (2019). Eye Tracker: An Assistive Tool in Diagnosis of Autism Spectrum Disorder. In S. K. Gupta, S. Venkatesan, S. P. Goswami, & R. Kumar (Eds.), *Emerging Trends in the Diagnosis and Intervention of Neurodevelopmental Disorders* (pp. 125–152). IGI Global. doi:10.4018/978-1-5225-7004-2.ch007

Wadhera, T., Kakkar, D., Kaur, G., & Menia, V. (2019). Pre-Clinical ASD Screening Using Multi-Biometrics-Based Systems. In D. R. Kisku, P. Gupta, & J. K. Sing (Eds.), *Design and Implementation of Healthcare Biometric Systems* (pp. 185–211). IGI Global. doi:10.4018/978-1-5225-7525-2.ch008

Waisman-Nitzan, M., Schreuer, N., & Gal, E. (2020). Person, environment, and occupation characteristics: What predicts work performance of employees with autism? *Research in Autism Spectrum Disorders*, *78*, 101643. https://doi.org/10.1016/j.rasd.2020.101643

Wali, L. J., & Sanfilippo, F. (2019, September). A Review of the State-of-the-Art of Assistive Technology for People with ASD in the Workplace and in Everyday Life. In *Conference on e-Business, e-Services and e-Society* (pp. 520-532). Cham: Springer. 10.1007/978-3-030-29374-1_42

Wandin, H., Lindberg, P., & Sonnander, K. (2020). Development of a tool to assess visual attention in Rett syndrome: A pilot study. *AAC: Augmentative and Alternative Communication*, *36*, 118–127. PMID:32791851

Wang, R. H., Sudhama, A., Begum, M., Huq, R., & Mihailidis, A. (2017). Robots to assist daily activities: Views of older adults with Alzheimer's disease and their caregivers. *International Psychogeriatrics*, *29*(1), 67–79. doi:10.1017/S1041610216001435 PMID:27660047

Warren, Z., Zheng, Z., Das, S., Young, E. M., Swanson, A., Weitlauf, A., & Sarkar, N. (2015). Brief Report: Development of a Robotic Intervention Platform for Young Children with ASD. *Journal of Autism and Developmental Disorders*, *45*, 3870–3876.doi:https://doi.org/10.1007/s10803-014-2334-0

Wechsler, T. F., Kümpers, F., & Mühlberger, A. (2019). Inferiority or Even Superiority of Virtual Reality Exposure Therapy in Phobias?—A Systematic Review and Quantitative Meta-Analysis on Randomized Controlled Trials Specifically Comparing the Efficacy of Virtual Reality Exposure to Gold Standard in vivo Exp. *Frontiers in Psychology*, *10*, 1758. doi:10.3389/fpsyg.2019.01758

Weech, S., Kenny, S., & Barnett-Cowan, M. (2019). Presence and cybersickness in virtual reality are negatively related: A review. *Frontiers in Psychology*, *10*, 158. doi:10.3389/fpsyg.2019.00158 PMID:30778320

Weiss, P. L., Rand, D., Katz, N., & Kizony, R. (2004). Video capture virtual reality as a flexible and effective rehabilitation tool. *Journal of Neuroengineering and Rehabilitation*, *1*(1), 12. doi:10.1186/1743-0003-1-12 PMID:15679949

Wender, R., Hoffman, H. G., Hunner, H. H., Seibel, E. J., Patterson, D. R., & Sharar, S. R. (2009). Interactivity influences the magnitude of virtual reality analgesia. *Journal of Cyber Therapy and Rehabilitation*, *2*(1), 27–33. PMID:20390047

Weniger, G., Ruhleder, M., Lange, C., Wolf, S., & Irle, E. (2011). Egocentric and allocentric memory as assessed by virtual reality in individuals with amnestic mild cognitive impairment. *Neuropsychologia*, *49*(3), 518–527. doi:10.1016/j.neuropsychologia.2010.12.031 PMID:21185847

Westphal, A., Dingjan, P., & Attoe, R. (2010). What can low and high technologies do for late life mental disorders? *Current Opinion in Psychiatry*, *23*(6), 510–505. doi:10.1097/YCO.0b013e32833d74d4 PMID:20717039

West, R. L., Welch, D. C., & Knabb, P. D. (2002). Gender and aging: Spatial self-efficacy and location recall. *Basic and Applied Social Psychology*, *24*(1), 71–80. doi:10.1207/S15324834BASP2401_7

Wherton, J.P. (2007). Technological opportunities for supporting people with dementia who are living at home. *International Journal of Human-Computer Studies, 56*, 65-66.

White, P. J. F., & Moussavi, Z. (2016). Neurocognitive Treatment for a Patient with Alzheimer's Disease Using a Virtual Reality Navigational Environment. *Journal of Experimental Neuroscience*, *8*(10), 129–135. doi:10.4137/JEN.S40827 PMID:27840579

Widmann, C. N., Beinhoffa, U., & Riepea, M. W. (2012). Everyday memory deficits in very mild Alzheimer's disease. *Neurobiology of Aging*, *33*(2), 297–303. doi:10.1016/j.neurobiolaging.2010.03.012 PMID:20392540

Wigfield, A., & Eccles, J. S. (2000). Expectancy-Value Theory of Achievement Motivation. *Contemporary Educational Psychology*, *25*(1), 68–81. doi:10.1006/ceps.1999.1015 PMID:10620382

Wiguna, T., Wigantara, N. A., Ismail, R. I., Kaligis, F., Minayati, K., Bahana, R., & Dirgantoro, B. (2020). A four-step method for the development of an ADHD-VR digital game diagnostic tool prototype for children using a DL model. *Frontiers in Psychiatry*, *11*, 829. Advance online publication. doi:10.3389/fpsyt.2020.00829 PMID:32973578

Willems, R. M., Özyürek, A., & Hagoort, P. (2007). When language meets action: The neural integration of gesture and speech. *Cerebral Cortex*, *17*(10), 2322–2333. doi:10.1093/cercor/bhl141 PMID:17159232

Williams, J. (2008). Children with disability grow into adults with a disability. *Developmental Medicine and Child Neurology*, *50*(3), 163. doi:10.1111/j.1469-8749.2008.00163.x PMID:18302633

Wilson, B. (2009). Evidence for the effectiveness of neuropsychological rehabilitation. *Neuropsychological rehabilitation: Theory, models, therapy and outcome*, 22-36.

Winstein, C. J., Stein, J., Arena, R., Bates, B., Cherney, L. R., Cramer, S. C., Deruyter, F., Eng, J. J., Fisher, B., Harvey, R. L., Lang, C. E., MacKay-Lyons, M., Ottenbacher, K. J., Pugh, S., Reeves, M. J., Richards, L. G., Stiers, W., & Zorowitz, R. D. (2016). Guidelines for Adult Stroke Rehabilitation and Recovery: A Guideline for Healthcare Professionals From the American Heart Association/American Stroke Association. *Stroke*, *47*(6), e98–e169.

Winterling, V. (2013). *Delaware Autism Program BT.* In F. R. Volkmar (Ed.), *Encyclopedia of Autism Spectrum Disorders* (pp. 854–856). Springer New York. doi:10.1007/978-1-4419-1698-3_381

Wolff, S. (2004). The history of autism. *European Child & Adolescent Psychiatry*, *13*(4), 201–208. doi:10.100700787-004-0363-5 PMID:15365889

Wolinsky, F. D., Mahncke, H., Vander Weg, M. W., Martin, R., Unverzagt, F. W., Ball, K. K., Jones, R. N., & Tennstedt, S. L. (2010). Speed of processing training protects self-rated health in older adults: Enduring effects observed in the multi-site ACTIVE randomized controlled trial. *International Psychogeriatrics*, *22*(3), 470–478. doi:10.1017/S1041610209991281 PMID:20003628

Woodyatt, G., & Ozanne, C. (1992). Breaking the silence in Rett Syndrome. *Nature Genetics*, *23*, 127–128. PMID:10508498

World Health Organization. (2007). *International Classification of Functioning, Disability, and Health: Children & Youth Version: ICF-CY*. World Health Organization.

World Health Organization. (2017). *Stroke: A global response is needed.* https://www.who.int/bulletin/volumes/94/9/16-181636/en/

World Health Organization. (2021). *International classification of functioning, disability, and health (ICF)*. Retrieved from https://www.who.int/classifications/international-classification-of-functioning-disability-and-health

Wright, M., & Palisano, R. J. (2017). Cerebral Palsy. In R. J. Palisano, M. N. Orlin, & J. Schreiber (Eds.), *Campbell's Physical Therapy for Children* (pp. 447-487). St. Louis, MO: Elsevier.

Wu, J., Cheng, H., Zhang, J., Yang, S., & Cai, S. (2021). Robot-Assisted Therapy for Upper Extremity Motor Impairment After Stroke: A Systematic Review and Meta-Analysis. *Physical Therapy, 101*(4), pzab010.

Xie, M. (2003). *Fundamental of Robotics: Linking Perception to Action.* World Scientific.

Yalom, I. D. (2002). *The gift of therapy : reflections on being a therapist.* Piatkus London.

Yee, N., & Bailenson, J. (2007). The Proteus effect: The effect of transformed self-representation on behavior. *Human Communication Research*, *33*(3), 271–290. doi:10.1111/j.1468-2958.2007.00299.x

Zamin, N., Norwawi, N. M., Nursyafira, Arshad, N. I., & Rambli, D. R. A. (2019). Make me speak: A mobile app for children with cerebral palsy. *International Journal of Advanced Trends in Computer Science and Engineering, 8*(S1), 368-373. . doi:10.30534/ijatcse/2019/5681.42019

Zellefrow, B., Shanaei, S., Salam, R., El Nasan, A., & Elzabadani, H. (2017). Halcyon – Assistive technology for Alzheimer's patients. *The British Journal of Psychiatry*, 375.

Zervogianni, V., Fletcher-Watson, S., Herrera, G., Goodwin, M., Pérez-Fuster, P., Brosnan, M., & Grynszpan, O. (2020). A framework of evidence-based practice for digital support, co-developed with and for the autism community. *Autism*, *24*(6), 1411–1422. https://doi.org/10.1177/1362361319898331

Zhang, L., Amat, A. Z., Zhao, H., Swanson, A., Weitlauf, A., Warren, Z., & Sarkar, N. (2020). Design of an Intelligent Agent to Measure Collaboration and Verbal-Communication Skills of Children with Autism Spectrum Disorder in Collaborative Puzzle Games. *IEEE Transactions on Learning Technologies*, 1–15. doi:10.1109/TLT.2020.3029223

Zhang, L., Fu, Q., Swanson, A. M. Y., Weitlauf, A. M. Y., Warren, Z., & Sarkar, N. (2018). Design and Evaluation of a Collaborative Virtual Environment (CoMove) for Autism Spectrum. *ACM Transactions on Accessible Computing*, *11*(2), 1–22. doi:10.1145/3209687

Zhang, M., Vallabhajosyula, R., & Fung, D. (2020). Emotional bias modification for individuals with attention deficit hyperactivity disorder: Protocol for a co-design study. *JMIR Research Protocols*, *9*(12), e24078. Advance online publication. doi:10.2196/24078 PMID:33355536

Zhang, X., Yue, Z., & Wang, J. (2017). Robotics in Lower-Limb Rehabilitation after Stroke. *Behavioural Neurology*, *2017*, 3731802.

Zhao, H., Swanson, A. R., Weitlauf, A. S., Warren, Z. E., Sarkar, N., & Member, S. (2018). Hand-in-Hand: A Communication-Enhancement Collaborative Virtual Reality System for Promoting Social Interaction in Children With Autism Spectrum Disorders. *IEEE Transactions on Human-Machine Systems*, *48*(2), 1–13. doi:10.1109/THMS.2018.2791562

Zhao, J., Sensibaugh, T., Bodenheimer, B., McNamara, T. P., Nazareth, A., Newcombe, N., Minear, M., & Klippel, A. (2020). Desktop versus immersive virtual environments: Effects on spatial learning. *Spatial Cognition and Computation*, *20*(4), 328–363. doi:10.1080/13875868.2020.1817925

Zhao, Y., Nonnekes, J., Storcken, E. J. M., Janssen, S., van Wegen, E. E. H., Bloem, B. R., Dorresteijn, L. D. A., van Vugt, J. P. P., Heida, T., & van Wezel, R. J. A. (2016). Feasibility of external rhythmic cueing with the Google glass for improving gait in people with Parkinson's disease. *Journal of Neurology*, *263*(6), 1156–1165. doi:10.100700415-016-8115-2 PMID:27113598

Zucchella, C., Capone, A., Codella, V., Vecchione, C., Buccino, G., & Sandrini, G. (2014). Assessing and restoring cognitive functions early after stroke. *Functional Neurology*, *29*(4), 255–262. doi:10.11138/FNeur/2014.29.4.255 PMID:25764255

About the Contributors

Fabrizio Stasolla, PhD, is an Associate Professor of Developmental Psychology at University "Giustino Fortunato" of Benevento.. His topic concerns the assistive technologies for children with multiple disabilities, developmental disabilities, autism spectrum disorders, Rett and Down syndromes, cerebral palsy. His interest deals with cognitive-behavioral interventions and alternative augmentative communication strategies for non verbal individuals. He teaches psychology of disabilities and rehabilitation to educational sciences students. The author works on PECS, VOCA, literacy process, ambulation responses, self-monitoring and self management of instruction cues to promote on-task behavior by persons with learning disabilities. He is coordinator of some research projects regarding the aforementioned themes. He his ad-hoc reviewer for 25 peer-reviewed Journals and he is in the editorial board of 5 peer-reviewed Journals. He is Associate Editor of the International Journal of Behavioral Research and Psychology.

* * *

Khalida Akbar obtained a PhD in 2016 from the University of Kwa Zulu-Natal and graduated as one of the youngest PhD graduates of the College of Law and Management Studies at the age of 26. Her PhD specialised in return to work and work reintegration post Acquired Brain Injury. After obtaining her PhD she works part-time as Cognitive rehabilitation specialist in the field of Acquired Brain Injury. Dr Akbar has been a Part-time lecturer at the University of Kwa Zulu-Natal for the past 7 years hand lectured in the discipline of Human Resource Management, Entrepreneurship, Public Governance and Industrial Organizational and Labour Studies. Dr Akbar has supervised honors students and is currently supervising Masters and MBA students. Dr Akbar has held positions previously as a graduate assistant, Masters in Commerce administrator, Teaching and Learning administrator, research assistant to the College dean of research for the College of Law and Management studies and research assistant to the College dean of research for the College of Agriculture, Engineering and Science .She continues to research as a Post-Doctoral Research Fellow at The Durban University of Technology in the faculty of Management Studies . She has attended and presented at international conferences, in South Africa, France, Germany, and Mauritius and as well as formed part of a joint research project with Germany from 2016 – 2018 and have had the opportunity to lecture and research in Germany Research Interests: Higher Education and Development, Disability, Brain Injury, Human Resource Management, Entrepreneurship and Management, Sharing Economies, Society and development and Managing Complexity.

Justine Belschner, PT, DPT, is a board-certified is a board-certified clinical specialist in pediatric physical therapy at Children's National Hospital in Washington, DC. Her clinical position allows her to treat on both the inpatient and outpatient side and she helps to staff the cystic fibrosis care clinic. She has been an investigator on numerous studies focused on leveraging home-based technology to enhance therapy for children with cerebral palsy. Dr. Belschner regularly presents her work at the annual meetings of the American Physical Therapy Association (APTA) and the American Congress of Rehabilitation Medicine (ACRM). She served as the Pediatric State Representative for DC for the Academy of Pediatric Physical Therapy and now is a serving as a district advocacy liaison for the Academy of Pediatric Physical Therapy. In addition to cerebral palsy, her clinical interests include vestibular rehabilitation, pelvic floor rehabilitation, cystic fibrosis, and traumatic brain injury.

Giulia Binaghi, MA, is a clinical and developmental psychologist. She earned her master's degree at the Catholic University of the Sacred Heart of Milan in 2017. She completed the post-graduate internship, in part, at the Catholic University dealing with the issues of bullying and cyberbullying, in part at the Auxologico Italian Institute where she dealt with obesity and eating disorders. Currently she works as a developmental psychotherapist in training and is running an internship at the developmental psychopathology department of the Niguarda Hospital in Milan. She received a master's degree in Psycho-diagnosis for adults and children in 2019 and works as a psycho-diagnostic and clinical psychologist in a private setting. She collaborates with psychologist counselors in the court and conduct protected hearings of minors. Additionally, she is a contract lecturer for the 'Psychology and Neurosciences' teaching of the second level master's degree in Applied Behavioral and Cognitive Psychology at Giustino Fortunato University of Benevento

Donatella Ciarmoli, MA, is a Junior Psychologist interested in severe to profound developmental disabilities, Cognitive-Behavioral Interventions, and Technology-aided programs to improve the independence and the quality of life in individuals with neurological disorders.

Elena Choong, MSBE, is a biomedical engineer at the U.S. Food and Drug Administration (FDA)/ Center for Devices and Radiological Health (CDRH). Ms. Choong has been with the FDA since January 2016 and has broad experience across the agency including the Center for Food Safety and Nutrition (CFSAN)'s Bioanalytical Division. Ms. Choong received both her bachelor's and master's degrees in biomedical engineering at The Catholic University of America in Washington, DC, and is currently a doctoral candidate in Health Administration at Capella University.

Jenny Downs leads child development and disability research programs at the Telethon Kids Institute in Perth. Her current programs include research on rare disorders including Rett syndrome, the CDKL5 Deficiency Disorder, MECP2 Duplication syndrome and Prader-Willi syndrome, as well as Down syndrome, autism and cerebral palsy which occur more frequently. Dr Downs led the development of a quality of life measure for children with intellectual disability, the Quality of Life Inventory – Disability. Her vision is that all children with developmental vulnerability or disability will live with reduced impairments and optimal quality of life, and that findings will be distributed equitably across the community.

Leila Goosen is a full professor in the Department of Science and Technology Education of the University of South Africa. Prof. Goosen was an Associate Professor in the School of Computing, and the module leader and head designer of the fully online signature module for the College for Science, Engineering and Technology, rolled out to over 92,000 registered students since the first semester of

2013. She also supervises ten Masters and Doctoral students, and has successfully completed supervision of 43 students at postgraduate level. Previously, she was a Deputy Director at the South African national Department of Education. In this capacity, she was required to develop ICT strategies for implementation. She also promoted, coordinated, managed, monitored and evaluated ICT policies and strategies, and drove the research agenda in this area. Before that, she had been a lecturer of Information Technology (IT) in the Department for Science, Mathematics and Technology Education in the Faculty of Education of the University of Pretoria. Her research interests have included cooperative work in IT, effective teaching and learning of programming and teacher professional development.

Yiannis Koumpouros (BSc, MSc, MBA, PhD) is an Ass. Professor in the University of West Attica, Department of Public and Community Health. He specializes in health informatics, e-health, m-health, telemedicine, assistive technologies, rehabilitation, users satisfaction assessment, and strategic management. Dr. Koumpouros serves as an expert for the European Commission in the e-health and m-health sectors, and as an evaluator of numerous R&D projects. He was responsible for the WHODAS 2.0 scale of cultural adaptation for the World Health Organization in Greece. Dr. Koumpouros has top-level managerial experience in the private and public healthcare sector (chairman of hospitals, member of the board of directors, business development and strategic management director, etc.). He was Chairman of several committees in the Ministry of Development, and was a regular member of the Consultative Technical Council (Ministry of Internal Public Administration and Decentralisation), etc. Dr. Koumpouros has published more than 70 papers in reputed journals and conference proceedings and has been serving as an editorial board member of repute. He has participated in more than 45 R&D funded projects in the field of healthcare and ICTs.

Kriti Mishra received her MBBS (2009) from Kasturba Medical College, India and MD (2014) in Physical Medicine and Rehabilitation from Christian Medical College, India. She received a University medal for receiving highest grades in MD. Post MD, she worked as a Senior Resident at AIIMS Jodhpur, India. During her tenure, she was involved in various research activities particularly related to neurodevelopmental disorders and studying the factors influencing the rehabilitation of these children in the given region. She also participated in various community awareness and outreach programmes related to disabilities and rehabilitation for these patients in surrounding areas. She also worked as an Assistant Professor and consultant in K.S. Hedge Medical Academy and its associated hospital, Mangalore, India. Currently, she is pursuing her academic interests in Public Health from University of London while continuing to do independent research work.

Laura Roche received her PhD in 2017 from Victoria University of Wellington, New Zealand. She is currently a lecturer in Special and Inclusive Education at the University of Newcastle, Australia. Laura's research focuses on applying behavioral intervention techniques to enhance communication skills for children with neurodevelopmental disorders and rare genetic syndromes.

Alberto Romano is a developmental therapist. He obtained a bachelor's degree in Developmental Neuropsychomotor therapy at the University of Pavia, a first-level University Master in Applied Behavior Analysis (ABA) at the University of Parma, and a Master's Degree in Rehabilitation Sciences at the University of Rome "Tor Vergata". He is a founder and member of the board of directors of SMART ONLUS (www.centrosmart.it) since 2016. It is a rehabilitation center for evidence-based pediatric rehabilitation in the field of behavioral sciences. Since 2017 he has carried out research activities as developmental therapist at the Movement Analysis and Robotics Laboratory (MARLab) of the Bambino Gesù Pediatric Hospital, Department of Neuroscience and Neurorehabilitation. He is a consultant and researcher for the Italian Rett Syndrome Association (AIRett) since 2013 and carries out weekly rehabilitation activities with children with neurodevelopmental disabilities. His main research interests concern the practice of pediatric neurorehabilitation, movement analysis, and the application of rehabilitation technologies.

Manon Maitland Schladen, MSE, PhD, is a senior researcher in the Department of Biomedical Engineering at the Catholic University of America in Washington, DC, where she serves as principal investigator on Project D3, Patient-centered outcomes to guide the design and implementation of technology in the home for neurological assessment, therapy, and assistance as well as co-principal investigator on Project R1, Home assessment of grasp development in infants at risk for fine motor delay. Dr. Schladen holds a concurrent appointment to the research faculty at the Department of Rehabilitation Medicine at the Georgetown University Medical Center. Her interests focus on using of technology to improve the delivery of rehabilitation interventions, foster greater self-efficacy among patients and enhance individuals' engagement with their health and therapeutic programs. Dr. Schladen conducts human factors research in the area of robotics, gamification, and machine learning-supported longitudinal monitoring for people with stroke, cerebral palsy, and non-specific infant motor delay. She recently completed a psychosocial research fellowship from the Craig H. Neilsen Foundation where she received training in advanced statistics and measurement. Dr, Schladen has published in a variety of peer-reviewed journals: most recently, Informatics, Technology and Disability and The Qualitative Report. She presents her research at the annual meetings of the Rehabilitation Engineering and Assistive Technology Society of North America (RESNA) and the American Congress of Rehabilitation Medicine (ACRM) as well as at the Applied Human Factors and Ergonomics (AHFE) International Conference.

Manish Shandilya is Assistant Professor at Amity University Haryana.

Jeff Sigafoos received his PhD in 1990 from the University of Minnesota. Since then he has held academic appointments at the University of Queensland, University of Sydney, and the University of Texas at Austin, He is currently a professor in educational psychology at Victoria University of Wellington in New Zealand. His research focuses on communication assessment and intervention for individuals with complex communication needs. He is co-editor of Evidence-based Communication Assessment and Intervention.

Michelle Stahlhut is a specialist in pediatric physiotherapy and work as a research physiotherapist at the Danish Center for Rett syndrome. At the center an interdisciplinary team focuses on optimal and lifelong health promotion and on enhancing the quality of life of those affected with Rett syndrome and their families. In her work Michelle Stahlhut aim towards the highest level of independence in each individual with Rett syndrome and to help them maintain this level so they can lead an active and healthy life.

Index

S

T

U

V

W

Ensure Quality Research is Introduced to the Academic Community

Become an Evaluator for IGI Global Authored Book Projects

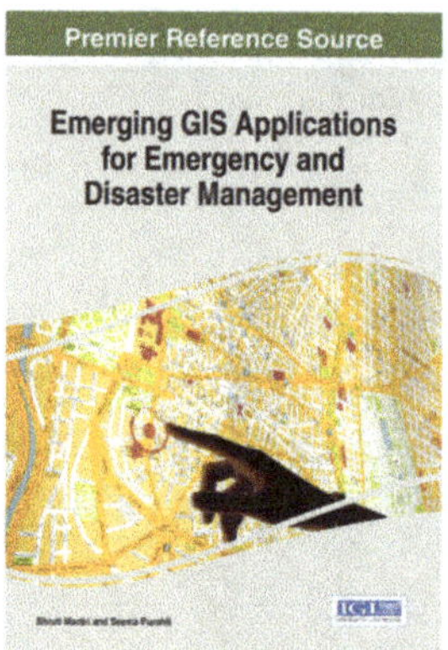

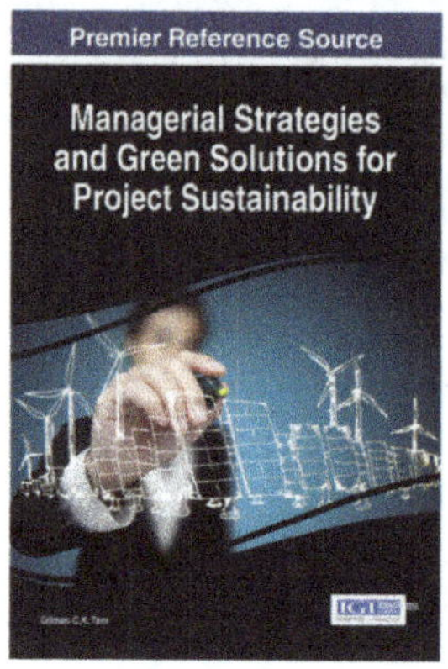

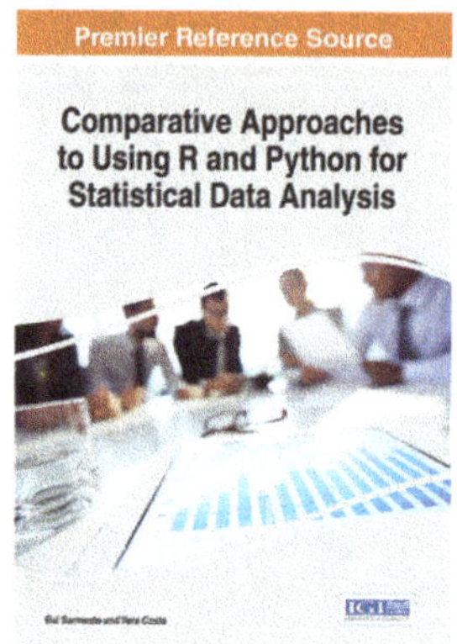

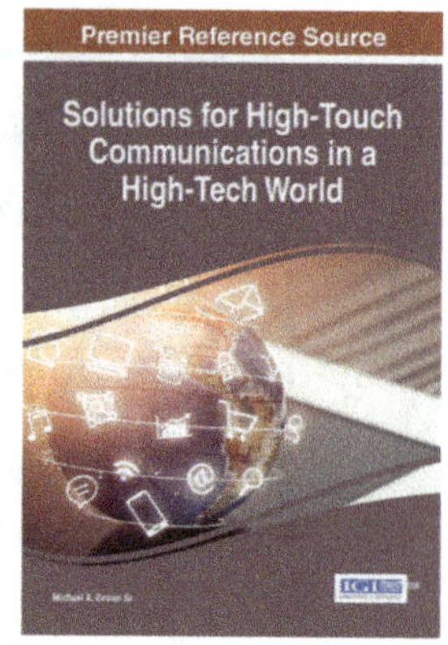

The overall success of an authored book project is dependent on quality and timely manuscript evaluations.

Applications and Inquiries may be sent to:
development@igi-global.com

Applicants must have a doctorate (or equivalent degree) as well as publishing, research, and reviewing experience. Authored Book Evaluators are appointed for one-year terms and are expected to complete at least three evaluations per term. Upon successful completion of this term, evaluators can be considered for an additional term.

If you have a colleague that may be interested in this opportunity, we encourage you to share this information with them.

IGI Global Author Services

Providing a high-quality, affordable, and expeditious service, IGI Global's Author Services enable authors to streamline their publishing process, increase chance of acceptance, and adhere to IGI Global's publication standards.

Benefits of Author Services:

- **Professional Service:** All our editors, designers, and translators are experts in their field with years of experience and professional certifications.
- **Quality Guarantee & Certificate:** Each order is returned with a quality guarantee and certificate of professional completion.
- **Timeliness:** All editorial orders have a guaranteed return timeframe of 3-5 business days and translation orders are guaranteed in 7-10 business days.
- **Affordable Pricing:** IGI Global Author Services are competitively priced compared to other industry service providers.
- **APC Reimbursement:** IGI Global authors publishing Open Access (OA) will be able to deduct the cost of editing and other IGI Global author services from their OA APC publishing fee.

Author Services Offered:

English Language Copy Editing
Professional, native English language copy editors improve your manuscript's grammar, spelling, punctuation, terminology, semantics, consistency, flow, formatting, and more.

Scientific & Scholarly Editing
A Ph.D. level review for qualities such as originality and significance, interest to researchers, level of methodology and analysis, coverage of literature, organization, quality of writing, and strengths and weaknesses.

Figure, Table, Chart & Equation Conversions
Work with IGI Global's graphic designers before submission to enhance and design all figures and charts to IGI Global's specific standards for clarity.

Translation
Providing 70 language options, including Simplified and Traditional Chinese, Spanish, Arabic, German, French, and more.

Hear What the Experts Are Saying About IGI Global's Author Services

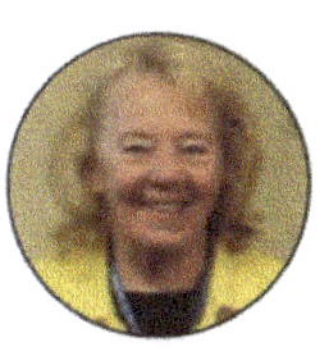

*"Publishing with IGI Global has been **an amazing experience** for me for sharing my research. The **strong academic production** support ensures quality and timely completion."* – **Prof. Margaret Niess, Oregon State University, USA**

*"The service was **very fast, very thorough, and very helpful** in ensuring our chapter meets the criteria and requirements of the book's editors. I was **quite impressed and happy** with your service."* – **Prof. Tom Brinthaupt, Middle Tennessee State University, USA**

Learn More or Get Started Here:

For Questions, Contact IGI Global's Customer Service Team at cust@igi-global.com or 717-533-8845

IGI Global
PUBLISHER of TIMELY KNOWLEDGE
www.igi-global.com

www.ingramcontent.com/pod-product-compliance
Lightning Source LLC
LaVergne TN
LVHW060300011026
849161LV00011B/2744
9781799874300